NATURE IN IRELAND
A Scientific and Cultural History

SENIOR EDITOR
John Wilson Foster

ASSOCIATE EDITOR
Helena C.G. Chesney

THE LILLIPUT PRESS
DUBLIN

First published in November 1997 by
THE LILLIPUT PRESS LTD
62-63 Sitric Road, Arbour Hill,
Dublin 7, Ireland.
E-MAIL: lilliput@indigo.ie

A CIP record for this
title is available from
The British Library.

ISBN 1 874675 29 5 (cased)
ISBN 1 874675 89 9 (paper)

*The Lilliput Press gratefully acknowledges the Heritage Council of Ireland (Dublin),
the Esme Mitchell Trust (Belfast), the Belfast Natural History and Philosophical Society,
the Arts Council of Northern Ireland, and the Department of the Marine (Dublin), for their
support of this publication.*

*Endpapers (cased edition only): Animals and people in north County Antrim, from
an anonymous and undated (probably early Elizabethan) manuscript map.
Orientation is south-south-west. [Public Record Office, London, MPF 88]*

Set in 10.5 on 13 Ehrhardt by Sheila Stephenson
Jacket design by Jarlath Hayes
Printed in England by Redwood Books

Contents

Illustrations

TEXT ILLUSTRATIONS

Preface

Nature in Ireland offers a history of the scientific and cultural examination of the landforms, flora, fauna and climate of the island. The subject of many of the essays is not nature itself but the study of nature. However, it has been thought valuable to the reader for the volume to begin with a survey entitled 'The Heritage of the Rocks', in which the geological formation of Ireland is presented as a founding narrative in the story of Irish nature.

Moreover, from those essays which recount the histories in Ireland of geology, cartography, botany, meteorology, mammalogy, entomology and ornithology, readers will incidentally accumulate a fair amount of knowledge about the geology and physical geography, topography, trees and flowers, weather, mammals, insects and birds of the island. In addition, there are histories of two major wild habitats – woodland and bogland – and one major cultivated mixed habitat, the demesne.

Nature in Ireland is a sizeable volume, but the histories of the disciplines that constitute natural history are necessarily short. Nonetheless, they are the vertebrae, as it were, of the book. The idea of the book suggested itself because the story of the systematic study of Irish nature has not been told in a coherent and compact form, a task the editors hope *Nature in Ireland* performs. That story is surely of intrinsic interest, a record of scientific accomplishment of value to naturalists (professional and amateur alike) inside and outside Ireland.

It will be of value also to historians and enthusiasts of Irish culture. The history of habitats, for example, is also unavoidably a history of culture and society, involving the utilization and exploitation of nature as well as its study. Nature and culture have traditionally been regarded as opposites, but the study of nature is the bridge between them.

The second task *Nature in Ireland* attempts to perform, then, is to rehouse natural history in Irish culture, from which it has effectively been evicted for a century or so. This can be done only when the systematic study of nature is put inside a cultural and intellectual setting broader than the history of scientific disciplines. This transgression of the boundary around the history of science is becoming commonplace in cultural studies elsewhere, but *Nature in Ireland* is the first sustained traffic in Ireland between the history of the sciences and the history of culture. It is hoped that the history of natural history can now be seen as a genuine field of Irish studies, here surveyed and ploughed but still fallow, awaiting seeding and cropping.

To see the study of nature as a cultural activity is to push inquiry beyond science into other kinds of histories – of invasion and conquest, of colonization and settlement, of utilization and exploitation, of immigration and emigration, of economics, ideas, institutions, sport, folklore, books, languages, literature, art, education, conservation, social structures, even politics and constitutions. It is also to push inquiry beyond the *study* of nature into the larger *perception* and *representation* of nature, ways of seeing and depicting nature (most obviously in art, illustration and literature). *Nature in Ireland* offers introductory perspectives on these histories, using natural history as a kind of panopticon.

Furthermore, to see the study of nature as a cultural activity is also to push inquiry back beyond the heroic days of modern British and Irish science in the seventeenth century of Bacon and the Royal Society, and the eighteenth century of the Enlightenment. The presence in Ireland of a large native population with an ambiguous relationship to the modern science of the newcomers, and the presence (and survival) of the Church of that population, with an equally ambiguous relationship to modern science, means that pre-scientific Irish attitudes towards nature have had to be taken account of, even if science managed largely in practice to ignore pre-scientific and non-scientific attitudes. *Nature in Ireland* offers a discussion of Celtic and classical notions of nature and their intersection during colonization with Tudor notions, at a time when the English were themselves developing modern scientific approaches to nature.

These Irish ambiguities might go some way to explaining why the history of science, including natural history, has been largely neglected by twentieth-century Irish cultural historians, who themselves share the wider hesitation in claiming Irish science for Irish culture. Such neglect was encouraged by the sundering of the sciences from the humanities, the classics and religion in Britain in the later nineteenth century, which left its legacy in Ireland too, with science being removed to the margins of culture (and cultivation). The debate provoked by the scientific data and theories of Lyell, Darwin and Wallace precisely implicated religion, the nature of humanity, and the educational curriculum: science was distanced by many as a threat and a species of philistinism.

Around the same time, scientists were distancing themselves through professionalization and specialization. It was in the 1860s that the British Association first entitled one of its sections 'Biology' (the word 'biology' was coined in 1819, 'scientist' in 1833, 'zoology' in 1818, 'geology' in 1795), and from that time onwards 'natural history' in the eyes of many scientists took on a quaintly amateur air. Meanwhile biology and other sciences withdrew into exclusive institutions and an increasingly technical language and methodology. Yet amateurism flourished. The 1860s saw the inauguration of the Belfast Naturalists' Field Club, signalling in Ulster, as such clubs signalled in Britain, the start of vigorous fieldwork carried out over decades by tremendously enthusiastic amateurs and part-time naturalists; the late Victorian period was the heyday of natural history, its energy and popularity. The scientific essays in *Nature in Ireland* translate science back into the language of natural history and are for 'lay' as well as professional readers, while the other essays attempt culturally to rehabilitate natural history.

Professionalization and specialization were a declaration of scientific independence from other, vested interests. The difference between Gerard Boate's *Irelands Naturall History* (1652) and Robert Lloyd Praeger's *The Natural History of Ireland* (1950) is the difference between a pre-Enlightenment concept of natural history, implicated in the economics and politics of plantation and development, and the modern concept of natural history as the classification and understanding of nature in its own right. *Nature in Ireland* attempts to close the gap between the two concepts.

Science prides itself on being international in method and procedure (although the study of nature at the level of data is national, regional or local, even if that data pertains to species that transgress the boundaries of nations). But culture too cannot be fully understood as an exclusively national or regional affair, and several essays in *Nature in Ireland* try to see nature study in Ireland inside international as well as Irish contexts.

Three recent issues have returned the science of nature to general culture, thereby generating the kind of awareness that informs *Nature in Ireland*. The global span of these issues demonstrates the growing internationalism of contemporary culture. One is the human threat to species and habitats; the term 'environmentalism' came into being in the 1950s and was joined in the following decade by the unscientific use of the term 'ecology' as a synonym for the natural environment ('oecology' was coined in the late nineteenth century). A second is the concept of animal rights (honed in the 1970s), involving the practice and theory of zoological gardens, wildlife management, and laboratory experiments on animals. The third is genetic engineering and cloning of animals and plants. Of these scientific, ethical, and even political issues, it is environmentalism that forms the backdrop to *Nature in Ireland*, and the penultimate essay in the book offers an Irish perspective on this vital subject.

But an intellectual development, oddly cognate with ecology, has probably been a more immediate stimulus. That is the emergence of cultural studies, pioneered by Raymond Williams and others, and founded on the notions that culture includes popular and material culture (not just 'high' culture), and that academic disciplines develop in cultural habitats and have social histories that influence practice, even in science. Moreover, disciplines are decreasingly seen as inhabiting intellectual compartments separated by bulkheads: dynamic interdisciplinarity has been central to cultural studies, and is central to *Nature in Ireland*.

This is not the place to rehearse the various historical meanings of 'nature', and readers are directed to Williams' trenchant account in *Keywords* (1988) of the shifting meanings and associations of what he calls 'perhaps the most complex word in the language'. Nature in Gilbert White's *Natural History and Antiquities of Selborne* (1789) meant the three kingdoms of the natural world, animal, vegetable and mineral, to which he added climate and the heavens. But 'nature' has also been defined by opposition, contrasted variously with 'the city', 'society', 'man' (humankind), 'art', and 'culture'. How these oppositions have in Ireland (as elsewhere) trafficked with nature fills – entertainingly and profitably, the editors hope – many of the pages of *Nature in Ireland*.

JWF

Vancouver, British Columbia/Portaferry, Co. Down, 1997

ACKNOWLEDGMENTS

The editors would like to thank the following for their help during the making of *Nature in Ireland*: Charles Bolding, Christine Cahoon, Robin Harbinson, Kenneth James, Paul Keegan, Dyane Lynch, Marshall McKee, Aodán Mac Póilin, Paula Marinescu, Frank Mitchell, Allison Murphy, Rowland Murphy, J.C. Nolan, Cormac Ó Gráda, Daniel O'Leary, Branko Peric, Wes Robertson, Brian Scott, Patricia Scott, Debbie Simpson, Peter Taylor, Gernot Wieland, Colin Wilkinson, Dominique Yupangco. Special thanks to Brendan Barrington of Lilliput for copy-editing the text and compiling the index.

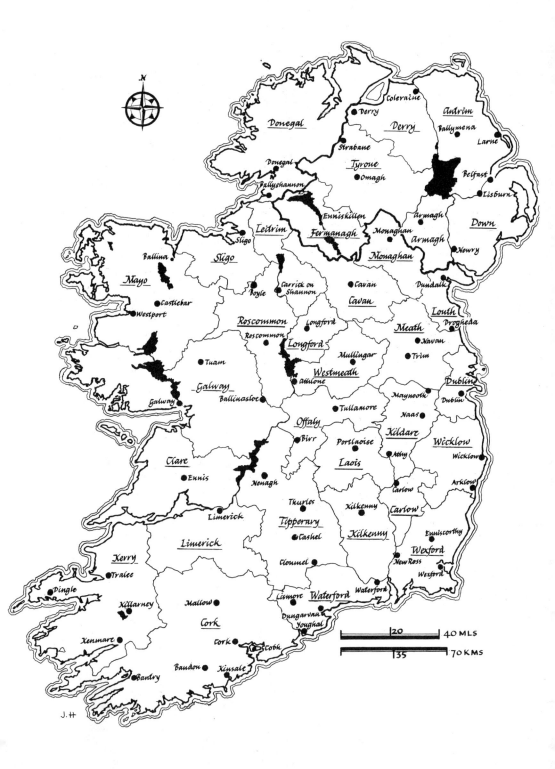

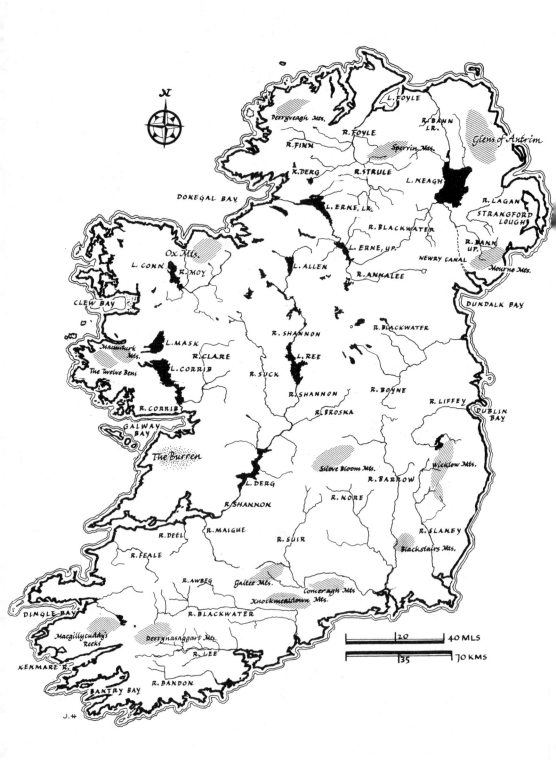

NATURE IN IRELAND

The Heritage of the Rocks

JOHN FEEHAN

Introduction

Ireland owes its natural distinctiveness to its unique geology more than anything else. We cannot, however, speak of the island of Ireland in the geological past, for it did not exist as such. The situation of this small island has been, at different times in the earth's past, a place where oceans were born and grew, and other oceans narrowed and ceased to exist; there have been mountains as great as those which bring the earth today closest to heaven, and rivers on the scale of the Niger, and deserts and great lakes. And glaciers such as those of Greenland today, not only during the most recent period of geological time, but in the most ancient as well, at the time our oldest rocks were taking shape. The story of man in Ireland occupies no more than nine or ten thousand years, whereas this story of the shaping of Ireland is spread across 2500 million years. The slow processes that moulded and shaped the earth in the distant past are at work with the same sure patience. Told in a few pages, the story of Ireland's shaping becomes a fabulous and magic tale. Run this story in time-lapse, and tens of millions of years become lines on a page, mere moments in the telling.

We can perhaps most usefully think of this island of Ireland as a jigsaw puzzle of rock, the various pieces having been put into place at different moments in geological time. Each piece records a different epoch in the shaping of Ireland, and more broadly in the shaping of Europe. Each opens a window on a different period in the earth's past, allowing us a glimpse of all those vanished worlds, different in almost every way from the familiar man-made face of Ireland today. And each part of this island, each piece of the jigsaw that is its geology, is unique, not only by virtue of the distinctive rocks of which it is formed, but because it has a distinct spirit, with which the rocks have much to do. The nature of the surface, the character of life on the surface, are profoundly influenced by the framework of rock beneath.

3

In particular, from the human point of view, the geological inheritance of an area has a determining influence on the soil, and hence not merely on the natural vegetation and its accompanying fauna, but on the possibilities for cultivation and the formation of pasture. It provides the raw materials not only for building the habitations of the human community, but for weaving the entire fabric of the cultural landscape. More locally it provides a precious resource of metals, which have always been an important factor in attracting human attention to different parts of the island at different times in the past.

The story of our understanding of how the jigsaw of Ireland was put together is itself a fascinating detective story, told later in these pages by Patrick Wyse Jackson, and at greater length elsewhere (Herries Davies, 1981, 1995).

Geologically, Ireland is still very much part of Europe; the waters that separate Ireland from Britain, and both islands from the European mainland, are a mere film on the continental shelf. The hundred-fathom contour extends westward from the Irish coast for between twenty-five and one hundred miles, before plunging rapidly to true oceanic depths of several thousand fathoms. A favourite description of the island as a whole is that it is basin-shaped. Indeed, viewed from the sea by a circumnavigating explorer it has the appearance of a mountainous country; but once the fringing barrier of mountains is penetrated, the island is low-lying and generally flat, the very middle being in the main a land of bog and lake.

The Beginning of Ireland

The first pieces of the framework of Ireland to be put in place occur in parts of the west and north-west. These oldest rocks, which are of late Precambrian age, comprise a complex sequence of now highly altered sedimentary rocks, together with a wide variety of rocks of igneous origin. The story they tell begins 700 million years ago, when these sediments were laid down in a rift-bounded sea not unlike the Red Sea of today. This sea, known as the Iapetus Rift, was at this time widening to what in later ages would become the Iapetus Ocean.

This complex of sedimentary rocks was folded and intruded by molten magma during the Grampian Orogeny (about 530-450 million years ago). The effects of heat and pressure exerted over long periods of deformation have changed the rocks into metamorphic rocks which often have a gnarled and twisted appearance, every fold and crystal of which is a clue to the decipherment of the pressures, temperatures and other changes to which they have been subjected over and over again through millions of years. These most complicated of the rocks of Ireland have fascinated students of geology from many countries, with the result that the geology of the island's most rugged and remote districts has the most voluminous literature (see Charlesworth, 1963, and Holland, 1981, for summaries of the earlier and more recent literature).

The shales and mudrocks were altered to mica schists, and the ancient sandstones became hard white quartzites. These quartzites dominate the landscapes in which they occur today: Nephin and Croagh Patrick in Mayo, Errigal in Donegal, the Beanna Beola in Connemara. The limestones have been transformed to marble, and where these outcrop, they give rise to bands of better farming land surrounded by the barren quartzites. The ancient volcanic rocks have been altered to dark, tough rocks called amphibolites. At times the ancient sediments were invaded from below by molten magma, baking and even dissolving the surrounding rocks; this magma slowly cooled to form granite, and many of these ancient granites were subsequently re-melted and now appear as banded gneisses.

Among the rocks of this age there is a formation called the Cleggan Boulder Bed. This is a tillite – a metamorphosed till, deposited by a melting glacier during a time of world-wide glaciation – and it follows abruptly on sediments of an earlier age of limestone deposition in a warm sea (the Connemara Marble). The sands that followed – the quartzites of the Beanna Beola today – are believed to have been blown from the boulder clays of the cold and lifeless landscape that emerged following the retreat of the ice. Some of the characteristic rock sequences are very widespread: for instance, the quartzites of the Beanna Beola, the Connemara Marble and the Boulder Bed have Scottish equivalents.

Life in the Beginning: The Lower Palaeozoic

The opening of the Cambrian period, 600 million years ago, saw the first great explosion in the oceans of life forms with hard parts that could – fortunately for us – survive as fossils in the rocks. In fact, there was incredible genetic and morphological diversity in the living world before this, but a geological record of these creatures – which are often bizarre by our stereotyped standards as to what an appropriate body plan should be – can survive only under exceptional conditions (Gould, 1991). At that time, 'Ireland' lay in the middle of an ocean in the southern hemisphere. To appreciate this apparent anomaly, it is important to realize that the earth's crust is not all of a piece. It is divided into a discrete number of solid crustal plates (the lithosphere) that float on the underlying asthenosphere, which has certain fluid properties. The boundaries between these plates are the places where most of the earth's geological activity is concentrated. Upwelling currents in the earth's mantle (which underlies the crust), powered by the natural heat

5

of radioactive decay in the rock material deep in the earth, cause slow movement of the plates at the surface. When two plates move away from each other, molten rock flows out to the surface as basaltic lava. On today's earth, for instance, the American and European plates are separating – as they have been doing since the opening of the Atlantic Ocean 210 million years ago – along a scar that runs down the middle of the ocean, reaching the surface in places like Iceland in the north Atlantic and Tristan da Cunha in the south. When two plates converge, on the other hand, the heavier plate (usually composed of denser oceanic crust) is forced to move underneath an overriding lighter plate (made of less dense contintental rocks) back into the asthenosphere. The jerking movements of the plates against each other, and the melting at depth of the subducted plate, give rise to intense earthquake and volcanic activity along these margins of subduction. The sediments, caught in the vice between the plate edges, are folded and heaved upwards, to create a range of high, young mountains. For example, where the eastward-moving Pacific plate disappears down the Nazca Trench beneath the continent of South America, the Andes rise skywards.

This brief outline of the key processes of plate tectonics is necessary for an understanding not only of the basic geological processes at work today, but of the early history of the earth. The same processes have shaped the earth's surface as far back as we can see into the geological past, from the time a crust first solidified on our newly born planet some four billion years ago.

So, in the beginning, Ireland's place on the earth's surface was in the southern hemisphere, and the basic underlying theme in its geological history for all the time since then has been a steady drift northwards to its present latitude on the surface of the earth.

Cambrian rocks in Ireland are mainly confined to the Bray area of Co. Dublin, but they are worth a special mention in a book on Irish life because of the presence in them of fossils of the burrows of bottom-dwelling sea creatures, Ireland's oldest life forms. The most famous of them is the enigmatic *Oldhamia*, now believed to be fossilized systems of radiating burrows; the creatures that made them, presumably soft-bodied, have not survived in the fossil record. The gleaming cone of the Great Sugarloaf in Co. Wicklow is made of Cambrian quartzites; the same hard rock forms the resistant promontories of Howth and Bray Head, stubbornly resisting the destructive action of the waves, while the softer slates and shales with which they alternate have been eroded away. It is this lithological accident of Ireland's Lower Palaeozoic heritage that has essentially been responsible for the hollowing out of the safe anchorage of Dublin Bay, with all the consequences this selective erosion has had for human history. But this is the way things always work. In countless ways, sometimes obvious, but usually requiring the geological eye to decipher the relationship, geology shapes human destiny.

These Irish Palaeozoic seas did indeed teem with the ancient life which gives them their name. There is a much better record of it in the sedimentary rocks of the second and third periods of the Lower Palaeozoic era, the Ordovician and Silurian. During this time the Iapetus Ocean, which then dominated the northern hemisphere, narrowed as the continental plates to the north and south converged. Ordovician and Silurian limestones, packed with fossils of the shellfish of ancient seas, are seen at Portrane on the Dublin coast and in the Chair of Kildare, but for the most part these rocks, which make up the foothills of the Leinster Chain, are unremarkable shales and greywackes. There is a wonderful shelly fauna in the Silurian rocks of Ferriter's Cove in the Dingle Peninsula; and in the Devilsbit Mountains in Co. Tipperary the scanty remains of *Cooksonia*, the world's first known land plants (*plate 1*), have been found.

The Rise and Fall of the Caledonian Mountains

The Iapetus Ocean finally closed around 450 million years ago, but the line of collision between the two crustal plates remained as an active scar for a very long time afterwards, with important consequences not only for geological history but for its impact on cultural opportunity as well. The period of mountain-building that followed the collision is referred to as the Caledonian Orogeny. The subducted sediments were bent into a series of great folds whose axes trend north-east/south-west – for instance in the Longford-Down massif between Cavan and Belfast, in the Sperrins, and in the rocks of the Leinster Chain. But the Caledonian Orogeny was not the first period of mountain formation in Ireland. The oldest rocks of the west and north-west had already been crumpled as still earlier continents collided, accompanied by extensive volcanic activity, to produce a range of once-great mountains that had been eroded to the very bone by Cambrian times. It was against the weathered remains of these mountains that the Cambrian sediments were laid down.

The already folded and twisted rocks of the old west and north-west were now refolded and further deformed, and the characteristic Caledonian north-east/south-west fold trend is often clearly dominant in these areas: in the Ox Mountains between Castlebar and Sligo for instance, where a granite core invades schists and amphibolites, and in the lines of fold and fracture in Donegal, such as the Great Glen from Gweebarra Bay to Sheep Haven. The folding was accompanied on a large scale by invasions of molten magma from beneath, which baked the earlier rocks they came into contact with to hard metamorphic rocks before slowly cooling to granite deep in the earth.

7

The erosion of all the ages since they cooled at depth has brought these granites to the surface, now flanked by dark Ordovician shales and older strata. The striking contrast between the granite and older sedimentary rocks is well seen in Glendalough, Co. Wicklow, about the Upper Lake, where the sheer walls of schist and shale abut on the granite spurs of Lugnaquilla. The Newry Granite was also intruded at this time; in some places (at Castlewellan for instance) it is full of bits of the sedimentary rocks it invaded. These Ordovician and Silurian rocks have been weathered to a highly irregular surface of small hills and glens over parts of Louth, Monaghan and Down.

The volcanic activity that accompanied these momentous events in the moulding of Ireland is most dramatically seen in what remains of a little volcano that erupted near Dingle, whose ash and agglomerate are exposed in the cliffs near Ballyferriter. Lambay Island, Co. Dublin, is all that remains of the neck of another worn Ordovician volcano, the once-famed green Lambay porphyry being the plug that slowly cooled in the choked vent. Vinegar Hill, which has earned an enduring place in Irish history as the last stand of the Wexford insurgents during the rebellion of 1798, is a volcanic cone, as are most of the smaller surrounding hills that you can see from its summit.

The great collision brought a new continent into existence. The ocean now lay far to the south-east, its fringing seas extending across the areas where Belgium and Devon are today. All the fury of the elements at high altitude was unleashed on the towering new mountains; enormous volumes of sand and other rock debris accumulated at the foot of the mountains and in the lake basins between; the lakes sank under this growing burden, so that eventually thicknesses of thousands of metres of sandy sediment accumulated. This onslaught continued for tens of millions of years, until eventually the new mountains were worn down to their roots and the southerly sea transgressed northwards across the vanishing continental mass. The sandy sediments that accumulated in these Devonian rivers and lakes became the rocks we now know as the Old Red Sandstone. It dominates the geology of Munster, and occurs in scattered patches in many other parts of the country. Its rocks are seldom suitable for the preservation of fossils, but at Kiltorcan in Co. Kilkenny fine sands and silts laid down in a quiet river backwater contain a splendid assemblage of seed ferns and other plants, dominated by *Cyclostigma kiltorkense*, which enables us to reconstruct, at least in outline, the first Irish terrestrial ecosystem of which we can get a clear glimpse. The concentration of sandy coasts north of the Dingle Peninsula is also a legacy of the debris of the Devonian sandstones of the peninsula, which were swept off the mountains into the sea and then round to the sheltered lee of the peninsula by wind and ocean currents.

Limestone Seas and Coal Swamps

The invading Lower Carboniferous sea eventually covered nearly the whole of the country. Limy muds, rich in remains of the sea life of the time, accumulated to great thicknesses on its floor (not unlike the seas of the Bahamas today) and became the Carboniferous limestone that now occupies nearly half of Ireland's surface. It has contributed more than any other rock to the character of the central part of Ireland. The Lower Carboniferous legacy is not entirely limestone; around Murlough Bay in Co. Antrim coal-bearing rocks, once the sediments of the coastal swamp forests that grew along the ocean's edge, outcrop in a sandstone sequence that extends from Dungannon to Lough Foyle, the shore deposits of the same ocean.

A gentle uplift marks the end of the Lower Carboniferous period, and on the coastal flats and deltas that replaced the seas swamp forests flourished, part of a vast forest network that extended across a wide area of the northern hemisphere. The vegetation of these forests, which probably covered the whole of the country at one time, was dominated by tree ferns, giant horsetails and clubmosses, their partly decayed remains forming coal seams between strata of coastal sandstones. Fragmentary remains of the plants that grew in the forests survive as fossils in the Coal Measures, and in the Castlecomer Plateau they have yielded a diverse fauna of early amphibians. In the Upper Carboniferous sandstones along the south Clare coast there is a petrified forest of standing trees that were engulfed and so preserved in ancient tidal sands.

The renewed uplift of the crust that followed at the end of the Upper Carboniferous period 300 million years ago led to the eventual weathering and erosion of this precious legacy once the rocks were exposed at the surface. Ireland was stripped of most of its Coal Measures, a circumstance that helped to deny it a role in the Industrial Revolution. But coal does occur at Castlecomer in Co. Kilkenny, Ballingarry in Co. Tipperary and Arigna in Co. Leitrim, and was exploited here and elsewhere in the past. Upper Carboniferous sandstones and shales dominate the landscapes of south Clare and the Laois-Kilkenny border, and in both places give rise to bleak, rushy plateaux because of the poor drainage of the underlying rocks.

Rocks, Rivers and Caves

One of the most striking geological contrasts in the country is that between Upper and Lower Carboniferous terrains, especially in the Burren of Co. Clare; north of Lisdoonvarna one steps abruptly from the dry, flower-rich grassland of the limestone on to the drab, wet rushland of the shale soils that succeed it. The juxtaposition of shales and limestone is responsible for the formation of Ireland's caves, because run-off flowing across the impermeable acid shales dissolves the limestone along the contact between the two kinds of rocks and continues its erosive work beneath the surface, accelerating the development of the karst landscapes that are characteristic of the limestone (Coleman, 1965; Tratman, 1969). So, today's active caves are mainly in north Clare and Fermanagh, where Upper and Lower Carboniferus rocks are in contact. Elsewhere the hollowing of the caves (such as those that provided homes for the fauna of Munster's late-glacial tundra) are more ancient; here the caves occur in limestone that is now some distance from once-adjacent shales.

The trend of the axes of the folds of the new mountains that came into being at the end of the Upper Carboniferous period (the Hercynian Orogeny) was predominantly east/west. The Carboniferous and Old Red Sandstone rocks of Cork, Kerry and Waterford were crumpled into a regular series of parallel ridges and valleys in the way a cloth pushed across a table would be, but farther north the folds are deflected by the north-east/ south-west trend of the earlier Caledonian mountains. The Carboniferous rocks in the crests of the folds were stripped away to reveal the Old Red Sandstone rocks beneath. These were more resistant to erosion, so that they now occupy the high ground, their weathered remains forming the backbone of the spectacular mountains of the south, covered today in moorland and blanket bog and, increasingly, with plantations of Sitka spruce. The sheltered and fertile valleys between are among the country's best grazing lands.

This simple pattern of east/west-trending sandstone mountains and ridges, separated by fertile valleys underlain by limestone, dominates the landscape of south and central Munster. As might be expected, most of the rivers to the east of the main watershed, which runs across the crests of the Boggeragh and Derrynasaggart Mountains, flow east/west along the valleys – great rivers like the Lee, the Upper Blackwater and the lower course of the Suir, and lesser rivers such as the Bandon and the Bride. But in the lower part of their course, the east-west rivers seem to defy this dominant trend by abruptly changing their course to flow southwards. This puzzling change is due to the persistent lines drawn on the palimpsest of the landscape *before* the east-west ridges and valleys had been etched out in their present form. The original course of the rivers draining the newly upheaved Hercynian Mountains had followed the ancient slope and flowed north-south; only later did the rapid course of erosion sculpt out the pattern of east/west-trending valleys and ridges, giving ever-greater prominence to the tributaries that flowed along them. In some instances the old north-south rivers were able to cut down rapidly enough to keep pace and retain their dominance – sometimes cutting across earlier structural trends to do so –

but in many cases they were beheaded and their function was taken over by their former tributaries. To the west of the watershed, the streams follow the floors of the valleys to flow into the Atlantic, but the former river valleys were later drowned by the invading sea. Inland, the lower lake of Killarney occupies the floor of one of these limestone valleys.

The flat limestone lowlands that stretch away northwards from the Munster mountains had been reduced long before the Ice Ages to a karstic plain, the denuded anticlines of older rocks rising here and there as inliers: islands of older strata in a sea of younger rocks. Most of Ireland's lakes are here – including the lakes on the Shannon, Lough Corrib, Lough Mask – occupying solution hollows in the limestone; Clew Bay is merely a drowned solution lake. One of the most magically evocative views in all of Ireland is that from the hill of Knockma at Castlehacket near Tuam in Co. Galway. Standing here and looking to the east on a misty morning it is not difficult to feel that you are viewing the landscape as it might have looked before the Ice Age: a flat plain that stretches away from you as it were forever. The abundance of ring forts dotted across this landscape bears testimony to the great length of time over which people have lived here and cultivated its soils. Much of the low ground is occupied today by the great raised bogs that grew up on the sites of the extensive network of shallow post-glacial lakes that dominated the landscape of central Ireland in the wake of the Ice Age. Most of the good farming land occurs on the rolling green hills of extensive glacial deposits between, which account for much of the topographical variation in the region. To the north-east the lowland is cut into two by the tumbled hills of the Longford-Down massif, running from Longford to Strangford Lough, which separate the limestone grasslands of Co. Meath from those surrounding Lough Erne.

Ireland's greatest river, the Shannon, rises on Cuilcagh, a scarp of Upper Carboniferous sandstone in Co. Fermanagh, before flowing south across the limestone, here and there expanded into lakes that at one time extended their fringes very much farther, especially to the east. At its southern end it has to cut its way across the more resistant rocks of the old anticlines near Killaloe in order to find its way out to the Atlantic. The Erne is similarly a river of the limestone country, but it is dominated by its lakes; Lough Oughter with all its islands is really a network of flooded tributaries. To the west, the limestone occupies higher ground, forming the spectacular cliff-and-scarp landscape of Sligo and Leitrim, where many of the country's rarest and most special plants shelter, and which was one of the areas favoured by the prehistoric builders of passage graves. Farther south the limestone again rises to high ground in the bare karst of the Burren, buoyed in this instance on a hidden stabilizing cushion of granite. Although it is one of the most remarkable areas of the country for plant and animal life, this is

a landscape whose form and surface today have much to do with the legacy
it has inherited from its early farming communities. After they were abandoned, the pastures of the Bronze Age were invaded by hordes of blue gentians and mountain avens, greatly extending their natural cover. This is a
classic instance of nature taking advantage of an opportunity provided by
human activities to achieve something it might not have achieved unaided.
If the Burren is Ireland's magic mountain it is not because it was ever the
wild world beyond the fields and gardens of man. It is a classic example of
the regenerative capacity of damaged ecosystems of which René Dubos
(1980) writes so elegantly, and which is such a recurring theme in Irish ecology:

Ecosystems possess several mechanisms for self-healing. Some of these are analogous
to the homeostatic mechanisms of animal life; they enable ecosystems to overcome
the effects of outside disturbances simply by re-establishing progressively the original state of ecological equilibrium. More frequently, however, ecosystems undergo
adaptive changes of a creative nature that transcend the mere correction of damage;
the ultimate result is then the activation of certain potentialities of the ecosystem
that had not been expressed before the disturbance.

The Mesozoic Era

During the Permian period, which succeeded the Carboniferous about 290
million years ago, the sea again extended its reach to Ireland, this time as
local embayments of an ocean to the south. Even these had retreated by the
Triassic period, which was characterized by a landscape of arid deserts and
lakes in which rock salt (which outcrops today at Carrickfergus, Co. Antrim)
and gypsum (at Kingscourt, Co. Cavan, and near Belfast) accumulated over
the ages. The lovely red sandstone – the sands of the ancient dunes – which
is the main rock type from this period, occurs mainly from Portadown to
Magilligan Point at the entrance to Lough Foyle, and it was widely used in
building, especially in the north-east of the island. These red sandstones lie
more often on top of Lower Carboniferous than on Upper Carboniferous
rocks, showing how extensively these latter had been eroded even by
Triassic times.

Only in the north-east were sediments laid down during the Jurassic
period, beginning about 190 million years ago. These are clays and shales,
and though they attract little notice of themselves, and are not widely
exposed at the surface, they have a dramatic impact in landscape terms.
These rocks are impermeable, and water percolating through the overlying
chalk and basalt produces a lubricated surface, which leads to extensive slid-
ing of the rocks above. Such landslips are a striking feature along parts of
the Antrim coast road, most obviously around Garron Point.

During the later part of the Cretaceous period, around 65 million years ago, the whole country was invaded by the shallow sea in which the pure white limestone called chalk was laid down. This originated as mud on the floor of the Cretaceous sea, and it has been important as a source of lime and for building; but it had a special importance for the first peoples of north-east Ireland because it contains a great abundance of flint nodules. This was a mineral more important than gold or silver to the people of the Stone Age, because from it they manufactured most of their tools and weapons. Flint is a legacy of the life of ancient seas, because it is derived from the glassy skeletons of the sponges that abounded in the Cretaceous ocean.

Only in the north-east has the chalk survived, protected under a capping of flood basalt. Highly fluid lavas poured from rifts in the earth's crust between 50 and 60 million years ago – at about the time the North Atlantic ocean began to open during the succeeding Eocene and Oligocene periods. The lavas poured quietly across the surface; there was little in the way of explosive volcanic activity. The basalt gives rise today to the high plateau scenery of Antrim and Londonderry, though today's plateau is but a remnant of a once-vast tableland. The thickness of the basalt is nearly nine hundred metres; originally it was more than twice as much. One of the early flows produced a vast lake of molten lava up to one hundred metres deep; as it cooled, the slowly freezing lava contracted and cracked into a solid honeycomb of rock, the great natural wonder of the world we know as the Giant's Causeway.

There were several lava flows, with long intervals between – long enough for the tops of the flows to become deeply weathered to red laterite in the tropical climate of the time. These laterites were a valuable source of iron and aluminium in the last century, but in a few places the laterites were baked by subsequent lava flows to a remarkably hard and even-textured rock called porcellanite. This is known to occur as small outcrops at only two places – Tievebulliagh mountain and Rathlin Island in Co. Antrim – yet in the Neolithic both occurrences of this very special rock were known and exploited for the manufacture and export of the finest axes of the late Stone Age, a demonstration of the intimate knowledge people had, even at this early stage, of the properties of rocks. Lough Neagh, famous for its eel fishery and the largest lake in these islands, developed along a rift valley in the basalt plateau, resulting from the depression of a segment of the crust between parallel fractures.

Two of the most dramatic landforms of the north-east are made of coarser lava that did not reach the surface, but cooled more slowly to a tougher rock called dolerite. Slemish, the mountain made sacred because of its association with St Patrick, is a dolerite cone, as is the dramatic peninsula of Fair Head. The vertical joints produced during cooling allow the agents of weathering to dislodge enormous blocks which tumble to the sea and maintain the sheer profile of the cliff. The magma, which later cooled to granite, and is today exposed in the splendid mountain country of the Mournes, was intruded at depth during this period of deep unrest some 65 million years ago.

The gleaming white chalk, overlain by dark basalt, gives rise to some of the most dramatic cliff scenery in the country along the coast from Red Bay to Larne in ·Co. Antrim. The Cretaceous sea floor was, in its turn, uplifted – a distant ripple of the crustal movements which lifted up the Alps and most of the mountains of southern Europe. These great mountains grew as the African tectonic plate began its unrelenting northwards push against Europe about 65 million years ago, a movement which continues to this day. In the millennia that followed, the soft chalk disappeared almost entirely from the rest of the country.

These earth movements separated Ireland from its continental continuations to the north and west, which now drifted away on new crustal plates, leaving this part of the crust at the north-western edge of the European landmass, then in the throes of upheaval as its southern mountains rose skyward. Through the rest of Tertiary time (Miocene and Pliocene periods), Ireland was a part of mainland Europe, sharing its flora and fauna, until the great upheaval of the Pleistocene – which so profoundly re-moulded the geological inheritance of all the preceding epochs – began a million and a half years ago.

The Ice Age and its Legacy

These geological events and processes, acting over hundreds of millions of years, have shaped the skeleton of the land of Ireland. But among the events that have most profoundly moulded the surface are those of the last two million years, during which the earth's northern hemisphere was gripped in the succession of cold climatic stages which we call the Ice Age. Each cold stage was separated from the succeeding one by an interglacial period during which climate returned to the warmer state we regard as 'normal'. Ireland lay near the southern margin of this great northern ice sheet, and at times was entirely covered by a blanket of glacial ice.

Each successive cold stage wiped the slate of the living landscape clean, leaving little or no evidence of the preceding glaciations or of the fauna and flora that had lived here in these warmer times. The last cold stage, called the Midlandian in Ireland, covered only the northern two-thirds of the island. To the south, much of Munster and south Leinster was frozen tundra, inhabited by animals that could tolerate its harsh demands: bear and hyena, wild cat and Arctic fox, mammoth, reindeer and lemming, whose remains are preserved today in the caves in which they sheltered, or into which their bodies were brought by predators or water. As warmer conditions returned, so too did the plants and animals. The first, cold-tolerant trees such as birch, willow and juniper were followed by the plant species less tolerant of cold. Broad-leaved forests of oak, elm and ash clothed the drift-covered lowlands, the undulations of the moraines and the steep slopes of the eskers adding a new dimension to the endlessly varied topography. The ecology of the forest varied with soil and topography from one region to another, and these evolved as the climate itself evolved. Open pinewoods flourished in the cooler west and on high ground everywhere by the time of the first farmers, between five and six thousand years ago.

The most dramatic animal that roamed the grasslands of Ireland in the late glacial period between 12,000 and 10,600 years ago was the giant Irish deer, the largest deer that ever lived. Although these magnificent animals lived throughout Europe, the densest populations seem to have been in Ireland. They were huge in every sense; they were up to two metres in height at the shoulders, and the enormous antlers of the stag had a span of as much as four metres and weighed up to thirty-five kilograms. Other grazing animals shared the rich post-glacial grasslands with the giant deer: reindeer and elk, very probably bears and wolves, lemmings, foxes and hares. The giant deer was exterminated by a sudden return to very cold conditions 10,600 years ago, which brought an end to the preceding warm period of the Woodgrange Interstadial. Almost all giant deer remains in Ireland have come from the clays underlying the raised bogs.

When the glaciers retreated they left a legacy of moraines and eskers, the rocky debris deposited by the melting glaciers. This impeded the natural drainage, and led to the formation of an extensive network of lakes, especially in the Midlands. It was on the shores of these lakes, and along the coast, only half a millennium after the retreat of the glaciers, that the earliest Irish human communities lived by fishing, hunting, and gathering wild plants. Much later, falling lake levels triggered the widespread development of fen, replacing reed-marsh and open water, and eventually leading to the development of the raised bogs. Much of the moraine consists of an unsorted mixture of everything from great boulders to fine clay; where clay predominated, poor drainage was the result, nowhere more so than where the pressure of slow-moving melting ice at the end of the last glaciation moulded it into the shoals of drumlins, which characterize the landscapes of Leitrim, Cavan and south Clare.

Eskers are one of the most distinctively Irish of landforms; the word *eiscir* is indeed one of the few words which the Irish language has bequeathed to the language of geology. These are the stranded beds of Ice

Age rivers that ran beneath the glaciers, or were deposited where these rivers emerged into the open at the snout of the glacier. Characteristically, they are long, sinuous, sometimes braided and generally steep-sided ridges of stratified sand and gravel. Because they were banked by walls of ice, the river beds were left as upstanding ridges when the ice melted.

The eskers of the Irish midlands, particularly perhaps those around Clonmacnois, are part of a chain known as the Esker Riada, which runs almost continuously in an east-west direction across central Ireland. Eskers provided natural trackways in older times, dry ridges raised above an otherwise wet and wooded landscape, and generally running at right angles to the overall direction of glacial retreat, although their direction may also reflect the line of former crevasses in the ice. The Esker Riada carried the great western road of ancient Ireland, the Slighe Mhór, westward from Clonard right across the midlands almost all the way to Galway. This natural feature was thus the greatest natural boundary line of ancient Ireland, dividing the country into two great divisions: Leath Chuinn and Leath Mhogha.

Once their cover of woodland was cleared, the eskers provided prehistoric farmers with well-drained, easily worked land, and they were farmed from a very early period. The abundance of archaeological features concentrated on them bears testimony to the antiquity of their fields. The Bronze Age settlement that has come to light at Clonfinlough, Co. Offaly, where Bord na Móna has removed the subsequent growth of peat, occurs on the lower slopes of the esker.

Beyond the agricultural advantages they provided, the eskers and related landforms were also of great strategic significance. They provided the Anglo-Norman invaders of the late twelfth century with ideal vantage points on which to erect their motte-and-bailey castles. Banagher, Shannonbridge and Athlone grew up at the only places in the south midlands where eskers crossed the Shannon, providing a short crossing and dry ground on which to erect a bridge or ferry. Clonmacnois is at the junction of the two most important arteries of communication in the midlands: the navigable Shannon, and the overland route that followed the eskers right across the midlands from Dublin. Even today, many quiet ancient roads in the country run along the crests or slopes of eskers.

The eskers and end moraines provided an abundance of ready-to-hand building material without the necessity of quarrying solid stone: cobbles for the paving of streets and courtyards, and sand for mortar and later for cement and even fertilizer. Sir Charles Coote (writing in his *Statistical Survey of the King's County* at the beginning of the nineteenth century) was impressed by the providential arrangement whereby a superabundance of the fertilizer that was essential to the reclamation of bogland was available right in the middle of the bogs themselves. Today the most obvious value of the eskers lies in the sand and gravel they contain, which is exploited for road-making and road-fill material, and in cement manufacture. Parts of the eskers still cling to their rich natural character, and they carry some of the most interesting and important woodland and grassland habitats in the country. The exploitation of the eskers for their sand and gravel has created numerous quarries whose exposed faces provide an ideal site for the burrows of sand wasps and sand martins, whose principal habitat they now are. The natural regeneration of abandoned quarries often provides an opportunity for species-rich natural grassland to extend its limited range.

The post-glacial rise in sea level flooded many of the U-shaped river valleys that had been hollowed out by valley glaciers, converting them to the finger-like fjords which are the most striking aspect of the south-west coast. Dingle Bay, the Kenmare River and Bantry Bay are all fine examples, but the finest of all is Killary Harbour between Galway and Mayo, ten miles long and half a mile wide. Wider bays like Galway Bay or Clew Bay, similar in form to the rias of Spain, are also subsidence features. In Galway Bay, the post-glacial rise detached the Aran Islands, which in Tertiary time had been part of the Burren. Clew Bay was a broad valley filled with drumlins at the end of the Ice Age; the rise in sea level submerged the drumlin hollows, leaving their island crests like a school of swimming whales.

The submergence of the east coast which finally made an island of Ireland 7500 years ago also created a series of fjords on that side of the island, features that reminded the invading Vikings in the tenth century of the coastline of their Norse homeland, and which they named in their own language: Carlingford, Wexford, Waterford, Strangford. Lough Swilly and Lough Foyle on the north coast are also submerged river valleys. Many of the rivers follow tortuous courses to the sea because glacial debris has made an obstacle race of their more natural courses. The associated wetlands constitute a network of habitats that are among the most important for wildlife.

The local ecological patterns that developed in Ireland in the wake of the Ice Age were shaped by a variety of factors. The character of the underlying geology was fundamental, because it determined the nutrient resources available and also topography. The legacy of the Ice Age profoundly modified this ancient inheritance of rock, because of the way it transported great amounts of till across country. These were moulded by post-glacial weathering to give new landforms, greatly altering the topography and the soil resources available to plants.

A second factor was Ireland's new situation on the globe: it was an island for the first time in its long history, and therefore more difficult of access to plants and animals on the European mainland. Ireland was an integral part of the European mainland throughout the Tertiary epoch. The fauna and flora had free access, unhindered by water. The rising sea level after the Ice Age first isolated Britain and Ireland as one large island, and then severed Ireland from Britain.

Climate and Habitat

Ireland's situation as a small island at the north-west of the European main-land, right in the path of the North Atlantic depressions moving in from the ocean, is largely responsible for its distinctive climate: cool in summer, wet and mild in the winter, with plenty of rainfall and modest amounts of sun. Two aspects of the temperate Irish climate are particularly important from an ecological perspective. First of all there is the high rainfall, a consequence of Ireland's island position at the north-western tip of the continent, exposed to the wet westerlies blowing in from the Atlantic. The heavy rainfall is especially characteristic of higher land in the west, often delaying spring and causing wet harvests in autumn, but providing constant moisture, which is conducive to the richness of the flora in this part of Ireland. Annual rainfall varies from 750 mm in the east to over 1300 mm along the western coasts, where there can be as many as 270 rain days in the year. Bright sunshine is correspondingly rare in the west: 1200 hours as against 1600 in parts of the east. Mean annual wind speed on the western coasts can be twice that of the sheltered midlands.

The sourth-west corner of the island is also in the path of the Gulf Stream, which is responsible for the mildness of the climate there. The few species of Irish flowering plants not found in Great Britain – plants such as the strawberry tree (*Arbutus unedo*), London pride (*Saxifraga spathularis*) and Irish heath (*Erica erigena*) – occur on this wilder and wetter side of the island. The warm, moisture-laden south-westerlies are responsible for the richness of the bryophyte (mosses and liverworts) and fern flora especially, which includes a significant number of south-western European species. The bryophyte flora of south-west Ireland is the most luxurious found in these islands, if not in the whole of Europe. The south-east of the island, out of the path of the Atlantic depressions and their rainfall, is drier and more continental in character than other parts.

Historical accident apart, biogeographic theory predicts that Ireland should have fewer species than its neighbouring island to the east because it is a smaller island stretched across fewer degrees of latitude. The principal British habitats lacking in Ireland are the chalk downs and lowland heaths of southern Britain and the high mountain habitats of northern Scotland – but geology and history also play a role in this difference in legacy.

The overall regional pattern of natural habitats is particularly reflected in the varying character of the woodlands, which is largely a response to the geological heritage of rock, the endowment of glacial sediment from the Ice

Age glaciers and the soils both of these produce, interacting with climate and topography. In early post-glacial times, hazel appears to have been especially characteristic of the north-east of the island, whereas pine was especially common all down the western seaboard. Oak was widely distributed and often dominant in the mature forests which came to dominate the land; elm, however, seems to have been common only on the eastern side of the country. Placename evidence helps us to pick out places where particular trees were especialy noticeable in later prehistoric times. Names like Youghal, Kyleanoe and Killinure (yew wood), or Mayo and Moynure (yew plain), indicate that yew *(iubhair* or *eo* in Irish) was prominent in the vegetation. (It is of interest to note the similarity of the English *yew* and the Irish *eo* or *iubhair,* indicating a common Celtic origin.) Oak placenames are especially common, especially as *doire,* an oak wood; more than 1300 townland names begin with the word in its various forms, and many others have it as an ending.

But within the different regions on the island there is much local variety, so that every district has its distinctive mosaic of ecotopes and habitats. Most importantly, interacting with this spatial variation there is the ongoing temporal dynamic of vegetation evolution, which it is easy to overlook because it pulses so slowly. The climate since the Ice Age has undergone a series of oscillations that have greatly influenced flora and fauna. The vegetation itself has also been dynamic, its patterns evolving in response to change, and particularly to climatic change and human influence. We are aware of its profound legacy in the past because the time frame is speeded up as we view the ages that have gone. But it will operate just as powerfully in the future.

The climate reached a warm and dry optimum 8000 years ago, at a time when Mesolithic or Middle Stone Age communities were settled throughout the island. The wet but still warm interval that followed favoured the development of fens and other wetlands, the fens in time generally developing into bogs. There was a reversion to cold and wet conditions around 2500 years ago, favouring the increased dominance of bog mosses (*Sphagnum*) on the raised bogs.

Human Impact on Irish Nature

The human influence on the natural life of Ireland has been pervasive. We now realize that there were human communities throughout Ireland probably within a few centuries of the retreat of the ice, long before the broadleaved forests or the peatlands had developed extensively. These communities probably had relatively little influence on the vegetation in pre-agricultural times, although the use of fire may have had a greater impact than we are now aware of. But once farming began between five and six thousand years ago, a new and selective influence was brought to bear. At different times, different ecological situations – different natural land-cover types – have been favoured for agriculture. It has often been observed that Neolithic farmers, with their tools of stone, favoured lighter lowland soils, which they identified from the prevalence of elm growing on them, thus precipitating the elm decline that so reduced the species in Ireland around 3800 years ago. The upland pinewoods provided grazing, perhaps assisted by burning, pressures that led in time to the erosion of their fragile soils at a time of worsening climate, and precipitated the spread of blanket bog. The sandy landforms of eskers and end moraines acted as natural routeways and provided strategic locations. Bronze Age prospectors sought those lands where the rocks yielded copper.

Oats are the cereal most favoured by the cool and wet climatic conditions that have prevailed in Ireland for most of its human history, but during the secondary climatic optimum that occurred between AD 1000 and 1400 wheat could thrive, making the country attractive to the Norman knights and farmers who valued land on the basis of its capacity to produce wheat. The coming of the Great Plague (1348-50), preceded by the wettest and coldest summers of the millennium, heralded the Little Ice Age, a time of long severe winters and short summers; the colony collapsed, and the growing of wheat was abandoned in northern Europe. This miserable climatic epoch lasted until the middle of the nineteenth century, the devastating potato famine of the late 1840s marking its end with human misery, as the plague had marked the beginning.

With the forward march of agriculture as the constant backdrop to human history, few wild species have actually disappeared altogether; but it is not only *numbers* of species or even the declining proportion of wild land to grassland or arable that matter. Agricultural inputs in earlier times were very low; there was no import of manure, no artificial fertilizer was used, there were no pesticides or weedkillers. The harvest was reaped with the sickle and the gleanings augmented the autumn supplies for birds and mammals. In terms of actual numbers of species, few that were present in earlier times are absent today – the opposite is much more the case – but there are great differences in the abundance and the extent of distribution of wild plant and animal species. Plants such as primroses and cowslips, orchids, and the flowers and mycoflora of grassland were vastly more abundant than they are today. As a consequence, there must have been a richer invertebrate fauna, with obvious consequences for the abundance of animals further up the food chains, such as birds and carnivorous mammals. There was no re-seeding or creation of artificial grassland; all grassland was semi-natural, and that is a habitat type which today is almost as rare as woodland. One has to

look hard in the Ireland of today to find the wonderful species-rich grasslands of the Middle Ages, although they do survive in odd, neglected corners. You get a glimpse of it in the neglected old fields of Connemara or the
Burren.

The same general conclusions hold for the abundance and diversity of
the larger animals, but here we are ascending the food chain, and the
absence of certain key species today that were present in the past is indication of the extent to which their habitat has contracted. The wolf was plentiful right through the medieval period; the difference in the attitude of people to the wolf at this time compared with the modern period – say after the
sixteenth century – is significant in environmental terms. It was tolerated up
to then, but after 1600 there was systematic persecution; in other words, as
land-use pressure built up, the woodland and scrub disappeared, until eventually *we could no longer find room for them*, and they were pushed over the
brink of extinction: an earlier and smaller-scale example of what is happening in the case of the African elephant or rhinoceros today. The wolf was of
course hunted earlier, but the important point is that the pressure on its
habitat was relatively low, and the human population too had been low.

Another of these key species is the bittern, whose magical booming call
echoed across the open land in many wetter areas of the country until the
early part of the nineteenth century. The bittern has not bred in Ireland
since about 1840; its disappearance is attributed to the extensive drainage of
the bogs and marshes in the early part of the nineteenth century, although
hunting is likely to have had an increasingly severe effect as populations
declined. Its occurrence and distribution in the earlier centuries is a reflection of the much greater extent of wetland. A third key species we might
note briefly is the golden eagle, which bred widely on the crags of the
mountains; as with the wolf, the rising tide of human pressure on land after
medieval times drove the bird from its last haunts in the corries. I met an
old man in Toor at the foot of Keeper Hill in Co. Tipperary some years ago
whose grandfather had 'looked the last eagle in the eye' on Coumaniller, a
corry lake on the hill.

The natural ecological patterns are thus intimately influenced by the
geological endowment, and particularly that of the Ice Age. The ways in
which the human community has exploited nature in Ireland, and the
opportunities for its survival and renewal, have been and continue to be
shaped by the heritage of the rocks. The unique patchwork landscape of
Ireland has resulted from more than nine thousand years of interaction
between man and nature on the island: but it echoes also a far more ancient
song of earth, which shaped land and sea and mirrors the making of stars.

People in earlier centuries may have been able to see history as cyclical,
ruled by the turning seasons, spring returning each year after the darkness

and want of winter to renew growth and hope. However, with the new eyes of those who no longer experience the wilderness – and can scarcely imagine what it was like – we can see, reviewing our history on this island, that it moves in one direction in two key respects. First of all, there has been a steady retreat of wild nature at the expense of fields since the beginnings of farming. This has accelerated with the rise in the human population; so little is now left that the retention of what remains must be a priority. Second, the march of technology, from stone axe to tractor, has provided the capability to destroy the remnants of the natural ecology in forest and bog and hedgerow with ever-increasing facility, so that the flame of the sword of the Angel posted at the gates of Paradise to prevent our return to an experience of the original wilderness, burns ever brighter. But with increased understanding and prosperity have come increasing awareness both of the value of lost nature and of the preciousness of what survives, and a realization that the power to heal is part of the power to change.

References

Coleman, J.C. 1965. *The Caves of Ireland*. Tralee: Anvil Books.

Charlesworth, J.K. 1963. *Historical Geology of Ireland*. Edinburgh and London: Oliver and Boyd.

Dubos, R. 1980. *The Wooing of Earth*. London: Athlone Press.

Gould, S.J. 1991. *Wonderful Life: The Burgess Shale and the Nature of History*. Harmondsworth: Penguin.

Herries Davies, G.L. 1981. 'The History of Irish Geology,' in C.H. Holland (ed.), *A Geology of Ireland*. Edinburgh: Scottish Academic Press.

Herries Davies, G.L. 1995. *North from the Hook: 150 Years of the Geological Survey of Ireland*. Dublin: Geological Survey of Ireland.

Holland, C.H. (ed.) 1981. *A Geology of Ireland*. Edinburgh: Scottish Academic Press.

Tratman, E.K. 1969. *The Caves of North-West Clare*. Newton Abbot: David and Charles.

Encountering Traditions

JOHN WILSON FOSTER

The Human Imprint

The impact of humanity on Irish nature is of such longevity and density that to refer to the Irish 'countryside' is to imply human presence as North American reference to 'the wilderness' or Australian reference to 'the outback' does not. For at least nine thousand years human beings have trod the island: it was in the Middle Stone Age that the first communities appeared. Yet for a long time, the human impact on land and wildlife would have been slight. The earliest sites discovered reveal an economy dependent on food-gathering, fishing and hunting. For three thousand years, it has been said, the Mesolithic people were 'passive exploiters of their environment, rather than active cultivators' (Ryan, 1987), the shift from food collection to food production occurring around 4000 BC.

Simple habitations, agriculture and modest clearances of the woods were followed over time by more complicated settlements, deforestation, land reclamation and improvement, and roadways. Habitats were shrunken, destroyed, created or otherwise altered. Yet even well into historical time, the impact would not have been serious: in the early Middle Ages (AD 500-1100) the population of Ireland is said to have been a mere half million (Richter, 1988).* Urbanization and major interventions in the natural (for example dams, reservoirs, waterways, railways, roads for horse-drawn traffic and then motor cars) lagged behind similar developments in Britain in their scale and number.

In addition to the kinds of impact noted above, which involved alterations of nature, the island has experienced historical episodes, including

---

* The history of early human presence on the island can be found in Evans (1957), Whittow (1974), Ryan (1987), Evans (1992) and Mitchell (1994). Certain essays in this volume (Feehan, Neeson, Foss and O'Connell) help to fill in modern details of the picture.

numerous wars and famines, that in greater or lesser degree impacted on plants and wildlife. I will return to famine elsewhere; as for war, I offer one particularly graphic example. 'After the great war in the seventeenth century,' wrote P.W. Joyce (1891), thinking presumably of the events of 1641 and the coming of Cromwell, 'wolves increased to such an extent, and their ravages became so great, as to call for state interference, and wolf-hunters were appointed in various parts of Ireland.' Joyce does not indicate the precise cause of the increase, but in any case it would have had at least short-term knock-on effects in the rest of the Irish ecosystem, the details of which are probably at this distance irrecoverable.

In 1864 George Parkins Marsh attempted in *Man and Nature* an ambitious account of the modification of physical geography in the modern world by human activity, and it can be consulted as a vast backdrop to what has gone on in Ireland. Among the human manipulations of the environment Marsh discusses are introductions of plants, quadrupeds and birds. Lever (1977, 1985, 1987, 1996) has recently brought the story up to date for naturalized and feral animals and birds. The result is that even when we decide what is natural and what is not, we might find it difficult to decide whether a particular species is native or foreign. The rabbit, for example, is not truly indigenous to Ireland or to anywhere in northern Europe, to which it spread after being transported from Spain to Italy by the Romans; it was taken to England in the twelfth century (White, 1968) and was first noted in Ireland a hundred or so years later (Fairley, 1984).

Despite the protracted humanizing of nature, our sense of the natural renews itself, through the reversion of the man-made to the feral (often by our neglect) or through our increasingly modest redefinition of what constitutes nature. Evans (1992) has claimed that the 'dominance of proudly independent scattered farms and the weakness of long-established village communities' at once lend historic unity to the Irish countryside and distinguish it from England. If this is the case, it suggests that the 'natural' may have survived longer in Ireland. Lennon believes that despite forest clearances, bog reclamations and nucleated villages of the medieval centuries, the landscape of early sixteenth-century Ireland was 'pristine and primeval'. In the next century appeared the plantation estates and the planned towns, yet except where agriculture, urbanization and industrialization later gained serious purchase (as in parts of Ulster), portions of the the island escaped deep human penetration. Even as late as 1974, Whittow could claim that 'Ireland retains landscapes which have all but disappeared in Britain', because most of the island was untouched by the Industrial Revolution during the hundred years after the middle of the eighteenth century.

Besides, the natural can reassert itself when human presence declines for economic and other reasons, as happened in the west of Ireland. Roy

Foster (1988) reminds us that 'in 1600 Ulster was synonymous with wildness and untamed Gaelicism' while Connacht in the west 'was characterized by economic activity and cultural vitality'; yet in later years the characterizations were reversed: north Armagh and south-east Antrim, for example, were by the early 1600s being landscaped and Big Houses being built.

The lessening of human presence in Connacht became the alarming depopulation of the early twentieth century. The flight from the land became a powerful literary motif, and in the 'waste places' of the west W.B. Yeats and his literary cohorts influentially located the mystical heart of Ireland. Indeed, Connacht became synonymous with 'real' nature in Ireland, and since it was part of the Gaeltacht or Irish-speaking remnant of the island, Gaelicism and nature reinforced each other in ways that were of ultimate benefit to Bord Fáilte (the Irish Tourist Board) later in the twentieth century. Ulster, a byword for wildness in 1600 (in the view of the English), ironically became for the native Irish – when the province was planted by Scots who farmed and wove and centuries later built factories and shipyards – a byword for the least 'natural' part of Ireland. From this, it could be a short step to the 'least indigenous', thus most politically dubious part of the island (Foster, 1991).

Nature and Colonization

The story of the study of nature in Ireland is therefore interwoven with the story of human presence and human perception of nature in Ireland. Moreover, to the extent that the human presence has made itself felt in waves, in the form of successive intrusions of cultures (including in historic times the Norse, Norman, English and Scots cultures), the Irish landscape and even its creatures and flora are a kind of palimpsest, superimposed forms that testify to the complex interaction of nature and human culture. (For example, see Fairley, 1984, and Sleeman in this volume, for successive introductions of mammals into Ireland.)

It was the most recent cultures to settle in Ireland, the English and the Scots, that initiated and developed the scientific, systematic study of nature. Roy Foster dates the beginning of modern Ireland to 1600, when resistance to the Tudor reconquest – begun in 1541 – was at a pivotal point, and Gaelic Ireland was about to succumb. What he calls the rich 'survey' literature of late Elizabethan observers gives us a picture of the contemporary Irish landscape. The most obvious difference between then and now is the extent of woodland: in 1600 the dense woods covered about an eighth of the island (Foster, 1988), and they sheltered wolves, pine martens, deer and wild boar (Neeson, 1991). The wolf did not become extinct in Ireland until around 1770, indicating the longevity of dense cover and sparse human settlement in sizeable areas of the island.

To the Elizabethans and Jacobeans, the density of the forests was to be deplored but also welcomed: welcomed because the forests could be profitably cut down to provide timber for English ships or serve the pipe-staving industry, deplored because they could conceal wolf and woodkerne (Irish soldier) alike. Cutting them down, as Queen Elizabeth decreed, destroyed shelter for the native enemies of the colonists (Neeson, 1991), who for several centuries after the first, fitful English incursions lived beyond the purview of cartography and the regimen of chronometry. Indeed, wolf and woodkerne were regarded as *being* alike. In *A View of the Present State of Ireland* (1596), the poet and colonial administrator Edmund Spenser has his dialogist Irenius recall the report that the Irish like the Scythians turn into wolves once a year, though 'Master Camden' (William Camden, 1551-1623, who published Giraldus Cambrensis's *Topographia Hiberniae* in 1602) supposed 'it was a disease called licanthropia, so named of the wolf, and yet [Irenius adds] some of the Irish do use to make the wolf their gossip' (Spenser, 1970; Ashton, 1890).* Of the 'natural Wild Irish', Laurence Echard in 1691 remarked that 'They pray for wolves, and wish them well, and then they are not afraid to be hurt by them' (quoted in Stevenson, 1920). These passages reveal as much about the Elizabethans' understanding of animals as about their understanding of the Irish; they are crude forerunners of what in our time, made scientific, became cryptozoology (see below). Incidentally, the woodkerne could also be likened to the eagle, both frequenting 'crafty' or 'uncivil' nooks beyond 'the Englishe pale', to quote John Derricke's *The Image of Irelande* in 1581 (Hadfield and McVeagh, 1994). Unless this was a merely verbal trope, our inference would be that the eagle – which could have been the golden or white-tailed eagle, or both – had by 1580 been driven out of Louth, Meath, Kildare and Dublin, the four shires of the Pale.

In 1685 William King – later to become Archbishop of Dublin – published 'Of the Bogs and Loughs of Ireland' in *Philosophical Transactions* (later included in *A Natural History of Ireland*, the 1726 expansion of Gerard Boate's 1652 *Irelands Naturall History*), in which he calls Irish bogs 'infamous' and equates extensive bogland with barbarity. Bogs covered about a quarter of the island in the sixteenth century and were densest in the central lowlands (Lennon, 1994). William Lithgow brightly complained in 1632 that 'there are moe Rivers, Lakes, Brookes, Strands, Quagmires, Bogs, and

---

* 'Gossips' were spiritual kindred though also, according to Sir John Davies in 1612 (1988, 171), secular allies capable of composing a 'confederacy' dangerous to the colonists. One is tempted to remark that Spenser's dialogue on the contemporary state of Ireland is answered three centuries later by the Irishman Oscar Wilde, in whose dialogue *The Critic as Artist* (1890) Eudoxus and Irenius become Cyril and Gilbert and in which there are pungent observations on the present degenerate state of England and the claim that it is the cultivated Celt who leads in art.

Marishes, in this Countrey, then in all Christendome besides; for Travelling there in the Winter, all my dayly solace, was sincke down comfort; whiles Boggy-plunging deepes kissing my horse belly; whiles over-mired Saddle, Body, and all; and often or ever set a swimming, in great danger, both I, and my Guides of our Lives: That for cloudy and fountayne-bred perils, I was never before reduced to such a floting Laborinth' (Hadfield and McVeagh, 1994). It would be interesting to speculate on the likely list, status and distribution of plants, insects, mammals and birds in the marshy expanses of sixteenth- and early seventeenth-century Ireland.

Like the woods, the bogs offered an advantage to resistant natives, who, King believed, deliberately built near them: the bogs 'are a shelter and a refuge to tories [dispossessed natives turned outlaws], and thieves, who can hardly live without them' (Carpenter and Deane, 1991). As Derricke had it in verse, bogs were the sites of reversion of native Irish introduced to the ways of the Pale: 'Yet doe thei loke to shaking Boggs,/scarce provying honest menne./And when as thei have wonne the Boggs,/suche vertue hath that grounde:/that they are wurse than wildest Karne,/And more in sinne abounde' (Hadfield and McVeagh, 1994). On the whole, bogs were to be regretted, though they were 'of some use' as fuel, especially, as King charged, 'we having very impolitickly destroyed our wood, and not as yet found stone coal' (Carpenter and Deane, 1991). Sir John Davies in 1612 thought that it had been a mistake for the English colonizers to estrange the native Irish (making it 'no felony to kill a mere Irishman in the time of peace'), to drive them into the woods and bogs (which became their synonym – woodkerne and bog-Irish) instead of bringing them in under English law (Davies, 1988).

For the Elizabethan colonists, the prospect (or actual view) of bogland from the English Pale was, as it were, the ground-level reality of Irish nature, very different from the colonial prospect (or anticipated view) of Ireland from England, a 'prospectus' of fine 'commodities' to which each country eyed for conquest and plantation was both reduced and magnified. Before the rational empiricism of Francis Bacon was applied in the later seventeenth century, there was no scientific vision or language available when the new in nature was contemplated or encountered. Spenser's vignette of Ireland in the early pages of his *View*, though it contains accurate observations, derives from pastoral, a favourite Elizabethan mode and vision:

And sure it is yet a most beautiful and sweet country as any is under heaven, seamed throughout with many goodly rivers replenished with all sorts of fish most abundantly, sprinkled with very many sweet islands and goodly lakes like little inland seas, that will carry even ships upon their waters, adorned with goodly woods fit for building of houses and ships so commodiously, as that if some princes in the world had them, they would soon hope to be lords of all the seas and ere long of all the world, also full of very good ports and havens opening upon England and Scotland, as inviting us to come unto them, to see what excellent commodities that country can afford, besides the soil itself most fertile, fit to yield all kind of fruit that shall be committed thereinto; and, lastly, the heavens most mild and temperate, though somewhat more moist than the parts towards the west. (Spenser, 1970)*

Davies opens his hardheaded ruminations on the long English campaign to subdue and 'civilize' Ireland with a comparable hymn to the Irish landscape. To these passages we might add Robert Payne's inventory of Irish wildfowl (c. 1589), which recalls similar contemporary claims of plenitude by New World explorers, and in which wildlife is a resource for sustenance and sport and evidence of a larger mercantile viability in the country to be colonized: 'There be great store of wild Swannes, Cranes, Pheasantes, Partriges, Heathcocks, Plovers, greene and grey, Curlewes, Woodcockes, Rayles, Quailes, & all other fowles much more plentifull then in England' (Hadfield and McVeagh, 1994). Colonization required the crying up of nature in such set pieces (which is not, of course, to deny their truthfulness: Ireland must indeed have teemed with wildfowl in those days, as did North America).

The colonizers at different times paint both an Edenic landscape and a fallen landscape (a 'desert' or 'waste'). This twofold depiction is both a cause and an effect of the deeply embedded European ambivalence about nature: nature is pristine and prelapsarian, innocent and good, but it is also sullied and savage, wild and unregenerate. If this ambivalence seems especially Protestant, we should remember that it was Protestantism that encouraged close attention to nature: the biblical licence for human dominion over nature and the Christian wish to admire the good created Earth could each be taken as jutification for scientific study.

The ambivalence towards nature found a specific venue in colonial Ireland. It was explained away partly on the racialist grounds that nature in Ireland was unregenerate because the nature of the Irish was unregenerate. And so for such a promising landscape to be *realized*, stern measures would have to be taken against its present undeserving custodians; to the colonial observer, nature's bounty is overlooked or squandered by the foolish, warlike native. The measures were politically as well as agriculturally wise: Davies was of the opinion that had the early colonizers built in the wooded and mountainous fastnesses, thereby reclaiming the land from its wildness, 'the Irish had been easily kept in order and in short time reclaimed from their wildness'; the English lords should have turned the mountains and bogs into deer forests, chases and parks as had happened in England.

---

* Spenser was the first English poet to make use of the Irish landscape, idealized depictions of which enliven *Colin Clouts Come Home Againe* (1591) and *The Faerie Queene* (1609).

When the stern measures are taken and the natives resist, as they did in 'the late wars in Munster', the 'most rich and plentiful country, full of corn and cattle' (Spenser, 1970), is reduced to penury, and we have the obverse image of what we might call 'commodity pastoralism', an elegiac version of King's bogland that centuries later haunted Scamus Heaney into poetry:

Out of every corner of the woods and glens they came creeping forth upon their hands, for their legs could not bear them. They looked anatomies of death, they spake like ghosts crying out of their graves, they did eat of the dead carrions, happy were they could find them, yea and one another soon after in so much as the very carcasses they spared not to scrape out of their graves, and if they found a plot of water cress or shamrocks, there they flocked as to a feast for the time, yet not able long to continue therewithal, that in short space there were none almost left and a most populous and plentiful country suddenly left void of man or beast. Yet sure in all that war there perished not many by the sword, but all by the extremity of famine, which they themselves had wrought.

(Spenser, 1970; cf. Heaney's poem 'Bog Oak' from *Wintering Out*, 1972)

In short, what Spenser and his contemporaries saw in Irish nature was in part real, in part preconceived through economics, literature and cosmology. They were vigilant and practical shapers of the world, but also sleepwalkers. We associate the Elizabethans with the Renaissance and identify them as ruthless, down-to-earth prosecutors of colonization in Ireland and the New World. But older ways of seeing nature survived into Bacon's day and even after, making the Elizabethan attitude to the natural world a hybrid creature.

Despite our usual notion of the Renaissance, it was then that 'the mind of man began seriously to sport with the fabulous' (White, 1984). *A Thousand Notable Things* (c. 1579) was a popular Elizabethan anthology of marvels similar to *The Book of Secrets* associated with the alchemical writer Albertus Magnus (1206-80, author of *The Marvels of the World* and *De Animalibus*) and printed in England in the sixteenth and seventeenth centuries. A Polish-Scottish physician named John Johnstone (or Jonston) published a book as late as 1650 called *Historiae Naturalis de Anibus*, widely read and translated into English in 1657 as *History of the Wonderful Things of Nature*, in which the harpy, phoenix and griffin are listed among its birds (Allen, 1951).

Travel had always been a source of wonders through travellers' tales (the archetypal narrative is by the figure known as 'John de Mandeville'), and since the Elizabethans were great explorers – colonization requiring such – their fascination with the remarkable should not be surprising. And travel (be it connected with Empire or not) and the marvellous have continued to be a powerful stimulus to natural history. In 1595 Sir Philip Sidney praised the poet for bringing forth, 'quite anew, forms such as never were in Nature, as the Heroes, Demi-gods, Cyclopes, Chimeras, Furies, and such like', refusing the narrow warrant of nature's gifts; the marvellous and the creative were for the Elizabethans connected (Sidney, 1970). But those who went fearlessly abroad to unknown or barely known regions reported sights that rivalled the poets' imaginings. And these reports were tenacious: one of the first papers delivered to the Royal Society (founded 1662), and by its president, re-told the venerable story of the generation of barnacle geese from shells adhering to Scottish trees (Allen, 1951).

The Philosophical Transactions of the Royal Society, which early had distinguished Anglo-Irish contributors, or 'correspondents', was a repository and clearing-house for the 'remarkables' of the known world and recorded its fair share of wonders and marvels along with the bizarrely misunderstood and grotesquely misperceived. The curiosity science was to require in turn required curiosities as its stimulus and object of attention. But the intensity of interest in those curiosities, even some of the curiosities themselves, derived from older belief systems. It has been claimed by the celebrated historian of science and magic Frances Yates that natural magic had as great an effect on early modern science as the traditional academic disciplines.

We have already seen evidence that the Elizabethan perception of Irish nature was a deeply cultural one. Ireland is a kind of 'Otherworld', the inhabitants of which are at best redeemably wild, at worst irredeemably brutish. Spenser and Sidney both pay respect to the reverence in which the Irish held their poets, but Sidney praised New World Indians for the same virtue (the Indians were frequently compared to the Irish by Elizabethans, even down to the kinds of trousers some Indian tribes wore) and the poetic bent was the exception that proved the rule of general barbarism and want of learning. Practical economic desire and literary daydream were the bifocal lenses through which the Elizabethans viewed Ireland, but the larger concept of the Earth and its inhabitants entertained by the Elizabethans derived as much from Renaissance cosmology as from a nascent Baconian science. (It derived especially from the scheme we know as the Great Chain of Being, with its hierarchies, microcosms and macrocosms; the Elizabethan world-view is explained in detail by Lovejoy and Tillyard.) The radical revisions of Copernicus, Kepler and Galileo were not generally accepted, even by astronomers, until after the first decade of the seventeenth century. And in the human portion of the Great Chain of Being, the Irish were thought to be a lowlier link than the English and certain other European peoples. But who in reality were the Irish and how did they perceive and understand the nature that surrounded them?

The Celtic View of Nature

Spenser's Ireland of cesses, folkemotes, carrows, rakehelly horseboys, churls, kernes, bards, bodrags, gallowglasses, mantles and glibs is an exotic culture to the modern-day Irish, and one that Celtic scholarship has since made more familiar by unravelling the complexities of Gaelic society and uncovering the buried treasures of its literature. Yet what the Celts appear to have believed about the world around them was not in some respects radically more peculiar to the modern understanding than what many Elizabethans believed.

The Celts were the Indo-European ancestors of the Irish, Scots, Welsh, Cornish, Bretons and early inhabitants of the Isle of Man; the evidence of their presence in Europe goes back to the Iron Age, around 1000 BC, and perhaps the early Bronze Age, about 1800 BC. They became the dominant people in non-Mediterranean Europe, expanding westwards, eventually as far as Ireland. They were no match for Roman organization and were overrun, save in Ireland which escaped Roman colonization. Celtic society in Ireland did not change until the coming of Christianity in the fifth century, and survived strongly for centuries after that.

Archaeological and literary research has shown that domesticated animals played a large role in the Celtic economy. Digs of early medieval sites suggest that the skins of red deer and seals were made into leather; the pelts of otter and marten were also used. Antler and bone knife-handles, bone pins, and antler combs have been recovered (Edwards, 1990). Fish and mammals were hunted for sport and livelihood (Joyce, 1913, II), and recovered bird bones indicate wildfowling (Edwards, 1990, 65). Joyce (1913, II) claims that wild as well as domestic animals were kept as pets: foxes, wolves, deer, badgers, hawks, crows and cranes (herons). Horses were war-steeds and drawers of chariots, and the images of animals and birds decorated Celtic war-gear. Such images were symbolic: the goose, for example, evoked alertness and aggression, the raven – presumably because it was a scavenger on the battlefield – was a prophet of battle outcome and symbolized pitilessness and carnage (Green, 1992). Ravens entered the early literature in symbolic guise: the enemies of the wounded Ulster champion Cuchulain (hero of the early medieval Red Branch cycle of stories) know he is dead when the Morigu (wargoddesses in the shape of crows) alight on his shoulders. The animal motifs of early Irish literature have been identified and arranged by Cross (1952).

Beyond custom and daily routine, animals were objects of sacrifice; they were omens or were the embodiments of human souls. Indeed, the metamorphosis of human beings into animals (often maidens into swans) is a recurring transaction in the saga literature and later folktales (Flower, 1947; Armstrong, 1958). The recurrence of metamorphosis amounts to a Celtic view of the natural world as deceptive, fluid, essentially formal rather than substantial, without fixity in the identity of species (but not, of course, evolutionary). Yet nature is not merely whimsical: there are formulas of shape-changing which carry the values of Celtic society. The succession of cultures on the island, the dictates of narrative interest in an oral culture, the advisability of concealment and disguise in a circumscribed and dangerous society – all might be cultural factors promoting the prevalence of transformations in Celtic nature (Foster, 1987). Celtic vision seems to be simultaneously dynamic (the creatures transformed) and stable (transformed creatures turning back into themselves). The whole business testifies less to organic notions of similarity – though swans can in their gracefulness and beauty be regarded as naturally feminine – than to an unseen dimension of life. Animals, birds and trees were links for the Celts to the Otherworld.

The pre-Christian, pre-scientific Celtic view of nature had its own coherence, which obviously does not harmonize with separable modern concepts of the utilization of nature (economy), the divinity of nature (religion), the imagery of nature (art and literature), and the autonomy of nature (natural history). One scholar has attempted to show that the cosmological, mythological and religious significance of nature for the Celts constituted a matrix of belief, not, as is commonly thought, a vague mysticism (Tymoczko, 1990). She does so by using as a case-study Old and Middle Irish terms for black birds. She finds that the Irish terms (*bodb, badb, dub, bran, fiach, fennoc, caoc, lon*) cannot be matched up with the species of dark birds to be found in Ireland, then or now: they are linguistic phenomena with a range of meanings that cut across and far exceed the semantic fields of modern scientific taxonomy. Indeed, 'black birds are central images expressing the Celtic world view' (Tymoczko, 1990). The Irish taxonomy is determined by 'visibilia' (much as early scientific taxonomy was to be), but 'what is seen is conditioned by what is believed and what is valued'; and colour is supremely valued.

Early Christian Nature

Certain early Irish narratives dramatize the confluence of the Celtic and Christian dispensations, which began in the fifth century AD. Flower (1947) has suggested that this confluence was in part a strategy by which Early Christian Irish historians could communicate with the best of pagan Ireland. One such story is the remarkable twelfth-century *Buile Suibhne* (*The Madness of Sweeney*). Just as pagan Ireland was being reincarnated (in part) as Christian Ireland, so Sweeney has been variously incarnated in Irish literature, famously in Flann O'Brien's novel *At Swim-Two-Birds* (1939) and Seamus Heaney's poetic translation *Sweeney Astray* (1983).

Sweeney is an east Ulster king who is turned into a bird-man by a curse from a saint whom he insults and is driven in madness to the tree-canopies where he makes mad beautiful verse. At one point Sweeney delivers a lyrical catalogue of praise to the Irish trees, shrubs and bushes he inhabits or frequents like a bird: the oak, hazel, alder, blackthorn, sloe-bush, watercress, saxifrage, apple, rowan, bramble, yew, ivy, holly, ash, birch, aspen (Jackson, 1971). This mellifluous registry is naturalistic evidence of the lushness of the twelfth-century Ulster countryside. But that lushness may have been an object lesson. In the Christian (or Christianized) story of Sweeney, spirit is separate from, and finally triumphs over, earthly nature. Nature can be observed but is a mere backdrop to the heavenly future: nature is condescended to in the religious aspect of the work and, in Sweeney's case, is the site of punishment, a wilderness bereft of human fellowship. One interpretation is that the monastic tradition of settlement felt itself threatened by the dynamics of nature (Knott and Murphy, 1966).

But the registry is also evidence of the necessity of the catalogue or formula to the Celtic and early Christian mind, which prevented incipient objective attention to the particularities of nature. Yet even the natural catalogues of the early literature cannot deaden the way nature lives and leafs afresh in the blasphemous Sweeney's hymns. Through the formulas of what the rhetorician calls 'aggregation', a device that became standard practice in eighteenth-century English poetry – the hardy cuckoo, the speckled fish, the swift herd, etc. – shines a reception of nature as a joyous inventory, and there are flashes of real observation in the anonymous poems of the ninth, tenth, and eleventh centuries that Jackson (1971) reproduces in translation from the Irish. From 'May-time':

Bees,* whose strength is small, carry with their feet a load reaped from the flowers; the mountain allures the cattle, the ant makes a rich meal ...

The corncrake clacks, a strenuous bard; the high pure waterfall sings a greeting to the warm pool; rustling of rushes has come.

It is little wonder that Matthew Arnold in the nineteenth century saw in Celtic literature a note akin to Romanticism, or that Celticism was a strand of Irish Romanticism in Yeats's time.

Nature in these early poems is vital, autonomous, at times inhospitable, yet familiar, utterly knowable and classifiable and without mystery, indeed condescended to, not from a Christian perspective of spiritual superiority, but from an unwittingly secular excess of the poets' human vivacity. This surplus of energy is a feature of Irish literature, from the medieval poems

---

* Isidore of Seville was of the opinion in his *Etymologia* (c. AD 615) that there were no bees in Ireland; Echard at the end of the seventeenth century remarks on how plentiful this insect is on the island (Stevenson, 1920).

in Jackson's selection to Oscar Wilde, James Joyce and Flann O'Brien – brio and bravura before nature that does not lend itself to a serious study or even serious depiction of landscape or its creatures. The Irish comic tradition bullies genially the world outside the supremely self-conscious ego (Mercier, 1962). The love of the exuberant catalogue has survived among Irish writers and reaches its apogee in the three writers I have just mentioned. The people of Early Christian Ireland never lived far from nature, save for the extremely pious who sequestered themselves in monasteries. But even the monasteries could be in remote locations (for example, Great Skellig beyond the craggy headlands of southwest Ireland) where subsistence required daily traffic with fish and wild birds, and practical knowledge of their ways. Elsewhere, nature was domesticated as cattle, pigs, sheep, goats, dogs and cats (de Paor, 1978).

The truly pious could betake himself to a solitary life in glen or on crag, where nature was virtually his furniture and drapery. Jackson reproduces a translation of an anchorite's wonderfully lyrical tally of the landscape and the creatures (some of them domestic) that delight his senses and his palate. This is God's menu, as it were, nature a divine bounty, the detailed accounting of which is both the exercise of relish and the arithmetic of gratitude. Flower (1947) explains the clarity of vision in early Irish Christian nature poetry as the effect of continual spiritual exercise which washed the monks' eyes miraculously clear (and perhaps we could add the peculiarly intense solitude of meditation as an aid to clear seeing). A blackbird is celebrated in the ninth-century lyric, 'Belfast Lough':

> The whistle
> of the bright
> yellow billed
>   little bird:

> Over the loch
> upon a golden
> whin, a blackbird
>   stirred
> (Montague, 1978)

This is naturalistic but also, in its spare, haiku-like quality, perfected.

Clarity of a different kind, one accompanying a famous complexity of design, is demonstrated in the artwork of Early Christian Ireland. It has been observed that 'the topic of Nature in the Middle Ages is pre-eminently a literary one in that the most explicit statements about nature and its various manifestations are found in literary works' (Roberts, 1982). But the visual representation of nature is also striking during that lengthy period. The Christian Church was a patron of Irish art through illuminated manuscripts.

One feature of these was stylized animal ornamentation, which played an important role in Irish decoration throughout the Early Christian period (Harbison *et al.*, 1978). The Book of Durrow (c. 670-80) was almost certainly a product of a Columban (Irish) monastery, even if it was brought to Ireland already painted. Rhythmically rendered animals decorate this manuscript of the gospels; one 'carpet' page (a whole left-hand page given over to ornamentation) with its animals painted in yellows, reds and greens (f. 192v), has been called 'a masterpiece of controlled animal ornament' (Harbison *et al.*, 1978, 44). There are snake-like legged creatures biting other bodies or their own limbs, and mammal-like creatures with exaggerated forelegs also biting their fellows to create the design.

The famous illuminated manuscript of the Four Gospels known as The Book of Kells (written and illuminated probably in Iona in the ninth century and brought unfinished to Kells, Co. Meath) frequently employs animals and weaves them into a vision of divine intricacy. The initials of paragraphs use animals and birds as ornamentation, and there are interlinear drawings of a variety of creatures, some fantastic (de Paor, 1978). Animals and birds are part of the larger design of natural and revealed Creation, at once themselves and allegorical.

It is the opinion of one scholar that what emerges from The Book of Kells is 'the hostility of Nature, its terrifying dangers' (Huppé, 1982). For example, the initial monsters, intertwining serpents and the menacing animal that greets the eye on one non-initial page of folio 19v are to be exorcised, according to this scholar, by the sacred Word. Etienne Rynne offers a different interpretation of the animals of the manuscript. Rynne agrees that 'strange, contorted, fighting, playing or otherwise, acrobatically cavorting men, animals, birds, fish, snakes or reptilian worms are undoubtedly the most common themes encountered in these initial letters', but sees the animal depictions as 'drolleries' and is not convinced of either their terrifying nature or religious symbolism. Those who ornamented the manuscript were 'artists who eschewed realism as unnecessary or undesirable, and who, most importantly, had a strong sense of humour which they were not afraid to allow stray into their marvellous work'. This interpretation accords with my characterization of early Irish poetry and later Irish fiction as exhibiting a surplus of imaginative vivacity. Whatever the merits of these readings of the vision of nature presented by The Book of Kells, it is clear that the natural world depicted there is very different from that of nature poetry by religious hermits.

Metalwork of the tenth century shows a further reconception or reconstitution of the animal kingdom, for both the artistic purpose of complex design and the religious purpose of respectful emulation of God's meaningfully convoluted Creation (natural theology of an early kind, we might say).

The supreme example is the Kells Crozier now in the British Museum (de Paor, 1978). In the eleventh and twelfth centuries appeared a proto-Romanesque art. Bronze-relief ornamentation of shrines display animal-interlace panels or even narrative scenes such as hounds pulling down a stag. Norse influence resulted in a change of style, but on occasion the Irish craftsmen reverted to a more native design when they zoomorphized what had tended to be foliate ornamentation (de Paor, 1978). A later Scandinavian style (Urnes) was more to the liking of Irish metalworkers, and the bronze Cross of Cong employs the forms of animals in a manner graphically described by Máire and Liam de Paor. There is a large animal head gripping in its jaws the bottom of the shaft; on the openwork cast gilt-bronze panels that adorn the back of the shaft and the arms is a zoomorphic interlacing; depicted on the front of the interlace is the Urnes combat theme, a struggle between quadrupeds and serpents, with the Urnes features of animal depiction: 'profile-heads of the beasts, with rolled-back lower jaws, swelling snout with moustache-lappet, bulging brow, pointed ear, and pointed ovoid eye' (de Paor, 1978).

Despite these depictions, there are many medieval Irish stories of what Helen Waddell, the noted Ulster scholar, called 'the mutual charities between saints and beasts' (Waddell, 1934): they virtually amount to a literary genre. In beginning his biography of St Francis as a 'nature mystic', the Ulster ornithologist and Anglican minister E.A. Armstrong devotes learned pages to the possibility that 'Irish ideas and practices influenced Francis and the Order' (Armstrong, 1973). In any case, the Irish stories are delightful. One of the best known concerns St Kevin (d. Glendalough, AD 618) whose hand outstretched to heaven was chosen by a blackbird for her nest. The bird laid eggs and hatched young before the saint would bring himself to move, for fear of disturbing it. Kevin's blackbird is quite a contrast with the fiercer black birds of the pagan Celtic sagas and the fiercer animals of the visual tradition.

In the Franciscan tradition, wild creatures are our brothers and sisters. In one story of St Ciarán, the animals that come to live with the saint are likened to his monks. Indeed, they can be chastised as if they were subordinates, as St Cainnic does the sea-birds and St Kevin the rook (Waddell, 1934). This was a common personification of nature: as late as 1545, the villagers of Saint-Julien in France beseeched the episcopal authorities to excommunicate the weevils that were ravaging the vines. There was a hearing and the decision was handed down that the weevils as God's creatures had equal rights to the earth's plant life (Anderson, 1995). However, the vast flocks of passenger pigeons that made havoc with the settlers' grain in Quebec in the 1680s were not so lucky: Baron de Lahontan records in 1687 that the bishop was forced to excommunicate the birds more than once, and in the light of the French episode it seems hardly a joke on the Baron's part (Lahontan, 1905).

Farmers' hostility to their enemies in nature is a far cry from the Franciscan attitude, but the mutual anthropomorphism is evidence that nature was not sufficiently 'other' to be objectively knowable as the New Science of the seventeenth century was to suggest it could be. In several saints' stories, for example 'St Ciaran and the Fox and Badger' and 'St Moling and the Fox' (Waddell, 1934), the fox is not just wily and deceitful as in later folktales, but is a potential apostate; perhaps the animal is a fugitive embodiment of fallen man, and perhaps displays the trickster element of the Christian Devil. There is even, one feels, an equation of domestication with godliness, as the renegade fox threatens to revert to the wild. (Early modern naturalists were more likely to equate domestication with degeneration of the species in question.)

Behind the allegorical suggestiveness of these saints' stories may lie the fable, in which God's creatures talk and act like human beings whose behaviour we are directed to find instructive. This moral conception of nature may have been Greek, but it survived into Christianity and lasted at least as late as the seventeenth-century divine Rev. Cotton Mather, and the natural theologians, for whom nature expressed God's wishes in a form different from his Word but as no less a text to be read and heeded.

In 1710 Fr Joseph Jouvency's survey of New France (Quebec) for his Jesuit superiors back in Paris described a bird that haunted Bird Island as having one of its feet armed with claws, the other webbed: with the latter it swam, with the former it seized and disembowelled fish (Thwaites, 1896). (The armed foot apart, the description suggests the great auk.) Earlier, in the 1520s, Gonzalo Fernandez de Oviedo reported from the West Indies a monstrous raptor with one webbed foot and one with talons (Allen, 1951). Earlier still, we find in *Topographia Hiberniae* (1188-1223) by Giraldus Cambrensis the Irish osprey with a similar bilateral asymmetry. This pathbreaking account of Ireland's natural history by an early visitor reveals the probability that these uneven birds are in this detail the product not of observation but of Christian doctrine in which God and the Devil are forever at loggerheads. Balance and symmetry are perfection and divine, imbalance and asymmetry are imperfection and demonic. Giraldus's Irish osprey swims (the real bird doesn't) but also dives and seizes its fishy prey (true): 'So does our old enemy see with his sharp glance whatever secret thing we do in the troubled waves of this world. And while with peaceful claw he approaches us airily through success in temporal things, still with grasping claw, bloody with its booty, he seizes and destroys our unhappy souls' (O'Meara, 1982). Many of the animals and birds Giraldus reports from Ireland have such lessons attached to their description.

Topographia Hiberniae is a kind of bestiary. Bestiaries were collections of animal observations cast in Christian morality, the best known in modern times being the twelfth-century bestiary translated and edited by T.H. White as *The Book of Beasts* (1984). Bestiaries report real observations (and therefore belong to the history of natural history) but fauna and landscape are refracted by a cultural lens (an intense and pervasive Christianity) through which few moderns now see. Through Giraldus, the approach to nature captured by the bestiary – full of the fantastic, the absurd, the true, and the instructive – entered Ireland and pioneered the survey of Ireland's geography, climate and fauna. In Giraldus can be seen the naturalistic and the allegorical in uneasy juxtaposition. The Elizabethan binary view of Ireland is perhaps traceable to this medieval double vision.

There is much that is accurate in Giraldus, for example the difference between Irish (hooded) and English (carrion) crows, the fact of female birds of prey being larger than their mates, the natural explanation of the absence of snakes in Ireland. There is much that is nonsense, for example cranes' ability to digest iron, but nonsense largely deriving from previous, including classical, sources. Certainly Giraldus finds much in Ireland and the Irish to his distaste, but he has points to make in their favour – the clemency of the Irish climate preventing poisonous creatures from living there, the healthiness of the native people and their great musicianship. And if he believes that many of the Irish animals are inferior to their British counterparts, that is hardly worse than Buffon's later (and similarly prejudiced) observation that New World animals were inferior in size to their European counterparts. This invidious comparison is repeated about Ireland four centuries after Giraldus by Echard: 'All living Creatures, besides Men, Women and Greyhounds, are smaller than ours in England' (Stevenson, 1920). When he reported on his travels in North Carolina in 1730-1, the Irishman John Brickell considered New World wildlife to be smaller in stature than Irish wildlife: a poetically just reversal of the prejudice against Ireland, if no more zoologically reliable (Brickell, 1969). The prejudice may be caused by colonialist arrogance or (in the case of Buffon) envy, but may also be caused by nothing more complicated than a traveller's homesickness and pride in his homeland.

The Irish natural wonders (a cow-stag, wolves whelping in December) and miracles (including St Kevin's blackbird) reported by Giraldus resemble both native Irish 'Mirabilia' or wonder stories (O'Meara, 1982) and medieval European books of 'Secrets' containing lore on the marvellous properties of real and imagined beasts and plants. In *Topographia Hiberniae*, the acceptance of the wondrous and the portrayal of a world composed by analogy and correspondence vie with the explicable and objective, and in doing so exemplify the human relationship to nature before and even after the rise of modern natural science. A sense of the marvellous survived into the natural theology and even modern naturalism of the eighteenth and nineteenth centuries. And it was, after all, Aristotle who said that all science begins with marvelling.

Nature in the Classical Tradition

Topographia Hiberniae was of course written in Latin. The first works in Latin known to have been written in Ireland were those by Patrick, and Latin began to be studied systematically in Ireland at the end of the sixth century (Richter, 1988). When the first schools were founded the medium of instruction was Latin, and it stayed that way until the eighteenth century throughout the various educational institutions: the monastic schools, the grammar schools, the Jesuit schools, the Royal schools of the seventeenth century, and the hedge schools (after the Battle of the Boyne). Formal classicism held sway in Ireland until the non-classical national schools of the nineteenth century (Stanford, 1976). Latin was the conduit of secular classical tradition as well as of Christianity.

There had been fitful pre-Christian contact between Ireland and the Classical world, but after Christianity the contact was one of ideas, including the ideas of Aristotle (384-322 BC) – the greatest naturalist of all time, as he has been called – and Pliny the Elder (AD 23-79). Classical learning remained in fugitive condition among the native Irish until the nineteenth century. Stanford records a German traveller in Ireland in 1843 meeting a Kerryman reading a manuscript in Irish containing treatises of antiquity, including 'the translation of a treatise by Aristotle on some subject of natural history!'

Pliny's collection of natural history fact and lore in *Historia Naturalis* would have had some impact on Irish students' ideas about nature. This astonishing magazine of truth and legend influenced Giraldus. White furnishes us with a genealogy of the bestiary that includes not only Pliny but Isidore of Seville, and these authors were those whose work, it is believed, Irish schools required their students to know (Stanford, 1976). Medieval Latin writers were translated into Irish, and the Irish knowledge of botany (for medical purposes) was partly derived from Latin compilations or Latin translations of Greek sources. *De Veneno* (*On Poison*) by Malachy of Ireland, written about 1268, drew upon classical sources for information about poisonous animals in Ireland (Stanford, 1976).

Classical natural history, which could be both scientific (in the modern sense), as with Aristotle, and pre-scientific, sat in Ireland alongside older, pre-classical and pre-Christian natural history.* Classicism overlapped with

---

*An account of classical science, including classical natural history, can be found in *Science in Antiquity* (1936) and *Greek Science* (1944) by Benjamin Farrington. The latter book sold a quarter of a million copies. Farrington was born in Cork in 1891 and educated at

modern science, and it is to be remembered that early modern scientific works were written in Latin. The earliest scientific work printed in Ireland was in this language, a medical treatise by Dermot O'Meara in 1619. The Royal Irish Academy, founded in 1785, was home to classical scholars as well as the new scientists. The chemist Richard Kirwan twice delivered papers to the Academy on classical subjects (Stanford, 1976). Heuvelmans, in his short history of cryptozoology, reminds us that the Irish naturalist Valentine Ball (1843-95) twice published on the identification of fabulous creatures of the early Greek authors, including the martikhora and the griffin.* One wonders if the switch to the vernacular by English scientists advanced their progress, and if correspondingly it inhibited the growth of science among the native Irish. Also, could the loyalty to classicism of the native Irish have enabled a resistance on their part to Baconianism, the new science, and other progressive elements of the Enlightenment?

The Folklore of Nature

In that fascinating compendium, *Pseudodoxia Epidemica* ('Vulgar Errors', 1646-72), Sir Thomas Browne collected for investigation numerous erroneous beliefs about the natural world. Some of them originated with, or were endorsed by, the classical authors and were therefore 'learned errors'. Some we recognize from Giraldus, for example that an ostrich – crane in Giraldus – can digest iron.** Some decorated the medieval bestiaries, some of them passed unharmed through the philosophical digestive systems of Aristotle and Pliny. These errors presumably would have been alive among the English and Irish of Browne's day. Some, for example the existence of the unicorn, can be found in the Bible. The importance of biblical natural history in Ireland is a subject that awaits investigation.*** The Judeo-Christianity of the Bible conveys certain attitudes to nature, including taboos; but how prevalent were these in modern Ireland? Did attitudes to animals and plants differ between the English and Scots Protestants and the native, Catholic Irish (qua Christians)? Did the popularity of the Bible among the more fundamentalist northern Protestants inhibit a scientific approach when their southern, broader-church Protestant co-religionists were starting modern science in Ireland?

University College Cork and Trinity College, Dublin, and was the author of numerous books. I am indebted to Seán Lysaght for this information.

* Cryptozoology, writes Heuvelmans, 'aims at a systematic search for unknown species of animals about which some testimonial and circumstantial evidence is available'.

** Oliver Goldsmith in his *History of the Earth and Animated Nature* (1774) moderated the claim: iron passes through the ostrich undigested but without harm to the bird.

*** The subject involves the lore of both Reformation England and the Middle East and,

By the same token, did the relative *un*popularity or inaccessibility of the Bible among many of the native Irish encourage the dominance of older, more pervasive, *un*biblical folklore about nature over empirical and systematic observations? Evans offers as the second distinctive and unifying feature of Irish rural culture (the first being the paucity of towns and tight-knit village communities) the persistence of 'certain attitudes towards the world and the otherworld, of traditional customs, beliefs and seasonal festivals which had often assumed the guise of Christian piety but which had their origins in the Elder Faiths of pre-Christian times' (Evans, 1992).* The 'Otherworld' has been an especially variegated and influential place in the Irish imagination from antiquity to modern times (Seymour, 1930; Foster, 1987). The remarkably well-appointed pagan version of the Otherworld – see, for example, the medieval Irish voyage-tales called *Immrama* – was Christianized without radical transformation and survived in modern Ireland in the vivid visions of heaven, purgatory and hell in modern Catholicism which amount to a spiritual natural history, counterparts of surveys of the natural world.** One wonders if this graphic and detailed concern about the next world drew energy away from the potential study of *this* world.

In the idea of the Otherworld the learned and vulgar are mingled, as are the pagan and the Christian. Likewise are they mingled in the fascinating story of the barnacle goose first told by Giraldus (see also Moriarty, 'The Early Naturalists', in this volume). The bird began life, it was thought, as an excrescence on fir-logs (or as fruit on a tree, in a Scottish version, Thorndike, 1941); it hung by its beak and metamorphosed into a goose. The larger implications of the story have to do with the factual process of metamorphosis: if a caterpillar into a butterfly, why not a natural protuberance – unrecognized as the barnacle shellfish by Giraldus – into a bird? They also have to do with the ancient belief in, and fear of, miscegenation and the monstrous, deviations from God's design or from 'nature' in its Aristotelian sense of directional growth: 'against nature' is Giraldus's phrase. For Giraldus the osprey and the barnacle goose were birds and yet not truly birds – they were bird-fish, birds of a twofold nature.

---

via the translators, classical lore. For biblical natural history, see Yehuda Feliks, *Nature and Man in the Bible: Chapters in Biblical Ecology* (1981).

* A rewarding two-volume survey of pre-Christian traditions in nineteenth-century Ireland, some of them involving attitudes to nature, can be found in *Traces of the Elder Faiths of Ireland* (1902) by W.G. Wood-Martin.

** A celebrated fictional rendering of the grimmest region of the Catholic 'Otherworld' is James Joyce's description of hell in *A Portrait of the Artist as a Young Man* (1916), in the guise of a sermon modelled after Pinamonti's *Hell Opened to Christians* (1688) and translated in Dublin in 1868. It is nothing less than a geology and topography of the nether world.

The story in its early version is an Irish one, and the birds became known as Hibernian geese (Ley, 1968). It was an Irish priest called Octavius (or Octavian) who swore to Konrad Gesner, the great German naturalist (author of *Historia Animalium*, 1551-8), that what Giraldus said of the goose was true (Ley, 1987; Allen, 1951). It was an Irish theologian's affidavit that convinced the early English ornithologist William Turner (c. 1500-68) that he had witnessed the generation of the geese from rotting ships (Thorndike, 1941). This should not be surprising, since pre-scientific classification and nomenclature were important to the religious; the nature of a creature dictated human relationship to it, including its edibility during and between fasts. Hence the significance of the *feet* of birds: webbed could mean edible during fasts, unwebbed inedible (Ley, 1987). This was natural theology of a precise and practical kind. In the early eighteenth century, Lahontan ironically commended the 'Doctors' who persuaded the popes to classify beavers, otters and sea-calves (seals?) as fish to eat during Lent, and Peter Kalm in his *Travels in North America* later in the same century wrote that the French in North America ate beaver on their fast days because 'his Holiness the Pope has, like many of the old zoologists, classified the beaver among the fishes, since he [the beaver, not the Pope!] spends most of his time in water' (Kalm, 1987). Like the Celts, pre-Enlightenment Catholics conceptualized and divided nature in ways that were later regarded as nonscientific.

The legend of the development of the barnacle goose was discredited by Aeneas Sylvius in the fifteenth century (Thorndike, 1941), apparently accepted by Gesner in the sixteenth century, and definitively discredited by Leonhard Baldner in the seventeenth century (Allen, 1951). The story of the barnacle shellfish-bird has been told by Heron-Allen (1928) – a correspondent of Oscar Wilde's – and its Irish contexts examined by Armstrong (1958). Armstrong reminds us that the belief in the barnacle (or brent) goose's being more fish than bird persisted among Irish Catholics into the twentieth century. The belief survived Oliver Goldsmith's contempt for this 'idle error'. Goldsmith (1728-74) produced in *An History of the Earth and Animated Nature* (1774) one of the first truly popular books of natural history. He was not a naturalist by training; he was a product of Trinity College, Dublin, and the classical tradition, and was the author of histories of Greece and Rome (besides, of course, his poetry).

The barnacle goose was only one Irish bird among many that were observed through a network of meanings and associations we might call folklore. In his immense collector's guidebook, *A Handbook of Irish Folklore*, Seán Ó Súilleabháin itemizes 'Goose (*cadhan, ean giughrainn,* barnacle-goose): as game; flesh of barnacle-goose eaten on Fridays ...' (1963). Several other species of bird have loomed large in the folklore, including the plover – '(*fideog, triollchán, pilibín miogach, saotharcán*): plover as weather-augur; belief

that these birds were introduced into Ireland by Brian Boru for use in war'
and, of course, the wren, once hunted in a St Stephen's Day ritual whose
European and Irish origins and distribution as a folk custom Armstrong
accounts for with his usual eloquent learning (1958). Ó Ruadháin's fully cited
brief survey, 'Birds in Irish Folklore' (1955), ought to be expanded and
updated for other Irish animals. The archives of the Department of Irish
Folklore at University College Dublin, previously the Irish Folklore
Commission, are a fund of information on folk natural history.

Ó Súilleabháin's *Handbook* is a ready reckoner, too, of Ireland's plant
lore, which would have had its roots in medicinal lore, both native – that is,
druidical – and introduced by the classical botanists and herbalists (Stanford,
1976). Individual plants may have curative properties or have attached to
them traditional explanations of their origin or nature. Corrigan has surveyed the Irish folklore of plant medicine but along the way gives us useful
information on the folklore of plants generally; he mentions A.T. Lucas's
work on gorse, *Furze: A Survey and History of its Uses in Ireland* (1960), as
the most extensive compilation of folklore relating to one species of plant.

Corrigan cautions that it is not always easy to establish definitively the
nativeness of Irish medical plant lore or to distinguish it from herbal lore
brought over by colonists. This caution would be less necessary in the case of
tree lore, which is voluminous in Ireland. As Ó Súilleabháin remarks, 'almost
every tree found growing in Ireland has a certain amount of traditional information associated with it'.

Named places, sometimes defined and identified by a natural feature (a
mountain, a bog, a strand, a river, a natural well, etc.), did not generate simply local lore, but also a topography intimately bound up with families, ownership, genealogy: the *dindshenchas*, the bardic lore of high places, constituted 'a kind of Dictionary of National Topography' (Flower, 1947). Places,
place lore, placenames: the landscape of Ireland was *seen* and *read* by the
Irish through powerful cultural lenses.

Placenames, for example, can be read as a venerable if patchy folk natural history, even in English, and Joyce (1891, 1893) believed that a century ago only one in thirteen Irish placenames was originally English. Irish
topographical names had been translated into English and often altered and
corrupted in the process; often the English version would imitate the pro-
nunciation rather than the written form of the Irish. Joyce thought that
Auburn, Goldsmith's deserted village, probably derived from a fanciful
adaptation of its old Gaelic name, *Aghanagrena*: the *achadh* or field of the
sun. (Some literary critics have identified Lissoy, Co. Westmeath, as the Irish
model for Auburn; others have suggested English models.) Working backwards, and drawing upon the scholarship of the seventeenth-century *Annals
of the Four Masters*, *The Book of Rights* (both translated by the nineteenth-

century scholar John O'Donovan) and the 'Field Name Books' (O'Donovan's interpretations of the placenames he collected during his Ordnance Survey work), Joyce classifies and annotates the origin and meaning of an immense number of placenames.

Many were inspired by animals: Keimaneigh, 'pass of the deer'; Kanturk, 'hill of the boar'; Feltrim, 'wolf-hill'; Clonbrock, 'meadow of the badger', etc. Joyce suggests that placenames can be used as rough guides to past distribution and status of these animals. Among bird-inspired names are Slieveanilra, Co. Clare, 'the eagle's mountain'; Tirfinnog, Co. Monaghan, 'the district of the hooded crow'; Balfeddock, Co. Louth, 'the townland of the plovers' (lapwings?); Cloonatreane, Co. Fermanagh, 'the meadow of the corncrake'. Joyce writes poignantly: 'The lonely boom of the bittern is heard more seldom year after year, as the marshes are becoming drained and reclaimed' (1893); the Irish name for the bittern was *bunnan*, commemorated in Mayo, Sligo and Kerry placenames. (The Irish for marsh is *curragh*, a word that names a flat grassy plain in Kildare that is the epicentre of Irish horse-racing culture but presumably named extensive marshland in pre-reclamation times.) Tree species gave rise to many placenames, but more interesting are topographical features (rock, valley, hollow, strand, spring, etc.): Lahinch derives from *leithinsi* (peninsula: literally, half-island). Perhaps more interesting still are Irish words that describe vegetation features and were the main grammatical element of a placename; the words suggest ways in which the Irish perceived, interpreted and arranged the landscape: *fásach*, a wild or uncultivated place; *scairt*, a cluster of bushes, a thicket; *muine*, a brake or shrubbery (chiefly occurring as 'money' in placenames); *gaertha*, woodland along a river, overgrown with small trees, bushes or underwood.

Given the daily ecological, economic, cultural, and even psychological importance of climate in a windswept north Atlantic island, it is hardly surprising that Ó Súilleabháin devotes pages to the folklore of the atmosphere, the weather and the points of the compass. Irish weather is infamously capricious (the ultimate shape-changer), spoiler of vacations, ensurer of the green landscape. Joyce offers several placenames that locate exposed or windy places, using the word *gaeth*, wind: Dungeeha, fortress of the wind; Drumnagee, hill-ridge of the wind.

In 1966 Richard Dorson, a respected American folklorist, wrote in his Foreword to *Folktales of Ireland*, edited by Sean O'Sullivan (Ó Súilleabháin): 'Who would know the national culture of modern Ireland must be aware of her folklore and folklorists.' Folklore and the collection of folklore have been ornaments of Irish culture, and the natural world figures largely in that lore. Folktales, like folksongs, are often local versions of international types and as local adaptations can include accurate observations of Irish nature, but can also be unreliable because ungrounded in Irish zoological and botanical reality. *The Types of the Irish Folktale* (Ó Súilleabháin and Christiansen, 1963) records eight hundred international folktales found in Ireland, but there is a comparative paucity of animal tales. Seals have figured prominently in Irish life and lore, to the extent of personification, 'the people of the sea' being a translation of one Gaelic name for them (Thomson, 1965). Flower (1944) reproduces a fine seal tale from Great Blasket island, where seals were of great economic benefit. The salmon, likewise personified, can be found both in the early Irish literature and in the oral tradition, associated with wisdom and immense longevity.

The perception and representation of nature that are implied or expressed in folklore are resilient vestiges of the ancient assumption of an intimate traffic between human beings and nature, and between the natural world and the supernatural world. Remnants of this venerable attitude can still be found, so that the pre-scientific relationship to nature has in fact persisted in Ireland and elsewhere. That persistence may account in part for the difficulty science has had in modern times in gaining cultural purchase on the island. Elsewhere I have attempted to demonstrate the emergence of a modern perception of nature from the elder folk perception, using the Irish-language peasant autobiographies of the Blasket Islands as a case-study (Foster, 1987).

The New Science and its Enemies

I have suggested that even among the Elizabethans and their successors, older ways of seeing and interpreting the natural world persisted.* Nevertheless, it would be foolish to deny the departure Baconian science represented. Mazzeo claims that 'the notion of gradual, continual progress, with no discernible limit, in a more or less linear ascent from an inferior condition, was unknown to mankind before the seventeenth century'. True, Christianity introduced an idea of progress but to a world beyond this one, while the thinkers of antiquity fused a theory of cyclical change and a theory of decay, even though the Greeks encouraged the cumulation of knowledge. Besides, Christianity exalted faith and belief above reason and accepted the Hebraic notion of the

---

* Natural history never quite lost its associations with folklore and antiquarianism, its penchant for the oddities of nature, the nooks and crannies of the Earth, which have served to attract professional naturalists as well as amateurs and enthusiasts. Attraction to the *wonders* and *curiosities* of nature succeeded to the fascinating *variations* of nature. As late as the middle nineteenth century, Thompson's *Natural History of Ireland* was enlivened by anecdotes of curious happenings, such as the living wigeon cut from the stomach of an angler fish or the severed head of a conger eel biting a hand (Thompson, 1849-56). Occasionally, Thompson can read like a descendant of Pliny.

degeneration of humankind. Although the expansion of knowledge between the fourteenth and sixteenth centuries (the period we call the Renaissance) involved in part a return to antiquity, Francis Bacon, in Mazzeo's words, 'did more than any other single individual to effect [a] reorientation toward the future by his eloquent denunciation of the notion of "ricorsi", of cycles'. Bacon saw the pre-classical period giving way to the classical period, followed by the modern period. The classical period and modern period (which included the Middle Ages) had contributed to science, but even Renaissance humanism 'did not emphasize useful scientific learning in their programs of renovation'. 'Bacon's radical departure from tradition,' Mazzeo writes, 'lay in his placing the amelioration of the human condition on the acquisition of useful knowledge, on the growth of man's mastery over his external environment.'

Ireland was in fact something of an early laboratory in which, not always knowingly, new ways of seeing the natural world were being generated and tested through the English colonizers' encounter with a largely pre-scientific society and a largely aboriginal countryside. Whereas folklore and earlier non-scientific views of nature were either content with the inexplicable or advanced unrealistic and fanciful explanations, the new scientists of the seventeenth century set their faces against the inexplicable and held at bay the supernatural. The three pillars of truth, as Browne (following Bacon) reminded the readers of *Pseudodoxia Epidemica*, are reason, authority and experience. Christianity when it conformed with these criteria assumed the form of natural theology, a pseudo-scientific overview of nature within which a scientific view could be as piercing as it liked.

In *Novum Organum* (1620), Bacon, pioneer of the new inductive science, wrote that correct scientific method 'leads with constant path through the woodlands of experience to the open country of Axioms'. (Much later, in the 1850s, John Cardinal Newman was to refer to science's 'exuberant sylva of phenomena' [Newman, 1982].) It is therefore apt for Salingar (1982) to begin with a settlement metaphor in describing Bacon's *The Advancement of Science* (1605) as 'a clearing of the ground'. Bacon is the essayist who wrote 'Of Plantations', and plantations such as those in Ireland usually required a radical clearing of the ground for building and sowing. Bacon preferred plantation 'in a pure soil; that is, where people are not displanted to the end to plant in others; for else it is rather an extirpation than a plantation' (Bacon, 1942). In Ireland it was a dispossession by the English (and later the Ulster Scots) when it wasn't an extirpation.

The clearing of the Irish landscape, like the first clearances in the English settlements of North America, occurred during the clearing away of Renaissance and pre-Renaissance mental lumber by the Elizabethan and Jacobean new philosophers. The rise of modern science coincided with the renewed colonization of Ireland and the colonization of British North America. To the British, the Irish, like the ancient Britons, were 'wood-born' and superstitious, and the woodland was the haunt of the irrational. Keith Thomas (1984) quotes Edmund Burke to the effect that only by being drawn out of the forests would men be led to civility. The alternative was to drive 'superstition' and 'irrationality' back into the dark woods from the clearings or 'Pale' that one's philosophy – or 'suns' – have established.

Two practical steps were necessary analogues to this intellectual expansionism. One was surveying and mapping of the 'benighted' territory preparatory to political 'reform' (in Elizabethan lingo, to 'plot' was both to survey and to devise radical political changes); the mapping of Ireland was a noteworthy episode in the early development of cartography. The other was cultivation of the soil. When Davies in 1612 suggested the steps required for the subduing of Ireland, he chillingly offered both a metaphor and a literal plan of action. 'For the husbandman must first break the land before it be made capable of good seed; and when it is thoroughly broken and manured, if he do not forthwith cast good seed into it, it will grow wild again and bear nothing but weeds: so a barbarous country must be first broken by a war before it will be capable of good government; and when it is fully subdued and conquered, if it be not well-planted and governed after the conquest, it will eftsoons return to the former barbarism.'

Many of the consequences of such thinking, of such metaphors, have been unhappy for the Irish. In historical hindsight the situation was made worse because the attribution of irrationality and ignorance was frequently itself irrational and ignorant, the colonists knowing next to nothing about the Celtic, Early Christian and classical traditions in Ireland. But these attributions accompanied the beginnings of the modern scientific study of nature, to which the Irish themselves were to contribute notably.

In the hundred years after the collapse of the Gaelic order in the early seventeenth century, the 'New Science', 'New Learning' or 'New Philosophy', as it has been variously called, gradually established itself in Ireland among those later to be referred to as the Anglo-Irish. Behind their science (or 'natural philosophy') lay the complex cultural dynamics of Protestantism, capitalism, colonialism, and urbanization.

Much of the native Irish intellect and learning went underground or overseas. Irish-born scholars engaged occasionally with medical science, rarely with natural history; their plight and accomplishments are explained in the pages of McGee (1857), Stanford (1976), Corish (1981), Leighton (1994) and Foster (1996), and in the Introduction to 'Naturalists Abroad' in this volume. Native Irish thought surfaced in Ireland two centuries later chiefly as Catholic apologetics, revival Celticism and Irish antiquarianism, and political republicanism. Anglo-Irish science developed far differently,

47

starting effectively with the Dublin Philosophical Society in 1683. The new-ness of the science has been questioned (Eamon, 1995; Hunter, 1995) and its links to older ways of thinking demonstrated (Thorndike, 1958). Until around 1680, Irish followers of the new science respectfully cited classical sources; however, this went out of fashion when Latin ceased to be the language of scientific publication (Stanford, 1976).

The Dublin Philosophical Society came into being when the city, already the second largest in the British Isles, was undergoing vigorous expansion. Dublin scientists early participated in the affairs of the Royal Society of London for the Improvement of Natural Knowledge and its organ, *Philosophical Transactions*, founded in 1665. Anglican Archbishop James Ussher of Armagh famously dated the age of the Earth from 4004 BC, but (lest this should be thought evidence of dogma) typified the tolerance of the New Learning. He was a driving force, financially aiding Samuel Hartlib (the German Puritan enthusiast for the New Learning) and the Dutchman Gerard Boate's *Philosophia Naturalis* (Dublin, 1641), which preceded Boate's economically motivated *Irelands Naturall History* (1652), 'the only scientific book in the modern manner relating to Ireland written before the Restoration' (Hoppen, 1970).

The activities of the Irish scientists helped to constitute the European Enlightenment, during which there was an attempt to substitute knowledge through experience for tradition and authority. This was not plain sailing; the New Learning in general and the Dublin Philosophical Society in particular had their enemies in Ireland, and the polemical situation resembled the hostilities between the 'Ancients' and the 'Moderns' in England. Hoppen has rehearsed the fierce and at base religious antagonism of Dudley Loftus (b. 1619), who saw in the new science 'sterile and useless learning' at the expense of the 'true and sublime'.

The most famous censure of scientific 'projectors' and 'virtuosi', abstract speculators and arcane experimenters, came from the pen of Jonathan Swift (1667-1745). Anglican and Tory scourge of the 'Moderns', Swift in Part Three of *Gulliver's Travels* (1726) satirized in the Academy of Lagado such bodies as the Royal Society and the Dublin Philosophical Society. The projects and experiments of the scientists offended against common sense and were worst when they attempted to apply themselves, to turn theory into practice. Swift saw practice as an almost inevitable degeneration from theory, be it political theory or scientific theory; and even when seemingly good, theory and science as abstract were offenders against right reason, not exponents of it, unless wit (intelligence, a sense of proportion, insight) mediated. Swift's attitude to the scientific bodies need not have been mere prejudice against science. Even naturalists thought that by Swift's time the Royal Society was not what it had been. The Swedish naturalist Kalm wrote in

1751 in his journal (and confirmed it in a letter to Linnaeus) that the Society 'has fallen into disrepute, even here in England, so that even the more sensible people speak of it with mockery'; Kalm thought the decline had set in around 1720.

In any event, Swift was philosophically wedded to the idea of decline: major and incontrovertible qualitative progress was a delusion of the 'Moderns', whereas the 'Ancients' were immeasurably our superiors and had themselves been cognizant of the decay in nature. Swift's contempt for the human being (not *animal rationale* in his eyes but merely *animal rationis capax*, an animal *capable* of reason) led him in irony to champion dumb creatures over the articulate and deceitful: at least the dumb creatures did not aspire out of pride and ambition to a higher rank than Nature had assigned them. At best, life was a modest proposal, a holding of the pale of reason against unnecessary degeneration.

Swift's vision was at odds with the optimism of the Enlightenment, the confident belief that science had established 'an impregnable basis of experimentally verified fact' and that man was now the master of his own destiny (Hampson, 1982). Gulliver by contrast is Man at the mercy of Fortune and natural forces. Yet the eighteenth century saw natural history issue in a coherent set of disciplines, attempt ambitious scientific classifications of the organic (and even inorganic) world, and become, through the notions of process and historicity, the 'history' of nature (Lyon and Sloan, 1981).

Swift and and his friend Alexander Pope were largely opposed to this particular spirit of the age. They believed, like those in the Middle Ages, that created Nature, from celestial powers to the mites, composed 'the great chain', and that every creature was by divine and static adaptation assigned its powers and place in an unchangeable hierarchy with humanity placed modestly on an 'isthmus of a middle state', halfway between the angels and the lowliest creatures. 'Nature to all things fixed the limits fit': humanity's attempts to transgress these limits had been proscribed by God, as John Milton reminded the readers of *Paradise Lost* (1667, 1674) when the Archangel Raphael warned Adam not to try to understand the stars, i.e. the divine edges of Nature off-limits to humanity. 'The proper study of mankind is Man', announced Pope in a statement of a humanism – part classical, part Christian – that would have put a cap on scientific inquiry. The attempts at transgression provided the theme, irony and savage humour of *Gulliver's Travels*. The undesirable state produced by pride and ambition balanced the undesirable state that was degeneration.

Yet Swift and Pope at least saw human beings as a link in the chain of creation, part of what Milton called 'the Scale of Nature', not special creations wholly outside it. Swift went further and saw mankind as animals; in *Gulliver's Travels* he brings to bear less a benign humanism than a painfully disabused biologism. Human beings are too animal-like to warrant their self-exaltation as semi-divinities, but too human (hairless, talonless, weak) to be adequate animals.

Moreover, the cosmic system of which this human animal is a part has, in Pope's *An Essay on Man* (1733), a Newtonian rather than medieval complexity. And the acceptance of limitation ('What can we reason, but from what we know?' asked Pope) could be regarded as the minimum requirement of that empiricism which Baconian method called for. Gulliver is the reader's middleman and is also a middle man in merit and intelligence, but his adventures expose him to the perils of Fortune and the hazards of extremes, be it of pride or power-hunger on one side or barbarism or degeneracy on the other ('Avoid extremes', Pope counselled); but his adventures are also his education in the hard school of experience.

Furthermore, Swift and Pope were believers in the government of right reason and believers in the pre-existence of order, and the science of their age could not have progressed without the use of reason to establish the concealed order of Nature. Of the scholastic Middle Ages, Pope remarked with disdain that 'Much was believed, but little understood'. (The superior Greeks and Romans inquired into things and pursued knowledge.) With Pope's claim that 'All Nature is but art, unknown to thee', Linnaeus would have agreed: both the numbers of species and their relationship were fixed, according to the great naturalist, and he saw his own task as revealing God's hidden design in Nature, i.e. his own classifications in the advancing editions of *Systema Naturae* from 1735 onwards. Pope and Swift thought the rules of Nature were already known to the 'Ancients', but would have agreed with the Swede that the rules had been 'discovered', not 'devised', that they were natural and not humanly imposed: 'Nature still, but Nature methodized', as Pope had it, as though anticipating Linnaeus by a few years.

And it is arguable that the familiar generalizing of eighteenth-century poets, the perception of life as genre, of nature in its aggregations (the 'silent bats', the 'vengeful snake', the 'glassy brook'), is due to their seeing nature as a taxonomy, a diversity of genera and species rather than individuals (Lemuel Gulliver is the 'type specimen' of the species *Homo brittanus*), indeed an early version of Linnaeus's binary nomenclature. To describe nature (and natural historians 'described' species when they formally identified them for the first time) is to demonstrate order and design, and both are good, indeed ideal rather than particular: hence the eighteenth-century partiality to the stylized pastorals of the classical poets. The phrases quoted above are from Goldsmith's *The Deserted Village* (1770), and the evocative opening of that poem, the description of Auburn as it once was, ideally should be, and *essentially* is despite the ruination, shows the attitude vividly.

Whatever is, is right, said Pope famously: surely whatever else was in his mind, he meant that whatever is allowed to enjoy its true nature is good; the idea of ever-threatening decay required its corollary of self-realization. If so, this Aristotelianism combined with its opposite, the Platonic idea of essences, by seeing essence in time, in process and growth, in a way that Linnaeus did too. The wrong was the degenerate or misshapen (in animal or work of art) and the misshapen or ugly could be the product of mal-adaptation, of nature's limits being transgressed. The monstrous was some-thing of a preoccupation of the time, and *Gulliver's Travels* exhibits it; Linnaeus too pondered the problem of the monster, since it flawed God's design and disrupted the idea of fixed species (Hagberg, 1952). The classi-cal natural historians, especially Pliny, were fascinated by the monstrous in nature. Man does not have a microscopic eye, said Pope in *An Essay on Man*, because it were idle for him 'to inspect a mite'; nor has he an all-sensitive skin 'to smart and agonize at every pore'. Earlier, in *An Essay on Criticism* (1711), Pope had written: 'Some figures monstrous and misshaped appear,/ Considered singly, or beheld too near'. Swift turned this possibility that had been rejected by right nature, maladapted perception, to literal account in *Gulliver's Travels*. Gulliver is cursed with an inhuman perception of mankind and animals: seeing them up too close and singly in the Brobdingnagian kingdom, too far away and in the aggregate in the Lilliputian empire. (But ironically the misperception enables Gulliver to see modern men *as they really are*: misshapen by pride and midget versions of their illustrious ancestors, and cumbersome creatures in animal bodies.)

It so happened that Aristotle was as great an inspiration to eighteenth-century naturalists as Newton, so that classicism was not in itself an imped-iment to natural history. But it did signal an ambivalence about science. In a different way from Swift and Pope, the Irish philosopher George Berkeley (1685-1753) transgressed the frame of the Enlightenment picture of nature. In his case it was through a subjective idealism and a Christian belief firmer and more explicit than Pope's and Swift's. He was a thoroughgoing empiri-cist but also a spiritualist; he was an amateur scientist (producing a treatise on the healthful benefits of tar-water) but copiously cited ancient scientists (Stanford, 1976).

Oliver Goldsmith, like Swift, Berkeley and Edmund Burke, was edu-cated at Trinity College, Dublin. He likewise traced his enthusiasm, one result of which was *An History of the Earth and Animated Nature* (1774), to his reading of the 'Ancients', especially Pliny, and described himself as hav-ing a taste rather classical than scientific (proven by the book's learned errors and system of classification). He was a tolerant member of the neo-classical reaction against modern science. Like a good neo-classicist, he was con-vinced of the radical difference between humanity and the animals, a belief deriving from the Great Chain of Being and Descartes. Yet like elder writers he allegorized animals, though in political rather than religious terms: many birds, for example, had 'a kind of republican form of government established among them', and the society of animals was debased by domestication, reducing them to servants or rebels (Thomas, 1984). The latter sentiment diverged from the medieval hermit poets and the Franciscan tradition, and also from the Judeo-Christian belief in humanity's divine right to dominate, domesticate and exploit the animal kingdom.

When, in *The Deserted Village*, he speaks of animals in these terms of political allegory, Goldsmith sets up complex and unsettling echoes of English government in Ireland, as of course does Swift in his famous Part Four of *Gulliver's Travels*, the voyage to the Country of the Houyhnhnms, when he speaks of human beings in terms of political allegory. In both writers, nature is simultaneously different from humanity (ironically so in Swift's case, and to the discredit of *Homo 'sapiens'*) and a parallel and therefore comparable kingdom, the moral lessons of which comparison are political for these Enlightenment writers where they were religious for the writers of the previous generations.

For Goldsmith, animals were like human beings; for Swift human beings were like animals, at worst Yahoos (who represent by turns mankind in general and the Irish in particular). In this regard, Goldsmith was a qualified Enlightenment optimist with his roots in classicism, Swift an anti-Enlightenment pessimist yet with similar rootage. The politicizing of animals (thinking of them as citizens of Nature: either subjects of an animal 'kingdom' or members of a civic society, whether republican or monarchic) and the scope of Goldsmith's histories and surveys (of England, Greece, Nature, the British Empire) are connected. Goldsmith 'clung to the notion that, with effort, an educated person could still command the whole field of knowledge and thereby become a citizen of the intellectual world. This was a classic ideal of the Enlightenment' (Deane, 1991). Hence the eighteenth-century attraction to collections, catalogues, classifications and cyclopedias. Natural history (in both senses: nature and its study) was, therefore, sufficiently expansive to attract Goldsmith and sufficiently like human history (in both senses: human nature and the history of mankind) to be a suitable object of Enlightenment civic concern.

In the notion that domestication degraded, Goldsmith was following Buffon, whom Goldsmith acknowledged as the chief begetter of *Earth and Animated Nature*. His attention to Buffon shows that Goldsmith was capable of absorbing and popularizing the latest scientific observations and data. Gilbert White may have thought in *A Natural History of Selborne*, published a year after Goldsmith's book, that swallows might indeed hibernate on stream-beds, but the Irish writer was convinced that British swallows migrate in the autumn to Africa (which they do).

Goldsmith's multi-volume work, like Buffon's multi-volume *Histoire Naturelle* (1749), which it in part adapted, was immediately popular, and it has been said that these two writers dominated popular natural history until Cuvier's *Animal Kingdom* early in the nineteenth century (Dance, 1990). They were adapted and edited frequently, Goldsmith's work as recently as 1990. Popular natural history is virtually a literary genre, and Cuvier was followed in England by such mid-Victorian naturalists as Philip Henry Gosse (a Plymouth Brother) and Rev. J.G. Wood, and in late Victorian and Edwardian Ireland by Robert Lloyd Praeger.

The first Irish edition of Goldsmith's work was printed in Dublin in 1776-7 in eight volumes with a hundred engraved plates by J. Lodge. The 'Advertisement by the Printer of the Irish Edition', James Williams, is worth quoting: 'In every endeavour I have used for promoting the Art of Printing in this kingdom, I have met with encouragement beyond my wishes; for I may with confidence affirm, that Hume's History of England [and other listed works] and other valuable books printed by me, are superior to the London Editions.'

This may be the occasion to remind ourselves that a study of the career of natural history in the Irish print trade is clearly wanted; David Cabot (in this volume) has given us a wide-ranging, introductory bibliographic survey of the printed works that would function as primary data in such a study. Dublin was an important publishing centre from the seventeenth century (Belfast a lesser and later centre), but it isn't immediately clear what percentage of important natural-history books published in Dublin were either 'cover' or 'pirate' editions of British or American books and what percentage were first editions. Nor is it immediately clear what impact on the Irish reading public important natural-history books published in Dublin had. A starting bibliography for the subject would include Hoppen (1970), Eager (1980, *s.v.* 'Printers and printing' and 'Publishers and publishing'), and Munter (1988).

Natural Theology

John Locke's philosophy, which dominated eighteenth-century thought in Britain, encouraged toleration, but this rational virtue was perhaps less difficult to contemplate in England than in Ireland where there was a seriously riven society. Two scholars analyze the qualified nature of Anglo-Irish membership of the Enlightenment like this:

The irony of the position was as follows: in an age that was moving away from belief in mysteries and belief in reason, away from the supernatural and towards the natural, Irish philosophers (though many of them were keen natural scientists and intellectually drawn to the new learning) found themselves forced into anti-

Enlightenment positions. They could not support toleration, sympathy for natural religion, or any form of anti-clericalism. The philosophical positions that went with such views – rationalism particularly – were equally suspect for them. Of course, such views emerged even in Ireland, and again one sees the paradox of the Irish situation: political and ecclesiastical establishment needs in Ireland led bishops and thinkers to attack the very ideas that seemed to be gaining ground elsewhere. These liberal ideas came to be associated in Ireland with the circle of writers connected with Lord Molesworth. By the 1720s, such views are to be found most clearly expressed in the work of Francis Hutcheson, who spent the years 1720-30 teaching at a dissenting academy in Dublin. Hutcheson went on to become the father of Scottish philosophy and a major inspiration for the American Revolution and constitution. (Berman and Carpenter, 1991)

Yet awareness of the inherent paradoxes in the Anglo-Irish position ought neither to condone neglect of the work in the natural sciences that was accomplished, nor to compel only a grudging recognition of these accomplishments, as is too often the case in Irish historiography.

The subject of toleration evokes religion in Ireland, and the relationship between the major Christian denominations and the rise of natural history is a complicated one. The requirement of the Reformation – as well as capitalism – for the emergence of scientific natural history is a thesis frequently put forward (Biese, 1905; Dillenberger, 1961). Almost all of the notable early European botanists professed a species of Protestantism. In Ireland, as in England, almost all of the seventeenth- and early eighteenth-century scientists were Anglicans; few were Dissenters or Catholics. Clerical figures like Ussher were drawn to academic modernity combined with a moderate religious Calvinism. Hoppen reminds us that the Established Church in Ireland was on average more Calvinistic than its parent, the Church of England. According to Calvinism, God had made man distinct from the animals by giving him intellect and reason. By using his power of observation and reason, and directing it upon nature, man could come to a greater understanding of God.

Nevertheless, Thomas Sprat, historian of the Royal Society, and others, warned against – as Sprat put it in 1667 – 'religious Men' who 'have multiplied upon us infinite Stories and false Miracles, without any regard to Conscience or Truth' (Ure, 1956). Yet Anglicans in England and Ireland remained largely sympathetic to the new science that some of them were helping to advance. Morrell and Thackray tell us that the blueprint for Samuel Taylor Coleridge's proposed 'clerisy' (or intellectual elite) in the early nineteenth century called for cultural leadership to be exercised by clergymen of the Established Church. At the time the British Association (successor to the Royal Society) got under way in 1831, all Oxford and Cambridge graduates and teachers were Anglicans. If there were some tensions appearing between science and religion, nevertheless the practice of science was, by a system of discrimination against non-Anglicans, largely an Anglican monopoly.

Morrell and Thackray write: 'In the 1830s Section A of the British Association became the familiar haunt of a group of Anglican, mainly clerical gentlemen committed to the placement of physical science within the dominion of mathematical analysis.' They then devote a paragraph to the Trinity College, Dublin, counterpart of the Cambridge programme, with Trinity being described as 'an outpost of English, and specifically of Anglican, culture from the time of its foundation'.

Natural history was containable within Protestantism by means of natural theology, which was highly compatible with Calvinism. '*Philosophy*', said Cotton Mather, the American divine and naturalist (and meaning by his term what we call science), 'is no *Enemy*, but a mighty and wondrous *Incentive* to *Religion*.' To the natural theologian, nature is wondrous but its wonders are studiable, collectable and explicable with diligence and science. Mather's *The Christian Philosopher* (1721) is one of the central manifestoes of natural theology, others being John Ray's *Wisdom of God Manifested in the Works of Creation* (1691), Nehemiah Grew's *Cosmologia Sacra* (1701), William Derham's *Physico-Theology* (1713) and George Cheyne's *Philosophical Principles of Religion* (2nd ed. 1715). But the attempt to deepen the understanding of God through a detailed appreciation of the marvels of nature is found as early as Konrad Gesner (1516-65) and as late as William Paley's *Natural Theology* (1802), the Ulsterman James L. Drummond's *Letters to a Young Naturalist* (1831), and Philip Henry Gosse's works in the Victorian period.* Linnaeus in the eighteenth century espoused a variety of natural theology.

In 1671 Ireland acquired its own natural theologian of stature, John Howe (1630-1705). Howe was a Presbyterian divine who came to Antrim Castle to become chaplain to Lord Massarene. In Antrim Howe wrote several treatises, worked for unity among Protestants (which he lived to see), and published the first part of *The Living Temple* in 1676, with its argument for the existence of God from the perspective of natural theology. The work has been called a Puritan *Summa Theologiae* and the first serious criticism of deism (Davies, 1963). The deistic deduction of the Creator from the created was a necessary component of natural theology, but insufficient for many

---

* A case of how classical natural theology was split in two after Darwin (God and nature worrisomely separable), yet lingered on, would be the attitude of J.P. Burkitt recorded by David Lack. Burkitt (b. 1870), the Co. Fermanagh inventor of scientific bird-ringing for the study of behaviour and age, told Lack: 'When I was doing the Robin I had pricks of conscience that I was really more interested in the created than the Creator' (Lack, 1959). Lack describes this ornithological pioneer as 'deeply religious' and a man 'who has spent his declining years reading his bible and working in his garden'.

natural theologians who could not accept the deistic belief in the adequacy of the Book of Nature as valid revelation. Howe's view of nature as 'nothing else but *divine art*' required rejection of Descartes's idea that animal bodies are machines. In Howe's opinion, the phenomena of organic growth, nutrition, propagation, spontaneous motion, and powers of sensation were sufficient to re-classify animals as God's creatures.

The closeness of Protestantism (especially, in Ireland, the Established Church) to science in the century before Lyell and Darwin is demonstrated practically in the subscriber list to John Rutty's pioneering *An Essay Towards a Natural History of the County of Dublin, Accommodated to the Noble Designs of the Dublin Society* (1772). Among the names are those of the bishops of Cloyne, Clogher, Waterford and Lismore, Dromore, Kildare, Limerick, Meath, Cork, and of the late Archbishop of Dublin. (The three hundred names appear to be overwhelmingly Protestant.) Rutty himself was a Quaker who revised in 1751 a history of the Irish Quakers by T. Wight and published *A Spiritual Diary and Soliloquies* in 1776.

The standard account of the disproportionate contribution Quakers have made to British natural history is by Raistrick (1968). The role of Quakers in natural history has been sufficiently significant for the Society for the History of Natural History (London) to have convened in Dublin in 1994 to investigate and celebrate it. Two explanatory factors in Quaker involvement in natural history from the eighteenth century to the present would be the congeniality of the Quaker worldview to nature and natural history, and the record of professional disabilities suffered by members of this sect, encouraging them by the archimedean principle of displacement to channel their energies away from the proscribed or discouraged professions to the profession of science. This second factor would perhaps offer the historical roots to Dissenter involvement in natural history in nineteenth-century Ulster, but the relative paucity of Catholic naturalists even when barriers against them came down would suggest that in the cases of Quaker, Dissenter and Catholic alike, worldview and system were paramount.

The Aesthetics of Nature

The design in divine Creation could be emulated by that in artistic creation: in *An Essay on Criticism*, Nature for Pope imparts life, force and beauty equally to the created world and the created work. The Anglo-Irish tradition was an exemplary demonstration of the understanding of this, as impressive in literature as in science.* The heyday of the tradition was the

---

* An historical overview of Anglo-Irish culture (though it stints on science) is *The Anglo-Irish Tradition* (1976) by J.C. Beckett.

eighteenth century, during which nature was 'methodized' by both the scientists and the writers. This was the positive 'hyphenation' of the Anglo-Irish tradition, whereas the philosophical and social self-contradiction Berman and Carpenter (1991) draw attention to is the negative hyphenation.

It is true that there was at the heart of the tradition an ambivalence about nature. Swift, in the guise of Tory pessimist and passive satirist, sees the prevalence of vices (deceit, pride, ambition), the degeneration of virtue and the greed for power ('the ambition of princes') as universal principles, deplorable but unavoidable, at least among modern mankind (the greed for power and commodities creates 'a modern colony' in a ruthless process that Swift summarizes in one scouring paragraph in Part Four of Gulliver's Travels). These principles, which play havoc with the colonized landscape, are the master themes of Gulliver's Travels. Yet Swift as reformer and active satirist leaves room both for improvement (as well as degeneration) and for indignation when improvement is not attempted. The irony is that his reform requires the colony to be bettered, not returned to the native people: it is the ruthlessness of colonization he objects to, not colonization itself.

In Part Three of his adventures, Gulliver is lowered from the flying island of Laputa (where the Court resides) to the island of Balnibarbi;. The capital, Lagado, 'half the Bigness of London', would seem to be Dublin: the people are in rags, look wild and have fixed eyes. The adjoining country-side, despite its excellent soil, is 'unhappily cultivated': Swift pondered the decline of Irish agriculture, due to the conversion of arable land into pasture (Swift, 1986). The belief of Gulliver's master Houyhnhnm is clearly Swift's: 'that all Animals [i.e. human beings] had a Title to their Share in the Productions of the Earth'. After all, as the maxim Swift draws on had it, 'Nature is very easily satisfied'. While scientists conduct absurd experiments in agricultural improvement, 'the whole Country lies miserably waste'. (A feral version of what Spenser and others regarded as the native wastes and deserts of the Irish landscape.)

In stark contrast is the designed estate of Gulliver's guide, with its productive farms, fertile countryside, delightful prospects: taste and judgment mediating (like wit) between science and reason, but threatened by what we today might call the centralized social engineering and applied science bureaucracy of Laputa. The Lord Munodi's estate is in disguise a magnificent demesne of the Anglo-Irish ascendancy. Swift saw the aestheticizing of landscape and the fruitful use of the earth as utterly compatible. Such estates were not outrageously ironic contrasts to the surrounding waste land, but models to be imitated, if government ('Princes') would permit and encourage it.

The people of Balnibarbi reappear, further sunk in barbarity, as the squalid Yahoos of Part Four of the book. Were they to represent the Irish and suggest a people beyond redemption not just because of misgovernment but also because of their own nature, Swift would be merely a latter-day John Davies. In his poem 'Holyhead', Swift describes Ireland as 'that slavish hateful shore ... the land I hate'. And in truth Swift retained some of the anti-Irish prejudices of the Elizabethans. But he was also an Irish patriot of a kind and believed that taste, judgment and political improvement were possible in Ireland: at the very least, art could civilize by example.

In 1723 Swift travelled through the south of Ireland and wrote a poem in Latin about the Carbery Rocks, 'Carberiae Rupes'; this appeared in 1735 in translation as 'Carbery Rocks in the County of Cork, Ireland' by William Dunkin (b. Dublin c. 1709), 'the most underrated poet of eighteenth-century Ireland' (Coleborne, 1991). The poem celebrates wildness and disorder but transforms them into a verbal representation of the picturesque, to which I will return. Fabricant (1982) has described Swift's real and imaginative landscapes as political and as characterized by forces of confusion and collapse, in contrast with Pope's orderly terrains. But there was depicted in Anglo-Irish poetry of the eighteenth century an orderly landscape symbolizing the allegedly calm polity established in Ireland by England; such poetic landscapes derived from Sir John Denham's famous long poem 'Cooper's Hill' (1642/55) and Pope's long poem 'Windsor Forest' (1713). Depictions of orderly landscapes were not the only dividend of stability: Hagberg reminds us that 'systematic botany did not advance until after the restoration of the Stuarts to the throne of England, and the termination of the long and bloody wars which distracted Europe. The influence of peace upon the progress of science was very great ...'.

Denham, as it happens, was born in Dublin in 1615 (where his father was the Chief Baron of the Exchequer and his mother the daughter of Viscount Drogheda), but he was taken to England when an infant. The poet's composition of his visual field from Cooper's Hill (on the Berkshire-Surrey border) became a model for similar poems. The poem embodies and celebrates in topography the social and political stability first achieved by Magna Charta at Runnymede (in the poet's line of vision) and consolidated by subsequent events in England.

There are Anglo-Irish counterparts of 'Cooper's Hill' and 'Windsor Forest', such as James Ward's 'Phoenix Park' (1718), that likewise use the landscape to represent wise English polity, to celebrate Tory peace and order after the Treaty of Utrecht and the Protestant ascendancy in Hanoverian Ireland. Like Windsor Forest, Phoenix Park was a spacious, variegated rural area within sight of the governing city of the island. 'In the period 1714 to 1760 Ireland had little or no political history', wrote Curtis (1950). 'At least in 1714, our country, after the unrest of a hundred and fifty years, reached an equilibrium which lasted for some fifty years. Unjust as was the established order, it gave peace and security for such gains as men could make or such education as their minds could take advantage of.' Potterton writes: 'Evidence, first of all of Ireland's peace and then of her prosperity in the eighteenth century, is supplied by the art and architecture of the time' (Harbison *et al.*, 1978).

'Cooper's Hill' established a long-lived poetic genre called 'topographical' or 'loco-descriptive' poetry (Aubin, 1936; Foster, 1970). These were long, spacious poems, which in the early stages of the genre exemplified the wider cultural shift from the Renaissance world picture – with its symbolic correspondences – to the classical concern with nature's measurable identities and differences, its visible characteristics. The rise of topographical poetry coincides with the acceleration of scientific surveying of the land, begun by the Elizabethans, which suggests that discipline's influence on the poetry (Foster, 1975/76) and a bridge between science and literature. There were in turn socio-economic spurs to the development of surveying: in England during the sixteenth and seventeenth centuries it was enclosure; in Ireland during the sixteenth and early seventeenth centuries it was conquest and colonization, and later in the seventeenth century the Cromwellian Settlement, during which Sir William Petty produced, in the so-called Down Survey, the first scientific mapping out of Ireland. Practical and theoretical map-making and surveying developed apace throughout the eighteenth century.

In Ireland during the eighteenth century several texts on surveying were printed, among them Robert Gibson's *A Treatise of Practical Surveying* (1752), Peter Callan's *A Dissertation on the Practice of Land-Surveying in Ireland* (Drogheda, 1758) and Benjamin Noble's *Geodaesia Hibernica* (Dublin, 1763).* Callan is unintentionally whimsical, setting out to rid Ireland of fraudulences and anomalies in surveying: his picture of the island swarming with dissembling surveyors is almost Dickensian. It is clear from his book, however, that surveying in Ireland was closely connected with the political land situation and the high incidence of confiscation, forfeiture and re-apportionment (Foster, 1974). Gibson's book, on the other hand, was a genuine contribution to the science and was the first English surveying text to be published in North America, where it passed through twenty-one editions (Richeson, 1966). (For a short history of Irish map-making, see Andrews in this volume.)

The rise of topographical poetry also coincides with the later development of English landscape gardening, one component in a cultural complex

---

*Surveying required instruments; for an account of the history of the telescope and of the quadrant, circumferentor and theodolite, see Daumas (1972). Dublin as the second British city in science as well as in size had its respected instrument-makers, for an account of whom consult Mason (1944).

that includes Whiggism in politics, Shaftesbury's philosophy in aesthetics and ethics – followed by *Inquiry into the Original of Our Ideas of Beauty and Virtue* (1725) by Francis Hutcheson (b. Co. Down, 1694) – and the cult of Italian landscape painting (Foster, 1975/76). The ideal was to balance art and nature, mind and feeling, reason and imagination, the balance to be achieved, among other places and mediums, in Anglo-Irish gentlemen's estates (demesnes). (The natural history of the demesnes is discussed by Reeves-Smyth in this volume.) Denham's and Ward's 'landscape of polity' gave way to the 'landscape of taste': the topographical locale is no longer the realm (achieved through blood, sacrifice and treaty) but polite human society (achieved through reason and artistic effort). Swift was not simply an angry depicter of a neglected Irish countryside that gainsaid English government on the island, but like Pope sought greater freedom in landscaping and was much interested in his friend Rev. Patrick Delany's demesne, 'Delville', at Glasnevin outside Dublin and nowadays part of the National Botanic Gardens.

Delany is credited by Malins with introducing the modern style of gardening into Ireland. Malins claims that the natural topography of Ireland was easily adaptable to the new style: 'In Ireland, where so much rolling, lake-begirt natural landscape was available, it was popular and cheaper to lay out a garden by making use of these natural advantages, rather than create Baroque *parterres* and elaborate *allées*.' In accordance with the fashionable significance attached to landscape, Delville became the centre of an artistic and intellectual coterie that attracted, among others, Swift, Tickell and Addison. The coterie, withdrawn for self-protection from the wider public, is imaged in the garden surrounded by walls, fences and less cultivated landscape (Foster, 1974). Letitia Pilkington recalled an occasion when she met Swift and Delany at Delville, and described the setting with exclamatory zest:

> Hail, happy *Delville*! blissful seat!
> The muse's best belov'd retreat!
> With prospects large and unconfined;
> Blest emblem of their master's mind!
> Where fragrant gardens, painted meads,
> Wide-op'ning walks, and twilight shades –
> Inspiring scenes! – elate the heart!
> Nature improved, and raised by Art,
> So Paradise delightful smil'd,
> Blooming and beautifully wild.
> (Fabricant, 1982)

The vistas and visual perspectives in these Irish cultivated estates, even more than in their English equivalents, were what I have called 'prospects of power' (Foster, 1974), specifically the political, social and economic power of the Anglo-Irish.

The criteria by which landscape was perceived and appreciated were being developed outside Ireland. Taste had early accommodated what was known after 1794 (when Uvedale Price's *Essay* appeared) as 'the picturesque', which Denham had already established but only as a minor motif. The instability Fabricant sees in Swift's Irish landscape is as much in the picturesque landscape of the imagination as in Swift's Ireland beyond the estate, beyond the Pale. The landscape of taste became the 'landscape of feeling' when the theories of Pope, Shaftesbury and Hutcheson gave way to Burke's *Enquiry into the Origin of Our Ideas of the Sublime and Beautiful* (1757), which took into account the feelings of individual men and nature's immensity independent of humankind. Burke stimulated a new generation of landscapers, who sought the picturesque qualities of roughness, irregularity and surprise.

Irish poets were especially equipped to capitalize on the fashionable search for remote and inspiring areas. The picturesque hand of time, in the guise of castles and abbeys, ruined or otherwise, was everywhere evident on the island: Killarney particularly inspired poems (Foster, 1974). These Anglo-Irish topographical poets, however, see the picturesque Irish landscape as complementing established order in Ireland, and merely play at the sublime, preferring instead to encourage English-style economic improvement of the land.

It can be said that the cult of the picturesque created modern tourism, which nowadays depends heavily on 'selling' the picturesque scenery of 'accessible' remote spots and of once-great landscaped demesnes seasonally open to the public. It was in the eighteenth century that places such as Killarney generated their modern reputation, and they did so partly through picturesque engravings, prints and etchings. Books of topographical prints became popular. Joseph Atkinson in his poem 'Killarney' (1798) counsels us to consult by way of compensation, should we be unable to get to Killarney, Jonathan Fisher's prints: Fisher published *A Picturesque Tour of Killarney* (1789) and *Scenery of Ireland* (1795). In twenty aquatints and six engravings, Fisher seeks in the former 'to lead the curious [who visit the Lake] to points of view, where the sublime and beautiful are most picturesquely combined; and which often might be hastily passed by, if the Painter's observation did not induce a more critical examination' (Foster, 1974). Other favourite haunts of the painter and etcher were the Giant's Causeway in Co. Antrim and Cashel in Co. Tipperary (Elmes, 1943).

Topographical painting depicted real scenes, whereas neo-classical landscape painting depicted either composite views out of the painter's head (imaginary views) or views merely suggested by reality or coloured by a school of sensibility (imaginative views). Thomas Roberts, George Mullins and William Ashford were among the eminent Irish eighteenth-century landscape painters. George Barret met Burke in Dublin and the latter advised him to paint in the Dargle Valley in Co. Wicklow (Potterton in Harbison et al., 1978). Barret's *Horses Watering* exemplifies Burke's concept of the beautiful, whereas *Stormy Landscape* displays the Burkean notion of the sublime (*plate 2*).

More informative than prints were the descriptions of tours in Ireland by doughty and industrious individuals. These mushroomed during the picturesque period, and included William Rufus Chetwood's *A Tour through Ireland* (1746), Richard Pococke's *Tour in Ireland* (1752), John Bush's *Hibernia Curiosa* (1768) and Arthur Young's famous tours in 1776, 1777 and 1778. Young bristles with practicality, but does permit himself this of Killarney (proving how standard such observations must then have been): 'Soon entered the wildest and most romantic country I had any where seen; a region of steep rocks and mountains .... There is something magnificently wild in this stupendous scenery, formed to impress the mind with a species of terror' (Young, 1892). Topographical poets, too, frequently fell into this rhetoric, which had once been fresh but eventually became the traveloguese of tourist operators.

Travel to picturesque places depended on the likelihood of personal safety, which in turn depended on political stability. There was in 1700, we are told (Hadfield and McVeagh, 1994), 'a greater sense of centralized control under the rule of Westminster than had existed in 1600. Under such stable conditions it was possible for what we now know as "travel writing" to develop within the British Isles.' (Both Swift and Goldsmith were travellers and exploited their travel in their writing.) Safety assumed, travel to picturesque regions still depended on such practical affairs as the state of transportation, the condition of the roads and the existence of road-maps. Road-books and road-maps began to appear in Ireland at the time interest in the picturesque was running high. According to Fordham (1923), there were no road-books in Ireland before 1647 when a surveyor produced one. Few followed until 1763. In 1778 George Taylor and Andrew Skinner published their pioneering and ambitious *Maps of the Roads of Ireland*, much used by subsequent topographers. It was not, however, until late in the century that road-books actually printed in Dublin began appearing, starting with William Wilson's *Post-Chaise Companion: or Traveller's Directory through Ireland* (1784). George Tyner's *Traveller's Guide Through Ireland* appeared in 1794, the same year as Price's *Essay on the Picturesque*. William W. Seward's directory, *Topographia Hibernica*, appeared the year after; it has a picturesque bias when treating Killarney, which he describes as 'astonishingly sublime' and which 'strikes the timid with awe' (Seward, 1795). But

Seward's book is useful as well as rhapsodic, and topographical poets and painters, as well as travelling sightseers, plainly availed of it.

Interest in the picturesque was maintained well into the nineteenth century, and in a sense its vocabulary and mode of perception were never totally abandoned. Despite the presence of the picturesque, the genre has nothing in common with genuine Romanticism, any more than does picturesque neoclassicism in painting, which likewise continued well into the nineteenth century through the brushes of James Arthur O'Connor and others. In his topographical poem 'Rosstrevor' (Newry, 1810), William Carr writes of 'ivy-mantl'd piles' and gothic grandeur and of the picturesque prospect from the top of the Mourne Mountains of Co. Down, this last an attempt no doubt to honour both the climactic situation in topographical poetry (the overview or survey from a hilltop) and the 'local pride' motif. Moreover, Carr's poem has many of the standard formulas, including a passing celebration of the recent Act of Union between Great Britain and Ireland *(his* Runnymede), without which Ireland 'must drooping then to gradual ruin tend' (Carr, 1810).

Poetry and Geology

Later in its career, the topographical genre fell under the sway of natural theology and the physico-theological movement, and many of the poets were clergymen–cum–amateur naturalists who created what we might call a 'landscape of divine phenomena'. The establishment of modern geology during what Von Zittel called the 'Heroic Age of Geology' (1790-1820) made the position of Christian scientists more difficult, particularly concerning the formation of the Earth's crust and the dating of fossils. One imagines that contemporary Ulster, with its contentious Protestant divines, would have been a hotbed for physico-theological debate. How far this was the case remains to be investigated, though meanwhile Livingstone in this volume has depicted the Ulster polemical scene during what we might call the 'Heroic Age of Biology' (i.e. the age of Darwin, Huxley and Wallace).

Certainly Ulster produced a large number of topographical poems during the heroic age of geology and the late flowering of the picturesque, which coincided (Foster, 1974). Few of these poems are of serious critical interest, but Rev. William Hamilton Drummond (1778-1865) published in *The Giant's Causeway* (1811) a work meant to be an epic poem but that is really a scientific mystery story, invoking a furious geological controversy. The action of water in the formation of the Earth's crust was held paramount by the 'Neptunists', headed by A.G. Werner (1750-1817), but they were opposed by the 'Vulcanists', whose chief theorist was James Hutton (1726-97). According to Hutton, the strata of the Earth's present crust are the debris of an antecedent Earth, worn down by the elements, carried into the oceanic abysses, and there laid horizontally down, fused and consolidated by subaqueous heat, and afterwards elevated to their present altitude, and broken and dislocated into their present form.

For both factions, the Giant's Causeway was a convenient case-study, an open secret of the Earth's subterranean workings. Drummond, a controversial essayist and sermonizer, was born in Larne, Co. Antrim and educated in Belfast and Glasgow, after which he became Pastor of the second Congregation in Belfast. He tells us that 'philosophers' began to attend to the Causeway, after a fifty-year respite, when in 1740 two beautiful engravings of the phenomenon came to public attention – an instance of the geological and the picturesque coinciding.

To Drummond, as topographical poet as well as amateur naturalist and clergyman, the Causeway was a microcosm of the Earth's crust and of God's handiwork, just as for Denham the Thames Valley was a microcosm of the realm. Like Denham, Drummond discusses the history and mythology of his locality in Book One, and in Book Two he describes the folkways of the area, a motif historians of topographical poetry call 'the genre sketch'.

In Book Three, Drummond versifies three main theories of the Causeway's origin – Neptunism, Vulcanism, and the vertical-force theory of Rev. William Richardson (1740-1820), an Irish geologist and rector of Moy – 'without having professed a decided attachment to any'. Irish geologists played a leading role in the formulation and application of Neptunism and Vulcanism. Three mentioned by Drummond are Richard Kirwan (1733-1812), the Galway chemist and geologist, author of *Elements of Mineralogy* (2nd ed. 1794-6), whose criticism of Huttonian theory involved him in a heated controversy and whom Drummond calls 'Neptunian KIRWAN, green Ierne's pride'; John Templeton (1766-1825), the Belfast botanist and meteorologist; and the unfortunate Rev. William Hamilton (b.1755), the Londonderry antiquarian and geologist whose *Letters Concerning the Northern Coast of County Antrim* (1786) professed a volcanic theory of the basalts, and who was assassinated (as a magistrate and clergyman of the Established Church) in 1797.

Drummond's poem was followed in 1819 by a poem of the same name from the pen of John McKinley. Like Drummond's, McKinley's poem is got up in the garb of a classical epic, further evidence of how the topographical poem, always partial to expansiveness, paradoxically belittled itself through bloated ambition and a purely mechanical notion of epic scale. McKinley follows Drummond in combining geology with a picturesque appreciation of the embattled capes, impending cliffs, and 'surge-scoop'd antres, thunder-splinter'd spires' of the Antrim coast.

The Huttonian theory towards which Drummond and McKinley inclined taught that geological formations succeed one another in an endless sequence of decay, upheaval and consolidation. The need for constant renewal accorded with the Christian belief that the present Earth is sinful and imperfect, while the geological concept of 'renovation' was evidence that God's benevolent hand was still upon the planet. Drummond would have differed from Hutton over the latter's majestically soulful claim that in the fate of the Earth's crust 'we find no vestige of a beginning – no prospect of an end'. The Christian poets preferred the notion of Doomsday (a catastrophic theory of geology brought to its final conclusion), and many of them used it as a convenient climax for their poems.

Of renovation, McKinley (though it could have been Drummond) writes:

> Hail, Renovation! thou whose plastic care
> Can worlds on worlds from age to age repair.

As a moral and spiritual notion, renovation was a bridge between science and Christianity. It also bridged these with political vision. Atkinson, exhorting hard-working Englishmen to come to Killarney, professes to desire to see the Irish, as a result, 'in their neat cots a renovated race'. In Atkinson can be heard a distant echo of Sir John Davies's recommendation of English models of order and productivity for Irish realities of disorder and waste. It is as if the original Anglo-Irish plantations were to be extended in missionary form to the native population.

From beginning to end, topographical poetry was a genre that promulgated the idea that things are always getting better. It was also a conservative genre that desired equilibrium and steady progress, harmony and moderation, states achievable only through vigilance (such as the poet's on his elevated position) and the will to check as well as to reform. Through its geology, nature exemplified the desirable Anglo-Irish vision of government and society in Ireland. Also, at the centre of the genre was the realization that equilibrium, steady progress, harmony and moderation paradoxically proceed from discord, excess and imbalance, as geology showed.

In *The Giant's Causeway* by Drummond, as in 'Cooper's Hill', certain climactic events propel the Earth and human society forward. But the prevailing concept of order-in-disorder (*concordia discors*) in nature and society was not always to hold unchallenged. The political and topographical prospects in loco-descriptive poetry stand opposed to those in the Romantic poetry that succeeded it, despite the fact that both poetries were inspired by the sublime and the beautiful. One sought nature cultivated, the other sought nature ideally without evidence of present or past cultivation; for one, nature was a vast homology for social and political order; for the other, nature was a vast freedom and otherness beyond the control of society and politics but yet instructive in being so. In Ireland, one poetry projected an essentially Anglo-Irish vision of plantation variously justified. The other was the anti-establishment English vision of Shelley and early Wordsworth and Coleridge, but it did not gain firm purchase in early nineteenth-century Ireland. Had it done so, it might have threatened culturally the stability of Anglo-Ireland (as its political version – quixotic rebellion – did in 1798), a stability reinforced by the culture of literary, economic and scientific topography, indeed by Anglo-Irish scientific culture itself.

References

Allen, E.G. 1951. 'The History of American Ornithology before Audubon.' *Transactions of the American Philosophical Society*. New Series. *41*: 390-591.

Anderson, K. 1995. 'Our Natural Selves.' *Times Literary Supplement*, 8 September.

Armstrong, E.A. 1958. *The Folklore of Birds*. London: Collins.

Armstrong, E.A. 1973. *Saint Francis: Nature Mystic. The Derivation and Significance of the Nature Stories in the Franciscan Legend*. Berkeley: University of California Press.

Ashton, J. 1890. *Curious Creatures in Zoology*. London: Nimmo.

Atkinson, J. 1798. *Killarney, A Poem*. Dublin: Porter.

Aubin, R.A. 1936. *Topographical Poetry in Eighteenth-Century England*. New York: MLA.

Bacon, F. [1620] 1855. *The Novum Organum*. Oxford: Oxford University Press.

Bacon, F. 1942. 'Of Plantations,' in *Essays and New Atlantis*. New York: W.J. Black.

Beckett, J.C. 1976. *The Anglo-Irish Tradition*. London: Faber and Faber.

Berman, D. and A. Carpenter (eds). 1991. 'Eighteenth-Century Irish Philosophy,' in Seamus Deane (ed.), *The Field Day Anthology of Irish Writing*, vol. 1. Derry: Field Day Publications.

Biese, A. 1905. T*he Development of the Feeling for Nature in the Middle Ages and Modern Times*. Rpt. [n.d.] New York: Franklin.

Boate, G. 1652. *Irelands Naturall History*. London: Hartlib.

Boate, G., T. Molineux [sic] et al. [1726] 1755. *A Natural History of Ireland in Three Parts*. Dublin: G. and A. Ewing.

Browne, Sir T. [1646-72] 1981. *Pseudodoxia Epidemica*. Ed. R. Robbins. 2 vols. Oxford: Clarendon Press.

Burke, E. 1757. *A Philosophical Inquiry into the Origin of Our Ideas of the Sublime and Beautiful*. London: Dodsley.

Bush, J. 1768. *Hibernia Curiosa: A Letter from a Gentleman in Dublin, to his Friend at Dover*. London: Flexney. 1769. Dublin: Potts and Williams.

Callan, P. 1758. *A Dissertation on the Practice of Land-Surveying in Ireland*. Drogheda.

Carpenter, A. and S. Deane (eds). 1991. 'The Shifting Perspective (1690-1830)' in S. Deane (ed.), *The Field Day Anthology of Irish Writing*, vol. 1. Derry: Field Day Publications.

Carr, W. 1810. *Rostrevor, A Moral and Descriptive Poem*. Newry: Murray.

Chetwood, W.R. 1746. *A Tour through Ireland*. Dublin: Wilson.

Coleborne, B. 1991. 'Anglo-Irish Verse 1675-1825,' in S. Deane (ed.), *The Field Day Anthology of Irish Writing*, vol. 1. Derry: Field Day Publications.

Corish, P.J. 1981. *The Catholic Community in the Seventeenth and Eighteenth Centuries*. Dublin: Helicon.

Corrigan, D. 1984. 'The Scientific Basis of Folk Medicine: The Irish Dimension,' in R. Vickery (ed.), *Plant-Lore Studies*. London: Folklore Society.

Cross, T.P. 1952. *Motif-Index of Early Irish Literature*. Bloomington: Indiana University Press.

Curtis, E. 1950. *A History of Ireland*. London: Methuen.

Dance, S.P. [1978] 1990. *The Art of Natural History*. New York: Arch Cape Press.

Daumas, M. 1972. *Scientific Instruments of the Seventeenth and Eighteenth Centuries and their Makers*. Trans. and ed., Mary Holbrook. London: Batsford.

Davies, H. 1963. *The English Free Churches*. London: Oxford University Press.

Davies, Sir J. [1612] 1988. *A Discovery of the True Causes Why Ireland was never Entirely Subdued*. Ed. J.P. Myers. Washington, D.C.: Catholic University of America.

Deane, S. 1991. 'Oliver Goldsmith: Miscellaneous Writings 1759-74,' in S. Deane (ed.), *The Field Day Anthology of Irish Writing*, vol. 1. Derry: Field Day Publications.

de Paor, M. and L. 1978. *Early Christian Ireland*. London: Thames and Hudson.

Dillenberger, J. 1961. *Protestant Thought and Natural Science*. London: Collins.

Drummond, J.L. 1831. *Letters to a Young Naturalist on the Study of Nature and Natural Theology*. London: Longman, Rees, Orme, Brown and Green.

Drummond, Rev. W.H. 1811. *The Giant's Causeway: A Poem*. Belfast: Archer & Wirling, Ward.

Eager, A.R. 1980. *A Guide to Irish Bibliographical Material*. Westport, Ct: Greenwood.

Eamon, W. 1995. *Science and the Secrets of Nature: Books of Secrets in Medieval and Early Modern Culture*. Princeton: Princeton University Press.

Edwards, N. 1990. *The Archaeology of Early Medieval Ireland*. London: Batsford.

Elmes, R.M. 1943. *Catalogue of Irish Topographical Prints and Original Drawings*. Dublin: Stationery Office.

Evans, E.E. 1957. *Irish Folk Ways*. London: Routledge & Kegan Paul.

Evans, E.E. [1973] 1992. *The Personality of Ireland: Habitat, Heritage and History*. Dublin: Lilliput Press.

Fabricant, C. 1982. *Swift's Landscape*. Baltimore: Johns Hopkins University Press.

Fairley, J. 1984. *An Irish Beast Book: A Natural History of Ireland's Furred Wildlife*. Belfast: Blackstaff.

Farrington, B. [1936] 1969. *Science in Antiquity*. London: Oxford University Press.

Farrington, B. 1944, 1949. *Greek Science*. Harmondsworth: Penguin.

Feliks, Y. 1981. *Nature and Man in the Bible: Chapters in Biblical Ecology*. London: Soncino Press.

Fisher, J. 1789. *A Picturesque Tour of Killarney*. Dublin and London.

Fisher, J. 1795. *Scenery of Ireland*.

Flower, R. 1944. *The Western Island, or The Great Blasket*. Oxford: Oxford University Press.

Flower, R. 1947. *The Irish Tradition*. Oxford: Clarendon Press.

Fordham, Sir H. 1923. 'The Road-Books and Itineraries of Ireland, 1647 to 1850, A Catalogue.' *The Bibliographical Society of Ireland 2*.

Foster, J.W. 1970. 'A Redefinition of Topographical Poetry.' *Journal of English and Germanic Philology 59*: 394-406.

Foster, J.W. 1974. 'The Topographical Tradition in Anglo-Irish Poetry.' *Irish University Review 4*: 169-87.

Foster, J.W. 1975/76. 'The Measure of Paradise: Topography in Eighteenth-Century Poetry.' *Eighteenth-Century Studies 9*: 232-56.

Foster, J.W. 1987. *Fictions of the Irish Literary Revival: A Changeling Art*. Syracuse: Syracuse University Press; Dublin: Gill and Macmillan.

Foster, J.W. 1991. *Colonial Consequences: Essays in Irish Literature and Culture*. Dublin: Lilliput Press.

Foster, J.W. 1996. 'Strains in Irish Intellectual Life,' in Liam O'Dowd (ed.), *On Intellectuals and Intellectual Life in Ireland*. Belfast and Dublin: Institute of Irish Studies and Royal Irish Academy.

Foster, R.F. 1988. *Modern Ireland 1600-1972*. London: Penguin.

Gantz, J. (trans.). 1981. *Early Irish Myths and Sagas*. Harmondsworth: Penguin.

Gibson, R. 1752. *A Treatise of Practical Surveying*. Dublin: Nelson.

Goldsmith, O. [1774] 1776-77. *An History of the Earth, and Animated Nature*. Dublin: J. Williams. 1990. Oliver Goldsmith's *History of the Natural World*. London: Studio Editions.

Green, M. 1992. *Animals in Celtic Life and Myth*. London: Routledge.

Greenblatt, S. 1991. *Marvelous Possessions: The Wonder of the New World*. Chicago: University of Chicago Press.

Greene, D.H. [1954] 1971. *An Anthology of Irish Literature*. New York: New York University Press.

Hadfield, A. and J. McVeagh. 1994. *Strangers to that Land: British Perceptions of Ireland from the Reformation to the Famine*. Gerrards Cross: Colin Smythe.

Hagberg, K. 1952. *Carl Linnaeus.* Trans. A. Blair. London: Jonathan Cape.

Hamilton, W. 1786, 1790. *Letters Concerning the Northern Coast of the County of Antrim … .* Dublin: Bonham.

Hampson, N. [1968] 1982. *The Enlightenment.* London: Penguin.

Harbison, P., H. Potterton and J. Sheehy. 1978. *Irish Art and Architecture from Prehistory to the Present.* London: Thames and Hudson.

Heaney, S. 1972. *Wintering Out.* London: Faber.

Heaney, S. 1983. *Sweeney Astray.* Derry: Field Day.

Heron-Allen, E. 1928. *Barnacles in Nature and Myth.* London: Oxford University Press.

Herries Davies, G.L. 1985. 'Irish Thought in Science,' in Richard Kearney (ed.), *The Irish Mind.* Dublin: Wolfhound Press.

Heuvelmans, B. 1984. 'The Birth and Early History of Cryptozoology.' *Cryptozoology 3*: 1-30.

Hoppen, K.T. 1970. *The Common Scientist in the Seventeenth Century: A Study of the Dublin Philosophical Society 1683-1708.* London: Routledge & Kegan Paul.

Howe, J. 1848. *The Works of the Rev. John Howe, M.A. as Published during his Life. Comprising the Whole of the Two folio Volumes, Edit. 1724. With a Life of the Author by the Rev. J.P. Hewlett.* 3 vols. London: William Tegg.

Hunter, M. 1995. *Science and the Shape of Orthodoxy: Intellectual Change in Late Seventeenth-Century Britain.* Woodbridge: Boydell.

Hutcheson, F. 1725. *An Inquiry into the Original of Our Ideas of Beauty and Virtue.* London: J. Darby.

Huppé, B.F. 1982. 'Nature in *Beowulf* and *Roland,*' in L.D. Roberts (ed.), *Approaches to Nature in the Middle Ages.* Binghamton, N.Y.: Center for Medieval and Early Renaissance Studies, State University of New York.

Jackson, K.H. 1971. *A Celtic Miscellany: Translations from the Celtic Literatures.* Harmondsworth: Penguin.

Joyce, J. 1916. *A Portrait of the Artist as a Young Man.* London: Egoist Press.

Joyce, P.W. 1891, 1893. *The Origin and History of Irish Names of Places.* 2 vols. 6th ed. Dublin: Gill.

Joyce, P.W. [1913] 1968. *A Social History of Ancient Ireland.* 2 vols. New York: Blom.

Kalm, P. [1770] 1987. *Peter Kalm's Travels in North America.* Trans. J.R. Forster. Revised, A.B. Benson. New York: Dover.

Knott, E. and G. Murphy. 1966. *Early Irish Literature.* London: Routledge & Kegan Paul.

Lack, D. 1959. 'Some British Pioneers in Ornithological Research, 1859-1939.' *Ibis 101*: 71-81.

Lahontan, Baron de. [1703] 1905. *Lahontan's New Voyages to North-America.* Ed. R.G. Thwaites. Chicago: A.C. McClurg.

Leighton, C.D.A. 1994. *Catholicism in a Protestant Kingdom: A Study of the Irish Ancien Regime.* Dublin: Gill & Macmillan.

Lennon, C. 1994. *Sixteenth-Century Ireland: The Incomplete Conquest.* Dublin: Gill & Macmillan.

Lever, C. 1977. *The Naturalized Animals of the British Isles.* London: Hutchinson.

Lever, C. 1985. *Naturalized Mammals of the World.* London: Longman.

Lever, C. 1987. *Naturalized Birds of the World.* Harlow, Essex: Longman.

Lever, C. 1996. *Naturalized Fishes of the World.* San Diego: Academic Press.

Ley, W. 1968. *Dawn of Zoology.* Englewood Cliffs, N.J.: Prentice-Hall.

Ley, W. 1987. *Exotic Zoology.* New York: Bonanza Books.

Lovejoy, A.O. 1936. *The Great Chain of Being.* Cambridge, Mass.: Harvard University Press.

Lyon, J. and P.R. Sloan (eds). 1981. *From Natural History to the History of Nature: Readings from Buffon and his Critics.* South Bend, Ind.: University of Notre Dame Press.

McGee, T. D'A. 1857. *The Irish Writers of the Seventeenth Century.* Dublin: James Duffy.

McKinley, J. [1819] 1821. *The Giant's Causeway, A Poem.* Dublin: J.J. Nolan.

Malins, E. 1973. 'Landscape Gardening by Jonathan Swift and his Friends in Ireland.' *Garden History 2.*

Marsh, G.P. [1864] 1965. *Man and Nature.* Cambridge, Mass.: Belknap Press.

Mason, T.H. 1944. 'Dublin Opticians and Instrument Makers.' *Dublin Historical Record 6*: 133-49.

Mather, C. [1721] 1968. *The Christian Philosopher: A Collection of the Best Discoveries in Nature, with Religious Improvements*. Gainesville, Fla.: Scholars' Facsimiles and Reprints.

Mazzeo, J.A. 1967. *Renaissance and Revolution: Backgrounds to Seventeenth-Century English Literature*. New York: Pantheon.

Mercier, V. 1962. *The Irish Comic Tradition*. Oxford: Oxford University Press.

Mitchell, F. 1994. *Where Has Ireland Come From?* Dublin: Country House.

Montague, J. [1974] 1978. *The Faber Book of Irish Verse*. London: Faber.

Morrell, J. and A. Thackray. 1981. *Gentlemen of Science: Early Years of the British Association for the Advancement of Science*. Oxford: Clarendon Press.

Munter, R. 1988. *A Dictionary of the Print Trade in Ireland 1550-1775*. New York: Fordham University Press.

Neeson, E. 1991. *A History of Irish Forestry*. Dublin: Lilliput Press.

Newman, J. Cardinal. [1873] 1982. *The Idea of a University: Defined and Illustrated*. South Bend, Ind.: University of Notre Dame Press.

Noble, B. (1763) 1768. *Geodaesia Hibernica, Or, An Essay on Practical Surveying*. Dublin: Author.

O'Brien, F. (1939) 1967. *At Swim-Two-Birds*. Harmondsworth: Penguin.

O'Meara, J.J. (trans.). 1982. *Giraldus Cambrensis (Gerald of Wales), The History and Topography of Ireland (Topographia Hiberniae)*. Dublin: Dolmen.

Ó Ruadháin, M. 1955. 'Birds in Irish Folklore.' *Acta XI Congressus Internationalis Ornithologici*. Basel: Birkhauser Verlag.

Ó Súilleabháin, S. [S. O'Sullivan]. 1963. *A Handbook of Irish Folklore*. Hatboro, Pa.: Folklore Associates.

O'Sullivan, S. (ed., trans.). 1966. *Folktales of Ireland*. Chicago: University of Chicago Press.

Ó Súilleabháin, S. and R.Th. Christiansen. 1963. *The Types of the Irish Folktale. Folklore Fellows Communications 78*: 1-347.

Pococke, R. [1752]. 1891. *Pococke's Tour in Ireland in 1752*. Dublin: Hodges, Figgis.

Price, U. 1794. *An Essay on the Picturesque: As Compared with the Sublime and Beautiful*. London: Robson.

Raistrick, A. 1968. *Quakers in Science and Industry: Being an Account ... of the Quaker Contributions to Science and Industry during the 17th and 18th Centuries*. Newton Abbot: David & Charles.

Richeson, A.W. 1966. *England Land Measuring to 1800: Instruments and Practices*. Cambridge, Mass.: MIT Press.

Richter, M. 1988. *Medieval Ireland: The Enduring Tradition*. Dublin: Gill & Macmillan.

Roberts, L.D. (ed.). 1982. *Approaches to Nature in the Middle Ages*. Binghamton, N.Y.: Center for Medieval and Early Renaissance Studies, State University of New York.

Rutty, J. 1772. *An Essay Towards a Natural History of the County of Dublin, Accommodated to the Noble Designs of the Dublin Society*. Dublin: by subscription.

Rutty, J. 1751. *A History of the ... People Called Quakers in Ireland ...* (Revised version of work by T. Wight.) Dublin: Jackson.

Rutty, J. 1776. *A Spiritual Diary and Soliloquies*. London: Phillips.

Ryan, M. 1987. 'History in the Landscape,' in F. Mitchell *et al.*, *The Book of the Irish Countryside*. Belfast: Blackstaff Press.

Rynne, E. 1994. 'Drolleries in the Book of Kells,' in F. O'Mahony (ed.), *The Book of Kells*. Dublin: Scolar Press.

Salingar, L.G. 1982. 'The Social Setting,' in B. Ford (ed.), *The New Pelican Guide to English Literature: 2: The Age of Shakespeare*. Harmondsworth: Penguin.

Seward, W.W. 1795. *Topographia Hibernica*. Dublin: Stewart.

Seymour, St J.D. 1930. *Irish Visions of the Other-World*. London: SPCK.

Sidney, Sir P. [1595] 1970. *An Apology for Poetry*, in W.J. Bate (ed.), *Criticism: The Major Texts*. New York: Harcourt Brace Jovanovich.

Spenser, E. [1596] 1970. *A View of the Present State of Ireland*. Ed. W.L. Renwick. Oxford: Clarendon.

Stanford, W.B. 1976. *Ireland and the Classical Tradition*. Dublin: Allen Figgis.

Stevenson, J. 1920. *Two Centuries of Life in Down 1600-1800*. Belfast: M'Caw, Stevenson & Orr.

Swift, J. [1726] 1986. *Gulliver's Travels*. Ed. P. Turner. Oxford: Oxford University Press.

Taylor, G. and A. Skinner. 1778. *Maps of the Roads of Ireland*. London: Authors.

Thomas, K. 1984. *Man and the Natural World: Changing Attitudes in England 1500-1800*. Harmondsworth: Penguin.

Thompson, W. 1849-56. *The Natural History of Ireland*. 4 vols. London: Reeve, Benham and Reeve; (vol. 4) Henry G. Bohn.

Thomson, D. 1965. *The People of the Sea: A Journey in Search of the Seal Legend*. London: Barrie and Rockliff.

Thorndike, L. 1941. *A History of Magic and Experimental Science*. Vol. 6: *The Sixteenth Century*. New York: Columbia University Press.

Thorndike, L. 1958. *A History of Magic and Experimental Science*. Vol. 7: *The Seventeenth Century*. New York: Columbia University Press.

Thwaites, R.G. 1896. *The Jesuit Relations and Allied Documents: Travel and Explorations of the Jesuit Missionaries in New France 1610-1791*. Vol. 1: Acadia 1610-1613. Cleveland: Burrows Brothers.

Tillyard, E.M.W. 1943. *The Elizabethan World Picture*. London: Chatto & Windus.

Tymoczko, M. 1990. 'The Semantic Fields of Early Irish Terms for Black Birds and their Implications for Species Taxonomy,' in A.T.E. Matonis and D.F. Melia (eds), *Celtic Language, Celtic Culture: A Festschrift for Eric P. Hamp*. Van Nuys, Ca.: Ford & Bailie.

Tyner, G. 1794. *The Traveller's Guide Through Ireland*. Dublin: Byrne.

Ure, P. (ed.). *The Pelican Book of English Prose*. Vol. 11: *Seventeenth-Century Prose*. Harmondsworth: Penguin.

Von Zittel, K.A. 1901. *History of Geology and Palaeontology*. Trans. M.M. Ogilvie-Gordon. London: Scott.

Waddell, H. (trans.). 1934. *Beasts and Saints*. London: Constable.

White, L. 1968. *Machina Ex Deo: Essays in the Dynamism of Western Culture*. Cambridge, Mass.: MIT Press.

White, T.H. [1954]. 1984. *The Book of Beasts: Being a Translation from a Latin Bestiary of the Twelfth Century*. New York: Dover.

Whittow, J. B. 1974. *Geology and Scenery in Ireland*. Harmondsworth: Penguin.

Wilde, O. [1890] 1989. 'The Critic as Artist,' in *The Writings of Oscar Wilde*. Ed. I. Murray. Oxford: Oxford University Press.

Wilson, W. 1784. *Post-Chaise Companion: or Traveller's Directory through Ireland*. Dublin: Author.

Wood-Martin, W.G. 1902. *Traces of the Elder Faiths of Ireland: A Handbook of Irish Pre-Christian Traditions*. 2 vols. London: Longmans, Green.

Yates, F. 1979. *The Occult Philosophy in the Elizabethan Age*. London: Routledge & Kegan Paul.

Young, A. 1892. *Tour in Ireland 1776-1779*. Ed. A.W. Hutton. 2 vols. London: Bell.

The Early Naturalists

CHRISTOPHER MORIARTY

The Irish 'Augustine'

In AD 655 an Irishman named Augustin wrote a treatise on miracles. By a happy accident some unknown medieval editor mistakenly included it in a collection of the writings of St Augustine. *De Mirabilibus Sacrae Scripturae Libri Tres* was printed as an appendix to the third volume of the collected works of St Augustine published in Paris in 1837. The text reveals that Augustin lived in Ireland in the seventh century. While that is all that is known of his life, the treatise tells much about his mind and shows a formidable intellect combined with an active interest in the living creatures that surrounded him.

Augustin was presented to Irish historians by Rev. William Reeves in 1861 and introduced to the world of naturalists by R.F. Scharff, Keeper of Natural History in the National Museum in Dublin, who published an account of the zoological work in the *Irish Naturalist* in 1921. Augustin's views on miracles are remarkable for their advanced thinking. He came close to Lyell's nineteenth-century theories which laid the foundation of modern geology. Augustin posited a world in which, after the initial Creation as described in the Book of Genesis, the landscape gradually changed its form. The relevance of his work in the context of natural history in Ireland is that he speculated on how the mammals, including amphibious species, survived Noah's Flood and made their way to islands after the waters had receded. This fundamental problem in zoogeography apparently received no consideration between the seventh and nineteenth centuries. Scharff observed in his *Irish Naturalist* article:

Augustine [*sic*] was puzzled how such animals as the otter and the seal fared during the flood. If a pair of each had been taken into the ark they could not have lived, he thinks, without an ample supply of water. If they remained outside where and in what manner did they survive the flood?

What next follows constitutes the most interesting part of Augustine's speculations, for it directly concerns the Irish fauna and its origin. Many pages of the *Irish Naturalist* contain discussions on this subject, and it has been the principal aim of the writers to show that many of the animals now existing in Ireland could only have reached the country by means of a former land connection with Great Britain. It is assumed also that the latter country was united by land with the continent. These ideas were considered as altogether modern, and it was never dreamt of that an Irish monk could have held those views more than a thousand years ago. Yet such is the fact.

Reflecting on Noah's Flood led Augustin to refer not only to his knowledge of the fauna of Ireland, but also to his observations of the sea and tides. He pointed out that we were all familiar with the rise and fall of the tides. The Flood was an exceptionally high tide which persisted beyond the normal length of time. But the destruction of all the animals, except those that entered the ark, gives rise to the problem of how they repopulated the islands after the waters receded.

'Who', Augustin asked, 'could have brought wolves, deer, forest pigs, foxes, badgers, little hares and sesquivolos to Ireland?' The reference to *sesquivolos*, incidentally, caused problems amongst lexicographers. W. D'Arcy Thomson, one of the very few writers who studied Augustin, showed in 1945 how a succession of transcriptions might have led to this word from an original *sciurulus* (squirrel). His view is supported by Anthony Harvey, editor of the Royal Irish Academy's forthcoming *Dictionary of Medieval Latin from Celtic Sources*. Although squirrels became extinct after the forest clearances of the seventeenth century, they had been abundant in the past. With the inclusion of otter and seal, Augustin listed a total of nine species of mammal in Ireland of which seven survive, while two, the wild pig and the wolf, have been hunted to extinction.

Augustin's explanation of the presence of land animals on islands again depends on his observations of nature. Perhaps the most remarkable of his achievements was to realize that after God had rested on the seventh day of creation, changes great and small continued to take place. He extended this observation to his interpretation of the miracles: they were natural events of such magnitude that they were recorded in the scriptures.

One of the less spectacular of these natural changes was the cutting off of promontories by the sea. It is tempting to speculate that Augustin had lived in the south-west of Ireland and seen some of the great promontories with their succession of large or small islands: perhaps the Dingle peninsula with the Blaskets. He accepts that such islands were formerly joined to the mainland and proceeds from this to postulate that Ireland and Great Britain once formed a great promontory and were separated from the mainland in the course of time – but not before the animals had safely arrived.

D'Arcy Thomson ends his essay with these words: 'I have heard it said that St Augustin [*sic*] did more than any other man to put Religion and Science asunder. I should be very sorry to think so; but certain it is that Theology and Natural Science, as we understand the latter, were far apart for St Augustin, but his Irish namesake held both in his hand.'

Where Augustin differed radically from all his known contemporaries, and indeed from the majority of pre-Renaissance European philosophers, was in his recording direct observations of nature and drawing conclusions from them. He was in this sense a modern scientist. Although *De Mirabilibus* is a commentary on the miracles recorded in the Bible, he supported his theory by examples from his own experience.

The scarcity of direct observation on nature in Christian philosophical writing is a continuation of a tradition already apparent in the Old Testament. In monotheistic religion, the priesthood may have felt that an interest in nature had undertones of animism. Whatever the reason, the scholars of the Church in Ireland devoted themselves mainly to learning and copying the scriptures. It may be mentioned in passing that the rule of the eighth-century St Maelruain of Tallaght extolled the learning and recitation of the Psalms because this prevented the monk from thinking.

Until the twelfth century, the Irish Church had held firmly to many of its own beliefs. We can only wonder whether Augustin was an isolated philosopher with original theories far removed from those of his fellows or whether his writing was a rare survival reflecting views that were widely held in heretical Ireland. Available evidence suggests the former. Modern writers including Ludwig Bieler (1963) and W.B. Stanford (1975) show that the Irish scholars concentrated on interpreting or analyzing the writings of past authorities. Indeed, this was the rule throughout Christendom. Even biographical writings were rare: the great majority of 'lives' of the saints were written to something of a formula to demonstrate the sanctity of the subject, and factual details are few.

Manuscripts were written and kept in the monasteries, and the monasteries were subject to the Rule of the foundation. Just how strict the rules were, and how obedience to a superior counted as a special virtue, is shown clearly in the Rule of St Columbanus, quoted by Bieler. This obsession with rectitude militates against scientific observation and its uncomfortable way of challenging the views of past authorities. The atmosphere of the monastery, therefore, would discourage the scientific approach of individuals such as Augustin, and philosophers who asked too many questions might have been very few. Furthermore, the writings of those who did deviate in this way were unlikely to have been widely copied and circulated.

Gerald of Wales

More than five hundred years were to pass after Augustin before the next surviving scientific treatise was compiled. Giraldus de Barri (Giraldus Cambrensis or Gerald of Wales) visited Ireland in the twelfth century and wrote *Topographia Hiberniae,* the second known work on our natural history. His references to the species of freshwater fish imply that he was in contact with extremely well informed and perceptive natives. Whereas birds are easily seen and it is possible to accept that his observations on them could have been entirely original, fishes, particularly fishes in lakes, are usually invisible. So it is hard to believe that, without expert local assistance, he could have come in contact with certain species in the course of a short visit in which he had many other duties. This suggests that, while written scientific observations on nature in Ireland remained extremely rare until the seventeenth century, many people were familiar with the names of a wide range of plants and animals and of the medicinal uses of many herbs.

Giraldus has fared better than Augustin in the eyes of posterity. His work was popular and he revised it many times. There have been several English translations, based on various revisions. In 1951 John J. O'Meara's translation of the earliest manuscript was published in Dundalk in a charming and scholarly volume with illustrations from a manuscript in the National Library of Ireland. And again, while Augustin comes down to us only in his writings, much is known of the life of Giraldus. He had a distinguished academic career and studied in Paris before coming in 1183 to Ireland where his family were among the successful invading warlords. The following year he joined the court of Henry II and in 1185 came to Ireland again as secretary to Prince John.

Topographia Hiberniae is a delightful, maddening work of genius. The genius lies in the acuteness of observation of wild creatures, which makes the *Topographia* a true work of science and allows a modern reader, with a minimum of care, to come to important conclusions on the nature of the fauna of twelfth-century Ireland. The charm is in the diversions into moralizing on animal behaviour, a legitimate form of interpretation of facts at the time. The maddening part is his credulity when it comes to tales of humans and the fact that, as O'Meara points out, Giraldus played to the gallery and with every revision of his work added more and more fantasy. Then, as now, fiction had greater popular appeal than science.

The second visit began in April 1185 and lasted until Easter of the following year. Giraldus travelled through Cork and Waterford and northwards to Dublin and Meath. He may have seen the Shannon and its lakes and certainly knew a great deal about the lakes around Mullingar.

The two paragraphs on fish merit quotation in full. I quote from O'Meara's translation with one small revision – he included identities for the three new fish species, suggested by the late Arthur Went, that I find difficult to agree with.

The sea, river and lake fish, and those that are missing

The sea-coasts on all sides abound sufficiently with sea-fish. The rivers, however, and the lakes are rich in fish peculiar to themselves, and especially in fish of three kinds, namely, salmon, trout, and mud-eels. The Shannon abounds in sea lampreys. They serve as luxuries for the rich. But some fine fish, found in other regions, and some magnificent fresh-water fish are wanting. I mean pike, perch, roach, gardon and gudgeon. Minnow, loach, bullheads, verones, and nearly all that do not have their seminal origin in tidal rivers are absent also.

Fish that are new and not found elsewhere

On the other hand the lakes of this country contain three kinds of fish that are not found anywhere else. There is one kind longer and more round than the trout. It has firm white flesh, and is pleasing to the taste. It is very like the tymal, except that the head is larger. There is another kind very like the sea herring in shape, size, colour and taste. A third kind is in every detail like the trout, except that it has no spots. These three kinds appear only in summer and never in the winter. In Meath, near Fore, there are three lakes near one another, of which each has one kind of these fish. Neither of the other two kinds ever approach it, even though the lakes communicate by a river that joins them. Moreover, if a fish of one lake is carried to the place and lake of another, it either dies or returns to its first home.

The first of these two passages is a very impressive statement. The absence of purely freshwater fish from Ireland at that time would be expected since it is highly unlikely that any of them could have survived the last glaciation. The first introductions of some of the species named are on record and the distribution of others supports the idea that they, too, were brought to Ireland by man. The final statement – 'and nearly all that do not have their seminal origin in tidal rivers are absent also' – shows clearly that Giraldus understood the problem of accounting for the migration of freshwater species across the Irish Sea.

The second paragraph suggests that Giraldus had good sources of information. He may, indeed, have seen the three fish species that he mentions but it seems unlikely that he could have captured them all on fishing trips without the aid of experienced local fishermen. His reference to the fish that resembles the tymal (grayling) is puzzling; it could perhaps have been a shad. The species 'very like the sea-herring' must be the pollan, long extinct from the Mullingar lakes though still found elsewhere in the Shannon basin. The unspotted trout sounds like a char, which was present in these lakes until the nineteenth century. Char are seldom unspotted, but their spots are pale and much less pronounced than those of the trout. After the perception comes an element of fantasy. Although it is possible that the species mentioned have strong homing instincts it is difficult to see how Giraldus or his contemporaries could have observed this behaviour in a lake.

Many of Giraldus's observations indicate changes in status of the fauna: 'This country above any other produces hawks, falcons and sparrow-hawks abundantly. These birds have been provided by nature with courageous hearts, curved and sharp beaks, and feet armed with talons, most suitable for catching their prey – and all to afford amusement to the nobles.' The splendidly anthropocentric theory of creation apart, the passage stresses the abundance of the birds of prey. Eagles, too, were plentiful: 'You will see as many eagles here as you will kites elsewhere.' Birds of prey are no longer plentiful in Ireland. Two factors brought about their decline. First, the importance of the amusement of the nobles: hawks and falcons were birds of great value in medieval times, in contrast to the situation in the nineteenth century when landowners generally brought about their destruction. Humans became serious predators of the falcons, whether hunting them for sale or in the interests of game preservation. Second, the habitat has changed greatly from a preponderance of forest to open spaces and a scarcity of trees, with consequent loss of refuge for hawks.

Giraldus's essential information on the crane is likewise accompanied by a delightful fantasy. In this and other tales Giraldus would have drawn on his knowledge of the bestiaries that used accounts of the habits of birds and animals – some credible, others far-fetched – to illustrate points of moral teaching. Bestiaries were popular throughout Europe in the Dark Ages. While the beasts in the Early Christian manuscripts of Ireland are largely used in decoration, some of the high crosses apparently used animal figures for doctrinal purposes. The High Cross at Moone in County Kildare has a particularly fine assortment. According to Giraldus, 'Cranes are so numerous that in one flock alone you will see a hundred or about that number. These birds, by a natural instinct, take their turns by night in watching the common safety, standing on one leg only, while in the other featherless claw they hold a stone. They do this so that if they should go to sleep, they will be wakened again immediately by the fall of the stone and continue their watch.' The flocking behaviour confirms that Giraldus indeed refers to the large migratory common crane, *Grus grus*, now a rarity in Ireland, rather than to the heron which, outside ornithological circles, is universally known as 'crane' in Ireland.

'Wild peacocks abounding in the woods' are likely to have been capercaillie, which survived until the seventeenth century. There is evidence, however, that true peacocks were imported, and Giraldus's description of the kingfisher's peacock colouring makes it clear that he was familiar with them.

The barnacle goose and the goose barnacle both seem to have been known to Giraldus. The goose barnacle, a crustacean that attaches itself to floating timber, must have been much more common in the days of wooden ships free from anti-fouling paint. Giraldus tells in detail of the wonderful metamorphosis from barnacle to bird. In this connection it is worth remembering that no European at the time had seen the breeding grounds of the goose *Branta bernicla* in Canada. Furthermore, the goose barnacle does look remarkably like a miniature black and white goose, its head buried in a piece of timber. Because of its supposed metamorphosis from a fish, bishops and religious men were permitted to eat without sin the flesh of the barnacle goose on days of abstinence.

The description of the osprey, now extremely rare in Ireland but likely to have been plentiful in the twelfth century, is very significant, as Giraldus stresses that he watched them himself. Indeed, St John's eagle in the ninth-century Book of Armagh is an osprey, gripping a salmon or trout in its talons (*plate 4*), and there are fishing eagles also in the eighth-century Book of Kells.

There are [Giraldus writes] many birds here of a twofold nature. They are called ospreys. They are smaller than the eagle, but larger than the hawk. One of their feet is armed with talons, open and ready to snatch; but the other is closed and peaceful and suitable only for swimming. It is a wonderful instance of nature's pranks. There is a remarkable thing about these birds, and I have often witnessed it for myself. They hover quietly on their wings high up in the air over the waves of the sea. In this way they can more easily see down into the depths below. Then, seeing with their sharp eyes through such a great distance of air and troubled water little fishes hiding below the waves, they dive down with amazing speed. While they enter and leave the water they control themselves by their swimming foot: but with their grasping foot they catch and carry off their prey. So does our old enemy see with his sharp glance whatever secret thing we do in the troubled waves of the world. And while with peaceful claw he approaches us airily through success in temporal things, still with grasping claw, bloody with its booty, he seizes and destroys our unhappy souls.

The passage on the 'kingfisher', based on observation at first hand, is one of the most impressive:

Here are found also those little birds which they call kingfishers. They are smaller than the blackbird, are rare, and are found on rivers. They are short like quails. They dive into the water in pursuit of very small fish on which they feed. While in all other respects they follow the nature of their type, here they are different in colour, but in that only. For they have a white belly and a black back. Elsewhere they are conspicuous in having a red belly, red beak and claws, and with bright shining wings and back like the parrot or peacock.

The bird so very clearly described in this passage is the dipper, not the kingfisher. Evidently Giraldus was familiar with the brilliantly coloured kingfisher from his travels in Britain. If he had seen both species together, he would not have made the mistake of believing that the dipper was an aberrant kingfisher. This suggests that the kingfisher did not appear in Ireland until after the twelfth century.

Swans were plentiful, but mainly in the north. Storks were rare and those that were seen were black. There were no black crows, or very few: 'What there are, are of different colours.' The remarkable distribution of the two forms of crow has persisted to this day. The black carrion crow, which is common in England and Wales, is extremely rare in Ireland and Scotland where its place is taken by the 'hooded' form. Partridges and pheasants were absent, as were magpies and nightingales. The first three are known to have been late arrivals and the nightingale is still unknown except as a rare migrant.

Giraldus lists most of the mammals known to have been in Ireland at this time, mentioning in particular the abundance of martens, which are 'hunted day and night, by means of fire'. He lists hedgehog, mole, polecat and beaver among the absentees. Possibly he overlooked the hedgehog since it is certainly less conspicuous than the kingfisher, but the species may indeed have been absent.

As for 'reptiles', Giraldus mentions that the lizard is present and quotes the legend of St Patrick's banishing the snakes, but with more than usual scepticism: 'Some indulge in the pleasant conjecture that St Patrick and other saints of the land purged the island of all harmful animals. But it is more probable that from the earliest times, and long before the laying of the foundation of the Faith, the island was naturally without these as well as other things.' Here, as in other places in the *Topographia*, Giraldus makes clear his awareness of the fact that a number of species of animals present in Great Britain are absent from Ireland. He seems, however, to have been more credulous of the wonderful and less inclined to seek explanations of phenomena than was Augustin. Nonetheless, he deserves full credit for his curiosity, his ability to identify birds and mammals and, above all, for his belief that these observations are worthy of being recorded in writing.

Roderic O'Flaherty

After Giraldus and his *Topographia*, nearly five hundred years were to pass before another observer of the same calibre would write on the Irish fauna. Roderic O'Flaherty was the owner of an immense tract of land in County Galway, west of the Corrib. Born in his father's castle in Moycullen in 1629, he died in poverty in 1718. A devout and scholarly man, his adherence to Catholicism cost him most of his possessions in the course of the succession of invasions and upheavals that characterized Ireland throughout the seventeenth century. In spite of his sometimes miserable existence, he was a prolific writer, his output including two major works: *Ogygia* (1685) in classical Latin, and *West or H-Iar Connaught*. The latter, written in English and unpublished in his lifetime, is the more interesting in the context of Irish natural history. My quotations are from Hardiman's edition of 1846, a work remarkable for the fact that its footnotes are about three times the length of the text. This edition was reprinted, with a new introduction by William J. Hogan, in 1978.

As Giraldus must have done, O'Flaherty relied to a great extent on first-hand information. The great difference between the two, however, was that O'Flaherty was a native with long years of experience of the country, its people and its fauna, while Giraldus based his observations on a relatively short stay. To a greater extent than Giraldus, therefore, O'Flaherty reflects the extent of local knowledge. In *H-Iar Connaught* he quotes a number of historical references, but the descriptions of the land, its antiquities and its mammals, birds and fishes all have the feel of personal observation. He mentions twenty-four species of fish, sixteen mammals, thirteen birds and ten invertebrates, most of the last named being edible shellfish. Systematic nature books were few at this time and therefore it seems most likely that the species named by O'Flaherty were well known to the people he met on his travels.

Fantasies are few. They include a charming tale of an eagle that dropped a golden ring, bearing a precious stone unknown to any lapidary, into the lap of the bountiful lady Margaret Joyce Fitz-John. Much more impressive is his account of the crocodile of Lough Corrib:

Here is one rarity more, which we may terme the Irish crocodil, whereof one as yet living, about ten years ago, had sad experience. The man was passing the shore just by the waterside, and spyed far off the head of a beast swimming, which he tooke to have been an otter, and tooke no more notice of it; But the beast it seems there lifted up its head, to discern whereabouts the man was; then diving, swom under water till he struck ground; whereupon he runned out of the water suddenly, and tooke the man by the elbow, whereby the man stooped down, and the beast fastened his teeth in his pate, and dragged him into the water; where the man tooke hold on a stone by chance in his way, and calling to minde he had a knife in his pocket, tooke it out and gave a thrust of it to the beast, which thereupon got away from him into the lake .... Old men acquainted with the lake do tell there is such a beast in it.

The tale is a perplexing one. The description does indeed sound like an encounter with an amphibious reptile rather than with a purely aquatic creature such as the Lough Ness monster. Although unlikely, it is not impossible that a crocodile, if released in Lough Corrib, could have survived at least for a summer. Could some merchant seaman from Galway have brought one home from Africa and released it in the Corrib? A more likely explanation could be that a traveller had witnessed an attack by a crocodile and had translocated the story to Lough Corrib. Traditional story-tellers usually give their accounts in the first person and from time to time move the scene of the action to some familiar place in their own neighbourhood.

On the more mundane creatures, O'Flaherty makes a list of mammals, including wolves, 'deere', foxes, badgers, hedgehogs, hares, 'rabbets', 'squirrells', 'martins', 'weesles', and the amphibious otter. Hedgehogs and rabbits, therefore, had arrived since the time of Giraldus. The weasel is absent from Ireland while the stoat is common; however, 'weasel' is the term widely used for stoat in Ireland (except by modern zoologists) and O'Flaherty was undoubtedly referring to the latter.

O'Flaherty's freshwater fish list is likewise an interesting statement on the species that were present in his time: 'The water streames, besides lamprey, roches, and the like of no value, breed salmons (where is recourse to the sea), eels, and divers sorts of trouts. There was never a pike or bream as yet encountered in all this countrey, nor in the adjacent parts of Mayo or Galway counteys.' The 'roche' (strictly speaking, the rudd) is surprising and may indicate a deliberate introduction. Pike and bream evidently were known to O'Flaherty, possibly from elsewhere in Ireland. The 'divers sorts of trouts' have been the subject of considerable controversy as to whether they represent true genetic races or simply develop in different ways according to habitat and feeding. In his essay on the trout of Lough Melvin, Andrew Ferguson (1986) makes it clear that the weight of evidence supports the existence of several races.

O'Flaherty's most intriguing comment on freshwater fish is a reference to the 'chop': 'Here is another kind of fish which hath recourse to the sea as the salmon, yearly to and from, they are called chops, and in Irish *trascain*, very like herrings, only that herring come not on freshwater.' The only reasonable identification is the pollan, but pollan have never been found in the Corrib catchment in modern times. However, although still plentiful in Lough Neagh the species is very rare in the Shannon lakes and could be approaching extinction. It seems likely that pollan lived in Lough Corrib in O'Flaherty's time. The pollan of Lough Derg migrate towards the sea and are caught, albeit in small numbers, in the nets set for eels at Killaloe. Similar nets have been used in the Corrib since the seventeenth century or earlier. The introduction of the pike, probably in the nineteenth century, could have dealt the pollan population a final blow.

The list of twelve marine fin-fish in *West or H-Iar Connaught* comprises eleven familiar species and one curiosity, the 'hawkfish'. O'Flaherty refers also to shellfish – 'oysters, scollops, cokles, muscles, razures, together with lobsters, crabs, shromps &c.' The first four named continue to be commercially significant and there are many references to the capture of razor shells until early in the twentieth century. O'Flaherty's zoology was sophisticated enough to separate molluscs and crustaceans. He refers also to the stranding of 'great whales, gramps, porcupisses, thunies' and frequently mentions the occurrence of ambergris on the shore.

O'Flaherty's bird lore includes the first extensive references to seabirds, which only rarely appear in poetry and sagas. In writing of birds he expands from time to time into observations on their habits: 'Here is a kind of black eagle, which kills the deere by grappling him with his claw, and forcing him to run headlong into precipices.' And again: 'Here the ganet soares high into the sky to espy his prey in the sea under him, at which he casts himself headlong into the sea, and swallows up whole herrings in a morsell. This bird flys through the ship's sailes, piercing them with his beak.' He repeats the barnacle legend and, in mentioning the permitted consumption of certain birds on fast days, tells of the cliff-nesting species and their importance in the economy of the islands: 'Here is a fowle that custom allowed to eat on fasting days, as cormorant feeding only on fish; as alsoe birds found in the high cliffts and rocks of Aran, which never fly but over the sea, which, with all other numerous sea birds, yield a great store of feathers.' The invertebrates mentioned by O'Flaherty include the pearl mussel and the medicinal leech. The pearl mussel is still plentiful in rivers west of Lough Corrib but the medicinal leech is considered extinct in Ireland and its presence at any time has been questioned.

O'Flaherty was one of the earliest writers to make a specific comment on the effect of climate on the flow of a river, in this case the Corrib in Galway:

It became suddenly dry in our own memory twice, first on Tuesday the 7th of September, anno 1647; the second time there was mighty great frost from the 28th November, 1683, to the 3rd of February, whereby the river was all congealed, only the rapid streame from the wood-key of the town to the sea. This stream suddenly stoped on Wednesday, the 23rd of January, from the night before to the night after; so as the channell was all along dry during this time, and though the frost continued as much after as before, yet the stream runned the day after and filled its channell, so continuing as usually before; soe alsoe it did after the 7th day of September the first time.

As Giraldus had done before him, O'Flaherty travelled extensively over a substantial part of Ireland. He had a considerable knowledge of the names and habits of animals. Most of this must have been passed on to him by word of mouth, indicating that he was not the sole possessor of such information. The rarity of systematic writing on nature – an average of one naturalist every five hundred years – is probably a reflection more of the outlook of medieval writers than of ignorance of nature and her ways. Scripture, theology and history were the basis of scholarship. Observation of nature was the exception.

Nature and Early Irish Law

Augustin, Giraldus and O'Flaherty are the only early names, indeed the only individuals, who have survived through history as writers on nature in Ireland and who based their work on original local observation. But there were two great classes of anonymous observers: the lawyers and the poets. They were not entirely distinct since legal poems were a feature of Old Irish.

A Guide to Early Irish Law by Fergus Kelly (1988) is a digest of the numerous pre-Norman legal tracts that have survived in various forms. Of particular interest in the context of the perception of nature is the classification of trees and bushes into a hierarchical system, the subject of an earlier paper (Kelly, 1976). This paper, entitled 'The Old Irish Tree-list', names twenty-eight trees and shrubs from an eighth-century legal tract entitled *Bretha Comaithchesa*. A ninth-century commentary on the list explains the economic basis for assigning the various species to their ranks. The species are divided into four orders of nobility, depending on their value to man and corresponding to the human social order. There is a scale of penalties for damage to the trees, commensurate with the status of the tree and the extent of the damage.

Compensation for the destruction of a 'noble of the wood' is equivalent to two and a half milch cows; for branch-cutting, a year-old heifer; for fork-cutting, a two-year old heifer; and for base-cutting, a milch cow. The next class is 'commoner of the wood', for which the compensation for destruction is one cow and, for branch-cutting, a sheep. For destroying a member of the 'lower division of the wood' you pay a year-old heifer and, for a 'bush of the wood', a sheep.

The seven nobles of the wood are oak, hazel, holly, yew, ash, Scots pine and apple. The oak is there because of its acorns and its dignity, acorns being important autumn fodder for pigs. The commentary includes some information on the use of oak bark in tanning leather and on the treatment required to protect from decay the wound made by stripping the bark. The cost of enough bark to tan a pair of woman's sandals is a cow-hide, and an ox-hide must be paid for the quantity required for a man's pair. The wound in the tree must be covered with a mixture of smooth clay, cow-dung and new milk until it is healed. Cow dung was a folk treatment for human injury and may have been a source of antibiotics.

The hazel, although small, provides nuts and rods. Hazelnuts have a long, almost mystical tradition because of their value as food. This could predate the Celtic people by many thousands of years, reaching back to the time of the Mesolithic hunter-gatherers. The legendary salmon of wisdom attained its knowledge by eating the nuts that fell from a hazel tree beside a well which fed the sacred River Boyne. Hazel stems were important in the construction of houses and fences and are still used in the River Bann to make wattle fences to guide migrating eels into nets.

The soft upper leaves of holly were fed to cattle at least until the second half of the twentieth century. Holly poles were used for the shafts of chariots. Yew is a noble tree because of 'its noble artefacts'; the wood is very hard and fine-grained and can be worked and polished to make vessels of many kinds. Frank Mitchell, in his *Shell Guide to Reading the Irish Landscape* (1986), mentions that the yew was prized for high-grade carpentry and that masters of yew-carving enjoyed a special social rank.

The ash and the Scots pine are obvious nobles. Like the oak, both grow to a splendid size. The ash provides 'support of a royal thigh and half-material of a weapon'. This poetic description probably refers to furniture-making and to the wood's use as the shaft of an iron-headed spear. The seventh noble is the apple, which is included not only for its fruit but also for its bark – but there is no reference to what the bark was used for.

The commoners of the wood form the next class. Sadly, they did not receive any explanation in the ninth-century gloss. Some have obvious uses, often of great importance; others seem to owe their position as much to their size as to anything. They would certainly all have had their place as firewood. The list begins with alder, which grows quickly and well in swamps which were impossible to cultivate and almost useless for grazing. Willow provides fine, tough stems for basket-making. Hawthorn and aspen have higher or lower status depending on whether you are using the eighth- or the ninth-century version of the tree list. Hawthorn since the eighteenth century has been of major importance as a hedge plant, forming a cattle-proof barrier. Hedges were fewer in ancient Ireland but it seems likely that hawthorn has long been used as a stockade bush. Like the hazel it has a high standing in folk belief and a solitary hawthorn will usually be treated with respect. Though my family had been suburban for several generations, I was told in childhood never to bring hawthorn flowers into the house.

The beautiful rowan tree (mountain ash or quicken), with its bright orange berries, is another species with strong folk traditions: it is believed to be capable of averting the unwelcome attention of the immortals. It grows, often out on its own, in poor soil on mountain sides, an ability which may have given it a special status. The remaining three commoners are birch, elm and wild cherry. Compared with oak, ash and pine, neither birch nor wild cherry is obviously noble. While the omission of the elm from high status might seem surprising, Frank Mitchell has shown that the elms became extremely rare about AD 500 and they may well have been scarce and also small at the time the law was drawn up.

The seven members of the 'lower division' are bushes rather than shrubs, and the list includes some such as arbutus, whitebeam and aspen, which can grow into quite substantial trees. The lowest class, the 'bushes of the wood', are small and bushy, but with more or less woody stems. They are a rather odd assemblage: bracken, bog-myrtle, gorse, blackberry, heather, broom and wild rose. Some, such as bracken and gorse, invade good sheep pasture but both were used as bedding and gorse provided a dye, as did bog-myrtle and broom. Blackberry is obviously a valuable plant and rosehips may also have been important as food.

The composition of the 'lower division' varies more than the other three classes amongst the writers of the various versions of the list. It extends to include such species as honeysuckle, ivy and rushes. The absence of many more species may well have been connected with the universal desire of lawmakers to put things in neat packages. The first three septets can be supported by logical arguments; the fourth group may have been given the same number in the interest of symmetry. Moreover, law that had to be passed on by word of mouth rather than in writing would have benefited by such rigid divisions.

Kelly's forthcoming book *Early Irish Farming* mentions the existence of gardens and the use of healing herbs. The gardens were associated more with the monasteries than with secular settlements and there is some evidence that they were herb gardens rather than vegetable plots. The names of the herbs grown are rarely given and there is much confusion over the identity of those that are mentioned. Practitioners nearly everywhere to this day conceal their knowledge of *materia medica* in coded prescriptions. Healers in the Dark Ages were no less enthusiastic about maintaining such professional secrecy and it is likely that details of herbal lore were kept to oral tradition amongst the initiates.

Nature in Early Irish Literature

From legal tracts we now turn to literature. Apart from the mammals mentioned by Augustin, the earliest Irish fauna list comes from an incident in the saga of Fionn Mac Cumhail. While written references to the exploits of Fionn and the Fianna go back no further than the eleventh century, and attempts to attach him to an historical figure associate him with King

Cormac Mac Airt, who reigned from AD 227 to 266, there is something about the stories that gives a hint of much greater antiquity. In contrast to the other great hero, Cuchulain, and his association with a pastoral society, the interests of the Fianna are primarily in the forest and associated with hunting. It is tempting to extend his time to that of the hunter-gatherers before the Neolithic revolution some five thousand years ago.

Be that as it may, the fauna list has no special claim to great antiquity and could easily have been extended by some scribe in the course of setting the tales down in manuscript. It has been quoted in a number of works, beginning with a paper by Sir William Wilde (1860) and subsequently by Lady Gregory in her *Gods and Fighting Men* (1904). Lady Gregory's translation includes a number of species, such as polecat and roe deer, unknown in Ireland. Fergus Kelly has kindly checked the Irish in the *Dean of Lismore's Book* (Mc Lauchlan, 1862) and his corrections lead to the conclusion that the compiler of the list was using his knowledge of the Irish fauna and shows no sign of influence by foreign writers or by travel abroad.

The story tells of how Fionn was abducted by the king of Tara and held to ransom, the ransom being a couple of each of the wild creatures of Ireland. Caoilte succeeded in capturing them all and, with great difficulty, confining them for just long enough to effect the release of Fionn – after which they all escaped and left the king no better off than he had been before. The list, with modern spelling of identifiable places and with the corrections suggested by Kelly, contains about fifty-five species. More than a simple species list, it has its elements of ecology and a definite consciousness of zoogeography.

Two ravens from Fiodh da Bheann, two wild ducks from Lough Sillane, two foxes from Slieve Cuilinn, two deer from Burren, two swans from blue Dobhran, two owls from the wood of Faradhruim, two martens from the branchy wood on the side of Druim da Raoin, two gulls from the strand of Loch Leith, four woodpeckers from white Brosna, two plovers from Carraigh Dhain, two thrushes from Leith Lomard, two wrens from Dun Aoibh, two herons from Corrain Cleibh, two eagles from Carraig of the stones, two hawks from Fiodh Chonnach, two sows from Loch Meilghe, two water-hens from Lough Erne, two grouse from Monadh Maith, two sparrow hawks from Dubhloch, two stonechats from Moycullen, two tomtits from MaghTuallainn, two swallows from Sean Abhla, two cormorants from Dublin, two wolves from Bricklieve, two blackbirds from the Strand of the Two Women, two hinds from Luachair Ire, two pigeons from Ceas Chuir, two pheatag from Leiter Ruadh, two starlings from green-sided Tara, two rabbits from Sith Dubh Donn, two wild pigs from Cluiadh Chuir, two cuckoos from Drom Daibh, two hawks from the Bright Mountain, two grey mice from Limerick, two otters from the Boyne, two larks from the Great Bog, two bats from the Cave of the Nuts, two badgers from the province of Ulster, two corncrakes from the banks of the Shannon, two wagtails from Waterford, two curlews from the harbour of Galway, two hares from Muirthemne, two deer from Sith Buidhe, two peacocks from Magh Mell, two eels from Duth Dur, two goldfinches from Slieve na nEun, two birds of slaughter from Magh Bhuilg, two bright swallows from Granard, two robins from the Great Wood, two rock cod from Cala Chairge, two porpoises from the great sea, two wrens from Mios an Chuill, two salmon from the waterfall of Mhic Muirne, two clean deer from Glenasmole, two cows from Magh Mor, two cats from the Cave of Cruachan, two sheep from bright Sidhe Diobhlain, two pigs of the pigs of the son of Lir, a ram and a crimson sheep from Ennis.

Nearly all the creatures named are indigenous but the rabbit is troublesome: it was introduced by the Anglo-Normans. Together with the domestic animals, it suggests that the writer (not necessarily the compiler of the original list) may have added a few whose omission he couldn't understand. The peacock is equally puzzling. The bird was known to an eighth- or ninth-century writer and may have been imported. However, the Irish word is appropriately *gesachtach* meaning 'screecher'; possibly it was the capercaillie, which is a surprising omission from the list.

Woodpeckers have long been extinct in Ireland, but their bones have been found in Iron Age rubbish heaps. The *pheatag* was translated as nightingale, a very unlikely native species at any time. The word sounds similar to *feadog*, meaning plover. The bird of slaughter appears to have no modern equivalent but the kite was abundant in medieval England and is likely to have been present in Ireland, too. Finally, the 'pigs of the son of Lir' begs for an explanation. The son of Lir was the sea god Manannan, the keeper of enchanted pigs that come back to life after being eaten.

Next in importance to the stories of the Fenian cycle, the poem *The Frenzy of Sweeney* is rich in the names of birds and beasts, trees and wild flowers. Sweeney, a warrior prince of Ulster, the story goes, insulted St Ronan and threw his beautiful psalter into a lake. In the act of dragging the saint out of his church, the erring warrior was interrupted by a summons to go and play his part in the Battle of Moira (AD 637). An otter brought the psalter back to Ronan who, in common with many a good saint, had little time for Christian forgiveness and cursed Sweeney, transforming him into an insane, winged creature and forcing him to travel almost endlessly throughout Ireland. St Moling, a less vindictive holy man, ultimately tamed Sweeney and gave him Christian burial in due course.

Several manuscripts of the tale of Sweeney exist, most of them relatively late but dated by their language at least as far back as the ninth century. Their importance in the present context lies in the fact that Sweeney, in between passages bewailing the misery of his fate, composed nature poems of startling beauty. They provide a substantial list of trees, flowers, birds and mammals – species familiar, evidently, to a person living in the wilderness. Among other subjects, he praises the trees of the forest. The following translation is by K.H. Jackson (1971):

Oak, bushy, leafy, you are high above trees; hazel bush, little branchy one, coffer of hazel nuts.

Alder, you are not spiteful, lovely is your colour, you are not prickly where you are in the gap.

Blackthorn, little thorny one, black little sloe-bush; watercress, little green-topped one, on the brink of the blackbird's well.

Saxifrage of the pathway, you are the sweetest of herbs; cress, very green one; plant where the strawberry grows.

Apple-tree, little apple-tree, violently everyone shakes you; rowan, little berried one, lovely is your bloom.

Bramble, little humped one, you do not grant fair terms; you do not cease tearing me till you are sated with blood.

Yew, little yew, you are conspicuous in graveyards; ivy, little ivy, you are familiar in the dark wood.

Holly, little shelterer, door against the wind; ash-tree, baneful, weapon in the hand of a warrior.

Birch, smooth, blessed, proud, melodious, lovely in each entangled branch at the top of your crest.

Aspen as it trembles, from time to time I hear its leaves rustling, and think it is the foray.

The poem is much more than a list of the trees and some flowers of the forest. The poet gives charming and accurate descriptions of them and mentions in passing the values of some and the habitats of others. It is interesting that the association between yew and churchyard has such a long history.

While the Sweeney poems probably form the most concentrated collection of nature poetry in early to middle Irish, there are many others. My survey was made in easily accessible translations and undoubtedly more species would be found in the course of a comprehensive study. But to a great extent the poets seemed to be concerned with a small number of familiar creatures. Modern English poetry, even if one includes conscious 'nature poets' such as Wordsworth, is no different.

My list of the plants and animals mentioned in Irish poetry totals thirty-one species of bird, thirty wild flowers, seventeen trees and ten mammals. Hardly any invertebrates appear, pride of place being given to the honey bee. Ectoparasites make one appearance in a satire against a twelfth-century monastery, tenanted by an unfortunate wandering scholar: 'But as multitudinous as the sands of the sea or as sparks of fire or as dew-drops on a May-morning or as the stars of heaven were the lice and the fleas biting his feet ...'.

The wild flowers are either edible or conspicuous and tend to be woodland, wetland or moorland species. Watercress is extolled by Sweeney and others as food. The foxglove is the most frequently mentioned of all. Besides its place in nature poetry it enters love poems in an allusion to the colour of a maiden's cheeks.

Of the birds, the blackbird appears more often than any other species – its song is praised by hunter and cleric alike – and the cuckoo comes a close second. Raven, swan, crane and heron, all large species, are next in importance. A raven appears on the base of the eighth-century North Cross of Ahenny in Co. Tipperary, pecking at a human corpse. On the tenth-century Cross of the Scriptures at Clonmacnois, the soul of the entombed Christ is represented by a bird that looks very like a wren.

The deer is usually introduced as the quarry of the hunt, as is the wild pig. But there are frequent gentler references to fawns and hinds. Enchanted hinds take a part in many legends, leading the hunters to further adventures. Stags appear on several eighth- to tenth-century crosses and pillars. Wolves are often mentioned, usually in the context of portraying the dangers of the wilderness. Hare, otter and fox make frequent appearances but marten and squirrel seem to be rare. The recognizable zoomorphic ornaments in the Book of Kells include wolf, otter, cat, hound, salmon and domestic cock.

The scarcity of seashore creatures is remarkable. Salmon and occasionally trout have a place in literature but sea fish are virtually absent until O'Flaherty lists a number of species found in Connemara. There are occasional references to seals and whales. The impression all through the poetry is of a people avoiding the seashore: forest and bog, river and lake seem to be where the Irish writers felt at ease.

The Problem of Folklore

In 1959 the seanachie Padraig Ann Conneely on Inisheer, the smallest of the Aran Islands, told me this tale: 'And you may not believe it, but there are sea cows and sea horses. I saw a cow and her calf walk down into the sea. And I took my boat and went out and looked down and saw them and they grazing on the seaweed.' Under the circumstances, I could have believed anything and attached no special importance to the story. Recently, my friend Gabriel King made a survey of turtle sightings around the Irish coast by interviewing fishermen. In Donegal he heard at first hand two accounts of sightings of walrus. To date this species has not been scientifically recorded in Ireland but the fisherman's accounts made me remember Padraig Ann's tale which, allowing for the storyteller's imagination, could very well describe a walrus.

The story illustrates the problem of using folklore in attempting to discover the extent of knowledge of nature in early Irish thought. Traditional storytellers usually speak in the first person and, as with O'Flaherty's Corrib crocodile, there is no way of knowing whether Padraig Ann had seen a sea-cow, whether he had been told about it at first hand, or whether he was reciting an old tradition.

88

There can be no doubting the antiquity of a great many folk tales but the details, including references to named species of plants and animals, cannot be verified. The rabbit was introduced to Ireland after the Anglo-Norman invasion. Reference to rabbits in a folk-tale dealing with a pre-Norman event implies nothing more than that storytellers have been familiar with rabbits in Ireland for nearly a thousand years. It is unlikely that any of them would know that rabbits came to Ireland in the wake of the Anglo-Norman invasion. Plants and animals in folklore therefore belong to a different chapter, perhaps to a different book.

Writing Nature

The widespread use of writing was introduced to Ireland by the Christians, but Christianity in the Dark Ages and for some centuries thereafter was less than enthusiastic about direct observation of nature. Respect for authority and conformity with the strict rules of religious orders was the accepted norm amongst the learned. The observational or experimental approach which leads naturally to questioning authority inevitably threatened the great institutions.

O'Flaherty was one of few to set down his knowledge of the world of nature. He had been educated by Alexander Lynch, whose school in Galway catered for the sons of nobles from all parts of Ireland. It is interesting to note that O'Flaherty was described by contemporaries as an historian and that his major published work, *Ogygia*, was strictly historical. *H-Iar Connaught* remained in manuscript until edited by the historian James Hardiman and published by the Irish Archaeological Society in 1846. O'Flaherty was highly respected by contemporary scholars, and those who visited him in his later years were shocked by his poverty. O'Flaherty was born a prince but lived to see most of his land confiscated and made over to Cromwell's supporters. In his lifetime authority had changed from a moderating influence to an oppressor and that may have encouraged him to turn to the study of nature.

Augustin's nature writings survived by accident. Giraldus revised his *Topographia* by adding fiction rather than by expanding on his original observations. O'Flaherty wrote down his description of western Connaught late in life and either did not attempt to have it published or failed to find a publisher. While these three writers provide clear evidence that a deep knowledge of nature was widespread amongst the people of Ireland, it also appears that the idea of setting down this knowledge in writing occurred to few. Even allowing for the destruction of manuscripts, there is no evidence that interest in the writing and copying of scientific observations compared in any way with the enthusiasm for the scriptures, for fiction and history, and for philosophy based on literature rather than experiment.

In this, the situation in Ireland was similar to that which prevailed throughout western Europe until the seventeenth century. Copernicus, Leonardo and Galileo were rare exceptions and not always popular with the civil and ecclesiastical establishment. By the time the Royal Society of London was incorporated in 1662, the days of a Gaelic Irish aristocracy had virtually passed away. The Royal Society was one of the first learned institutions to encourage observation and experiment rather than the acceptance of past writings. It is therefore not at all surprising that such studies are so rare in the Gaelic tradition. With the penal laws militating against higher education amongst the native – and largely Catholic – population, the next phase in the development of studies of natural history in Ireland was to be carried forward largely by the settlers and their descendants.

References

Bieler, L. 1963. *Ireland: Harbinger of the Middle Ages*. London: Oxford University Press.

Ferguson, A. 1986. 'Lough Melvin: A Unique Fish Community.' *Royal Dublin Society Occasional Papers in Irish Science and Technology 1*.

Gregory, A. 1904. *Gods and Fighting Men*. London: John Murray.

Harvey, A. (ed.) [forthcoming]. *Dictionary of Medieval Latin from Celtic Sources*. Dublin: Royal Irish Academy.

Jackson, K.H. 1971. *A Celtic Miscellany*. Harmondsworth: Penguin.

Kelly, F. 1976. 'The Old Irish Tree-list.' *Celtica 11*: 107-24.

Kelly, F. 1988. *A Guide to Early Irish Law*. Dublin: Dublin Institute for Advanced Studies.

Kelly, F. 1997. *Early Irish Farming*. Dublin: Institute for Advanced Studies.

Mc Lauchlan, T. 1862. *The Dean of Lismore's Book*. Edinburgh: Edmonston and Douglas.

Mitchell, F. 1986. *The Shell Guide to Reading the Irish Landscape*. London: Michael Joseph/Country House.

O'Flaherty, Roderic. [1684, 1846] 1978. *West or H-Iar Connaught*. Ed. J. Hardiman, Rpt. with Introduction by W.J. Hogan. Galway: Kenny's Bookshop.

O'Meara, J.J. 1951. *The First Version of the Topography of Ireland by Giraldus Cambrensis*. Dundalk: Dundalgan Press.

Reeves, W. 1861. 'On Augustin, an Irish Writer of the Seventh Century.' *Proceedings of the Royal Irish Academy 7*: 516-19

Scharff, R.F. 1921. 'The Earliest Irish Zoologist.' *Irish Naturalist* 30: 128-32.

Stanford, W.B. 1975. *Ireland and the Classical Tradition*. Dublin: Figgis.

Thomson, D'Arcy Wentworth. 1945. '*Sesquivolus*, a squirrel: and the *Liber de Mirabilibus S. Scripturae*.' *Hermathena 45*: 1-7.

Wilde, W. 1860. 'Upon the Unmanufactured Animal Remains Belonging to the Academy.' *Proceedings of the Royal Irish Academy 7*: 181-211.

Fluctuations in Fortune:
Three Hundred Years of Irish Geology

PATRICK N. WYSE JACKSON

The origins of geology as a science in Europe lie in the early eighteenth century, when it developed out of the widespread interest in natural history, particularly in minerals and mining. From the 1600s mining methods became more advanced and came to be widely known across Europe through the writings of Agricola and others. In Germany, institutions were established to promote scientific thought, and mineralogical studies advanced rapidly from the 1700s onwards. In these islands, the first formal societies that promoted science were established from the mid-1600s, with the Royal Society (1660) and the Oxford Philosophical Society (1683) in England and the Dublin Philosophical Society (1683) in Ireland.

The development of Irish geology owes as much to the collective efforts of various learned societies, government agencies and universities as to the individual men, and latterly women, who have carried their hammers and packs across Ireland's countryside. While a number of societies and groups – such as the Dublin Philosophical Society, the Physico-Historical Society and the Geological Society of Dublin/Royal Geological Society of Ireland – have come and gone, others, including the Royal Irish Academy, the Royal Dublin Society, the Geological Survey of Ireland, and Trinity College, Dublin, have remained active in geology for over one hundred and fifty years.

Early Geological Investigations in Ireland, 1683-1750

In Ireland, the first formal geological investigations were carried out by members of the Dublin Philosophical Society, 1683-1708 (Hoppen, 1970). William Molyneux was the main force behind the establishment of this society, where he was joined by men such as the cartographer Sir William Petty and the anatomist Allen Mullen (Kelly, 1992). Through papers published in *Philosophical Transactions of the Royal Society of London*, various aspects of

Ireland's geology were examined by members of the Dublin Philosophical Society. Probably for the first time, two gems of Irish geology were described in print – the Giant's Causeway (*plate 4*) by the Rev. Samuel Foley and Thomas Molyneux (brother of William) in 1694 and the Giant Irish deer by Thomas Molyneux in 1697.

In 1744 the Physico-Historical Society of Ireland was established in Dublin to survey the natural resources of the country (Herries Davies, 1979). It employed several people, including Charles Smith and the botanist Isaac Butler, who were to survey each county, collect botanical and geological specimens, and write an account of their findings. Reports appeared for only four counties: Cork, Down, Kerry and Waterford. The Cork volume by Smith was accompanied by a map that portrayed the east-west trending synclinal valleys floored with limestone. It was the first attempt to depict the solid geology of any portion of Ireland (Herries Davies, 1983). Though the Physico-Historical Society of Ireland lasted only a dozen years, many of its aims were later pursued by the Dublin Society.

Development of Mineralogical and Geological Studies, 1750-1824

From the mid-1700s mineralogy became a focus for serious scientific study, and from it the science of geology developed (Laudan, 1987). Ireland, and in particular Dublin, became an important centre for mineralogical and geological studies, ranking close to centres of excellence such as Freiburg and Edinburgh. There were three main reasons for this: the establishment of various institutions that promoted these studies, such as the Royal Irish Academy, the Dublin Society (later the Royal Dublin Society) and the Belfast Literary Society; the international stature of Irish scientists; and the debate on the origin of basalts, centred on the Antrim coast, which was of fundamental importance to the development of geological thought in Europe.

The Royal Irish Academy was founded in 1785 for the study of sciences, 'polite literature' and antiquities (O'Raifeartaigh, 1985). It elected its members from the noble, clerical and academic circles of the day and rapidly built up an important library and museum. Geological problems were among those tackled by members, and many papers on such topics were published in the Academy's *Transactions*. This journal was published from 1798 until 1907 and copies were sent to similar learned institutions in Europe, thus allowing for a rapid diffusion and exchange of ideas. The Academy also developed a museum that contained important archaeological material and some geological specimens and became the official repository for treasure trove found in Ireland. Many years later the geological collections were incorporated into the collections of the Dublin Society; they are now in the National Museum of Ireland.

Perhaps the most influential member of the geological fraternity at the time was Richard Kirwan (*plate 14*), a Galway-born chemist and geologist and President of the Academy from 1799 to 1812 (McLaughlin, 1939-40; Burns, 1985). Through his book *Elements of Mineralogy* (1784) he became one of the most influential mineralogists of his day. In it he coined the term 'Calp' for a flinty grey limestone quarried near Dublin. In later life Kirwan became a noted eccentric who disliked flies so much that he paid his servants for each corpse presented to him. He also disliked replying to correspondence and had his door-knocker removed each evening at seven o'clock to deter further visitors. He died in Dublin while engaged in the practice, common for the time, of starving a cold (Somerville-Large, 1975).

Within the pages of the *Transactions* were published a suite of papers dealing with a controversy that began at the end of the eighteenth century: the origin of granite, basalt and other igneous rocks. One school of thought, the 'Neptunists' or, to use a contemporary term, 'watermen', believed that these rocks were precipitated from water – a view held by the German mineralogist Abraham Gottlib Werner and his students in the Freiburg School of Mines. Kirwan also followed the theories of the Neptunists. The other group, variably known as 'Vulcanists' or 'firemen', according to the rock types in which they were interested, argued that the rocks were the products of volcanoes and other igneous phenomena (Herries Davies, 1981). These men included the Rev. William Hamilton, a Fellow of Trinity College, Dublin, who wrote an important and influential memoir entitled *Letters Concerning the Northern Coast of the County of Antrim* (Dublin, 1786). In 1790 he became rector and a local magistrate of Clondevaddog, an isolated parish in Co. Donegal, but was brutally murdered seven years later after local unrest which culminated in the uprising of 1798.

The debate was centred around the basaltic Giant's Causeway in County Antrim, which made Ireland one of the more important sites for resolving it. In the late eighteenth and early nineteenth centuries, the Giant's Causeway drew many visitors from Britain and some from continental Europe, including John Wesley in 1778, John Whitehurst in 1783, Abraham Mills in 1787-8, Humphry Davy in 1806 and Jean-François Berger in 1811 (Herries Davies, 1978; Siegfried and Dott, 1980; MacArthur, 1990). Its unusual character had been widely advertised by Frederick Hervey, Bishop of Derry and fourth Earl of Bristol, and by Susanna Drury, who won a commission of £25 from the Dublin Society in 1740 to paint views of the Causeway. Her gouaches were subsequently engraved and distributed widely, thus bringing the area to the attention of many travellers and scientists (Anglesea and Preston, 1980; Anglesea, this volume).

Both factions in this geological conundrum felt that they could explain the formation of the basalts according to their principles. The Neptunist or

Wernerian view was reinforced by the presence of marine shells called ammonites – thought to be in basalt occurring at Portrush, County Antrim –
which were first described in 1803 by the Rev. William Richardson, a vociferous 'waterman' (Herries Davies, 1985). However, detailed examination of
the ammonites by Sir James Hall and John Playfair in Edinburgh revealed
that they were present in a sedimentary rock that had been baked by hot
basalt close by, giving it a similar appearance to that basalt (Playfair, 1802).
These conclusions were confirmed by the Rev. William Daniel Conybeare
and Jean-François Berger in 1816. This piece of evidence was critical, and
swung the scales in the favour of the Vulcanists. Additional evidence came
from observations made in Italy of active and extinct volcanoes – especially
Vesuvius, which had erupted in the 1790s – and from a suite of Italian volcanic specimens presented to the Museum of the Academy by one of its
members, the Rev. George Graydon, who had personally collected them so
as to demonstrate the similarities between Antrim and the Italian areas
(Wyse Jackson and Vaccari, 1993; Vaccari and Wyse Jackson, 1995).
Another paper of note was that by a Scottish civil engineer, Alexander
Nimmo, which described the geology of offshore Ireland (Nimmo, 1825;
Wyse Jackson, 1996). Some 140 years later this area was to become well
known, thanks to feverish exploration for oil and gas.

The Dublin Society and Other Institutions

The Dublin Society was established in 1731 to promote agriculture and sciences in Ireland. It did so by offering premiums to members to carry out research, organizing county statistical surveys, acquiring specimens for its
museum, and acting as a forum for discussion, debate, and study (Berry,
1915; Meenan and Clarke, 1981; Mollan, 1990). In 1786 Donald Stewart,
appointed as Itinerant Mineralogist, studied the geology of various parts of
the country and collected specimens for the Society's museum (Stewart,
1799). The museum's large and important collection contained 7331 mineral
specimens assembled by the German mineralogist Nathanael Gottfried
Leske (1751-86), which had been purchased in 1792, largely thanks to the
efforts of Kirwan, for the huge sum of £1350 (the equivalent of approximately £35,000 today). The acquisition remains geologically the most important ever made by an Irish museum. It stimulated considerable geological
activity by members who made mineral collections for themselves, many of
which ultimately found their way into the museum or other institutions.

Between 1801 and 1832 the Dublin Society published the results of
county statistical surveys of twenty-three counties, each of which gives some
geological information. Of particular note are the volumes on Wicklow
(1801) by Robert Fraser, Kilkenny (1802) by William Tighe, Londonderry

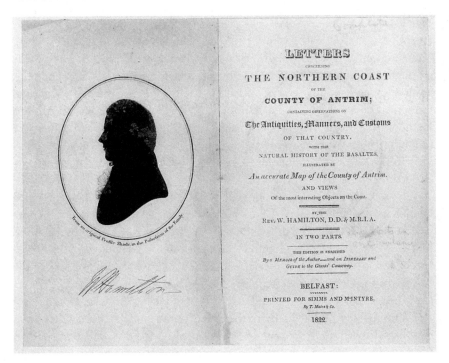

(1802) by George Vaughan Sampson and Cork (1810) by Horatio Townsend, all of which contained highly advanced geological maps (Herries Davies, 1983).

Richard Griffith, who went on to make a profound contribution to Irish geology (Herries Davies and Mollan, 1980), was engaged to report on the Leinster coalfield in 1809, and was appointed as Mining Engineer in 1815. He surveyed and mapped various other coalfields, including those of Connacht (1818) and counties Tyrone and Antrim (1829). The Dublin Society attempted to instigate a geological mapping scheme for the whole country, but this did not happen until it was officially carried out by the Geological Survey, and unofficially by Griffith.

In order to promote geology further, the Dublin Society decided in 1812 to appoint a Professor of Mineralogy. The position was first offered to Robert Jameson of Edinburgh, who had visited Dublin in 1797 to study the Leskean collection (Sweet, 1967). Jameson accepted the post but later rescinded his acceptance, so the job went to the German-born mineralogist Sir Charles Lewis Giesecke. He is best known for his collection of minerals acquired in Greenland in the early years of the 1800s (Praeger, 1949), for which he was knighted by the Danish king, and for appearing in the first performance of Mozart's *The Magic Flute* in Vienna in 1791 (Whittaker, 1991). Many of his Greenland specimens were hijacked at sea and eventually ended up in Scotland. Others were deposited in Copenhagen, many were donated to the Dublin Society Museum (Monaghan, 1993), and some have recently turned up in Trinity College, Dublin (Wyse Jackson, 1996a). Giesecke rapidly learned English so that he could lecture on mineralogy. He catalogued the collections (Giesecke, 1832) and made several collecting trips around Ireland, adding many specimens to the Dublin Society Museum. Giesecke also arranged for material to be exchanged with foreign institutions including the Royal Institution, Vienna, and the German Goethe Institute (Hennig, 1951; Waterhouse, 1933).

In Cork from 1790, Thomas Dix Hincks, a Unitarian minister, instigated lectures on 'general and useful knowledge'. As a result of this work, the Royal Cork Institution was founded in 1802 (Pettit, 1976). It soon ran a botanic garden and employed four professors, one of whom lectured in natural history, and another of whom was the accomplished chemist Edmund Davy, a nephew of Sir Humphry, who himself had collected geological specimens in Co. Donegal in 1805 and 1806 for use in his lectures at the Royal Institution in London (Davis, 1985; MacArthur, 1987). The Royal Cork Institution was later assimilated into the Queen's College, Cork.

During this period in Belfast, a small number of learned bodies were established that rapidly became the cultural focus for the north-east part of the country. These never attained the recognition accorded their Dublin counterparts, probably because their membership was drawn from the middle and working classes, but nevertheless they were important in the development of the study of geology in that city. The Belfast Reading Society (later the Belfast Library and Society for Promoting Knowledge, properly known as the Linen Hall Library), which was founded in 1788, possessed a collection of fossils. The Belfast Literary Society, founded in 1801 (Anon., 1902), also kept a small cabinet of minerals, many of which were possibly collected by its first president, James McDonnell, who was the geological mainstay of the society and who read several papers to it (Doughty, 1980). Both of these small collections were passed on to the Belfast Natural History Society in the 1830s. This society was established in 1821 by James Lawson Drummond in association with others including the zoologist Robert Patterson and Hincks of the Royal Cork Institution (Deane, 1924; Nesbitt, 1979). Soon collections of geological and other materials were made, and these laid the foundations for the present Ulster Museum. In 1831 James Bryce, a schoolmaster in Belfast Academy, published a catalogue of their collections, which were assembled for 'the cultivation of the science generally' (Bryce, 1831). The work of the Belfast organizations played an important role in fostering an interest in the natural sciences among the population of a city where few people had access to formal education (Nesbitt, 1979).

Ordnance Survey and Geological Survey Mapping

From the 1820s onwards, for over six decades, Ireland was an important centre of scientific research through the work of men such as William Rowan Hamilton, the mathematician and inventor of quaternions; the physicist Humphrey Lloyd; the astronomers William Parsons, third Earl of Rosse, who built a telescope with a 72-inch reflector at Birr, Co. Offaly, and Robert Stawell Ball, the Astronomer Royal; the seismologist Robert Mallet; and the geologists Rev. Samuel Haughton and Sir Richard Griffith (Wyse Jackson and Wyse Jackson, 1992). Geological study in Ireland flourished: primary mapping of the solid geology of the country was initiated and completed; a strong and influential geological society was very active; geology was formally recognized as a university subject; and many of Ireland's geologists, professional and amateur, attained a high international profile.

In 1809 the Commissioners of Bogs began their mammoth task of surveying Ireland's boglands. Soon afterwards, in 1824, the Ordnance Survey under Lieutenant-Colonel Thomas Colby began to survey the country and produced the first large-scale topographical maps. The scene was set for geological and economic mapping of the country. At first the Ordnance Survey staff collected topographical and demographical information, as well as geological specimens and observations (Herries Davies, 1974). It published a volume entitled *Memoir of the City and North Western Liberties of Londonderry. Parish of Templemore* (1837), which included a geological map. Unfortunately, collection of information for such a memoir stretched resources, and no further parish reports appeared. However, another report emanated from the Ordnance Survey when Joseph Ellison Portlock, together with Thomas Oldham and a staff of more than thirty, produced in 1843 a map and a bulky memoir entitled *Report on the Geology of the County of Londonderry, and of Parts of Tyrone and Fermanagh* (Seymour, 1944). The geological data collected during this work was for the first time plotted on the large-scale six-inches-to-the-mile maps which had only just been published. Portlock was an engineer who spent considerable time in Ireland on the basic measurement or triangulation of the country, very often in harsh conditions. In 1828 he overwintered 1200 feet up on Slieve League. For his efforts Portlock was rewarded by being sent to Corfu, where he supervised the installation of fortifications. He remained there until 1849, after which he spent some time in Britain before retiring to Dublin in 1862. Portlock was a highly regarded member of the geological fraternity; he was a Fellow of the Royal Society and President of the Geological Society of Dublin, and also became a Major General in the army. Today his palaeontological collections, many of which were collected by Patrick Doran (of Glassdrummond,

Co. Down) and James Flanagan, are largely housed in the British Geological Survey and the Ulster Museum (Tunnicliff, 1980) and remain an important research asset for modern geologists. While Flanagan continued to earn his salary collecting fossils for the later Geological Survey, Doran became one of the first itinerant mineral collectors and dealers in Ireland. Many of his specimens found their way into collections, including those of the Royal Dublin Society, the Belfast Natural History and Philosophical Society, and the British Geological Survey (Cleevely, 1983).

Two years after the publication of Portlock's Londonderry memoir, the Geological Survey was established under the general directorship of Thomas de la Beche and the local directorship of Henry James. For the next forty-five years the officers of the Geological Survey in Ireland were engaged in producing a geological map of the country. Their first published maps depicted the geology of various counties at a scale of one inch to two miles. The geological colours that indicate the various rock types were hand-painted on to base maps of the Index sheets to the Townland Series. Five such maps appeared: Wicklow (1848), Carlow (1849), Kildare (1849), Wexford (1851) and Dublin (1851), this last at a scale of one inch to one and a half miles. The problem facing the geologists was that there were no maps at the preferred scale of one inch to one mile. They had to wait a number of years before such maps became available from the Ordnance Survey. The first geological map at this scale was published in 1856, accompanied by a memoir that contained an account of the geology depicted on the map. The Geological Survey was to produce a total of 205 such map sheets and memoirs before its task was completed (Herries Davies, 1983, 1995). The importance of the Geological Survey to Irish geology at this time cannot be overstated. In men such as Edward Hull, Joseph Beete Jukes, George Henry Kinahan, George Victor Du Noyer and Thomas Oldham, it employed some of the most eminent geologists to work in Ireland. Du Noyer was a fine geological artist, and his field sheets and notebooks are liberally adorned with quick but perceptive sketches (Archer, 1993, 1995; Coffey, 1993). Oldham did not remain in charge of the Survey for very long, and in 1850 he removed himself and his new wife to India to take charge of the new Geological Survey of India, based in Calcutta. Over the next twenty years he succeeded in persuading many Irish geologists to join him there.

Oldham was replaced by Jukes, an Englishman born near Birmingham, who appointed an additional ten men to the Geological Survey and began an ambitious regime of field-mapping. From 1850 to 1870 an average of about a thousand square miles was covered per year, and from 1856, the one-inch-to-one-mile maps were published. By 1860 the maps for most of Munster and south-east Leinster were published, by 1869 maps of all of Leinster and east Galway were available, and by 1890 geological mapping of the whole country had been completed. The mapping programme did not always proceed smoothly, however; there were frequent clashes of personality and opinion. The most serious of these was that between Hull, who had replaced Jukes as Local Director in 1869, and Kinahan, who resented Hull's appointment. This infighting led to numerous delays in the publication of maps and memoirs. In addition, Hull's revisionist interpretation of some of the geology of southern Ireland was questioned by his team, and subsequently, in the period 1903 to 1912, the areas affected by Hull's work were resurveyed.

The conditions endured by the geologists were not always pleasant. Salaries were low: Jukes earned £575 as Director in 1865, while an Assistant Geologist was paid twelve shillings per day (Herries Davies, 1983). In addition, the geologists mapped in typical wet Irish weather and moved from field station to field station, which did not allow them to put down roots. In some cases the adverse conditions led to a breakdown in health, and a few geologists actually succumbed while surveying: Frederick Foot and William Benjamin Leonard were drowned; Frederick William Egan died after being thrown from a car; Jukes, while in Kenmare on a tour of inspection, fell down a flight of stairs and never fully recovered; Joseph O'Kelly died of bronchitis; and Du Noyer died of scarlet fever in 1869. Altogether, of the thirty-two men who worked for the Geological Survey between 1845 and 1890, seven died while in its employment (Herries Davies, 1983).

The end result of the work of the Geological Survey was the publication of a series of maps of the highest standard which for many parts of Ireland remained until very recently the only available geological maps. The one-inch-to-one-mile geological map of Ireland is a lasting testament to the labours of the thirty-two geologists employed by the Geological Survey of Ireland in this period.

Richard Griffith's Unofficial Geological Survey of Ireland

From the 1830s Richard Griffith was engaged in compiling a geological map of the country. Griffith, who had studied under the eminent mineralogist Robert Jameson in Edinburgh, came under the influence of George Bellas Greenough, who encouraged him to start this task. Griffith had started collecting geological information during his period of employment with the Dublin Society and as Engineer to the Office of Public Works. His geological activity received a boost in 1830 when he was appointed Commissioner for the General Valuation of Rateable Property. As such he employed many surveyors, who were instructed unofficially to make geological observations. Indeed, Patrick Ganly, one such employee, spent almost all his time mapping geology and returned frequent missives to Griffith containing his results. By another stroke of fortune, Griffith was appointed as one of the

Commissioners of Railways in 1836 and persuaded his fellow members of the great importance of a geological map of the country as an aid to planning for the rapidly expanding railway network. Griffith's first map was published in 1838 at a scale of one inch to ten miles, and this was followed a year later by his splendid map executed at the scale of one inch to four miles. This map, and its various versions produced up to 1855, represents one of the milestones of Irish geology and remains one of the finest geological maps ever produced (Herries Davies, 1977, 1983). While the map owes much to Griffith's own efforts, its genesis owes more to the geological observations made by Ganly (Archer, 1980), one of which deserves special mention. In 1856 Ganly published a short paper in the *Journal of the Geological Society of Dublin*, in which he illustrated the 'structure of strata' and demonstrated how the shape of rippled sandstone could be used to determine the original attitude of strata. His comments on what is now termed cross-stratification remain fundamental to geologists today (Wyse Jackson, 1995).

The Body Geologic

The university geologists, their colleagues in the Geological Survey, and amateur geologists such as Lord Talbot de Malahide, William Willoughby Cole (later the 3rd Earl of Enniskillen), and the Rev. Maxwell Henry Close, were brought together through their membership of the Geological Society of Dublin and its successor, the Royal Geological Society of Ireland. The Society, which was the third such body devoted to earth sciences in the British Isles, had been founded in 1831, largely due to the efforts of Bartholomew Lloyd, the Provost of Trinity College, Dublin (Herries Davies, 1965). This Society acted as a forum in which geological opinions could be voiced and published in the pages of its *Journal*. It formed its own museum (M'Coy, 1841), which in 1844 was given to Trinity College in return for permission to hold its meetings there. By Royal Charter it became the Royal Geological Society of Ireland and remained active until 1890.

The Society met once a month between November and June and as many as five papers were read at each meeting; nearly half were subsequently published. In the pages of the *Journal* many important papers appeared: William Hellier Baily on fossil plants from the classic site at Kiltorcan, Co. Kilkenny (Herries Davies, 1990); John Ball on the glaciation of Kerry (Herries Davies, 1990a); Maxwell Close on glacial striations near Dublin; Ganly on determining the way-up in strata; Griffith on the subdivision of the Carboniferous rocks in Ireland; Haughton on geological time; Hull on the microscopic nature of granites; Oldham on the Cambrian rocks at Bray; Kinahan on Irish economic geology; and Jukes on river valleys in southern Ireland. Oldham's and Kinahan's papers are of special significance. The work by Kinahan on the economic geology of Ireland was published in several papers which made up the eighteenth and final volume of the *Journal*. It contained information on the quarries of Ireland and described the rocks that were extracted from them. It remains a very important source for those interested in building materials. The paper by Jukes, read to the society on 14 May 1862, explains the curious nature of some rivers in Munster, most notably the River Blackwater, which flows due east until it reaches Cappoquin, where it turns through ninety degrees and flows due south to Youghal. The prevailing view at the time was that the landscape had been shaped by marine currents and waves during recent submergence. Jukes recognized the pivotal role of fluvial action in moulding present features and said that the drainage system adopted by these rivers was independent of the underlying geological structure. The Blackwater south of Cappoquin was a survivor of an old north-south system founded on the young southward-dipping surface, but above Cappoquin it was a younger river that extended itself westwards by headward extension along the older grain of the landscape (Herries Davies, 1985a).

Another influential member was Robert Mallet, an engineer who had a large ironworks in Dublin (Cox, 1982). Mallet, who served as President of the Geological Society of Dublin and its successor on three occasions, was interested in the mechanisms of earthquakes and conducted experiments on Killiney beach to see how seismic waves moved through the sand. He compiled a seismic map of the world and was the first to measure the epicentre of an earthquake (Cox, 1985). He is today rightly regarded as the 'father of seismology' (Dean, 1991).

The British Association for the Advancement of Science was founded in York in 1831. Four years later it met in Dublin under the presidency of Bartholomew Lloyd. This meeting generated a great deal of attention, much of which was beneficial to Irish geologists. Many of the eminent British geologists attended, including Sir Roderick Murchison, the Rev. Adam Sedgwick and William Smith. Smith, who was a surveyor, had found lasting fame as the author of the first large-scale geological map of England and Wales, which he published in 1815. At the 1835 meeting he was conferred with the degree of Doctor of Laws – his only academic accolade (Herries Davies, 1969). Since 1835 the Association has met in Ireland ten times – in Belfast in 1852, 1874, 1902, 1952 and 1987; in Cork in 1843; in Dublin in 1857, 1878, 1908 and 1957 (Morrell, 1990) – and has helped to generate enthusiasm among the native scientists.

After the 1835 meeting Murchison and Sedgwick, together with Charles Lyell, John Phillips (Smith's nephew), Phillip de Malpas Grey Egerton, Louis Agassiz (an expert on fossil fishes) and Griffith, met at Florence Court, near Enniskillen, Co. Fermanagh, the home of William

Willoughby Cole. Cole, together with Egerton, had accumulated one of the finest collections of fossil fishes in these islands, which was housed in its own museum in one of the pavilions at Florence Court (Herries Davies, 1970a). Such geological collecting did not impress Cole's father, who referred to it as being 'damned nonsense' (James, 1986). Many of the specimens were collected in the company of Egerton, and as the fish were often preserved as two halves on a split slab, it was customary for the two friends to keep one half each. Just before his death Cole sold his collection to the British Museum (Natural History) in London, where his specimens were eventually reunited with those of Egerton.

University Geology

The teaching of geology was placed on a firm footing in the 1840s when several chairs were founded in Irish universities. The oldest is in Trinity College, Dublin, where the chair was established in 1843; those in the Queen's Colleges followed in 1849. In Trinity College, geology had been taught from the 1770s onwards (Wyse Jackson, 1994). Whitley Stokes lectured on natural history from the early 1800s and published two fine catalogues of minerals in the University Museum (Stokes, 1807, 1818). Although a classics scholar, William Fitton was interested in the geology of the Dublin area and as an undergraduate was arrested in the Dublin mountains while engaged in fieldwork. His crime was possession of a dangerous weapon – his geological hammer! (Herries Davies, 1983). Fitton, who produced a fine memoir on the geology of the region based on his, and the late Walter Stephens's, observations, was an early member and President (1827-8) of the Geological Society of London, and through his writings in the *Edinburgh Review* raised the profile of geology in the British Isles (Stephens and Fitton, 1812; Woodward, 1907).

From 1777 Trinity College actively acquired geological specimens for its museum, which had been founded by William Hamilton (Wyse Jackson, 1992) and which was used for teaching. The most important acquisitions were the minerals purchased in 1823 from the Right Honourable George Knox, one-time Member of Parliament for Dublin University, and the Carboniferous fossils donated by Sir Richard Griffith in 1845. The Chair at Trinity was established in December 1843 and was offered to, and accepted by, John Phillips, Professor of Geology at King's College, London, and later at Oxford. Phillips thought he would be offered the additional post of Local Director of the Geological Survey, but in this he was disappointed. He resigned and returned to England – it was potentially a great loss for Ireland. He was succeeded by Thomas Oldham, who concurrently held the Geological Survey position. From 1851 until 1881 the Professor of Geology was the Rev. Samuel Haughton, a very able scientist whose interests were wide-ranging. He is remembered for his estimates of the age of the earth, which ranged from 2298 million years to 200 million years, his work on animal mechanics, his opposition to Charles Darwin's views and his invention of a humane method of execution by hanging (McMillan, 1988; Wyse Jackson, 1992a; Spearman, 1990).

In 1849 Chairs of Geology were established in the Queen's Colleges of Belfast, Cork and Galway. Two able palaeontologists – Frederick M'Coy and William King – were appointed to Belfast and Galway, and a noted mineralogist, James Nicol, was appointed to the Cork chair. Nicol spent only four years in the position, during which time he published a manual of mineralogy, but he wrote little on the geology of Ireland and was succeeded by Robert Harkness in 1853. King, who was born in north-east England (Pettigrew, 1979), is remembered as the author of the important monograph *The Permian Fossils of England* (1850) and as a principal contributor in the debate over Eozoön, which had been regarded as an early fossil but was shown by King to be composed of inorganic material (Harper, 1988). M'Coy had a chequered career in Ireland; while still very young he was appointed Curator of the Geological Society of Dublin, the collections of which he catalogued (M'Coy, 1841). However, he fell out with the Society and was then employed by the Geological Survey for a short time before resigning in 1846 (Herries Davies, 1983). M'Coy then spent a number of years working in Cambridge, before moving to Belfast. He produced monographs on the Carboniferous (1844) and Silurian (1846) fossils of Ireland, based on material collected by Richard Griffith's valuation surveyors, that represent with little doubt the most important palaeontological publications ever produced in Ireland (Wyse Jackson and Monaghan, 1994). In general the descriptions are short, but they are accompanied by accurate lithographs executed by Du Noyer. It is now acknowledged that in these works more new species were described than can be justified by the material; nevertheless they remain, together with the original specimens now in the National Museum of Ireland, important to present-day palaeontologists as sources of many valid fossil groups. M'Coy resigned his chair at Queen's in 1854 and took up the position of Professor of Natural Science in Melbourne, Australia, where he took on additional official positions (Vallance, 1978) and was knighted in 1891. However, after his departure from the British Isles his research output declined and the promise of his early career in Ireland was left largely unfulfilled.

Decline of Irish Geology, 1890–1922

In 1890 the final map in the Geological Survey's mammoth series of one-inch-to-one-mile maps was published. Immediately the Survey's staff was trimmed; the Dublin office was kept open with a skeleton staff who worked with decreased funding. Mapping of solid geology was no longer a priority; the general consensus was that everything was known of Ireland's geology. Nevertheless, during the period 1890 to 1922 the Geological Survey of Ireland carried out some important work, particularly in the area of glacial geology. Much of the impetus for this project came from George William Lamplugh, who took charge from 1901 to 1905. Lamplugh, who became Assistant Director of the Geological Survey of England and Wales, was a glacial geologist of considerable influence whose ideas were based largely on field observation (Penny, 1966). Together with men such as William Bourke Wright, James Robinson Kilroe, Herbert Brantwood Muff, Henry J. Seymour, Sidney Berdoe Neal Wilkinson and Alexander M'Henry, Lamplugh surveyed the glacial deposits, revised the solid geology of the major metropolitan areas, and produced maps and *Memoirs* of Dublin (1903), Belfast (1904), Cork (1905), Limerick (1907) and Londonderry (1908).

After 1905 the Irish section of the Geological Survey became an autonomous entity under the directorship of Grenville Arthur James Cole. During the next twenty years, the Geological Survey of Ireland produced a number of *Memoirs* on economic topics: the intrabasaltic rocks of Antrim (1912), the geology of the Ballycastle Coalfield (1924), and the mines and mineral deposits of Ireland (1922). Solid geology was not neglected; Clare Island (1914) and the Killarney region (1927) were surveyed. Possibly the most important publication of this period described rocks from the seabed of the Porcupine basin off the west coast of Ireland, representing an early examination of the geology of an area that recently has been the focus of considerable exploration in the search for hydrocarbons (Cole and Crook, 1910).

The slow demise of the Geological Survey coincided with a general decline in Irish geological fortunes. The Royal Geological Society of Ireland had for a number of years prior to 1890 been affected by falling membership, resulting in financial difficulties which caused delays in publishing parts of the *Journal*. This in turn probably resulted in further non-renewed memberships. Finally, in 1894, the Society ceased to exist, having stopped meeting four years earlier. It was another sixty-five years before another such body donned its tattered mantle.

It is to the credit of both the Royal Irish Academy and the Royal Dublin Society that they continued to provide a channel through which Irish geologists could publish their research findings. During this period the monthly journal *The Irish Naturalist* appeared. This acted as a catalyst for naturalists, particularly those associated with the Field Clubs, and enabled them to publish their research findings (Wyse Jackson and Wyse Jackson, 1992). However, it was a 'popular' journal and precious little of geological note was published, other than a few papers by Grenville Cole.

In some of the universities, the appointment of academics to geological positions was not, in hindsight, beneficial. Excellent researchers such as Haughton, William Johnston Sollas, an expert on fossil sponges and a keen field geologist in Trinity College, and Andrew Leith Adams, a medic, palaeontologist and cave explorer in Queen's College, Cork, were replaced by men such as John Joly in Trinity and Marcus Hartog in Cork. Although Joly was undoubtedly one of Ireland's greatest scientists, he was largely interested in physics and radioactivity (Dixon, 1934, 1941; Nudds, 1986). Field geology did not enthuse him, which is probably why few geologists of note graduated from Trinity College during his tenure of the Chair of Geology and Mineralogy from 1897 to 1933 (Wyse Jackson, 1992a). Joly is perhaps best remembered for his pioneering work in colour photography (Coonan, 1991) and for developing a method of treating cancer with radium. His geological work included research into the age of the earth and the relationship between radioactivity and geology (Nudds, 1986).

Hartog was Professor of Natural History in Queen's College, Cork (which became University College in 1909) from 1882 to 1909 and then became Professor of Zoology until 1921, but in that time he published only one geological paper. The major university geologist of note in Ireland at this time was Grenville Cole, who was Professor of Geology at the Royal College of Science for Ireland in Dublin as well as Director of the Geological Survey of Ireland. Cole was small in stature, but had unlimited energy. He was a prolific author, with over five hundred publications to his name, and an advocate of field studies, which he stressed were of fundamental importance for an understanding of geology. He was also a keen tricyclist and later bicyclist who together with his wife made frequent excursions deep into Europe (Wyse Jackson, 1989, 1991). He played an important role in the development of geography in Ireland, urging its adoption as a university subject (Herries Davies, 1977a).

In 1902 and 1908 the British Association for the Advancement of Science visited Belfast and Dublin respectively, and while these meetings attracted many scientists of note and undoubtedly raised the interest of those in Ireland, they failed to arrest the slow erosion of interest in geology in Ireland. There were at this time a number of amateur geologists who made important contributions to Irish geology. The majority hailed from the Belfast area, where they had come under the influence of Ralph Tate and later the Belfast Naturalists' Field Club. Two women, Sydney Mary Thompson (Madame Christen) [*plate 4*] and Mary Andrews, collected information on glacial erratics which was presented to the British Association. Joseph Wright was a Quaker grocer of Belfast who became an expert on microscopic foraminifera, particularly those recovered from Cretaceous strata in north-east Ireland, and from glacial boulder clays as far afield as Canada and the Arctic (Wilson,

1987). Robert John Welch, another amateur naturalist, was the foremost photographer of the period; his photographs of geological phenomena plants, scenery, ships and shipbuilding, and prehistoric monuments (*plates 11, 15*) appeared in many important publications as well as popular handbooks produced by railway companies (Evans and Turner, 1977). He spared no effort in getting the best image and would spend considerable time setting up his heavy equipment before shooting. He developed and printed all his own photographs, the clarity of which would defy many modern photographers. Welch's photographs were all the better for keen perception of his subjects. He made the study of molluscs his prime natural history pursuit and was awarded an honorary MSc by Queen's University (Praeger, 1949). Over five thousand of his photographic plates are now in the Ulster Museum, as are the many photographs of geological interest that he presented to the British Association (Turner, 1979; Hackney, James and Ross, 1983; McKenna, 1990). The Irish prints in the Ulster Museum number 638, of which Welch contributed over half. Others were taken by Grenville Cole, William Gray (a Belfast naturalist), Mary Andrews and Professor Sidney Hugh Reynolds.

Reynolds, who was Professor of Geology at Bristol University, was one of the few England-based geologists who worked in Ireland around the turn of the century. Together with Charles Irving Gardiner, he comprehensively mapped various Ordovician and Silurian rocks in Ireland and published nine papers reporting their findings, which were important at a time when the relationship between rocks of the two geological periods was first being understood. After 1922 Reynolds and Gardiner ceased their Irish work and turned their attentions to matters in Britain.

Another blow to the geological community came in 1922 when the new Irish Free State government decided to take over the geological galleries of the Museum of Science and Art for use by clerical workers. The scientifically and historically important collections of Irish and foreign geology, acquired over nearly two centuries, were put into storage where they remained for many decades, and only today are they beginning to be seen again.

Why did geology decline from the 1890s? There are a number of reasons: the completion of the Geological Survey mapping programme; the constant emigration of competent geologists and geology graduates, which increased after 1922 as many Protestants left Ireland; and the effects of the First World War, when at least three budding Irish geologists were killed along with thousands of other young men on the fields of France.

Irish Geology in the Doldrums 1922-60

While geology in official government institutions was not regarded as of national importance, the universities continued to train geologists. Many of these graduates of Trinity College, Dublin, Queen's University, Belfast, and the University Colleges of Cork, Dublin and Galway emigrated soon after graduation and found geological work in various parts of the globe. Few stayed at home because there were no employment opportunities, either economic or academic, in Ireland. Between the 1920s and the 1950s university geology was dominated by a handful of academics: Louis Bouvier Smyth in Trinity College, John Kaye Charlesworth in Queen's University, Belfast, Henry B. Seymour in University College Dublin and Isaac Swain in University College Cork, each of whom largely operated as one-man departments. With the exception of Charlesworth these leading figures of Irish geology did not publish a great deal and consequently were not well known beyond Ireland's shores.

Charlesworth, a Yorkshireman, was appointed as Professor of Geology at Queen's University, Belfast, in 1921 and thus became the first to hold the Chair since M'Coy's departure in 1854. He wrote extensively on the Pleistocene of Ireland and of other areas and his work culminated in 1957 in the bulky two-volume *The Quaternary Era* (Williams, 1973; Wilson, 1972). Smyth, who was a quiet, unassuming man, is remembered for his work on coral faunas from the Lower Carboniferous rocks and for a fine and meticulous stratigraphical description of Hook Head, Co. Wexford (Farrington, 1954). Swain, a Quaker, published only a handful of papers during his tenure in Cork as Professor of Geology and Geography from 1908 to 1944.

In the 1940s some of the university departments were enlarged through the employment of further academic staff. At the same time the first postgraduate students were enrolling in the universities. This period marks the slow climb of Irish geology out of the trough in which it had languished during the period between the two world wars. Through the 1950s geological graduates still found most employment opportunities abroad, although more stayed in Ireland – initially, at least, to carry out postgraduate research. It was during this period that William Edward Nevill of Trinity College was awarded the first doctorate in Irish geology in 1951. From 1951 to 1992 over two hundred higher degrees have been awarded in geology on the basis of research theses: ninety-four from Trinity College; sixty-three from Queen's University, Belfast (since 1969); twenty-eight from University College Dublin; twenty-two from University College Galway; and twenty from University College Cork. These postgraduate theses have added considerably to our present knowledge of Irish geology.

The Renaissance of Irish Geology from 1960

Since the early 1960s the state of Irish geology has improved enormously. There are a number of reasons for this: increased staffing in universities, discoveries of major base metal and hydrocarbon deposits in Ireland, confidence in the merits of exploration, and the development of professional and semi-professional associations to cater to the expanded geological community.

Without exception, staffing in the five university geological departments has increased, the research output has diversified and, in consequence, the number of publications has jumped. Such research has been of immense value in increasing the sphere of knowledge pertaining to Ireland's geological structure and has been published in international and Irish earth-science journals such as the *Scientific Proceedings of the Royal Dublin Society*, the *Proceedings of the Royal Irish Academy* and the *Irish Journal of Earth Sciences*. The last of these journals was established in 1978, published by the Royal Dublin Society until 1983 and by the Royal Irish Academy since then. It maintains a link between geologists working in Ireland today and some of the pioneers of nearly two hundred years ago who presented geological findings to these two bodies.

The second factor in the revitalization of Irish geology was the realization and subsequent confirmation that Ireland possessed significant deposits of economically viable resources, both onshore and offshore. In 1960 the government of the Republic of Ireland passed the Petroleum and Other Minerals Development Bill, which allowed for the exploration of parts of Ireland and its surrounding continental shelf. New techniques, such as gravity measurements and seismic profiling (the method first used by Robert Mallet on Killiney beach nearly one hundred years before), were employed for geological exploration. In 1961 the first significant find – large reserves of base metals at Tynagh, Co. Galway – was announced. Exploration by various mining companies continued throughout the 1960s and further base metal deposits were discovered at Navan, Co. Meath, and Gortdrum, Co. Tipperary, which like Tynagh were brought into production, as were deposits at Avoca, Co. Wicklow, and Silvermines, Co. Tipperary. More recently, base metal deposits have been discovered at Lisheen, Co. Tipperary, and Galmoy, Co. Kilkenny.

The search for oil and gas in Ireland from the early 1960s was prompted by the discovery of gas in the Netherlands. Initially exploration and drilling were carried out onshore in Leitrim and Fermanagh, but soon interest was focused on the continental shelf. Such exploration was controlled at government level by the provisions of the Continental Shelf Act of 1968, and in 1971 a large gas field was discovered in the north Celtic Sea Basin, twenty-five miles south-west of Kinsale, which now supplies much of the Republic of Ireland's domestic demand for natural gas.

The increasing importance of economic geology was reflected in the foundation of the Irish Association for Economic Geology (IAEG) in 1974, which aimed to advance the practice of economic geology, provide information regarding mineral and hydrocarbon exploration and production, and promote the exchange of ideas and information through field excursions and meetings. IAEG produces an annual review and has published two fine volumes, *Geology and Genesis of Mineral Deposits in Ireland* (1986) and *The Irish Minerals Industry – A Review of the Decade* (1992).

While the credit for discovery of many of the hydrocarbon and metal deposits must go in part to the exploration companies, the university geological departments and various government agencies played an important role as well. The Geological Survey of Ireland has embarked on compiling a new series of geological maps of the country, at the scale of 1:100,000, that will complement maps recently produced by the Geological Survey of Northern Ireland.

The last factor in the renaissance of Irish geology was the foundation of the Irish Geological Association – the modern-day successor of the Royal Geological Society of Ireland. This was established with the encouragement of Robert George Spencer Hudson, who was Professor of Geology at Trinity College, Dublin, from 1961 until his death in 1965. He had been Professor of Geology at Leeds and later worked in the Middle East before coming to Dublin. Hudson became an authority on Carboniferous stratigraphy and coral faunas. He fostered in his students a love of research and field geology (Jackson, 1966). The Association, which brings together professional and amateur geologists from all parts of the island, organizes lectures and field excursions, an annual research meeting at which new findings are presented, and an annual geology day at which the general public is invited to participate in a wide range of geological activities such as field trips and museum visits.

Despite its small size, Ireland has made important contributions to the study of glaciation and glacial geology. Early writings included those of Richard Prior, who described an esker in 1699, and Charles Smith, who was the first to describe a drumlin swarm as 'basket of eggs' topography in 1744 (Herries Davies, 1966, 1970). Indeed the words 'drumlin' and 'esker' are derived from the Irish language – *druim* meaning back and *eiscir* meaning a ridge (Quin and Freeman, 1947). As we have seen, John Ball and Maxwell Close in the nineteenth century made important observations on glaciation, and Ireland was well known throughout Europe for the Giant Irish Deer *Megaceros giganteus*, which had become extinct at the end of the last glaciation ten thousand years ago, and of which many skeletons were found beneath a raised bog at Ballybetagh, Co. Dublin. But the study of the glacial geology only developed a measurable popularity following the efforts of the Royal Irish Academy, which brought Knud Jessen to Ireland from Denmark in the 1930s. After these visits various native students of the Irish Pleistocene emerged, most notably Anthony Farrington, a graduate of University College Cork and subsequently Resident (later Executive)

Secretary of the Royal Irish Academy (Mitchell, 1990), Frank Mitchell and William A. Watts of Trinity College, Dublin, and Francis Millington Synge of the Geological Survey of Ireland, who together made major advances in our knowledge of the effects of the last glaciation in Ireland. Today glacial geologists and botanists have their own organization, the Irish Association for Quaternary Studies.

In the last thirty years geology in Ireland has been thriving. Great advances in our knowledge of the island's geological structure have been made. History will relate which aspects of research made in this time will have had the greatest effect, but perhaps among them may rank the following: the research carried out on the Donegal granite by Wallace Pitcher and others from Liverpool; the research by Bernard Leake and colleagues from Glasgow on the complex geology of Connemara; the collection and analysis of the vast volume in geological data derived from offshore Ireland and from the exploration for metals onshore; research on Lower Palaeozoic rocks and fossils which has yielded much information on the palaeogeography of Ireland; the work on thermal maturation of the Upper Palaeozoic rocks by researchers in Trinity College, Dublin; advances made in structural geology which have contributed greatly to understanding Ireland's underlying geology; the work carried out by Mitchell and others which has opened our eyes to the complexity of the last Ice Age and the greening of Ireland after the ice had melted; and finally the work *A Geology of Ireland* (Holland, 1981), a synthesis of much of this recent knowledge into a comprehensive and usable book.

In 1856, after a three-week visit to Ireland during which he suffered from the enveloping mists of the Dingle peninsula, the Director of the Geological Survey, Sir Roderick Murchison, returned to England and declared 'that the geology of Ireland is the dullest which I am acquainted with in Europe. If St Patrick excluded venomous animals he ought to have worked a miracle in giving to the holy isle some one good thing under ground.' A great deal has happened in Irish geology since.

References

Anglesea, M. and J. Preston. 1980. 'A Philosophical Landscape: Susanna Drury and the Giant's Causeway.' *Art History 3*: 252-73.

Anon. 1902. *The Belfast Literary Society 1801-1901*. Belfast: Belfast Literary Society.

Archer, J.B. 1980. 'Patrick Ganly: Geologist.' *Irish Naturalists' Journal 20*: 142-8.

Archer, J.B. 1987. 'Science Loners: The *Journal of the Geological Society of Dublin* and its Successors,' in B. Hayley and E. McKay (eds), *Three Hundred Years of Irish Periodicals*. Mullingar: Association of Irish Learned Journals/Lilliput Press.

Archer, J.B. 1993. 'Geological Artistry: The Drawings and Watercolours of George Victor du Noyer in the Archives of the Geological Survey of Ireland,' in A.M. Dalsimer (ed.), *Visualizing Ireland: National Identity and the Pictorial Tradition*. Faber and Faber: Boston and London.

Archer, J.B. 1995. 'Field Folios: Du Noyer's outdoor geological artistry,' in F. Croke (ed.), *George Victor Du Noyer 1817-1869: Hidden Landscapes*. Dublin: National Gallery of Ireland.

Berry, H.F. 1915. *A History of the Royal Dublin Society*. London.

Bryce, J. 1831. *Tables of Simple Minerals, Rocks and Shells; with local Catalogues of Species, for the use of the Students of Natural History in the Belfast Academy*. Belfast: Simms and M'Intyre.

Burns, D.T. 1985. 'Richard Kirwan: Chemist, Mineralogist, Geologist and Meteorologist, 1733-1812,' in R.C. Mollan, W. Davis, and B. Finucane (eds), *Some People and Places in Irish Science and Technology*. Dublin: Royal Irish Academy.

Cleevely, R.J. 1983. *World Palaeontological Collections*. London: British Museum (Natural History).

Coffey, P. 1993. 'George Victor Du Noyer 1817-1869.' *Sheetlines 35*: 14-26.

Cole, G.A.J. and T. Crook. 1910. *On Rock-Specimens Dredged from the Floor of the Atlantic of the Coast of Ireland, and their Bearing on Submarine Geology*. Dublin: Geological Survey of Ireland.

Conybeare, W. and J.-F. Berger. 1816. 'On the Geological Features of the North-eastern Counties of Ireland.' *Transactions of the Geological Society of London 3*: 121-222.

Coonan, S. 1991. ' John Joly's Irish Tricolour.' *Technology Ireland 23* (6): 18-21.

Cox, R. (ed.). 1982. *Robert Mallet, F.R.S., 1810-1881*. Dublin: Institution of Engineers of Ireland and the Royal Irish Academy.

Cox, R. 1985. 'Robert Mallet: Seismologist, Materials Scientist and Engineer, 1810-1881,' in R.C. Mollan, W. Davis, and B. Finucane (eds), *Some People and Places in Irish Science and Technology*. Dublin: Royal Irish Academy.

Davis, W. 1985. 'The Royal Cork Institution,' in R.C. Mollan, W. Davis, and B. Finucane (eds), *Some People and Places in Irish Science and Technology*. Dublin: Royal Irish Academy.

Dean, D.R. 1991. 'Robert Mallet and the Founding of Seismology.' *Annals of Science 48*: 39-67.

Deane, A. 1924. *The Belfast Natural History and Philosophical Society Centenary Volume 1821-1921*. Belfast: Belfast Natural History and Philosophical Society.

Dixon, H.H. 1934. 'John Joly 1857-1933.' *Obituary Notices of the Royal Society of London 3*: 259-86.

Dixon, H.H. 1941. *John Joly: Presidential Address to the Dublin University Experimental Science Association*. Dublin: Dublin University Press.

Doughty, P.S. 1980. 'Collections and Collectors of note 33: James M'Donnel, M.D. (1762-1854).' *Newsletter of the Geological Curators' Group 2*: 465-6.

Evans, E.E. and B.S. Turner. 1977. *Ireland's Eye: The Photographs of Robert John Welch*. Belfast: Blackstaff Press.

Farrington, A. 1954. 'Louis Bouvier Smyth.' *Proceedings of the Geologists' Association 65*: 90-1.

Foley, S. 1694. 'An Account of the Giant's Causeway in the North of Ireland.' *Philosophical Transactions of the Royal Society of London 18*: 170-5.

Gabbey, W.A. 1985. 'William Molyneux: Astronomer and Natural Philosopher, 1656-1698,' in R.C. Mollan, W. Davis, and B. Finucane (eds), *Some People and Places in Irish Science and Technology*. Dublin: Royal Irish Academy.

Giesecke, C.L. 1832. *A Descriptive Catalogue of a New Collection of Minerals in the Museum of the Royal Dublin Society to which is added an Irish Mineralogy*. Dublin: Graisberry.

Graydon, G. 1816. 'On the Dykes of Monte Somma, in Italy.' *Transactions of the Geological Society of London 3*: 233-5.

Hackney, P., K.W. James and H.C.G. Ross. 1983. *A List of Photographs in the R.J. Welch Collection in the Ulster Museum, Volume 2: Botany, Geology, and Zoology*. Belfast: Ulster Museum.

Hamilton, W. 1786. *Letters concerning the Northern Coast of the County of Antrim*. Dublin.

Harper, D.A.T. 1988. 'The King of Queen's College: William King D.Sc., First Professor of Geology at Galway,' in D.A.T. Harper (ed.), *William King D.Sc. – A Palaeontological Tribute*. Galway: Galway University Press.

Hennig, J. 1951. 'Irish Minerals in the Vienna Collections.' *Irish Naturalists' Journal 10*: 195-6.

[Herries] Davies, G.L. 1965. 'The Geological Society of Dublin and the Royal Geological Society of Ireland 1831-1890.' *Hermathena 100*: 66-76.

[Herries] Davies, G.L. 1966. '"Basket of Eggs" Topography.' *Journal of Glaciology 6*: 466.

[Herries] Davies, G.L. 1969. 'The University of Dublin and Two Pioneers of English Geology.' *Hermathena 109*: 24-36.

[Herries] Davies, G.L. 1970. 'Early Discoverers 28: Richard Prior's 1699 Description of an Irish Esker.' *Journal of Glaciology 9*: 147-8.

[Herries] Davies, G.L. 1970a. 'The Palaeontological Collection of Lord Cole, Third Earl of Enniskillen (1807-1886), at Florence Court, Co. Fermanagh.' *Irish Naturalists' Journal 16*: 379-81.

[Herries] Davies, G.L. 1974. 'First Official Geological Survey in the British Isles.' *Nature 249*: 407.

[Herries] Davies, G.L. 1977. 'Notes on the Various Issues of Sir Richard Griffith's Quarter-inch Geological Map of Ireland, 1839-1955.' *Imago Mundi 29*: 35-44.

[Herries] Davies, G.L. 1977a. 'The Making of Irish Geography II: Grenville Arthur James Cole (1859-1924).' *Irish Geography 10*: 90-4.

Herries Davies, G.L. 1978. 'Geology in Ireland before 1812: A Bibliographic Outline.' *The Western Naturalist 7*: 84-99.

Herries Davies, G.L. 1979. 'The Making of Irish Geography IV: The Physico-Historical Society of Ireland 1744-1752.' *Irish Geography 12*: 92-8.

Herries Davies, G.L. 1981. 'The Neptunian and Plutonic Theories', in D.G. Smith (ed.), *Cambridge Encyclopaedia of Earth Sciences*. Cambridge: Cambridge University Press.

Herries Davies, G.L. 1983. *Sheets of Many Colours: The Mapping of Ireland's Rocks 1750-1890.* Dublin: Royal Dublin Society.

Herries Davies, G.L. 1985. 'Astronomy, Geology, Meteorology', in T. O'Raifeartaigh (ed.), *The Royal Irish Academy: A Bicentennial History 1785-1985*. Dublin: Royal Irish Academy.

Herries Davies, G.L. 1985a. 'Cappoquin, County Waterford', in R.C. Mollan, W. Davis, and B. Finucane (eds), *Some People and Places in Irish Science and Technology*. Dublin: Royal Irish Academy.

Herries Davies, G.L. 1990. 'Kiltorcan, County Kilkenny,' in R.C. Mollan, W. Davis, and B. Finucane (eds), *More People and Places in Irish Science and Technology*. Dublin: Royal Irish Academy.

Herries Davies, G.L. 1990a. 'Lough Doon, County Kerry,' in R.C. Mollan, W. Davis, and B. Finucane (eds), *More People and Places in Irish Science and Technology*. Dublin: Royal Irish Academy.

Herries Davies, G.L. 1995. *North from the Hook: 150 Years of the Geological Survey of Ireland.* Dublin: Geological Survey of Ireland.

Herries Davies, G.L. and R.C. Mollan. 1980. *Richard Griffith: 1784-1878*. Dublin: Royal Dublin Society.

Holland, C.H. 1981. *A Geology of Ireland*. Edinburgh: Scottish Academic Press.

Hoppen, K.T. 1970. *The Common Scientist in the Seventeenth Century: A Study of the Dublin Philosophical Society 1683-1708*. London.

Jackson, J.S. 1966. 'Robert George Spencer Hudson 1895-1965.' *Scientific Proceedings of the Royal Dublin Society Series A, 2*: i-ix.

James, K.W. 1986. *'Dammed Nonsense!' – The Geological Career of the Third Earl of Enniskillen.* Belfast: Ulster Museum.

Kelly, P. 1992. 'From Molyneux to Berkeley: The Dublin Philosophical Society and its Legacy,' in D.S. Scott (ed.), *Treasures of the Mind: A Trinity College Dublin Quatercentenary Exhibition*. London: Sothebys.

Laudan, R. 1987. *From Mineralogy to Geology: The Foundations of a Science 1650-1830*. Chicago and London: University of Chicago Press.

MacArthur, C.W.P. 1987. 'Mineralogical and Geological Travellers in Donegal 1787-1812.' *Donegal Annual 39*: 39-57.

MacArthur, C.W.P. 1990. 'Dr Jean-François Berger of Geneva (1779-1833): From the Travelling Fund to the Wollaston Donation.' *Archives of Natural History 17*: 97-119.

McCabe, R.A. 1992. '"Learned to a Miracle": James Ussher (1581-1656),' in D.S. Scott (ed.), *Treasures of the Mind: A Trinity College Dublin Quatercentenary Exhibition*. London: Sotheby's.

M'Coy, F. 1841. *A Catalogue of the Museum of the Geological Society of Dublin*. Dublin: Hodges and Smith.

M'Coy, F. 1844. *A Synopsis of the Characters of the Carboniferous Limestone Fossils of Ireland*. Dublin: Dublin University Press.

M'Coy, F. 1846. *A Synopsis of the Characters of the Silurian Fossils of Ireland*. Dublin: Dublin University Press.

McKenna, G. 1990. 'Geological Photographs of the British Association for the Advancement of Science.' *Geology Today 6*: 157-9.

McLaughlin, P.J. 1939-40. 'Richard Kirwan.' *Studies 28*: 461-74, 593-605; *29*: 71-83, 281-300.

McMillan, N.D. 1988. 'Rev. Samuel Haughton and the Age of the Earth Controversy,' in J.R. Nudds, N.D. McMillan, D.L. Weaire and S.L. McKenna Lawlor (eds), *Science in Ireland 1800-1930: Tradition and Reform*. Dublin: Trinity College, Dublin.

Meenan, J. and D. Clarke (eds). 1981. *RDS: The Royal Dublin Society 1731-1981*. Dublin: Royal Dublin Society.

Mitchell, G.F. 1990. 'Anthony Farrington, Geomorphologist and Quaternary Geologist, 1893-1973,' in R.C. Mollan, W. Davis, and B. Finucane (eds), *More People and Places in Irish Science and Technology*. Dublin: Royal Irish Academy.

Mollan, R.C. 1990. 'Royal Dublin Society,' in R.C. Mollan, W. Davis, and B. Finucane (eds), *More People and Places in Irish Science and Technology*. Dublin: Royal Irish Academy.

Molyneux, T. 1694. 'Some Notes upon the Foregoing Account of the Giants Causeway, Serving to further illustrate the Same.' *Philosophical Transactions of the Royal Society of London 18*: 175-82.

Molyneux, T. 1697. 'A Discourse concerning the Large Horns frequently found under Ground in Ireland, concluding from them that the Great American Deer, call'd a Moose, was Common in that Island.' *Philosophical Transactions of the Royal Society of London 19*: 489-512.

Monaghan, N.T. 1993. 'Sir Karl Ludwig Metzler-Giesecke (1761-1833), Royal Mineralogist, Greenland Explorer and Museum Curator,' in E. Hoch and A.K. Brantsen (eds), *Deciphering the Natural World and the Rôle of Collections and Museums*. Copenhagen: Geologisk Museum.

Morrell, J. 1990. 'The British Association in Ireland', in R.C. Mollan, W. Davis, and B. Finucane (eds), *More People and Places in Irish Science and Technology*. Dublin: Royal Irish Academy.

Nesbitt, N. 1979. *A Museum in Belfast: A History of the Ulster Museum and its Predecessors*. Belfast: Ulster Museum.

Nimmo, A. 1825. 'On the Application of the Science of Geology to the Purposes of Practical Navigation.' *Transactions of the Royal Irish Academy 14*: 39-50.

Nudds, J.R. 1986. 'The Life and Work of John Joly.' *Irish Journal of Earth Sciences 8*: 81-94.

O'Raifeartaigh, T. (ed.). 1985. *The Royal Irish Academy: A Bicentennial History 1785-1985*. Dublin: Royal Irish Academy.

Penny, L.F. 1966. 'Early Discoverers XXIV: George William Lamplugh (1859-1926).' *Journal of Glaciology 6*: 307-9.

Pettigrew, T.H. 1979. 'William King (?1808-1886) – a Biographical Note.' *Newsletter of the Geological Curators' Group 2*: 327-9.

Pettit, S.F. 1976. 'The Royal Cork Institution: A Reflection of the Cultural Life of a City.' *Journal of the Cork Historical and Archaeological Society 81*: 70-90.

Playfair, J. 1802. *Illustrations of the Huttonian Theory of the Earth*. Edinburgh.

Praeger, R.L. 1949. *Some Irish Naturalists: A Biographical Notebook*. Dundalk: Dundalgan Press.

Quin, E.G. and T.W. Freeman. 1947. 'Some Irish Topographical Terms.' *Irish Geography 1*: 85-9.

Richardson, W. 1803. 'Account of the Whynn Dykes in the Neighbourhood of the Giant's Causeway, Ballycastle, and Belfast.' *Transactions of the Royal Irish Academy 9*: 21-43.

Richardson, W. 1806. 'On the Volcanic Theory. Part 3. Arguments against the Volcanic origin of Basalt, derived from its Arrangement in the County of Antrim, and from other Facts observed in that Country.' *Transactions of the Royal Irish Academy 10*: 87-107.

Seymour, H.J. 1944. 'The Centenary of the First Geological Survey made in Ireland.' *Economic Proceedings of the Royal Dublin Society 3*: 227-48.

Siegfried, R. and R.H. Dott, Jr. 1980. *Humphry Davy on Geology: The 1805 Lectures for the General Audience*. Madison: University of Wisconsin Press.

Somerville-Large, P. 1975. *Irish Eccentrics*. London: Hamish Hamilton.

Spearman, T.D. 1990. 'Samuel Haughton: Mathematician, Geologist, Anatomist and Physiologist – 1821-1897', in R.C. Mollan, W. Davis, and B. Finucane (eds), *More People and Places in Irish Science and Technology*. Dublin: Royal Irish Academy.

Stephens, W. and W. Fitton. 1812. *Notes on the Mineralogy of Part of the Vicinity of Dublin*. London: William Phillips.

Stewart, D. 1799. 'The Report of Donald Stewart, Itinerant Mineralogist to the Dublin Society.' *Transactions of the Dublin Society 1*: 1-142.

Stokes, W. 1807. *A Catalogue of the Minerals in the Museum of Trinity College*. Dublin: W. Watson.

Stokes, W. 1818. *A Descriptive Catalogue of the Minerals in the Systematic Collection of the Museum of Trinity College Dublin*. Dublin: [Dublin] University Press.

Sweet, J.M. 1967. 'Robert Jameson's Irish Journal, 1797.' *Annals of Science 23*: 97-126.

Tunnicliff, S.P. 1980. *A Catalogue of the Lower Palaeozoic Fossils in the Collection of Major General J.E. Portlock, R.E., LL.D., F.R.S. &c*. Belfast: Ulster Museum.

Turner, B.S. 1979. *A List of Photographs in the R.J. Welch Collection in the Ulster Museum, Volume 1: Topography and History*. Belfast: Ulster Museum.

Vaccari, E. and P.N. Wyse Jackson. 1995. 'The Fossil Fishes of Bolca and the Travels in Italy of the Irish Cleric George Graydon in 1791.' *Museologia Scientifica 4*: 57-81.

Vallance, T.G. 1978. 'Pioneers and Leaders – a Record of Australian Palaeontology in the Nineteenth Century.' *Alcheringa 2*: 243-50.

Waterhouse, G. 1933. 'Goethe, Giesecke, and Dublin.' *Proceedings of the Royal Irish Academy 41C*: 210-18.

Whittaker, A. 1991. '*The Magic Flute* cast: Geological Correlations with Mozart.' *Terra Nova 3*: 9-16.

Williams, A. 1973. 'John Kaye Charlesworth C.B.E., Hon. D.Sc. (Belf.), D.Sc. (Leeds), Ph.D (Breslau), M.R.I.A., F.R.G.S., F.G.S.' *Royal Society of Edinburgh Year Book 1972-73* (unpaginated).

Wilson, H.E. 1972. 'John Kaye Charlesworth, 1889-1972.' *Irish Naturalists' Journal 17*: 209-10.

Wilson, J. 1987. 'Joseph Wright, F.G.S., 1834-1923.' *Irish Naturalists' Journal 22*: 169-80.

Woodward, H.B. 1907. *The History of the Geological Society of London*. London: Geological Society.

Wyse Jackson, P.N. 1989. 'On Rocks and Bicycles: A Biobibliography of Grenville Arthur James Cole (1859-1924), Fifth Director of the Geological Survey of Ireland.' *Geological Survey of Ireland Bulletin 4*: 151-63.

Wyse Jackson, P.N. 1991. 'The Cycling Geologist.' *Cycle Touring and Campaigning* (June-July): 26-7.

Wyse Jackson, P.N. 1992. 'The Geological Collections of Trinity College, Dublin.' *The Geological Curator 5*: 263-74.

Wyse Jackson, P.N. 1992a. 'A Man of Invention: John Joly (1857-1933), Engineer, Physicist and Geologist,' in D.S. Scott (ed.), *Treasures of the Mind: A Trinity College Dublin Quatercentenary Exhibition*. London: Sotheby's.

Wyse Jackson, P.N. (ed.). 1994. *In Marble Halls: Geology in Trinity College, Dublin*. Dublin: Department of Geology, Trinity College.

Wyse Jackson, P.N. 1995. 'Patrick Ganly (1809-1899) and the Discovery of Evidence of Way-up in Rocks on the Dingle Peninsula.' *The Kerry Magazine 7*: 8-9.

Wyse Jackson, P.N. 1996. 'Alexander Nimmo's *On the Application of the science of Geology to the purposes of Practical Navigation* (1825): An Early Investigation of the Nature of Offshore Geology.' *Earth Sciences History 15*: 167-71.

Wyse Jackson, P.N. 1996a. 'Sir Charles Lewis Giesecke (1761-1833) and Greenland: A Recently Discovered Mineral Collection in Trinity College, Dublin.' *Irish Journal of Earth Sciences*.

Wyse Jackson, P.N. and N.T. Monaghan. 1994. 'Frederick M'Coy (*c.* 1823-1899): An Eminent Victorian Palaeontologist and his Synopses of Irish Palaeontology of 1844 and 1846.' *Geology Today 10*: 231-4.

Wyse Jackson, P.N. and E. Vaccari. 1993. 'Volcanoes and Straw Bonnets: The Graydons of Burrishoole.' *Cathair na Mart: Journal of the Westport Historical Society 13*: 90-101.

Wyse Jackson, P.N. and P.S. Wyse Jackson. 1992. 'The Irish Naturalist: 33 Years of Natural History in Ireland 1892-1924.' *Irish Naturalists' Journal 24*: 95-101.

The Kingdom of the Air:
The Progress of Meteorology

BRENDAN MCWILLIAMS

The Best of Times, the Worst of Times

Outsiders, and indeed we Irish ourselves at times, are apt to take a somewhat jaundiced view of Irish weather. John Burke of *Burke's Peerage* fame,
writing around 1880 and comparing Ireland to the island of Great Britain,
tells us: 'In climate there is little difference, other than that more rain falls,
as the country is more mountainous and exposed full to the westerly wind,
which blowing from the Atlantic Ocean prevails during the greater part of
the year. This moisture, as it has enriched the country with large and frequent rivers, and spread out a number of fair and magnificent lakes, has on
the other hand encumbered the island with an uncommon multitude of bogs
and morasses.'

If one subscribes to this despondent school, one can at least find conso-
lation by recalling that there have been times when things were considerably
worse. Climates change over the centuries, and even more so over millennia,
and the average temperature of Ireland has risen and fallen at various periods in our history to produce weather patterns very different, at times, from
those familiar to us now.

Fifteen thousand years ago the earth was in the throes of the last Ice
Age. Glaciers extended over much of North America, as well as Scandinavia,
Britain and Ireland. When this Ice Age ended about ten thousand years ago,
it was followed by a sudden warming, and by 5000 BC the average temperature in these parts was about two degrees Celsius above its present level. As
the great accumulation of ice over northern Europe gradually melted, the level of the sea rose by fifty metres to give to our island a shape not too dissimilar from that defined by its present coastline.

There was a short, sharp shock about three thousand years ago: a
change to much colder conditions took place over a relatively short period
around 1000 BC, and the drop in average temperature was accompanied by a

general increase in storminess and rainfall. But this deterioration lasted for a mere millennium; by the early centuries AD, the climate was not significantly different from that which we know today. This trend towards warmer weather continued through the Dark and Middle Ages, and by the time of the Viking settlements the average temperature over Ireland had again increased to about one degree above present-day values. Our ancestors enjoyed conditions unusually congenial for this island, and across the channel the Normans, newly arrived in the south of England, drank wine from English vineyards (Lamb, 1982).

Even then, however, Irish weather was not totally benign. It was during this period that there occurred a disaster remembered in both song and story as 'St Maury's Wind' – a violent storm that reached Dublin on the feast of that saint on 15 January 1362. A contemporary chronicler described it as 'A vehement wind, which shook and threw to the ground steeples, chimneys and other higher buildings, trees beyond number and divers belfries and the bell tower of the Friars Preachers' Church in Dublin' (Dixon, 1954). This unwelcome event was the subject of a long poem by one John Harding – a work, it must be said, that is appreciated more for its antiquity and the information it contains than for artistic merit or the author's rhyming skill:

> In that same yere was on Saint Maury's day
> The greate winde and earthquake marvelous,
> That greatly gan the people all affraye,
> So dredfull was it then, and perelous,
> Specially the wind was so boisterous,
> That stone walles, steples, houses and trees
> Were blown doune in diverse farre countrees.
>
> (Dixon, 1954)

Harding's narrative extends to some considerable length. His reference to earthquakes, incidentally, should not be taken literally: it was common at the time for observers to assume that a coincident earthquake was responsible for the violent vibrations often experienced during severe gales.

Coping with a 'Little Ice Age'

Perhaps St Maury's Wind was the beginning of the end of that climatic golden age. In any event, during the next few centuries conditions once again became colder and often wetter, and the period from about 1450 to 1850 is remembered as the 'Little Ice Age', which reached its peak in the freezing decades of the 1690s. The summers were short, the winters long and severe, and average temperatures were a degree or more lower than before or since. The winter scenes with copious amounts of snow depicted by artists of the time contrast sharply with even the worst conditions we experience now. (See, for example, the paintings of Hendrick Avercamp, often used on Christmas cards; the images of the frozen Thames in the late seventeenth century portrayed by Abraham Hondius; and 'Hunters in the Snow' by Brueghel the Elder, a scene painted in the very severe winter of 1564/65 that started a whole new artistic tradition.)

The cold weather infused itself into the spirit of the times. In 1786, for example, the leader-writer of *Faulkner's Dublin Journal* was moved to proclaim: 'The pernicious custom of throwing snowballs has arrived at an intolerable height. No less than a dozen decent persons have been desperately wounded by stones and brickbats wrapped up in these missile weapons of barbarous amusement.' And in the following year, the *Dublin Chronicle* was more provocatively vociferous on the same subject: 'A gentleman passing through Marybone Lane was hit by a fellow in the face with a large snowball, upon which he immediately pulled out a pistol, pursued the man, and shot him dead. Those deluded persons are therefore cautioned against such practices, as in similar circumstances they are liable, by Act of Parliament, to be shot without any prosecution or damage accruing to the person who should fire.' Nonetheless, there was a good side to the colder weather: during the long winters, ice-skating was very much in vogue, and the populace could disport themselves upon the frozen rivers in a way that is impossible today (Dixon, 1954).

Towards the end of the Little Ice Age, on 6 January 1839, there occurred another storm of sufficient magnitude that folk-memories of its great ferocity still survive: *Oíche na Gaoithe Móire* – 'The Night of the Big Wind'. Retrospectively, it is clear that the 'Big Wind' was caused by a very deep depression that originated on the Atlantic and passed eastwards just to the north of Ireland and Scotland. But at the time more sinister forces were feared to be at work. Some saw the storm as a precursor of the Day of Judgment, a sharp reminder on the part of the Almighty of the wrath of God which may await mankind when the final trumpet sounds. Others were of the view that the Freemasons were behind it, that they had called the Devil out of hell and failed to get him back again. And others again blamed the fairies: their notion was that the English fairies had invaded Ireland, and that the indigenous Little People had to raise a ferocious wind to blow them out again.

Be all that as it may, it can be argued convincingly that *Oíche na Gaoithe Móire* was the worst storm ever to have affected Ireland; certainly the damage to life and property was exceptional by any standard (Shields and Fitzgerald, 1989; Carr, 1991). Dublin after the storm was described as resembling 'a sacked city'. The Liffey rose many feet to overflow the quay walls, and the splendid avenue of elms that graced the main thoroughfare of the Phoenix Park was completely levelled. In Loughrea, Co. Galway, 103 houses were destroyed, and great distress was caused to the farming community throughout the country by the loss of virtually all their cattle fodder. More than a hundred people died, either crushed by falling masonry or swept away in the floods that accompanied the raging winds. One of the incidental consequences of the storm was the total collapse of the price of lumber, as what had previously been a valuable commodity became practically worthless overnight through over-supply (Shields and Fitzgerald, 1989).

A few years later there occurred another weather-related disaster whose scars Ireland still bears. By the middle of the nineteenth century the potato, for various reasons, had become virtually the sole means of nourishment of the vast majority of the population of Ireland. If anything were to happen to cause a failure of this crop, the result would be disaster. And that is precisely what occurred in 1845 with the Great Famine.

Although a great many social and political factors contributed to the strange and terrible events of 1845 and thereafter, the immediate cause was a specific combination of meteorological conditions. The weather during the years leading up to 1845 was ideal for the spread of potato blight, a fungal disease that thrives only when high temperature and very high relative humidity coincide. For the fungal spores to infect the potato plant, three conditions must prevail over an extended period: the leaves must be wet, the relative humidity must exceed 90 per cent, and the temperature must be greater than 10°C. Such weather was a frequent visitor to northern Europe in the early summer of 1845. The blight first appeared in Belgium in late June, and by mid-August it had spread to northern France and southern England. By September 1845 it had reached Ireland. On continental Europe and in Britain the following summers were dry and hot, so the blight died out; but in Ireland the weather was abnormally wet and warm, and the blight was enabled to thrive for several years (Bourke, 1993).

A Not Unpleasant Land

The warm conditions that facilitated the potato blight heralded yet another change in thermal direction on the island: from 1850 to the middle of the present century the average temperature over Ireland gradually increased, the total rise over the period amounting to about half a degree Celsius. From the late 1940s, and continuing to the end of the 1970s, the average showed a small but persistent tendency to fall, and this cooling has been followed during the 1980s and early 1990s by a certain ambiguity of trend – something of an anomaly in a period when the rest of the world has been inclined to panic about global warming.

Nowadays we live on an island whose temperature averaged over the year is in the region of 10°C. The prevailing westerly winds that blow from the Atlantic take their temperature from the warm waters of the North Atlantic Drift that bathes our coast. They moderate the heat of summer and, even more importantly, they temper the severity of winter. The average temperature ranges from about 5° in the coldest month, January, to the pleasant warmth of July and August when we enjoy an average of near 16°. The national average rainfall is about 1100 millimetres; local rainfall varies from about 3000 mm per annum in some mountainous areas of the west to 800 mm or thereabouts in the vicinity of Dublin. The sun shines unobscured by cloud for some 1700 hours per year in the vicinity of Carnsore Point, Co. Wexford, in the extreme south-east, while the the national mean is somewhat lower – 1300 hours or thereabouts (Rohan, 1986).

There are some who will claim, with understandable hyperbole, that parts of the extreme south-west of Ireland enjoy a Mediterranean climate. The winters, after all, are very mild, frost is rare – rarer than in parts of the south of France – and a number of sub-tropical plants, like fuchsia and laurel, flourish in the region. But there are differences too. Irish summers are dull and damp by comparison with the south of France, and the average temperatures even in the warmest months are well below Mediterranean levels. A common criterion for asserting the existence of a Mediterranean climate is a thriving population of olive trees – and there are very few olive trees in County Kerry.

I rather like the way in which the Irish climate was summed up by Austin Bourke, former Director of the Irish Meteorological Service. His verdict was: 'If each country in the world could temporarily detach itself from its climate, and if the various climates were placed on show in a public place, then we Irish would without question be trampled underfoot in the headlong rush of those who wished to take ours in place of theirs.' Recognizing, however, that our regime is not without its drawbacks, Bourke goes on: 'The place of the climate in our economy is much like that of the reliable husband and good provider in the domestic scene: a little lacking perhaps in superficial glamour and gaiety as compared with some foreign Lotharios, but constituting a steady support whose contribution is not really appreciated until it is withdrawn' (Bourke, 1974).

Meteorology Looks Up

Before the days of weather forecasts, our ancestors strove hard to cope with, and make sense of, the climatic mixture they inherited. Our national saint, for example, being a man of many talents, had his own unique ways of coping with the meteorological vicissitudes of Irish life:

Saint Patrick, as in legends told,
The morning being very cold,
In order to assuage the weather,
Collected bits of ice together;
He gently breathed upon the pyre,
And every fragment blazed on fire!

(orig. unkn.)

The laity, however, had to use more orthodox methods. By observing the elements and the passing seasons very closely, they evolved rules of thumb by
which they could guess at what the future had in store for them. Their interpretation of a red sky, for example – a sign of good weather in virtually
every culture since biblical times – was tempered to the Irish climate:

Dearg anuas, fearthainn is fuacht;
Dearg anoir, fearthainn is sioc;
Dearg aníos, fearthainn is gaoth;
Dearg aniar, tuineadh is grian.

Red high up, rain and cold;
Red in the east, rain and ice;
Red low down, rain and wind;
Red in the west, fine weather and sunshine.

The significance of the location of the red, it seems, is merely to tell you
what other unpleasantness one may expect with the inevitable rain; only in
the western sky can a touch of crimson be observed with any optimism.

The behaviour of birds was also carefully watched. A flight of swallows, for example, was invariably a sign of rain, or as it was put: *Is tuar*
fearthainne ealt ainleog. A robin, on the other hand, could be either good or
bad, depending on his early-morning mood. *Má bhíonn an spideóg faoi thor*
ar maidin beidh sé ina lá fhliuch, ach má bhíonn sí ar an ghéag is airde, is í ag
gabháil cheoil, beidh sé ina lá mhaith: rain is on the way if the robin hides beneath a bush at morningtime – but if he sings from the highest branch in
the vicinity, a pleasant day can be expected.

Long-range forecasting, it seems, was the preserve of the cuckoo – a
situation which some might say has changed little in the intervening years:
Nuair a sheinneas an chuach ar chrann gan duilleóg, díol do bhó is cheannaigh
arán – 'When the cuckoo sings on a tree without a leaf, sell your cow and
buy bread.' The theory is that if the trees have not developed leaves before
the cuckoo comes, you will not have sufficient grass to feed your cow; you
should dispose of it and stock up with bread and other foods instead (Ó
Muirgheasa, 1976).

And Myles na gCopaleen (Flann O'Brien) has passed on yet another
useful tip. The narrator of his 1941 novel *An Béal Bocht* tells us that on the

night that he was born, his father sat with his friend Mháirtín Ó Bánasa atop the hen-house and observed the darkening sky: '*Féach gur olc an tuar é, a Mháirtín*', he said, '*go bhfuilid na lachain imeasc na neantóg*' – It is a woeful sign when the ducks go in among the nettles.

Our forefathers also had appropriate stories to explain periods of the year which seemed to be out of step with the smooth progression of the calendar. For example, the history of the Bó Riabhach (the brindled cow of Irish legend) should be a salutary tale for all of us: she complained too much about the weather, and came to a sad and nasty end as a result. Once upon a time, it seems, at the beginning of April the Bó Riabhach began to complain about the harshness of the previous month; March was piqued, and resolved to teach the Bó a lesson. March duly borrowed three days from April, and these were so wet and cold and stormy that the Bó Riabhach drowned in the ensuing floods. In Irish these borrowed days at the beginning of April are called *Laethanta na Bó Riabhaí*, and they are renowned for the frequent harshness of their weather.

But then a touch of belated wintry weather was not necessarily something bad:

> *Sioc soineann an earraigh*
> *Is é a líontas fearrantaí le stór;*
> *B'fhearr cith cloch shneachta i dtús an Aibreáin*
> *Ná leathadh an aigéin de ór.*

(Shields, 1986)

or roughly translated:

> Bright frosts in spring will never fail
> To bring more crops than the fields can hold;
> An early April shower of hail
> Is better than half a sea of gold.

The Pioneers of Meteorology

There was a healthy disdain in ancient times for weather forecasting:

> *Ná creid sionnach agus ná creid fiach*
> *Agus ná creid comráite mná;*
> *Pé moch no déanach a eiríonn an ghrian*
> *Is mar is toil le Dia a bheidh an lá.*

(Shields, 1986)

> Do not believe the fox or deer
> Nor women talking together;
> Be it early or late the sun may appear,
> Only God can dictate the weather.

But there were those who did not take such advice too literally, and who tried over the centuries with the best means at their disposal to build our understanding of the elements on more logical foundations. As the scientific Renaissance developed in Europe during the seventeenth century, slowly but surely its effects began to manifest themselves in Ireland. Meteorology began to develop as a science as experimental techniques were used to unravel the tangle of Nature's secret ways.

Robert Boyle, the seventh son – and fourteenth child – of the first Earl of Cork, was not a meteorologist per se, but he laid much of the basic groundwork for atmospheric studies. Boyle was born at the family seat, Lismore Castle, in 1627, and like many affluent young men of his time spent some years travelling on the continent of Europe. He came across the work of Galileo Galilei in Florence, and this appears to have whetted his appetite for scientific matters. In any event, he devoted most of the rest of his life to the study of physical phenomena. Boyle settled eventually in Oxford, and in his laboratory he succeeded in constructing air pumps that were more efficient than any that existed at the time. One of the most striking qualities of air – indeed of any gas – is its compressibility: a given amount of it can be squeezed into a smaller and smaller volume when sufficient pressure is applied. Or as Boyle himself put it: 'There is a spring, or an elastic power, in the air in which we live' (Wolfe, 1968). Boyle discovered that a *quantitative* relationship existed in these circumstances: provided the temperature remains constant, the reduction in volume experienced by a gas is exactly proportional to the amount of extra pressure applied to it. 'Boyle's Law', enunciated in 1662, became one of the fundamental cornerstones of physics; it was also a first step in understanding the dynamics of the atmosphere and is one of the basic formulae used today in numerical weather prediction. Robert Boyle also dabbled in barometers and thermometers, and made important contributions to the development of both.

Meanwhile, there were other ways of studying the weather than by carrying out experiments in a laboratory. Accurate observation of the elements themselves was also seen as a potentially fruitful avenue of enquiry, and a near contemporary of Robert Boyle, William Molyneux of Trinity College, achieved a lasting place in meteorological history by becoming Ireland's very first scientific weather observer.

Molyneux was born in 1656. His interests throughout his life were wide, and indeed he was no stranger to political controversy: only a few months before he died in 1698 he wrote *The Case of Ireland's Being Bound by Acts of Parliament in England, Stated,* a tract which attracted sufficient attention for it to be condemned by the London Parliament for being 'of dangerous tendency to the Crown and to the people of England'.

The late seventeenth century was an era of rapid development in the field of scientific instrumentation, and the potential of these new instruments for gaining an insight into the behaviour of the atmosphere quickly became apparent. Molyneux was discouraged, however, by the difficulty of acquiring them: 'I am living in a kingdom barren of all things,' he lamented in 1681, 'but especially of ingenious artificers; I am wholly destitute of instruments on which I can rely.' But the situation did improve. In March of 1684 Molyneux was able to begin a 'Weather Register' at Trinity College, which for the first time in Ireland included readings of barometric pressure. By 2 June of that year he had compiled enough material to present a paper to the Dublin Society on 'The Observations of the Weather for the Month of May, with the Winds and the Heights of the Mercury in the Baroscope'. He sent a copy of his May Register to Oxford University where it remains to this day, preserved in the Bodleian Library (Simms, 1982).

In May of the following year Molyneux handed over the exacting task of keeping weather records for Dublin to St George Ashe, later to become Provost of Trinity, and Ashe maintained the continuity for another year or so. This series of observations – although it lasted only for the two-year period 1684-6 and only a small fragment of it survives – is regarded as one of the most important milestones in the history of Irish meteorology.

Even as great advances were made in methods of meteorological observation, much about the weather and its causes remained open to pure speculation, and much of this speculation was wildly off the mark. Like many intellectuals of the time, George Berkeley (1685-1753), Bishop of Cloyne and one of the more influential philosophers of his day, had an interest in the weather. Berkeley wrote to his friend Tom Prior in Dublin:

The bulk, situation and motions of the earth are given, and the luminaries remain the same; if the weather proceeded only from such fixed and given causes, the changes thereof would be as regular as the vicissitudes of the days or the return of eclipses. To me, however, it seems that the causes of the variable winds are the subterranean fires which, constantly burning but altering their operation according to the various quantities or kinds of combustible material they happen to meet with, send up exhalations which, diversely fermenting in the atmosphere, produce uncertain variable winds and tempest. To me also it seems that nitrous exhalations produce cold and frost, and that the same causes which produce earthquakes within the earth produce the storms above it.

Berkeley's theories notwithstanding, others, with or without instruments, carried on the Molyneux tradition of direct observation of the weather. Dr John Rutty was born in Wiltshire in 1697 and moved to Dublin in 1724 after qualifying as a medical doctor. His detailed weather records compiled over the succeeding half-century are perhaps our greatest source of information on

Irish weather in the mid-1700s: *The Weather and Seasons in Dublin for Forty Years* was published in 1770, and is all the more valuable in that besides Rutty's own carefully compiled daily observations, it includes data from other weather diaries to which he had access at the time. The result is a comprehensive and detailed pen-picture of Irish weather from 1716 to 1766.

Rutty was not just an observer of the elements; he was a thinking meteorologist who put the data he collected to good use for the advancement of the science. Much of his interpretation was directed at showing that astrology or astronomy were not reliable predictors of the weather. He claimed that his long series of observations demolished 'the vulgar error of great rains at the equinoxes, showing that storms are far more frequent at other times of the year'. Any attempt to use astronomical occurrences to forecast the weather should, he said, 'be ridiculed as equally practicable and useful as fixing a sundial on a weather cock' (Rutty, 1772).

Then there was Richard Kirwan. Kirwan was born to a well-to-do family in County Galway in 1733 and, as was the custom of the time, he was sent to the Continent to complete his education. In due course he entered a seminary at Poitiers to be trained as a Jesuit but, the story goes, his elder brother was killed in a coffee-house duel in London, and Kirwan was obliged to abandon his vocation and return to Ireland as head of the Kirwan clan. One can only speculate as to how happy Kirwan might have been as a member of the Jesuits. But his commitment must be suspect: not long after his return, he found it expedient to adopt the Protestant faith so as to be able to preserve the family estates intact. In due course he qualified as a barrister, but since he enjoyed financial independence, he was able to devote his life to chemistry, mineralogy and other branches of science.

Meteorology was one of Kirwan's special interests. He made a number of original contributions to the science, publishing them in the *Transactions of the Royal Academy*. Indeed many of his ideas anticipated twentieth-century concepts: he evolved a theory of air masses, and classified them as 'polar', 'tropical' and 'marine' – ideas familiar to today's weatherpeople. One of his less enduring theories was that when air from the equator reached the poles it combusted, thus causing the *aurora borealis*. Kirwan also tried his hand at forecasting, using climatological information to predict the coming season: the story goes that his forecasts were so popular and well respected that farmers delayed their sowing until they knew the details of his latest prognostications.

But Kirwan is best remembered for the long series of weather observations he made in the garden of his house in Cavendish Row in Dublin. Others, as we have seen, had kept weather diaries, but Kirwan's observations were the first to be compiled in Ireland with the aid of a wide range of accurate instruments. Excellent records survive from 1787 to 1808, giving readings from a barometer, thermometers, a rain-gauge, and an anemometer of singular design built by Kirwan himself. The premises in Cavendish Row could well lay claim to having been Ireland's first modern weather station (Ryan, 1821).

The Captors of the Wind

While Richard Kirwan in his declining years was carefully noting the daily changes in the weather at Cavendish Row in Dublin, Sir Francis Beaufort was sitting at his desk at the Admiralty in London. It was Beaufort who devised the Beaufort Scale of Wind Force, which has survived to this day with only cosmetic changes and which is still in use throughout the world for the dissemination of wind forecasts for shipping.

Beaufort was born in 1774 into a family of French Huguenot origin in County Louth, where his father, Dr Daniel Augustus Beaufort, was the rector of a local church. At the tender age of fourteen the young Francis embarked on a naval career, his family having paid the not inconsiderable sum of a hundred guineas to enable him to do so. In due course he crowned a distinguished career by becoming Hydrographer to the Royal Navy and being knighted.

Before the invention of instruments that could measure the speed of the wind accurately, people used to guess at it – and then describe it. For hundreds of years such descriptions were purely subjective; Beaufort's great achievement in 1803 was to provide a means by which assessments could be carried out in a standardized way, so that everyone knew exactly what was meant. For the lower range of his thirteen-point scale, Beaufort took his cue from the descriptive terms traditionally used by sailors. Force 0 was a calm, Force 1 a 'light air', and Force 2 a 'slight breeze'. But for the stronger winds, he realized that he had to define his scale in terms of some well-known yardstick, just as a standard measure might be used to determine the length or weight of another object. The criterion he chose was the full-rigged battleship or 'man-o'-war' of his day. He described the winds by the effect they might have on such a vessel – and in particular the amount of sail it could carry in high winds without getting into trouble. The criteria used to define the Forces of the Beaufort Scale have been adapted over the years, but in essence the scale has changed little from that produced by the Irish Admiral almost two hundred years ago (Friendly, 1977).

The Beaufort Scale was a notable advance for the marine community, but in scientific circles the ambition was to put a number on the wind, to measure its speed accurately in miles per hour. The Rev. Thomas Romney Robinson fulfilled this need. Robinson was born in Dublin in 1792 and spent many years at Trinity College. In 1821 he forsook the groves of academe and moved to Enniskillen to fulfil his priestly duties in a rural setting. Science and religion, however, mixed easily for Robinson. So it was that in 1823 he assumed the Directorship of Armagh Observatory, and it was from there that he made his name as one of the foremost men of science of his day. While astronomy was his forte, meteorology was his second string, and he is chiefly remembered as the inventor of the 'rotating cup anemometer', the familiar whirling instrument for measuring the wind.

He completed his first working model in 1846, and it was almost identical to the instrument we know today. The anemometer is based on the principle that wind exerts more pressure on the concave side of an open hemisphere than it does on the convex surface. A bar mounted on a vertical axis and fitted with two such hemispheres – one at each end and facing in opposite directions – will rotate with the wind because of this pressure differential, and the speed at which it rotates is related to the wind speed. All you have to do is count the revolutions or arrange for the variations in the wind speed to be recorded on a chart. Modern instruments have four 'cups', and can be seen whirling around at airports and at many weather stations (Middleton, 1969).

The Admiral's Legacy

Although men like Molyneux and Kirwan had dabbled in the science, and by the middle of the nineteenth century regular weather observations were being carried out at many places on these islands, organized meteorology aimed at practical objectives did not exist at that time. Then came the 'Royal Charter Storm'. October 1859 was a very stormy month, and over two hundred vessels, large and small, were wrecked in the waters around Britain and Ireland in the last ten days of the month. Among them was the Royal Charter.

On 25 October 1859, the steamship Royal Charter called at Cobh – then Queenstown – in County Cork. It had left Melbourne, Australia, just two months before and was on its way to Liverpool with 430 passengers and crew, and a cargo of £500,000 in gold bullion. The stay in Cork was brief, and the vessel left Queenstown later that day on the final leg of its long voyage. At 3 a.m. on the 26th, a vicious storm drove the ship ashore near Moelfe on the north-east coast of the isle of Anglesea. Within five hours the ship had been dashed to pieces; a few of those on board were saved, but over four hundred persons perished in the wreck (Booth, 1970).

It was as a result of the publicity given to this tragedy, and the storm that caused it, that the head of the 'Meteorological Department' of the British Navy, Vice-Admiral Robert FitzRoy, was charged with organizing a system of 'storm warnings', which were to be sent over the newly invented electric telegraph to threatened coastal areas. It was the beginning of shipping forecasts as we understand the term today.

FitzRoy organized a network of forty weather stations around the Irish and British coastlines, which provided him with daily weather reports by telegraph. His forecasting methods were primitive by today's standards, but he was a practical man at heart. He produced the required forecasts, and instituted a system of warnings that began in February 1861. When gales were expected, warnings were telegraphed to forty ports and harbours around the country, and within thirty minutes appropriate signals were prominently displayed on shore to relay the word to passing ships. The signals were of a semaphore type: a cone pointing upwards indicated a northerly gale; a drum or cylinder warned of successive gales from many directions; and other patterns had meanings which quickly became standard and widely understood (Mellersh, 1968).

One of FitzRoy's new weather stations was on Valentia Island in County Kerry, chosen because it was the landing place of the transatlantic cables and therefore had a direct onward telegraphic link with London. At eight o'clock on the morning of 8 October 1860, the very first Irish 'real time' weather observation was transmitted from Valentia. Weather reports have been coming in a continuous stream from that part of the country ever since, albeit not from precisely the same spot.

The new observatory was at first a very modest undertaking. It occupied a rented house on the narrow strait that separates Valentia Island from the rest of Kerry, and from there the routine flow of observations continued until March 1892. It was in that year that Valentia Observatory moved across the sound to its present site on the mainland near the town of Cahirciveen, retaining its traditional name – the name by which, somewhat confusingly, it is still known.

Its new home was Westwood House, theretofore the residence of one Captain Needham, the local agent of Trinity College, which was at that time a very prominent landowner in the area. Westwood was purchased for the not inconsiderable sum of £1400, and in the succeeding years was decked out with the impressive array of scientific instruments that was in due course to make Valentia Observatory one of the most important meteorological and geophysical observatories in all of Western Europe (O'Sullivan, 1992).

Meteorology Comes of Age

As meteorology developed and forecasting techniques improved over the succeeding decades, the focus was almost entirely on safety at sea. In the twentieth century, however, the science gained a new and exciting customer in the shape of the aviation industry. To say that this new activity was weather-sensitive is an understatement: in the early 1920s the average life expectancy of a professional pilot was a mere four years, and a great many of the fatal accidents were related to bad weather. Indeed, it was the clear need to provide accurate weather information for transatlantic aviation that led to the formal establishment of an Irish Meteorological Service in 1936, and aviation dominated the activities of the new body during the following twenty-five years.

After World War II, or the Emergency as it was known in the Republic of Ireland, the Service broadened its activities. In 1948 it assumed responsibility for the weather forecasts broadcast by Radio Éireann, which had previously been supplied from London. In 1952 it began to supply forecasts to the daily newspapers, and by 1961 it was able to co-operate with Radio Teilifís Éireann in the presentation of the daily weather forecast on television. In the mid-1970s meteorology in Ireland might be said to have come of age by entering the computer era, initially employing the new machines for communications purposes, and shortly afterwards using computers for the new technique of numerical weather prediction. Today, Met Éireann, as the Irish Meteorological Service is now known, has a staff of some 250 people at sixteen locations around the country.

These weather installations are scattered over Ireland like currants on a cake, distributed more or less evenly over the surface of the island. Their *raisons d'etre* are various. Meteorological Offices at the main airports, for example, provide a wide range of facilities to civil aviation. The Central Analysis and Forecast Office at Glasnevin in Dublin makes weather forecasts, statistical information on the climate, and specialist advice available to the media, to industrial and commercial interests, and to a variety of clients in the public and private sectors. Meanwhile at Valentia Observatory, a wide range of geophysical observations is carried out: the observatory performs upper-air measurements, using a *radiosonde* attached to a hydrogen-filled balloon to obtain values of pressure, temperature and humidity many miles above the earth; it monitors variations in the earth's magnetic field over Ireland and carries out precise measurements of the radiation coming from the sun; and it operates a seismograph, which detects and records tiny vibrations that may have their origins in earthquakes halfway around the world.

Other weather stations around the country are less comprehensive in their scope, but no less vital in their role. Those at Malin Head, Belmullet, Clones, Claremorris, Birr, Rosslare, Kilkenny and Mullingar provide regular hourly reports throughout the twenty-four hours of the weather in their vicinity, and similar observations are carried out at Aldergrove in Northern Ireland. These reports, combined with similar information from all over the world, are the raw material of tomorrow's weather forecasts.

But the weather knows no geographical or political boundaries; the weather systems that affect Ireland today may have originated hundreds, or even thousands, of miles away a day or two ago. To produce the daily Irish weather forecast it is necessary to have not just reports from Irish weather stations, but similar information in 'real time' from virtually every other country in the world – a massive international co-operative effort co-ordinated by the World Meteorological Organization (WMO) in Geneva.

Times have changed since FitzRoy's day, when the observations were laboriously tapped out in the Morse code. Nowadays computers do a great deal of the work. WMO's Global Telecommunications System is a world-wide network of communications channels dedicated entirely to the international circulation of meteorological information. The 'trunk circuit' of the network, its main artery, is arranged around three World Meteorological Centres at Washington, Moscow and Sydney, and on its long meandering journey it passes through Tokyo, New Delhi, Cairo, Prague, Offenbach and Paris. It reaches its closest point to Ireland at Bracknell in England, through which weather information from Ireland speeds its way around the world in under an hour, as Irish weather reports join thousands of other observations in a vast river of data in perpetual motion around the globe. But in return the lines begin to hum in the opposite direction: forecasters in Ireland receive their payback in the form of a deluge of weather reports from every corner of the world.

The Age of Technology

Until about thirty years ago, weather forecasts were produced in much the same way as Admiral FitzRoy had assembled the material for his famous storm warnings. The weather observations were plotted on a chart with special symbols; then, noting the pressure values plotted for each station, the forecaster would draw the 'isobars', or lines joining points of equal pressure, and these would outline the anticyclones and depressions in the area of interest. Other information on the chart would allow the forecaster to identify the positions of the fronts or rainbelts. Then, using skill, experience and scientific knowledge, he or she would try to anticipate the future positions of these various features, and from this infer the likely sequence of the local weather.

Nowadays, much of this work has been taken over by computers. 'Numerical weather prediction' is based on a description of the behaviour of the atmosphere in terms of mathematical equations. Scientists know that air – as a gas – obeys certain physical laws: it expands, for example, at a certain rate when heated by a given amount. It is also possible to describe mathematically the ways in which energy changes from one form to another – from heat into motion, or vice versa.

Armed with the equations that specify these processes, and given the values of pressure and temperature at a certain spot in the atmosphere, we can calculate expected values of these parameters at some future time. If the same operation is carried out by computer for hundreds of points on the weather chart, a new weather map for some future time can be constructed. The computer moves forward step by step, hour by hour, until it arrives at a forecast four or five days ahead of the original observations.

The models used in numerical weather prediction are very complex, and are continually being refined and improved to reflect the behaviour of the real atmosphere with greater accuracy. Although the human weatherperson is still better than the computer as regards very-short-range forecasting, he is no match for the machine when it comes to predictions for several days ahead. The forecaster's expertise now lies in the skilful interpretation of the computer products; he or she must translate those mysterious lines on the chart produced by the computer into a description of the weather that will be meaningful to the person on the street.

Perhaps the most spectacular development in modern meteorology has been the advent of the satellite picture. Although a snapshot of the current cloud pattern does not provide a clear vision of the future, at least the forecaster can see where the fronts and the various depressions lie at a specific instant. When artificial satellites became a fact of life some forty years ago, someone had the idea that if a satellite's speed in an orbit over the equator were to be synchronized exactly with the rate of rotation of the planet, a spacecraft would appear to be fixed in space – a trick that can be achieved by launching the satellite in such a way that it ends up 32,000 kilometres above the equator. For meteorologists the arrangement has the advantage that successive pictures received from such a spacecraft at, say, half-hourly intervals, are taken from the same vantage point, and can therefore be combined to form a 'movie' of the evolving weather situation.

But there are also more sophisticated uses to which satellite pictures can be put. Ways are being developed of obtaining numerical values of temperature, wind and rainfall from the satellite images, and these data can then be used, along with the conventional ground-based observations, as input for the numerical models processed by computer.

In the case of rainfall, for example, the brightness and the texture of cloud patterns on a long series of satellite pictures is compared with the rainfall intensity measured by conventional rain-gauges within the satellite's field of view. The relationship between the two is then used to interpret future satellite images, so that rainfall amounts over a large area can be estimated with reasonable accuracy.

Temperatures can be obtained from infrared satellite pictures. Since these images are produced by infrared radiation rather than by the visible light of conventional pictures, the brightness of any part of the image is proportional to the temperature of the object in view. If the height of any cloud in the picture is known, the temperature at that level can be estimated. Winds at upper levels in the atmosphere are measured by comparing two satellite pictures taken, say, thirty minutes apart. The distance travelled in that time by a number of distinctive features of the cloud pattern is observed; if it is assumed that the cloud moves at the speed of the wind – often a reasonable assumption – then the wind speed at that level can be calculated.

Not all these clever techniques have been perfected; indeed scientists are still somewhat disappointed with the accuracy of many of the values they obtain. But much of the data obtained is useful, particularly over large areas of the globe where conventional observations are very sparse, and a great deal of effort is being invested in perfecting the techniques. As they improve, so too should the accuracy of our daily weather forecasts.

The Key to the Kingdom

Meteorology in Ireland has come a long way since William Molyneux began it all three hundred years ago. The tradition has been carried on by Rutty, Kirwan, Beaufort and FitzRoy, and many others, to culminate in the forecaster of the 1990s gazing at a collage of multicoloured hieroglyphs on a computer screen, his work as an individual backed up by the simultaneous effort of at least a thousand colleagues around the globe. This aspect of the science was recognized in the middle of the last century by the English art critic John Ruskin, no mean meteorologist himself:

There is one point in which the science of meteorology differs from all others. A Galileo or a Newton by the unassisted workings of his solitary mind may discover the secrets of the heavens, and form a new system of astronomy. A Davy in his lonely meditations on the crags of Cornwall, or in his solitary laboratory, might discover the most sublime mysteries of nature and trace out the intricate combinations of her elements. But the meteorologist is impotent alone; no progress can be made by the enthusiasm of the individual, because it is necessary that the many should think, observe and act simultaneously, even though separated from each other by vast distances – on the greatness of which, indeed, may well depend the ultimate utility of their undertakings.

Ruskin went on to encapsulate in a single paragraph the utter fascination of the science: 'He whose kingdom is the heavens can never meet with an uninteresting space or exhaust the phenomena of an hour; he is in a realm of perpetual change, of eternal motion, of infinite mystery. Light and darkness, cold and heat, are all to him as friends of familiar countenance – but of infinite variety of conversation; and while the geologist yearns for the mountain, the botanist for the field, and the mathematician for the study, the meteorologist is a spirit of a higher order than any, and rejoices in the kingdom of the air.'

References

Booth, B.J. 1970. 'The *Royal Charter*.' *Weather 25*: 550-3.

Bourke, A. 1974. 'The Climate of Ireland as a Natural Resource' [1972 Kane Lecture]. *Administration 21*: 365-83.

Bourke, A. 1993. *'The Visitation of God'?: The Potato and the Great Irish Famine* [Ed. J. Hill and C. Ó Gráda]. Dublin: Lilliput Press.

Burke, J. c. 1880. 'The Conquest of Ireland,' in *Half Hours of English History*, ed. C. Knight. London: Frederick Warne & Co.

Carr, P. 1991. *The Big Wind*. Belfast: White Row Press.

Dixon, F.E. 1953. 'Weather in Old Dublin.' *Dublin Historical Record 13*: 94-107.

Dixon, F.E. 1954. 'Weather in Old Dublin.' *Dublin Historical Record 15*: 65-73.

Friendly, A. 1977. *Beaufort of the Admiralty*. London: Hutchinson.

Lamb, H.H. 1982. *Climate, History and the Modern World*. London: Methuen.

Mellersh, H.E.L. 1968. *FitzRoy of the Beagle*. London: Hart-Davis.

Middleton, J. 1969. *The Invention of the Meteorological Instruments*. Baltimore: Johns Hopkins.

na gCopaleen, Myles. [1941] 1975. *An Béal Bocht*. Dublin: Dolmen Press.

Ó Muirgheasa, E. (ed.). 1976. *Seanfholail Uladh*. Baile Atha Cliath: Oifig an tSolathair.

O'Sullivan, John. 1992. *Valentia Observatory: A History of the Early Years*. Dublin: Meteorological Service.

Rohan, P.K. 1986. *The Climate of Ireland*. Dublin: Meteorological Service.

Rutty, J. 1770. *A Chronological History of the Weather and Seasons, and of the Prevailing Diseases in Dublin; With the Various Periods, Successions, and Revolutions, during the Space of Forty Years; With a Comparative View of the Difference of the Irish Climate and Diseases, and Those of England and Other Countries*. London: Robinson and Roberts.

Rutty, J. 1772. *An Essay Towards a Natural History of the County Dublin*. Dublin: Author.

Ryan, R. 1821. *Biographical Dictionary of the Worthies of Ireland*. London: John Warren.

Shields, L. 1986. 'Popular Weather Lore in Ireland.' *The Irish Meteorological Service: The First Fifty Years*. Dublin: Meteorological Service.

Shields, L. and D. Fitzgerald. 1989. 'The Night of the Big Wind in Ireland.' *Irish Geography 22*: 31-43.

Simms, J.G. 1982. *William Molyneux of Dublin*. Dublin: Irish Academic Press.

Wolfe, A. 1968. *History of Science, Technology and Philosophy in 16th and 17th Centuries*. London: George Allen and Unwin.

Woodland in History and Culture

EOIN NEESON

Early Irish Woodland

Natural or wild woodlands are now all but extinct in Ireland. True, some regenerated remnants of ancient woodland, generally scrub, are to be found here and there, but there is some doubt that even these are truly natural, some experts taking the view that they are more likely to be the residue of medieval or later forests which were at one time cultivated.

Like animals, trees may be classified in two broad groups, wild and domesticated (or natural and cultivated), with sub-divisions that extend to individual species. The point is that we take the use of woods, of timber and of wood products by man from beyond the dawn of history so much for granted that we tend to overlook the fact that the relationship between these two living organisms, man and tree, is no less complex and intimate than the relationship between man and animals.

After the last Ice Age, during which it is unlikely that any tree species survived in what became Ireland, the detritus from the retreating ice-cap provided a foothold for plant colonization. Ferns and other primitive organisms took hold and were followed by what would, for thousands of years, become the dominant species in a thickly forested environment – first dwarf birches and willows, then alder, pine and the dominant oak and elm. These were later reinforced by ash, whitebeam, cherry, poplar, apple, holly, prostrate juniper, arbutus and yew. Compared with the rest of Europe it was a restricted range of trees, due, it is thought, to the inundation that separated Ireland from the Continent between ten and twelve thousand years ago, roughly a thousand years before the arrival of man. 'European trees, like beech, lime and horse-chestnut, though perfectly at home in the Irish climate, never reached us until they were introduced from abroad in the seventeenth and eighteenth centuries' (Ross, 1980). But the native growth was sufficient to provide dense forest cover. 'It is hard for us', says Mitchell

(1976), 'to picture the majesty and silence of those primeval woods, that stretched from Ireland far across northern Europe.'

From the very earliest times there was a profound relationship between trees and political and economic development in Irish society. It began with the arrival of the first settlers – Mesolithic people (meaning those who used implements of stone and other natural substances) – between eight and ten thousand years ago. Evidence of human activity at Mount Sandel near Coleraine in County Derry has been carbon-dated to around nine thousand years ago (Woodman, 1981; Mitchell, 1976). Self evidently these people were already sufficiently skilled to build sea-going boats. Since boat-building is a derived skill, it follows that they were also experienced woodworkers. With their arrival began the association in Ireland between man and the woodland environment.

At first the impact of man on this environment was small. These Mesolithic people were hunter/fishers and gatherers, their use of wood being for their crafts – house-building, tool- and weapon-making – and for fuel. But between five and six thousand years ago these earliest settlers were joined by Neolithic farmers and the decline of forest cover accelerated. The newcomers began to clear woodlands for tillage and grazing. At that time Ireland presented a mosaic of different woodland types, depending on local soil and climatic conditions: mixed broadleaf (oak, elm and ash) on the lowlands and sheltered valleys, pines, birch and willows on poorer soils. Alder, nowadays small and confined almost entirely to watery areas, was at that time a forest tree, sometimes reaching great size. Extensive areas were cleared by felling, by deliberate fire and by grazing stock. While stone buildings of various sorts survive from this and later periods, by far the vast majority of dwellings, as in the rest of Europe, were built with timber. Places like Newgrange, and later monastic sites, were, when inhabited, surrounded by virtual townships of wood and wattle buildings. Celtic people began to arrive about 800 BC, and they appear to have brought with them a new relationship with trees, namely tree-veneration. These 'Irish' Celts do not seem to have given special veneration to the oak as did their continental cousins, but gave pride of place instead to the ash. Perhaps this is yet one more indication that the dominant Irish Celtic people did not come directly from Gaul, but, as tradition holds, via the Mediterranean, through Spain. At all events there is no evidence to suggest that the oak was worshipped or had any uniquely traditional significance in Ireland (Neeson, 1991; Joyce, 1920). The ash is what was usually meant when a *bile* or venerated tree was referred to.

Certain trees were associated with specific characteristics and emotions – the birch with love (birch-wreaths being a common love-token), the hazel with wisdom, and so on. The derivation of certain names from trees is interesting: MacCuill (Son of Hazel), MacCairthin (Son of Rowan), MacIbair

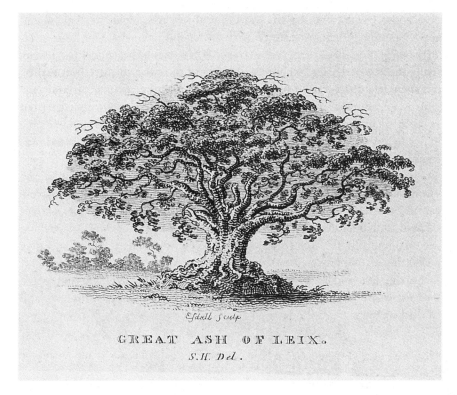

GREAT ASH OF LEIX.

S.H. Del.

(Son of Yew), MacCuilin (Son of Holly), to name a few. The common Irish word for a tree was and still is *crann* (crown). A wood is *coille* (kill or kyle), *fid* (in this context meaning sacred place or place of refuge, usually associated with the yew) or *doire* (*dirra*), specifically an oak wood. In some rural districts the branches of a rowan tree may still be placed over doors of houses and byres to deter witches and fairies alike.

So important were trees in the Gaelic/Celtic world that they are listed in the Brehon Law tracts. The Brehon Law is the ancient legal code of Ireland, 'the oldest specimens of Irish learning that have been preserved' (MacNeill, 1921). These laws accumulated over many centuries and were eventually written down. They purported to legislate for every possible contingency. In the Celtic social order there were four classes and, no doubt indicating their importance to society, trees were classified on a stratified basis (four classes with seven species to a class), replicating, according to their economic importance, the social order. This was probably determined by their average size and the use to which the timber or fruit were put. There were also laws and penalties appropriate to each class and species – e.g. the penalties (*dire*) for trees in the 'noble' group were five *scot* or two and a half milch cows, or the equivalent; for cutting a branch, a year-old heifer (Kelly, 1976).

Some species of native trees died out quite early, including the elm and the Scots pine. The elm suffered what Mitchell (1976) describes as a 'catastrophic decline' about the year AD 500. By the seventh century it had virtually disappeared. The Scots pine is thought to have vanished even earlier, but there is a difference of opinion about that. But disappear it certainly did and those examples we have today are descendants of ones imported from Scotland in the eighteenth century. By AD 300 not only were the Scots pine and elm gone or going, the ash was also under threat and bogland was beginning to increase.

Gradually man controlled and began to utilize the natural forest and woodland resources in Ireland for pasturage and agriculture, destroying forest land to make room for fields, flocks and herds. Forests were also sources of food and provided the raw materials for building, cooking (household utensils) and fighting (weaponry). Nevertheless, the extent and regenerative properties of the native forests were so great and powerful that, in spite of inroads of this and more intense kinds over the following thousand years, the greater part of the country even as late as the twelfth century was still clothed in trees.

Woodland and Medieval Ownership

Throughout all this time wood was an inescapable part of daily life everywhere. Timber was an even greater economic essential than is oil today. It was a raw material of incredible versatility in a non-technical society. Not until the extended use of coal in the nineteenth century did the now almost unimaginable dependence of communities in developed nations on woodland products began to change.

In Ireland, there was another vital aspect of woodlands that pitched them – willy-nilly – into the same bed as political and military activity. In spite of the vastness of the woodlands, in spite of their general indestructibility over millennia, in spite of the multiple uses of wood, man did not conceive ideas of possession and title until he had cut most of them down and converted the land to other uses. And it was this question of possession and title that was to become of fundamental importance in Ireland and that is vital to any appreciation of the conflict between native and imported cultures over many centuries.

Before the Norman period there was a considerable timber trade. The Danish kingdom of Dyfflynarskiri (Dublin) exported timber to treeless Iceland, Faeroe Islands and elsewhere. Dublin, Cork, Waterford, Limerick and other settlements throughout the country all had mainly timber buildings. Shipbuilding was carried on extensively at that time, as Brian Boru's fleet of over three hundred ship indicates. Tomar's Wood, near present-day

Phoenix Park, where Brian Boru was killed, is an example of a Danish woodland. The nature of Tomar's tenure is not known, but it most likely conformed to Irish law. Danish law, even in Danish holdings, did not always run, established Irish law evidently being generally found more convenient. That situation changed with the Norman invasion in 1169.

The Normans had conquered England in 1066 and the Norman laws of ownership and title that were introduced there were very different from those obtaining in Ireland. Prior to the Norman Conquest Britain was neither a unified nor a homogeneous state as, by and large, was Ireland. Britain was divided amongst the Norse, Northumbrians, Angles, Saxons and other lesser groups such as the Friesians and Jutes, that had proliferated after the collapse of the Roman Empire. It was, therefore, a relatively easy target for a powerful invader (and was one that Brian Boru himself had in mind). The Norman impact on Ireland 103 years later was different. It was an invasion, not a conquest. They came as allies of an Irish nobleman (Dermot MacMurrough, King of Leinster), and not as conquerors. In the interval between the Norman Conquest of England and the Norman invasion of Ireland, Ireland had suffered from internal struggles for power and was weaker and less unified that it had been under Brian Boru. Norman enclaves sprang up and shaky internal alliances struck an uneasy balance. Critical was the law of the land or, as it transpired, laws of land. The Normans, within their enclaves large and small, tended to proceed according to Norman ideas, while the inherent Irish legal system was, of course, well established.

Villlages were infrequent in Ireland, but there were other settlements which were sometimes as large as medieval towns. The monastery of Clonard, for instance, had more than three thousand students at one time with all the tutors, servants and necessary support required. It was probably a settlement of not fewer than ten thousand people. Accordingly, the reliance on timber would have been comparable to that of similar populations anywhere in Europe. and was underwritten in Irish law.

In England, the Normans had introduced the notion of 'forests' (a term that simply meant a large area of land, not necessarily all wooded) as areas where a special law applied. It was called Forest Law. Common Law was a second leg to the Norman legal body. Where the writ of Forest Law ran, Common Law did not, and vice versa. So important was Forest Law that at one time it applied to more than one third of all England. It was more rigorous, in both its strictures and in its penalties, than Common Law. Both were grounded in the concept of the absolute ownership of property and land. But no such concept existed in Irish law, or in Irish thinking, so far as land and consequently woodland was concerned.

The Norman idea of title to land, including woodland, was quickly in conflict with Irish law and Irish landholders. And perhaps it is well to point out that the Brehon Law (long since committed to writing) was a comprehensive and, for the time, sophisticated code, derived from ancient oral tradition. In the Celtic oral legal system 'maintenance of customary law was not due to the power of any central authority, but in fact rested on its own venerability, ritual potency and popular acceptability' (Powell, 1980).

The Irish idea of land title was very different from the Norman one of absolute ownership, and this much facilitated the Normans. When an Irish lord or king donated land to one of his subjects, he gave not ownership, but dominion subject to recall. Therefore the Irish nobleman who 'gave' land to a Norman was allowing a rescindable dominion in trust. When he learned that the Norman thought otherwise and was prepared to fight for it the Irish lord fought back, or agreed to the Norman authority under what he saw as duress. 'The feudal invaders believed that they were acquiring a rigid, complete and perpetual ownership of the land from the zenith to the uttermost depths – an ownership more complete than that of any chattel – an ownership that they imagined to be self-existing even when the person in whom it should be "vested" was, for the time being, unknown and unascertained' (MacNeill, 1921).

Under Irish law woodlands were usually common land with (in general) rights in common in each *tuath*. The tuath was the people and, by extension, the territory ruled by a king on a pyramid base – king, nobles and free commoners. There were also slaves and others, such as refugees, without status, collectively known as *fudirs*. The king was elected from within the kin of his predecessor, and it was possible to rise or fall within the social structure; for instance, a family lost the right to be considered for kingship if one of its members was not elected within five generations. In general, timber was a communally owned resource with some specific rights, regulations and penalties as to usage and abuse.

In Irish law, 'title' – for want of a better word – was essentially one of land and was vested in the tuath. As we have seen, in general it could be given only in trust to individuals. But, so far as we know, ownership of standing timber on titled land was vested in the people of the tuath as a resource through the title owned by the tuath (or sept, the extended clan or tribe). By and large, all timber was owned by all the people. When land was owned individually it was usually the gift of the king (from his sept's title), but the recipient had obligations in respect of maintenance extending to both trees and worked timber. The 'lordship' of land, as MacNeill puts it, belonged to the political rather than to the economic order and it was essentially the use of the land that was granted, not outright ownership of it.

The Norman system of forests and forest law in England produced enormous revenues for both crown and landowners. And so the concept of Forest Law and management they brought with them to Ireland was, like that of the Tudor freebooters who came later, persuasively economic.

The conflict of legal and economic systems that followed the Norman settlements encouraged political confusion and corruption and contributed to the decline of the already internally demoralized Gaelic order. It was during the medieval period that Irish forests in Norman hands were first frequently used as a source of timber supply for the English market – and of course as a source of profit for the Normans – leading to the 'el dorado' aspect of Irish woodlands, which was exploited to the extreme during the Tudor and Restoration periods.

Apart from its use as fuel, one of the chief uses of timber in Ireland was for building purposes. Since a majority of buildings was of clay and wattle, hazel was an important tree crop. Until its extraordinary and sudden devastation in a matter of only forty years at the end of the seventeenth century, it accounted for some 30 per cent of all tree species and, up to then, was one of the few trees that appears to have been purposefully cultivated and propagated, in this case mainly for wattling.

Roads and bridges, as well as houses, were among the artifacts made from wattling, as the name Baile Atha Cliath (the Ford of the Wattles) clearly demonstrates. That it was more than a simple ford in the generally accepted sense of the term is evident from the depth and span of the River Liffey as calculated for that time. Whole townships were built of wattling, though planking was also extensively used. We are told by Joyce (1920) that the hostelry or inn built at Rahane in AD 749 was of boards, and required over a thousand of them. According to Joyce the most commonly used timbers were deal, oak and yew.

Principles of profitable forest management were developed in France and were brought to England by the Normans who later tried to introduce them to Ireland, but with a similar lack of success as they experienced with Forest Law. Even if the will were there, Irish law did not provide the means to formulate a national economic policy, and Norman law could not provide an Irish one. Moreover, the optimum market for timber was England, where the demand was great and growing.

Tudor, Stuart and Commonwealth Exploitation

In spite of forest management and controlling legislation there was a timber shortage in England by Tudor times. Henry VIII's Forest Act (1543), a new Charter of the Forest, was prompted by two factors that had changed the national policy with regard to timber and woodlands. The first of these was the national requirement for shipping. This expanded as England embarked on its explosion of colonization, trade and statecraft which gave her such a powerful influence on the world stage for the next four hundred years. The Atlantic challenge by such as Drake, Raleigh and Frobisher led to a contest for the balance of power in Europe and control of the Atlantic trade routes. The second was the disclosure of corruption on a vast scale in forest administration, with a consequent grievous shortage of native timber suitable for naval requirements. Prompted by these two factors, the change of national policy in England was to have drastic and enduring effects on Irish woodlands.

At a time when sail moved the goods of the world, Ireland occupied a dominant geographic position. The prevailing winds were westerly, from the Atlantic. Whoever held Ireland had England open before them, and so as a jumping-off ground for an invasion of England Ireland could not be bettered. The strategic factors in the Tudor consideration of a conquest of Ireland were obvious. Ireland was close, it was self-sufficient, it possessed troops and, above all, it had long been hostile and resistant to England. That these things were as evident to the Tudors as they were to the Spanish, the French and the Irish, history leaves us in no doubt. The English determined to secure Ireland before it became just such a jumping-off place for an attack on themselves.

The exploitation and reduction of Irish woodlands was a natural consequence of Tudor military action and the policy of settlement – plantation – that accompanied it. In the political and social confusion that existed in Ireland throughout the fifteenth and sixteenth centuries, it was impossible for such an innovative idea as forest management to develop, much less be put into practice. Gradually forests in Ireland became what Norman Forest Law and the fractured political state of that country had prevented English forests from becoming five hundred years before the Tudor conquest: gathering places of opposition. Woodlands, in addition to being the wooden *el dorado* for the English, now became important rallying places and strongholds for the Irish – hence the common use in Ireland of the word 'fastness' to describe them. Elizabeth I, well aware of the two aspects mentioned above, expressly ordered the destruction of all woods in the country to deprive the Irish of this shelter (Brewer and Bullen, 1970).

Precautions were taken against threats to the settlers. Wolves and woodkernes, who inhabited similar ground, were bracketed together and there were rewards for both, described in 1610 by Lord Blennerhasset as the most serious dangers to colonists. He 'recommended periodic manhunts to track down the human wolves to their lairs.' (McCracken, 1971). But the principal method employed by the Tudors to conquer and subdue Ireland was systematic plantation on a vast scale. With the planters (variously called settlers or supplanters) who came after the statesmen and soldiers, came English timber speculators. While there was often friction between these elements about the uses to which Irish timber should be put, they held two views in common: namely that the forests should be exploited for profit and that they should not provide the Irish with a defence capability. The first plantation was in Laois/Offaly. Then, in Munster alone, more than half a million acres were forfeited and made available to colonists. A similar acreage was planted in Ulster a generation later. In all, of the two million acres comprising Ireland, something in the order of a million and a half were planted.

The systematic devastation of Irish woodlands followed rapidly on the unexpected defeat of the combined Irish and Spanish forces at Kinsale in 1601. As a result the substantially forested Ireland of 1600 had by 1711 become a treeless wilderness and a net importer of timber. 'They had not left wood enough to make a toothpick in many places ...', according to the Chevalier de la Latocnaye in *A Frenchman's Walk Through Ireland* (1798).

Thus was introduced a pattern that accelerated dramatically during the sixteenth and seventeenth centuries, when forests were felled indiscriminately for profit and because they were refuges for Irish soldiers (hence the coinage of the term 'woodkerne'). Whereas the Normans had acclimatized to a considerable degree and adopted, or partly adopted, some Irish customs, including native laws, the Tudor conquistadors neither sympathized with nor attempted to understand what they considered primitive customs, rather than laws, of savages. The opposition to the Tudor Conquest throughout the sixteenth century enlarged the role of forests as strongholds for the Irish. They became dominant features – as Elizabethan directives indicate – for both Irish leaders and English colonists: for the one, secure rallying places, for the other, places of fearful ambush – and also of vast potential wealth. They remained an important strategic feature until the end of the seventeenth century.

Great numbers of 'undertakers' – English or Scots planters on forfeited lands who 'undertook' certain developments, or acquired a franchise to do so – spread across Ireland throughout the sixteenth and seventeenth centuries, felling woodland at an incredible rate. So profitable was timber that it was often the case that the amount for which an estate was bought was recovered in full from the sale of the timber, thus 'making the feathers pay for the goose', as the contemporary phrase had it. In order to mislead the English authorities as to the true worth of Irish woodlands, reports such as the following disingenuous example (from Co. Down) were submitted by undertakers who had no wish to see their vast profits taxed or diverted elsewhere: 'Whereas any woddes do signify in these plattes ye underwoodes as hazle, holye, alder, elder, throne, crabtree and byrch with such Iyk, but no great hoke, nayther great buylding timber, and the mountayne top ys barynge save onlye for firres [furze] and small thrones [thorns].'* At the same

---

*Note in State Papers Office, London, accompanying map of Co. Down dated 1566. Cf. McCracken, 1971.

time, officials were submitting reports from all over the country commenting on the incredible quantity and quality of the timber to be found.

The English government became so alarmed at the obvious financial and material losses to the exchequer that it had Irish woodlands surveyed by one Philip Cottingham in 1608 and again in 1623. He first surveyed Wexford and part of Waterford and then part of Connacht. The essence of Cottingham's reports was that the country abounded in timber, mainly 'noble oaks' fit for shipbuilding, that were, instead and contrary to the law, being riven up to make staves for barrels. One need only consider the goods that it was then necessary to barrel to realize that this was a far more profitable enterprise.

While Irish forests were being despoiled and not replanted under the effects of the twin policies of profit and prevention of their use by native armies, profound political changes in England in the sixteenth and seventeenth centuries affected forests and economics there. New laws were introduced concerning the predominant place of timber in the national economy. The extent to which between 1550 and 1862 the political and economic fortunes of nations depended on a continuing supply of timber is hardly realized today. As Robert Greenhaugh Albion (1926) wrote, 'The relationship of ship timber to sea-power gave it [timber] an importance far above ordinary articles of commerce .... In all the maritime nations of that period, the preservation of ship timber was the chief aim of forest policy.' It was an era of international maritime rivalry, of great wooden ships and of colonization, a major aim of which was to secure fresh woodland resources. There was a clear relationship among sea-power, timber, and economic and political dominance. That being so, coupled with the abundance of forests and cheap timber and the absence of any forest policy in Ireland, it is not to be wondered at that the settlers and undertakers exploited the situation to the hilt.

So while Ireland was conquered and colonized by the Tudors primarily for strategic reasons, the relationship between timber and economic dominance also played a profound part in subsequent historical development. In that sense, policy in Ireland was a prototype for basic English policy in the colonization of Canada and New England, namely to secure the timber supply. One of the inducements offered to the City of London Guilds, for instance, for participation in the plantation of Ulster was the availability and abundance of wood for housing. In 1610 each planter was given two hundred good oaks to make timber for such buildings as he wished to erect (McCracken, 1971). Even as late as the nineteenth century, when replanting had been in progress for more than eighty years, the effects of the deforestation were obvious and another French visitor was able to write: 'The most striking thing on first sight of the Irish landscape is the total absence of trees of any kind. They are seen only in private parks' (Grousset, 1887).

Among the Munster planters were Walter Raleigh and Edmund Spenser. The latter wrote in *The Faerie Queene*:

> Whylom when Ireland ...
> ... that is soveraine Queene profest
> Of woods and forests, which therein abound,
> Sprinkled with wholsom waters, more than most on ground.

(Spenser, 1679)

Raleigh received twenty thousand acres, which he later sold to Richard Boyle, Earl of Cork, one of the greatest exploiters of all, for £1500 – only one third of which was paid.

In addition to the almost continuous warfare that turned Ireland into one vast battlefield from the Tudor conquest and throughout the Stuart and Commonwealth periods, woodland despoliation for profit continued. After the civil war in England, which caused much damage to the forests of that country, Cromwell turned his attention to Ireland, and not only in the military sense; he 'did not fail to grasp the important commercial question of the value of the still existing Irish forests' (Lyons, 1883).

From the mid-seventeenth century onwards industrial development began to reduce forests very rapidly. There was scarcely a conceivable industry in which furnaces, each of which consumed huge quantities of timber, were not active, often both day and night. The iron industry was unquestionably the major industrial predator of Irish woodlands at this time. The use of iron, and not only for cannon and other weaponry, was increasing everywhere. It took the entire crop of a one-acre coppice of oak to provide one ton of charcoal, and it took two-and-a-quarter tons of charcoal to make one ton of iron. With the raw material costing so much less in Ireland, Irish iron could be marketed very competitively. The demand for ships and houses and for barrel staves increased. The manufacture of furniture and of household utensils – plates, mugs, dishes, bowls, tankards, ladles, pails, forks, handles and so on – required considerable quantities of wood. But the greatest demand on woodlands was for fuel. Throughout most of Europe in the sixteenth and seventeenth centuries technological advances had brought with them such huge increases in the consumption of wood that whole nations were forced to become borrowers to finance production – and vast fortunes were made as a consequence, not least from the woodlands of Ireland.

There is another disheartening aspect to the forest devastation of the seventeenth century. Although I am not aware of any detailed historical study of the relationship, it is clear that the destruction of the woodlands had a profound impact on associated wildlife. Some species which subsequently disappeared – the wolf, different species of eagle and other birds of prey, the wild cat and other creatures – were undoubtedly affected by the gross alteration of habitat, but to what extent is not clear.

In spite of the explosion of timber use throughout Europe during these centuries, England was not to the forefront of forestry development. Where England lagged, Ireland received no consideration and timber continued to go up in smoke and out of the country as fast as it could be brought to the furnaces and the ships. At the beginning of the seventeenth century most exported timber went to France and Spain. According to McCracken (1971), the forests of Cork and Kerry 'were used to cask nearly all the wine that France and (to a lesser extent) Spain would produce'.

But the vast amount of staves exported for this purpose cannot have compared with the incalculable amount used for staves for other purposes. The woods of Glenconkyne and Killetra in Tyrone and Derry, earmarked by the crown to provide timber only for the proposed plantation of Derry by the City of London Companions, were wiped out by the stave trade; the amount of timber cut and exported for staves would have built the cities of Derry and Coleraine several times over. Even the East India Company, which had bought the woods along the Kinsale river for its shipbuilding illegally used more of this timber for pipe-staves than it did for the intended purpose. Because of protectionist prohibition on the export of live cattle from Ireland to England, Irish exporters turned to salted provisions, with a consequent increase in the demand for barrels.

Following the great fire of London in 1666 the demand for Irish timber for building purposes there increased. Together with building demands at home – small half-timbered, English-style towns and villages were quite common in seventeenth-century Ireland – this placed additional demands on supplies. After the London fire a law was passed prohibiting the building of houses in Dublin from wood, which was, in any case, now scarce and expensive. This extraordinary decline in Irish timber resources in little more than one hundred years seems to have had related social effects.

While debarking trees for tanning was forbidden in 1628 and 1634, it seems less likely to have been a conservation measure than an attempt to reserve the timber for other purposes, for which debarking would render it useless. Legislation intended to offset this was eventually introduced. But the effect was the opposite. The Act encouraged landowners to deprive the peasantry of essential firing and building materials, which they themselves then exploited. In 1698 legislation to grow more trees was introduced. It was the first of seventeen Acts which were belated and inadequate so far as halting the destruction of the previous hundred years was concerned, and which were intended more to protect England's strategic and economic requirements than to protect Irish timber sources.

Between 1680 and 1700 (Mitchell, 1965) there was a remarkable and inexplicable nationwide decline in hazel growth. It is, however, possible to suggest a plausible reason for this sudden decline. Hazel was the tree most used for wattling and was, therefore, in great demand in Ireland for traditional building of all kinds. In 1705 the use of saplings for wattling was forbidden. This was, presumably, part of the Anglicization policy which outlawed Irish usage and custom. The rapidity of the decline and the time at which it occurred also suggest that the law was little more than a legal convenience enabling the hazel woods to become what was now scarce – fuel timber. In any event the practical effect was to deprive the rural population of its customary building material, prevent its cultivation and provide an additional short-term source of industrial fuel. To the problems resulting from the lack of earlier compulsory re-planting and preventive legislation was added a rapidly growing population, now without the traditional means of building. It may be from then that the mud and sod huts that so disfigured the landscape and the social order of the period proliferated. Some experimental planting occurred about this time, but it was, of course, confined to the great estates, giving rise to what I have elsewhere called 'Estate Forestry' (Neeson, 1991).

Reafforestation 1765-1845

There is no doubt that there were extensive forests in Ireland before 1600, and there is no doubt that these were gone by 1800. The descendants of the planters who had effectively deforested the country often inherited large estates of confiscated and treeless land. During the eighteenth century planter owners became suffficiently secure and confident to seek to improve their bare lands with trees. Afforestation had become a minor craze in England, where modern ideas of silviculture and management had at last been imported from the Continent. Some Irish landowners also began to appreciate the importance of applying principles of forest management. So began elementary timber management.

Landowners devoted time and money to planting, seeding and growing. Books about woodlands and timber growing were published, not least one in 1794 by Samuel Hayes, owner of the well-wooded estate at Avondale in Co. Wicklow: *A Practical Treatise on Planting, and the Management of Woods and Coppices*. It is not without interest that from then Avondale was to feature significantly in forestry development up to the present day. Hayes, a member of the Irish House of Commons, was also a founder member of the Botanical Gardens in Dublin.

The Dublin Society, which later became the Royal Dublin Society, encouraged tree planting and between 1766 and 1806 some 25,000,000 trees were planted as a result of this encouragement. In 1765 planting premiums and medals were introduced for certain species, but the practice was open to abuse and was later abandoned because of corruption. Obviously, while they did some good in improving the situation, these schemes were insufficient and were clearly elitist, being of little concern to the ordinary people and the exploitation of centuries had left devastation too great to be repaired by private means. By 1801 there were still only 132,000 acres of woodland in the country. The Act of Union in 1800 made the situation worse rather than better, one by-product being Parliament's reduction in votes-in-aid to the RDS. One larger consequence of the Act was the linking of a rich country with one that was poor as a result of trade restrictions, exploitation and repression by the former. London now became the capital, attracting Irish landlords from their estates and, instead of prospering, the country became steadily more impoverished as rent-capital drained from it.

Apart from its requirements for building, staving, fuel and ship-building, wood still remained an all-pervading commodity in a society lacking such modern items as plastic, paper-bags, wire, tinfoil, reinforced concrete and so on. Raffia bags, cane baskets, buckets, casks and mugs were produced on an incredible scale. Timber merchants proliferated, over 150 of them in Dublin alone between the years 1750 and 1800, some of them women. One, Bridget Moss, after the death of her husband in 1758, ran her yard in Golden Lane until 1786 (McCracken, 1971). Yet in spite of difficulties, planting continued privately and by 1845 the woodland acreage had increased to 345,000.

But a new, interesting, and enduring element was strikingly evident. While most early estate planting was for shelter belts, orchards and avenues, it progressed to the planting of acorns in compliance with commercial and strategic requirements. Then it began to include other species – ash, beech, sycamore and elm. For instance, the elms that graced the canal banks in Dublin (until most of them were felled because of Dutch elm disease in the 1970s) were planted in order to provide conduits for the city's water system. Finally larch and other conifers, most of them 'exotic' or non-native species, began to appear.

From Shipbuilding to Silviculture

It is generally, and incorrectly, believed that Irish woodlands were devastated in order to provide timber for shipbuilding. The provision of timber for this purpose was an important element of English policy and did contribute to the general destruction of Irish forests, but, as we have seen, it was by no means the principal cause. A ship of the line took about five years to build and a 74-gun ship consumed about two thousand large trees of about two tons each, the equivalent of clearing a woodland of fifty acres of wellgrown timber. Throughout the Elizabethan period and until the decline of timber ships, Irish timber went for shipbuilding to England, but ships, usually small

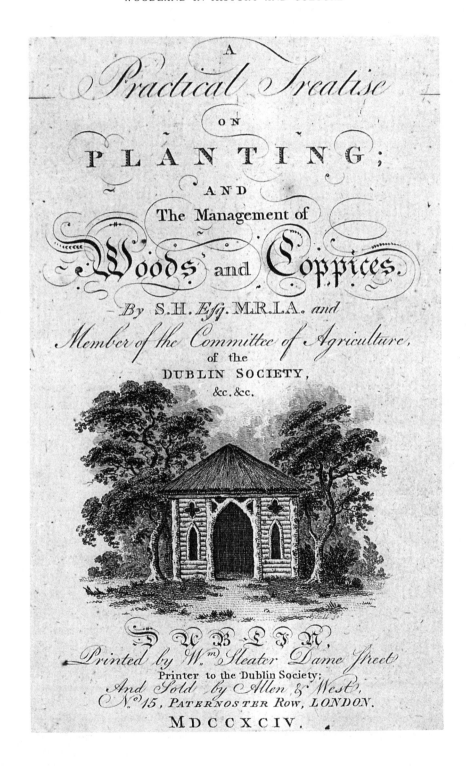

A

Practical Treatise

ON

PLANTING;

AND

The Management of

𝔚𝔬𝔬𝔡𝔰 and ℭ𝔬𝔭𝔭𝔦𝔠𝔢𝔰.

By S.H. *Esq.* M.R.I.A. *and*

Member of the Committee of Agriculture,

of the

DUBLIN SOCIETY,

&c. &c.

𝔇𝔘𝔅𝔏𝔦𝔑,

Printed by Wᵐ Sleater Dame Street

Printer to the Dublin Society;

And Sold by Allen & West,

№ 15, PATERNOSTER Row, LONDON.

MDCCXCIV.

merchant ships, were also built in Ireland. In 1613 the East India Company built ships of five hundred tons burden at Dundaniel in Cork, and Sir Arthur Chichester wrote: 'The Irish build very good ships .... Many of our English merchants choose to build here, for foreign trade especially; their oak is very good and they have a very good store of it' (Brewer and Bullen, 1970). Chichester also reported that the woods of Shillelagh, Co. Wicklow, were sufficient for the King's ships for twenty years. More than five hundred ships totalling 23,500 tons are known to have been built in Ireland between 1778 and 1800. But this, of course, did not begin to compare with the shipbuilding output of England.

The four main shipbuilding families in Dublin in the late eighteenth century were the Kinches, the Murphys, the Kehoes and the Cardiffs and, in 1778, they faced a strike from workers who threatened to emigrate unless their wages were brought into line with the wages of their English counterparts at three shillings a day. The shipyard of Ritchies flourished in eighteenth-century Belfast, and laid the keel of the shipbuilding tradition for which that city became famous.

Some smaller types of Irish vessel survived into the twentieth century, notably the small trading and fishing boats that very often serviced coastal towns when provision by road was both difficult and expensive. Of these the Connemara Hooker is probably the best known. But there were many similar vessels, with local variations, from Mayo to Kinsale. Towns such as Arklow on the east coast, adjacent to an abundant timber supply, produced a tradition of shipbuilding in the forty- to eighty-foot class that still survives. One of the last wooden vessels built in Arklow was the training ship *Asgard* which was so successful in the international tall ships' races.

By and large English oak was reserved for naval use, but during the nineteenth century imported timber replaced oak for shipbuilding in many countries, not only because oak was very scarce but also because imported timber was cheaper. It also became clear that other species besides oak were suitable commercial timber for most purposes. Thus the first great blow to the oak forests and the oak trade was struck. In the eighteenth and nineteenth centuries species of North American conifer were introduced which proved to be extraordinarily versatile. This was at a time when the British navy outnumbered the combined navies of the rest of the world and when the financial year had closed on what was 'without doubt the maximum timber purchase by the English navy on record' (Albion, 1926) and shortly after the navy commissioners in Britain had proposed a system of providing adequate supplies of oak for the navy 'indefinitely'.

The second blow was also delivered from America when in March 1862, a two-day battle took place in the 'Hampton Roads' that separated Newport from Norfolk in Virginia, between the iron-clads *Monitor* and

Merrimac, respectively Union and Confederate ships. The battle altered fundamentally the whole course of naval architecture and helped to end traditional ship and naval design. It also helped to bring to an end Britain's four hundred-year-old forest and economic policy, based mainly on the cultivation of oak, as it was immediately realized that unless the navy converted to iron-clads, then its role as a great sea power was over. 'We have learned what if two months ago any man had asserted he would have been scouted as a lunatic; we have learned that the boasted navy of Great Britain, when opposed to iron vessels, is useless as a fighting navy' (Parliamentary Debates, 1862, clxvi).

The first Irish forest policy coincided with this sudden demise of oak as the basic economic forest crop. Before the nineteenth century was out conifers would be accepted as more economically viable than broadleaves and would become the dominant tree crop.

Few subjects have given rise in recent years to so much ill-informed controversy and comment as has forestry. Even those who should know better still argue that conifer plantations are the brain-child of State forest services dedicated to planting commercial softwoods only, to the exclusion of hardwood species. That is far from being correct. There were, and are, powerful economic arguments in favour of conifer planting. Hardwoods continue to be planted both South and North, though for practical reasons not on the same scale as conifers. In recent years there appears to be some evidence that large-scale conifer plantations can be environmentally detrimental. But Michael Viney's defence of the conifer position is unequivocal: 'the kind of land available for planting and the prevailing appetite of the world's timber industry both demand softwood. Ireland has, in fact, been very lucky in this coincidence of potential and demand. Even if we could afford to wait for the hardwood trees ... they just wouldn't grow on the kind of land we can spare for forestry' (Viney, 1966). While one might not entirely agree with this wholeheartedly pragmatic espousal of conifers, the facts Viney states are broadly correct.

Conifers were introduced initially towards the end of the eighteenth century in accordance with the new thinking on afforestation in Europe. It was a process that accelerated when the oak forests of Britain were rendered virtually commercially useless. At no time did conifers supplant existing native hardwoods, by then all but extinct. Today there are more hardwood plantations and more hardwood trees growing in this country than at any time since the mid-seventeenth century. It is, of course, not enough.

Paradoxically, because of the earlier devastation experimental woodland development in Ireland was feasible. New ideas and techniques could be used without disrupting established traditions. Hence the early interest in conifers. For the obvious reason that there was no oak left, the effects of the 'oak-crisis' on Ireland were less dramatic. But its demise in England as a commercial timber coincided with the emergence in Ireland of a positive attitude to, and incipient policy on, forestry. The opportunity then presented itself to encourage afforestation according to new principles of management and silviculture with conifer as the dominant species. Douglas fir and Sitka spruce were shown to respond favourably in the Irish climate and yield large volumes.

Afforestation and Politics

However, this revived interest in forestry by the landowning elite came to be seen by the deprived peasantry and smallholders not as a means of reviving a natural national capital asset, but as yet another means of depriving them of the use of land rightfully theirs. Not unnaturally this helped entrench an enduring hostility on the part of the smallholder towards afforestation. Forestry meant landowners and gentry and, for the majority of the people, 'landowners' and 'gentry' meant 'foreigners' and 'grabbers'. The Famine devastated and halved the population of about nine million and helped strengthen the hunger for rights, prominent among these being the right of ownership of land. At the same time arose land agitation and the movement towards justice for rights of the smallholder, a movement continued in the Land Acts that, paradoxically, were to prove nearly disastrous for woodlands. The nineteenth century also saw a powerful resurgence of the spirit of national self-determination, chiefly among the Catholic population. Republican and social ideas were spread – again ironically – through the imposed medium of English. Mutilation and cutting of trees became a common form of protest. General hostility to woodlands amongst the farming community, although the reasons for it altered, did not diminish significantly for almost a century.

Once again new laws, the liberalizing Land Acts, encouraged timber clearance at an alarming rate. The Land Act of 1881 enabled land to be transferred from landlord to tenant, complete with standing timber. Both new owners and vendors found it convenient to sell plantations for additional cash – the feathers, this time, not only paying for the goose, but also increasing its value, landlords selling for additional profit before the sale of land, new owners selling after purchase to recoup some of their outlay. With the passing of the Land Act of 1903 land transfers took place on a greater scale than ever and much timber was sold to travelling sawmills. Some 874 official sawmills were active, and the woodland area in the country, estimated at a mere 1.5 per cent of the total land area, was shrinking ruinously, what was left being of indifferent material.

It was against such a background of political and land agitation, and in the aftermath of starvation, that the early fumbling steps in cohesive national managed forest planning emerged.

In the years between 1889 and 1900 decisive events took place affecting the fortunes of Irish woodlands. In England, German experts who had served in the Indian Forest Service began to put new thinking about afforestation to work. The problem was that the new thinking indicated the need for new forests and action at government level. The idea of state forestry was thus conceived. In England only old forests in private hands were available, but Ireland offered a suitable testing ground for experimentation. Land and labour were cheaply available.* It would also be good for Irish woodland development. The so-called Knockboy Experiment of 1889 to 1898 resulted. It was the first attempt at state afforestation, in the modern sense, in these islands and it was a fiasco that might have halted reafforestation in Ireland there and then. Fortunately it did not. Although it failed, it was a failure with important positive features. It focused political and administrative attention on afforestation in general and on state afforestation in particular.

The problem with the experiment was divided into three parts. Firstly, the land in Co. Galway, though recommended by the Irish Land Commission, was unsuitable; secondly, it was planted and replanted over ten years with a mixture of unsuitable species that failed; and finally, wholly inadequate research was undertaken. Unfortunately, the whole project had been the subject of a prolonged and bitter controversy between two forestry specialists, one a German, William Schlich, and the other a Dane, Daniel Howitz.

In spite of these difficulties, forestry was now seen as an important, even vital resource, and interest in it did not flag. Planting continued elsewhere and by 1914 some foreign species of conifer had reached a size and age that demonstrated both their value as timber trees and their ability to grow successfully on poor land. These successful species were mainly Sitka spruce, Douglas fir, the giant silver fir, western red cedar and Japanese larch. In 1899 the Department of Agriculture and Technical Instruction (DATI), with responsibility for forestry, was formed. But, just as matters seemed ready to progress, two major difficulties followed hard on the heels of one another.

The first of these was World War I, which considerably reduced nineteenth-century plantings. The second was the coming into existence, in 1922, of Saorstát Éireann (The Irish Free State). In 1904, before either of these, DATI bought Samuel Hayes's and Parnell's old home at Avondale and established a forestry school there. It opened in 1906 with, as its head, A.C. Forbes. In 1908 a national commission issued a seminal report on Irish forestry which (in both its correct and incorrect interpretations), was to have

---

* Day-wages for 'an ordinary labourer' in England, Scotland, Wales, and Ireland in 1883 were, respectively: 2/6d-4/-; 2/4d-3/4d; 2/4d-2/10d; 1/6d-1/10d.

a profound effect on the future of Irish woodlands. The 1908 Report recommended a comprehensive national scheme of forestry to be carried out
under the direction of the State with the object of creating not less than one
million acres of woodland in eighty years. This national scheme was envisaged as consisting of about 25 per cent state woodlands, the remainder private or local authority forest.

Land was bought in Tipperary and Wexford. But a major and lasting
difficulty was how to persuade farmers to plant trees on marginal – or any
– land, when trees provided no return for fifteen years and then only a
minuscule one, with profit a further thirty to forty years ahead.

The diffficulty of providing the vast funding required to start afforestation on such a scale also emerged early on. By 1914 the government had
acquired a mere 15,000 acres of the projected 50,000 and the First World
War was to reverse some of the progress that had taken place. Forbes became
responsible for timber supply and control in Ireland. Avondale was closed
and 30,000 acres of woodlands were felled. The strategic importance of timber stock was emphasized when David Lloyd George later declared that
Britain had come closer to losing the war for lack of timber than for lack of
food.

After the executions following the 1916 Easter Rising the explosion of
nationalist feeling, both political and military, included forestry, which was
seen – sometimes in an over-enthusiastic and uninformed way – as a kind
of national panacea that would solve a multitude of social and economic
problems. By 1918 it was clear that events were in train that, come what
might, would affect the future of the country. In 1919 a new Forest Act
came into effect in the United Kingdom. It incorporated, amongst other
matters, a new forest policy based on the modern concept of state forestry
first undertaken in Ireland. Implementation of the Act in Ireland was
delayed, and then shelved, because of the War of Independence, the coming into being of Saorstát Éireann and the Civil War.

Woodland since 1922

In accordance with the provisions of the Treaty of December 1921, on 1
April 1922 matters affecting woodlands and forestry were handed over either
to the Provisional Government (which functioned between the signing of the
Treaty and birth of Saorstát Éireann) or to the Government of Northern
Ireland. There were then less than 250,000 acres of woodland in Saorstát
Éireann and about 44,000 in Northern Ireland, mostly in private hands.
From then on, in both parts of Ireland, woodlands developed mainly as state
enterprise with the emphasis on commercial conifer production, but
broadleaf planting was not ignored and Ireland now contains more hardwood

than at any time since the seventeenth century. The most pressing problem was, as always, finance, but there were others, many of them unforeseen. It would have been unrealistic to expect fledgling governments, beset with more immediate concerns, to make available massive funds on a long-term and incalculable basis for initial afforestation on the scale proposed.

But neither was forestry neglected. In the South a programme of piece-meal land acquisition and planting became, for over two decades, such policy as existed. Conflicts would arise with the Departments of Agriculture and Lands over land, with landowners who owned private forests, and with farmers who did not and who preferred to run mountain sheep than to grow trees; between proponents of conifers and those of slow-growing but more attractive broadleaves; between private and state forestry; and, ultimately, between the bureaucratic dynamic responsible for woodland development and the increasing requirement for commercial marketing.

Almost by definition, therefore, the progress of woodland development depended to a disproportionate extent on the energies and goodwill of individuals who were prepared to take immediate problems by the throat and shape the future. In sequence these were Forbes, Senator Joe Connolly, Otto Reinhardt, Seán MacBride, Erskine Childers and Henry Grey – three officials and three politicians. In the North David Stewart and Kenneth F. Parkin took comparable roles.

Most of the powerful landowners, who were the mainspring of woodland activity under DATI (and who held 84 per cent of the country's woodland), belonged to the old British tradition. In the South, following the establishment of Saorstát Éireann, this contributed to a lack of adequate co-operation between them and the new government.

Other than acquiring land and planting – which led to such anomalies as the acquisition and planting of totally uneconomic plots, some during World War II as small as half an acre – no recognizable long-term forest policy emerged either in the South or in the North, in both cases due in the main to circumstances and financial restrictions. Encouragement of private forestry, though advocated strenuously by Connolly, Forbes and Reinhardt, was neglected. In spite of that, the largest stocks of mature timber in the country were still in private hands. Although the State holding was then 102,960 acres, mostly young timber, World War II found the country with no useful source of mature timber other than these privately held stocks, which, by the end of the Emergency (World War Two) had suffered a reduction from 84 per cent to a mere 16 per cent of the small total. In the North things were slightly different, but little better.

In 1948 the Minister for External Affairs of Saorstát Éireann, Seán MacBride, galvanized afforestation by introducing a vastly expanded planting target (from an existing 5000 acres a year to 25,000) with the object of the

South's becoming self-sufficient in timber by the year 2000. He threw his considerable talents and weight behind this enterprise. A forest survey of the country was carried out by the International Food and Agricultural Organization in 1950. Its recommendations endorsed the expanded programme and from then on – with some hitches – woodland development acquired a new significance.

Two main conflicts dominated these later years. Firstly, that between sheep and trees so far as farmers were concerned and, secondly, that between the bureaucratic architects of the afforestation programme and the increasing need for a commercial marketing dynamic as timber matured. The latter problem was not seriously addressed until the mid 1980s (after which a decision was taken in the Republic to form a semi-state forest authority, hence the forest board, Coillte Teoranta). The former problem was resolved by events rather than by decisions. Forestry is, overall, more profitable than sheep-raising, and while the return to forestry was much delayed, co-operative 'tree-farming' programmes helped resolve the dilemma.

Also in the 1980s private owners of a new sort, co-operative investors, saw rapidly developing forestry as a suitable investment medium and initiated what the State might wisely have done long before, namely co-operative enterprises with farmers and the landowners. Simultaneously, substantial EC grants for afforestation became available and were another notable feature in eliminating the sheep/tree conflict.

While the actual area was comparatively small, by 1979 Ireland had the largest and most rapidly expanding forest area per capita in Europe. The area of woodland, as a percentage of the total land area, is about the same (a little over 5 per cent) both South and North. There are 76,000 hectares (172,970 acres) of woodland in Northern Ireland, 16,000 hectares (39,536 acres) of which are privately owned. It is intended to reach an ultimate woodland target of 120,000 hectares – 90,000 state owned, 30,000 privately owned – in Northern Ireland. The Forest Service of the Department of Agriculture in Belfast has also placed a lot of emphasis on conservation and educational programmes over the past ten years. An increasing proportion of broadleaf trees is being planted – about 50 per cent of all private planting in 1991, for instance. In the South, Coillte Teoranta as of 1997 owned some 430,000 hectares, or just over a million acres, of which over 95 per cent was under woodland. The government plans to plant an additional 500,000 hectares of woodland over the next thirty-five years or so, principally in the private sector. Such a target, if achieved, would result in woodlands being about 10 per cent of the total land area North and South. While such an increase would nevertheless still mean that Ireland had the smallest percentage in Europe of land under trees, it would also provide a base for a comprehensive and economically viable timber industry capable of producing about ten million square metres of timber a year. Strikingly, in spite of hazards, obstacles and a misinterpretation of the report's recommendations, the target set by the 1908 Report of the Commission on Forestry for the country as a whole was not only met, but was surpassed, and within the time limit of eighty years, albeit in a fashion inconceivable to those who produced the report.

Dendrology, the science of trees, like so much else to do with managed woodland, has been to a considerable extent a matter of practical evolution as much as academic discipline. An important development has been dendrochronology, the fixing of dates by the comparative study of the annual growth of tree rings. Dendrochronology is particularly useful in archaeology.*

And so we have come full circle, from a country very largely covered by natural woodland, through one virtually denuded of tree cover, to one in which virtually all woodlands are cultivated as a crop and in which forestry is tree-farming. Accordingly, producers, whether private or state, will, as with other crops and stock, to the best of their ability select and cultivate the species which will generate maximum return. Hence today's emphasis on conifers. A hundred and fifty years ago, for the same reason, the emphasis was on oak. In time the requirement may again alter. Over-use of conifer species in certain types of land may be counter-productive in some respects. For instance, it is held that conifers can excessively acidify certain soils and waters with unsatisfactory ecological results, but this is challenged. It may be that more broadleaf woodlands would look more attractive (at least for most of the year), but how economically viable would they be? It may be, given the vast life-cycle of trees compared with other crops, that these questions, both environmental and economic, will resolve themselves satisfactorily in time.

What seems of overriding importance is that we recognize that trees are living organisms of vast consequence with which mankind in many critical ways has built up a domestic and dependent relationship, similar to that he has with some animals. As with many animal and fish species, man is reducing stocks of trees world-wide. This is comparable to the destruction undertaken in Ireland during the seventeenth and eighteenth centuries. The consequences, if it continues, will be incalculably more horrendous. Deprived of

---

* In dendrochronology, a composite picture of tree growth is assembled by 'matching' overlapping tree rings in similar timber, usually oak and pine, from earlier timbers from suitable sources, such as old buildings, ancient wooden objects, or those incorporating wood. This new science has furnished much additional data to Irish archaeological artifacts and sites and was pioneered in Ireland by Jon Pilcher and Michael Baillie of Queen's University, Belfast. The modern science of trees is adding to our knowledge of our early culture, in which trees played such an important part – H.C.G.C.

the contribution of woodlands to the welfare of all its creatures, the world would be an altogether different, barren, inhospitable, and perhaps uninhabitable, place.

References

Albion, R.G. 1926. *Forests and Sea Power: The Timber Problems of the Royal Navy 1562–1826.* Cambridge, Mass.: Harvard University Press.

Brewer, J.S. and W. Bullen. 1970. *Calendar of State Papers (Carew MS).* London: Longman Green.

Grousset, P. (1887) 1986. *Ireland's Disease: The English in Ireland.* London: Routledge. Facs. ed.Belfast: Blackstaff.

Hayes, S. 1794. *A Practical Treatise on Planting, and Management of Woods and Coppices.* Dublin: Dublin Society.

Innes, A.D. 1929. *England under the Tudors.* London: Methuen.

Joyce, P.W. 1920. *A Social History of Ancient Ireland.* Dublin: Gill.

Kelly, F. 1976. 'The Old Irish Tree List.' *Celtica 11:* 107-24.

Latocnaye, Chevalier de la. [1798] 1985. *A Frenchman's Walk through Ireland.* Belfast: Blackstaff Press.

Lecky, W.E.H. 1892. *History of England in the Eighteenth Century.* London: Longman Green.

Lyons, R.D. 1883. 'Re-Afforesting of Ireland.' *The Journal of Forestry.* February, pp. 656-69.

McCracken, E. 1971. *The Irish Woods Since Tudor Times.* Newton Abbot: David and Charles.

MacNeill, E. 1921. *Celtic Ireland.* Dublin: Lester; London: Parsons.

Mitchell, F. 1965. 'Littleton Bog, Tipperary: An Irish Vegetational Record.' *Geological Society of America, Special Paper 84.*

Mitchell, F. 1976. *The Irish Landscape.* London: Collins.

Neeson, E. 1991. *A History of Irish Forestry.* Dublin: Lilliput.

Powell, T.G.E. 1980. *The Celts.* London: Thames and Hudson.

Ross, R.I. 1980. *Irish Trees.* Dublin: Eason and Son.

Spenser, E. 1679. *Works of Edmund Spenser.* London.

Viney, M. 1966. 'Forestry.' *The Irish Times,* 12 October 1966.

Woodman, P.C. 1981. 'A Mesolithic Camp in Ireland.' *Scientific American 245:* 120-132.

Botany in Ireland

DONAL SYNNOTT

Beginnings

The scientific recording of the Irish flora began in the troubled seventeenth century. One Richard Heaton is usually credited with the first reports of Irish plants, giving exact locations in which they had been found. Heaton was born in the picturesque hamlet of Hooton Pagnall in Yorkshire in 1601. He may have developed a taste for botany while a scholarship student at Cambridge from 1620, graduating in Arts in 1624 and taking the oath for his Master's degree in 1627. He probably remained at Cambridge for another year for further studies in theology, which led to his ordination. In an England where civil war was brewing between loyalists and parliamentarians and where post-Reformation religious fervour informed much of the politics of the day, Heaton was loyalist and High Church.

Through his neighbour Richard Hutton, lord of the manor at Hooton Pagnall, Heaton met Sir Thomas Wentworth and became chaplain of Wentworth's Life Guard of Horse. Wentworth came to Ireland in July 1633 as Lord Deputy. In August of that year Heaton was appointed prebendary of Iniscattery, an island in the Shannon estuary near Kilrush, and in September he was appointed to the Rectory of Birr, Co. Offaly, in the Diocese of Killaloe. Travel between the two places would have brought him close to the botanically interesting territory of the Burren and his records (in How's *Phytologia*, 1650) include three plants from there: mountain avens (*Dryas octopetala*), which he noted 'makes a pretty shew in the winter with his rough heads like Viorna'; spring gentian (*Gentiana verna*) from the 'Mountains betwixt Gort and Galloway' [Galway]; and dwarf juniper (*Juniperus nana*) from rocks near Kilmacduagh. There is one plant record from the Dublin area, 'The small spring starred Hyacinth (*Scilla verna*), at Rings-end neere Dublin'. The remainder are from the Midlands: winter-green (*Pyrola rotundifolia*) from 'a bogge by Roscre in the King's County';

long-leaved sundew (*Drosera anglica*), described as being 'plentiful in a Bogge near Edenderry'; and 'Wild white hellebore with dark red flowers' (*Epipactis helleborine*), from Lysnegeeragh, the property of Thomas Medhop, who was to become Heaton's father-in-law when Heaton married Grizell Medhop, about the year 1645 (Walsh, 1978).

Heaton attaches an Irish name to one of his discoveries: 'soon-a-man-meene: in English, The juyce of a faire Woman: In a Wood near Edenderry. I referred it to the *Rubus Saxatilis*. But the berries of this plant were yellow.' This first record of the stone bramble (*Rubus saxatilis*) for Britain or Ireland indicates at least a passing interest in Irish names of plants. Though Irish was the language of the vast majority of the people, Heaton would have been an exception if he had learned it, since most of the English Protestant clergy in Ireland at the time did not know the language (Walsh, 1978). It might have been on the basis of this one published Irish plant name that Caleb Threlkeld attributed his manuscript list of Irish names to Heaton: 'As to the Irish names, I copied them from a Manuscript, which bears great authority with me, and seems to be written sometime before the civil Wars in 1641, and probably by that Revd. Irish Divine, Mr. Heaton' (Threlkeld, 1726). However, later commentators have discredited Threlkeld's opinion as to the origin of the important, but no longer surviving, manuscript (Mitchell, 1974; Nelson, 1988; Walsh, 1978).

Heaton has been described as 'a devoted husband and father, a devout cleric, perhaps ambitious, certainly one to fight for his rights and a wealthy man at the time of his death' (Walsh, 1978). Certainly he was systematic and selfish in his pursuit of property. He was equally assiduous in protecting his claim as the discoverer of Irish plants when he complained to William How that his record of 'Ros solis [*Drosera anglica*] ... was sent to John Parkinson by an acquaintance, Mr Zanchie Silliard, an apothocarie of Dublin, as though it were his own record'. Parkinson's report that *Arbutus unedo* had been 'of late dayes found in the west part of Ireland' might be attributable to Heaton (Nelson, 1988), but it is unlikely that Heaton would have allowed such an interesting record to pass anonymously in view of his concern about the *Drosera anglica* record. In any event the strawberry tree was known to at least some gardening enthusiasts already, for living trees had been sent from Ireland to England as early as the latter portion of the sixteenth century, as is evident from the following passage in the 1586 *Calendar of State Papers* (Scully, 1916):

You shall receive herewith a bundle of trees called the wollaghan tree [a name described by Scully in his flora of Kerry as a fair phonetic rendering of the Irish name, ulla caithne] whereof my Lord of Leicester and Mr Secretary Walsingham are both very desirous to have some, as well for the fruit as for the manner of bearing, which is after the kind of the orange, to have blossoms and fruit green or ripe all the year long, and the same of a very pleasant taste, and growing nowhere else but in one part of Munster, from whence I have caused them to be transported immediately unto you ....

A further two Irish plant records may be attributed to Heaton: St Patrick's cabbage (*Saxifraga spathularis*) and Irish spurge (*Euphorbia hyberna*), since they both occur in How's *Phytologia* (Praeger, 1909).

The rebellion of 1641 and the temporary ascendancy of the native, Catholic Irish were a cause of great concern to the Protestant population and to the loyal English then resident in Ireland. It is likely that Heaton abandoned Ireland in that year for the relative safety of his native Yorkshire. By 1643 he was to find himself again in a threatened minority group, for he had nailed his colours firmly to the royalist mast when civil war broke out in England and loyalist Yorkshire was in the hands of the parliamentarians. Heaton continued to record interesting plants in England, but though he returned to Ireland at the Restoration in 1660 to reclaim his lands and properties, he made no further contribution to Irish botany. Although Heaton's botanical contribution is small, a mere eight to twelve records of Irish plants, it is a highly significant one – his were the first botanical reports of Irish plants to go into print, and they give an indication of the diversity and potential interest of Ireland for the botanist.

In the meantime the upheavals in Ireland continued and after a few years of supremacy following the Confederation of Kilkenny the hopes of the native Irish were finally shattered by the arrival of Cromwell. He had secured England, Scotland and Wales for Parliament and could now turn his efficient attention to the subjugation of the Irish. The Cromwellian campaign left no mark on Irish botany, although the description of the Burren made by a Cromwellian officer is often quoted. He reported that it was a savage place, yielding neither water enough to drown a man, nor wood enough to burn a man, nor soil enough to bury a man. Of course the turmoil of the campaign and the dreadful state of relations between natives and settlers that continued in its aftermath did nothing to encourage the pursuit of botanical exploration among the few persons who might have been inclined in that direction.

The Seventeenth Century

We know nothing of any botanical observations in Ireland from 1641 until the 1680s. The Dublin Philosophical Society provided a forum for scientific discussion from its founding in 1683 to its eventual disbandment, after two revivals, in 1708. William Molyneux, older brother of Thomas, is generally credited with founding it and certainly was one of the principal figures in its early deliberations. Most of the Society's meetings were devoted to experiments of various kinds; one even included conjuring tricks by a visiting German entertainer. The study of natural history was among its aims, though the only surviving records of botanical meetings refer to a detailed treatise on the germination of the bean and a report of an unexpected growth of poppies in a tilled field in Donegal which was attributed to spontaneous generation. The Society does not appear to have promoted investigations of the Irish flora.

One prominent member of the Society with an interest in botany was a colourful and tragic character, Dr Alan Mullen, a native of Ulster and graduate of Trinity College, Dublin. He is credited with finding the beautiful red alga, *Delesseria sanguinea* (Threlkeld, 1726). Mullen is remembered for his work on the anatomy of the eye and for a celebrated account of the dissection of a circus elephant that had been burned to death. He was forced to leave Dublin for London after an 'indelicate love affair'. On his way to Jamaica – where he hoped no doubt to make his fortune – in the company of the Earl of Inchiquin and possibly also James Harlow, plant collector for Arthur Rawdon, he died at Barbados, 'from the effects of intoxication' (Hoppen, 1970).

In 1684, at the age of twenty-two, Arthur Rawdon inherited the baronetcy created for his father George, who at the Restoration of Charles II in 1660 had been awarded lands at Moira, Co. Down, for services rendered before 1649 (Nelson, 1981). Charles II died in 1685 and was succeeded by the Catholic James II. When James began appointing Catholics to positions of authority, Protestant opinion united behind William of Orange in his claim to the English throne and opposed James's interests in Ireland. Sir Arthur Rawdon led armed opposition to the Jacobite forces and earned himself the popular nickname 'Cock of the North' for his bravery and persistence. Although he fled to Derry and was prominent among the Protestant commanders there, signing the Declaration of Union in March 1689, he was not in Derry during the long siege of the city in that year and appears to have taken no further active part in the war. The Williamite victory at the Boyne was consolidated in the following year by a bloody victory at Aughrim, a battle in which some five thousand men were killed and which is echoed in botanical literature by the gruesome reference to a plant found growing on skulls that had been brought 'from Aghrim field' to Dublin's Custom House Quay in large butts (Threlkeld, 1726). The identity of this hideous plant has not been established; it has been claimed variously as a lichen (Knowles, 1929), a fungus (Jones in Edwards, 1992) and a moss (Synnott, 1984). It was apparently in use as a salve and Edwards gives a reference to the fact that most of it in use in England came out of Ireland. Burial of the dead at Aughrim seems to have been perfunctory and the collection of skulls was apparently not a difficult task some years later if they could be obtained in such quantities as to fill 'large butts'.

The Williamite wars brought another plantsman to Ireland: Gédéon Bonnivert, a member of King William's troop of horse, who botanized close to where he was stationed, around Belfast, Dublin and Limerick. Some of his records were published by Leonard Plukenet, a physician who was Queen's botanist and Superintendent of Hampton Court Gardens (Nelson, 1988; Desmond, 1994).

A century of relative stability was to follow the Williamite victories. The 'old Irish' were defeated. The Catholic landowners were replaced or were loyal to the Crown. Landowners could now develop their estates without fear of war or challenges to their ownership. At Moira Arthur Rawdon built one of the first greenhouses in Ireland and then set about creating a garden of exotic plants. This was to have important consequences not only for the future of horticulture in Ireland, but also for the progress of Irish botany, for it brought William Sherard to Moira for a period of three years beginning in 1690. Rawdon was a friend and correspondent of Sir Hans Sloane, a fellow County Down man only two years his senior, whose collections were to form the nucleus of the British Museum collections. Sloane had collected plants in Jamaica. Rawdon was also interested in Jamaica and employed James Harlow, who had already collected in America for the Chelsea Physic Garden, to collect living plants there. Harlow succeeded in bringing an astonishing one thousand living specimens out of Jamaica to Moira. They were packed in twenty cases, each containing fifty specimens, and were landed at Carrickfergus in April 1692 (Nelson, 1981). It appears that many of them survived at least for a time.

William Sherard, who was to found the chair of botany at Oxford, was at Moira during this time, perhaps as tutor to Rawdon's family or as Rawdon's guest. There can be little doubt that he enjoyed the company of a man so interested in gardening and botany, although he was to complain later to Sir Hans Sloane, on whose recommendation he had gone to Moira, that in Ireland 'I lost three years and a half of my life ... which would have been much better spent elsewhere'; as late as 1715 he complained to Sloane that he was owed a substantial sum of money when he left Rawdon's service, a debt that was never paid. Nevertheless, Sherard made a useful contribution to Irish botany, collecting plants about Lough Neagh, the Mourne Mountains, the Boyne mouth, Wicklow and Dublin. The records are of the rare and the curious; for example, the Boyne mouth records are for dodder (*Cuscuta epithymum*) and the rayless form of the common ragwort (*Senecio jacobea* var. *discoidea*), while in the Murrough of Wicklow Sherard collected the now rare and decreasing oyster plant (*Mertensia maritima*). In addition to the flowering plants and ferns Sherard also collected mosses, lichens and fungi.

Sherard was a friend of Thomas Molyneux, who had also studied medicine at Leiden. There Molyneux bought a large volume of dried plants that had been prepared by one Antoni Gaymans, and on his return to Dublin he had the plants annotated and further identified by Sherard. This most interesting and significant collection of plants only came to light in 1958 when it was offered for sale to the National Museum. It was in the library of Moore Hall in Monasterevin, which had been the seat of the Earl of Drogheda. How the volume came to be at Monasterevin is not known but perhaps Thomas Molyneux gave it to the Earl as a gift. The 'worthy gentleman' who sent plants to Caleb Threlkeld (1726) from Monasterevin was perhaps the same Earl. The house and its contents, including the Molyneux volume, was later the property of Count John McCormack, the celebrated Irish tenor, who lived there in the 1930s and 1940s.

In late 1693 or early 1694 Sherard returned to England. Rawdon died in 1695. In August of 1696 three Dublin doctors – Patrick Mitchell, Francis Vaughan and Nathaniel Wood – went to Wexford to take the waters (Mitchell, 1975). Wood and Vaughan both corresponded with the English botanist John Ray about Irish plants; Vaughan wrote to him: 'Sir, Dr. Wood, Dr. Mitchell and I have resolved to be as curious as our leisures will permit in making a collection of what plants this kingdom affords, we have begun this summer at Wexford, where we casually meet to drink the medicinal waters.' They collected some 280 plants, which they hoped to augment as opportunity arose (Mitchell, 1975; Nelson, 1993). Also in 1696 was published the second edition of Ray's *Synopsis Methodicae*, a work which was to provide a model for the first Irish flora, that of Caleb Threlkeld, which included many of Sherard's records.

The Welsh botanist and naturalist Edward Lhwyd paid two visits to Ireland in 1699 and 1700 (Lhwyd, 1712). He collected plants in Antrim, Sligo, Connemara, the Aran Islands, the Burren and Kerry. He included Irish names of plants in his report, giving further proof that the Irish-speaking population had an awareness of the flora and had accommodated it in their language, and emphasizing the hiatus between the indigenous plant knowledge in the oral tradition and the new scientific approach that relied on written records. The written record was for the most part being made by an elite group of English-speaking botanists who often communicated their plant finds and descriptions in Latin; they were ignorant of the Irish tongue, though sometimes aware of the considerable botanical content of the native language. Efforts to correlate Irish plant names with scientific and English plant names would be made by succeeding generations of botanists, mostly with ease though occasionally with regret that some of the earlier manuscripts mentioned in the botanical literature were not extant.

Lhwyd was aware of the records made by Richard Heaton from How's *Phytologia*, for in recording *Dryas* from Ben Bulben he mentions Heaton's previous record from the Burren. He also met with William and Thomas

Molyneux in Dublin and discussed a projected 'Natural History of Ireland' which apparently came to nothing. However, it is interesting to know that the idea was being talked about more than a century before the Belfast naturalist John Templeton began assembling materials for such a work.

The Eighteenth Century

No complete list of the Irish flora had as yet been published. Apart from the small number of Irish records in How's *Phytologia* and Ray's *Synopsis*, there was no account of the Irish flora as a whole. Many native speakers could probably have given a good account of the flora of their own areas using the Irish names of the plants. But this would have been meaningless to the scientific and English-speaking world, and unless accompanied by voucher specimens would have had little value as a botanical record. The few specific records made during the seventeenth century were of rare or unusual plants; common plants were completely ignored as far as the written record goes. In those days knowledge of plants and where they grew was widespread in the community, as they were collected and used in medicinal preparations. Those of the recently arrived English planters and their followers who knew anything of plants would have found that much of the flora was not greatly different from that of their homeland. 'So that although we are not the same Nation of Men, who dwelt here a thousand Years ago, yet the spontaneous Plants are the same they were in the time of the Danes and Bryan Boro ...' (Threlkeld, 1726). As a result, for more than two decades into the eighteenth century the most recently produced list against which the status or interest of plant occurrences could be measured was Ray's *Synopsis* (1696).

John Ray was the son of a blacksmith and herbalist. He had gained a sizarship at Cambridge, where he distinguished himself and remained for twelve years. His contribution to natural history and to the scientific thought of the seventeenth century was considerable and his influence on the conduct of botany in the succeeding century was decisive. Part of Ray's design was to produce a list of the British flora giving localities for each of the plants and crediting the collectors or those who had reported them. To this end it was very successful for Great Britain, but the Irish content depended on a very few contributors, chiefly Heaton, Lhwyd and Sherard, since Ray himself did not visit Ireland. Although it contained several Irish plant records, mostly of the rare and the curious, it was hardly an account of the Irish flora. Such an account was soon to be provided, however, in Caleb Threlkeld's *Synopsis Stirpium Hibernicarum*, published about the same time as Jonathan Swift's *Gulliver's Travels*.

Threlkeld came to Ireland in 1713. He was pleasantly surprised to find that the weather was milder than that of his native Cumberland. He commented (*Synopsis* 1726): 'Anno 1713. March 26. I saw Snow upon Skiddaw in Cumberland, but when landed in Ireland, April 3d. Good Friday, no Appearance of either Frost, or Snow, since which time, I never saw so many Days of Snow here, as I have of Weeks in Cumberland.' But he was not so enthusiastic about the state of botany in Ireland. He wrote:

The only Reasons I know why this branch of Learning has been dormant in Ireland, and no publick Advances made towards its illustration are that the Wars and Commotions have laid an Imbargo upon the Pens of the Learned, or Discord among the petty subaltern Princes has render'd perambulation perilous, least they should be treated like spyes, as I was once myself at Tinmouth-Castle near Newcastle upon Tyne, the year of the Union 1707, because I clamboured up the rocks, and kept not the High-road.

Threlkeld had already acquired some skill in botany before coming to Ireland:

I began to follow the natural bent of my mind thirty years ago (when I pursued a Philosophy course in the University), in viewing plants and acquainting myself with the skillful in Botany when we made sallies out into the Fields and Fells; and afterwards when settled, I used to wander through the Woods and Dales with two books, Mr Ray's Methodus emendata ... and his Synopsis Stirpium Britannicarum; by which simpling became easy and pleasant, and the discovery of an uncommon plant gave a particular relish to that pleasure, so that from a miscellany of the piquant, and the Agreeable, an harmonious satisfaction affected the mind.

He trained as a physician and would therefore have studied medicinal plants but his natural curiosity extended his study to the flora as a whole. He was familiar with the botanical literature since the works of How and Ray were available to him as models of what was required for the study of Irish plants. He was aware of the necessity for a stable system of naming plants, though he betrays his conservatism in a somewhat arrogant attack on Ray and the editor of the third edition of Ray's *Synopsis* for their growing realization that there was more to variation in the dandelion tribe than that due to soil and climate:

It is odd, that in Mr. Ray's first edition of his Synopsis, he has three sorts, in his second Edition four Sorts, in the third Edition five Sorts; and if we get another Edition, some unheeded Gash in a brilliant Fancy, may add a sixth Species, etc. which I look upon as confounding, rather than advancing true Knowledge, which appears to me as ridiculous, as to say, that a Scotch Runt differs specifically from an English Ox, or a Manx Tit from an Irish Coach-horse.

Along similar lines, he favoured standardization of botanical nomenclature:

... for variety of names confounds the learner, and I could heartily wish for my part all Botanists would agree to the names used by Dr Caspar Bauhin in his Pinax, which was forty years in the Loom ... Nothing I think happens worse to the Art of Botany, than that, which daily befalls it, which is, That any Author of a Plant long since described, and rightly named, may arbitrarily coin a new Name without any Advantage or Necessity.

Threlkeld understood the necessity of recording localities for his plants so that his readers could find them for themselves. He repeated the records made by earlier botanists, sometimes with acknowledgment and sometimes without. Some passages from Ray's *Synopsis* are translated from the Latin without acknowledgment, though it is unlikely that Threlkeld wished to pass them off for his own since he must surely have assumed a knowledge of Ray's work in at least some of his readers.

Realizing that a bare botanical list would be of interest to very few, and displaying good commercial sense, Threlkeld included the medicinal virtues of the plants: '... a bare Nomenclature without the Usefulness of the Plant would please few Buyers ... I desire this Treatise may be of use to such as cannot obtain the Advice of the Experienced ... I hope the reader will find his Time well employed, and the Buyer his Money well laid out, in getting Knowledge of Simples.'

Another feature of Threlkeld's book that gives it popular appeal is the inclusion of vernacular names in both English and Irish. His English names display a mixture of those in everyday use, perhaps in his native Cumberland or more widely in England, indicating in names such as 'purple-spiked willow-herb' and 'bastard nigella' the bookishness that was to become a feature of the development of English plant names as used by botanists. In Ireland the accumulated lore and familiarity with the plants was recorded in its language as the tradition was oral rather than written.* Richard Heaton had earlier recorded one Irish plant name and Edward Lhwyd had included Irish names for plants, but Threlkeld had in his possession a list of Irish names that he prized. Threlkeld added some further Irish names from his own research or from information given by correspondents but he must have been a little disappointed in the amount of material he could add to the manuscript list, for he commented: 'I could not find any living Persons could come near this M.S. either for Number or Exactness of Names, among all those I conversed with viva voce.'

Although Threlkeld's book must have been useful to those interested in the study of botany in eighteenth-century Ireland, its importance was lost sight of and underestimated by some commentators. S.A. Stewart, writing

---

*A recent standard list of English names attempts to provide an alternative and precise system of nomenclature tied to the botanical system. This often results in unnatural and odd-sounding word combinations, such as 'reflexed saltmarsh-grass' and 'intermediate lady's-mantle' (Dony et al., 1986).

for his introduction to the *Flora of the North-east of Ireland*, describes it as 'very deficient in localities', and complains that it 'partakes more of the character of an herbal than a flora' (Stewart and Corry, 1888). From Stewart's northern Irish perspective Threlkeld's book is disappointing since it contains few plant records for that part of the country. In contrast, the Dublin area is well represented in the list of localities from which plants are reported, and Colgan in *Flora of the County Dublin* (1904) has this to say on the history of botanical exploration in Dublin:

While the *Synopsis* must always have a special value and interest for students of Irish botany, the literary qualities of the book recommend it to a much wider circle of readers. Nothing, indeed, could be farther removed from a bald scientific catalogue than the piquant medley of herbal and homily in which this medical missionary from Cumberland delivers himself of his opinions on botany, medicine, morals, theology, witchcraft, and the Irish Question.

Little progress with publication of the Irish flora was made for the next half century, but that is not to say that no progress was being made with the study of plant distribution. In 1744 the Physico-Historical Society was founded in Dublin with the purpose of 'promoting an enquiry into the ancient and present state of the several counties of Ireland'. Its first meeting was held in the Lords Committee room of the Parliament House in College Green, now the headquarters of the Bank of Ireland. The Society commissioned Isaac Butler to report on the natural history of several Irish counties including Longford, Westmeath, Meath, Louth, Dublin, Wicklow, Wexford, Tipperary and Cork. Butler died in 1755, at Bull Alley, Patrick Street, Dublin. An obituary notice stated that he 'gained such a knowledge in Botany that he not only collected simples for the curious and officinals for the sick, but also taught several tyroes in Pharmacy to know most of the indiginous vegetables' (Colgan, 1904). A copy of Threlkeld's *Synopsis* in the Royal Irish Academy has several manuscript plant records attributed to Butler. They include the Downpatrick record of *Galium cruciata*, still rare in Ireland, and *Orobranche hederae* from Castlebellingham, which could still be seen there in the 1970s. Colgan believed that Butler had a wider knowledge of the Irish flora than many of his contemporaries, one of whom, a John Smith, placed a notice in *The Freeman's Journal* of 26 April 1766, offering his services: 'John Smith of Elbow Lane, Meath Street, Botanist, collects and preserves the true great Water-dock, the true Mountain Valerian ... and many other useful and medicinal Plants. He perambulates the Fields with Gentlemen, who are willing to be instructed in the useful Science of Botany.'

Charles Smith's *The Ancient and Present State of the County of Waterford* (1746), and corresponding volumes for Cork (1750) and Kerry (1756), were also published 'with the approbation of the Physico-Historical

Society' (Scully, 1916). Although they contain many errors there is a useful botanical element to them. The Kerry book, for example, contains some seventy-eight plants which are first records for the county. It is not known whether Smith knew the plants himself or relied on reports sent by others. Scully accepted the accuracy of the records since many of them, including the rare *Lathyrus japonicus*, were still to be found at the places mentioned or had been seen subsequently by reputable botanists.

The Physico-Historical Society did not survive for long, but the materials collected by members of the Society for a book on County Dublin, on which Butler had worked, were eventually published in 1772. Its author was John Rutty, an English physician who settled in Dublin in 1724. It was in many ways a backward-looking book, for although some 230 pages are given over to botany, it added only twenty-eight species to the Dublin flora and it used the old polynomial system of plant nomenclature, even though the binomial system adopted by Linnaeus in his *Species Plantarum* had been introduced in Hudson's *Flora Anglica* ten years previously.

Patrick Browne, a Mayo-born medical man and botanist who knew Linnaeus and was later respected for his contribution to the knowledge of the flora of the West Indies, collected plants in Mayo and Galway in 1788. These survive with his notes in the Linnaean Society in London and include Irish names of the plants collected in those localities. Browne does not, however, seem to have had any influence on the subsequent development of Irish botany.

By the end of the eighteenth century Dublin had developed into the second city of the Empire. The Royal Dublin Society founded a Botanic Garden at Glasnevin in 1795, mainly through the influence of John Foster, Speaker in the Irish Parliament, who had developed a collection of exotic plants at Collon in County Louth. Walter Wade was appointed Keeper of the Gardens and charged with developing the plant collections. The heady period of 'Grattan's Parliament' was shaken by the agitation of the United Irishmen for full Irish independence, culminating in the rebellion of 1798, which was swiftly suppressed. Robert Brown, who was to make such an impression on the botanical world, came to Ireland as physician with the British army and made notes on the botany of the country as he travelled around with a substantial botanical library (Nelson, 1992a).

The Nineteenth Century

The Act of Union of 1800 was a watershed in Irish political affairs but scarcely affected the progress of botanical studies in the country. Walter Wade, who had published a volume on the Dublin flora complete with modern Linnaean and vernacular names and with several new localities for plants, understood what was required in botanical studies. As well as fulfilling his duties in regard to the development of the Botanic Gardens he continued his researches into the Irish flora and in 1804 produced a catalogue of Irish rare plants. His intention to produce an illustrated flora of Dublin was not fulfilled though some part of his design survives (Nelson and McCracken, 1987).

Meanwhile Belfast had been growing in size and importance. John Templeton had been cultivating plants at his home in Cranmore, near Belfast, and studying both native and exotic plants. While still a young man his reputation as a botanist came to the notice of Joseph Banks, who offered to take him to New Holland (Australia) and promised a good salary and a large grant of land. Templeton, whose personal circumstances enabled him to devote his full time to his scientific interests, declined the offer. Praeger (1949) commented on his lack of curiosity about other places and attributed it to his wide natural-history interests, for which he found adequate material about his native place. He was the first discoverer of *Rosa hibernica* and was awarded the premium of five pounds offered by the Royal Dublin Society for the discovery of a new Irish species. The moss *Funaria templetonii* was named by James Smith in his honour and Robert Brown dedicated the Australian genus *Templetonia* to him. Although his projected 'Natural History of Ireland' was never brought to fruition, Templeton's contribution to Irish natural-history studies is an outstanding one. As a mark of his standing he was made an honorary member of the Belfast Natural History Society at its foundation in 1821. His example inspired a love of nature in those who knew him and his influence on the progress of natural history went well beyond his own considerable contribution. He was the first of a number of diligent and accurate naturalists from Belfast who have kept knowledge of the flora of the north-east of Ireland abreast of developments in Britain and often in the vanguard of Irish studies on the subject. The continuity of botanical expertise in Belfast, beginning with Templeton and continuing through the Natural History Society and later the Belfast Naturalists' Field Club, and inspired by such enthusiasts as William Thompson, Samuel Alexander Stewart, Robert Lloyd Praeger and Patricia Kertland, to name but a few, has been a dynamic influence on the development of botanical studies in Ireland.

Ulster was fortunate too in drawing the attentions of three Scotsmen who were major contributors to the development of botany in Ireland. Thomas Drummond, who was chiefly interested in mosses, was the first Curator of the Belfast Botanic Garden. Hooker named the genus *Drummondia* after him. David Moore, formerly Muir, came to Ireland to work for the Ordnance Survey in the 1830s. He has left a twelve-volume *Hortus Siccus* or dried collection of plant specimens collected from Antrim and Derry during his work for the Survey, together with notes from his work on the Derry flora. The Survey, although intended to be extended to the whole country, did not continue for more than a few years, but enabled Moore to make an important contribution to the botany of the north-east and to establish himself as one of the leading botanists of his day. He had been assistant to James Townsend Mackay at the Trinity College Botanic Garden and, on the resignation of Ninian Niven, became Keeper of the Dublin Society's Botanic Gardens at Glasnevin in 1838. The third important Scottish contributor to the botany of Ulster was George Dickie. Born in Aberdeen, Dickie came to Belfast in 1849 as Professor of Botany at Queen's College, returning to his native city in 1860 to take up the Professorship of Botany in the new University of Aberdeen. Dickie produced a *Flora of Ulster* (1864) that embraced all of the province and also included parts of Louth and even Sligo and Mayo.

In Dublin at the Botanic Garden many native plants were being cultivated by John Underwood, resulting in seven hundred native species and varieties being included in his 1804 *Catalogue* of Glasnevin plants. Mackay, Curator of the Trinity College Gardens, took the next step in cataloguing the Irish flora. Walter Wade's *Catalogue* (1804) had consisted of rare plants only; Mackay expanded the list to include all the known flora of the country. *Flora Hibernica* (1837) was a full list of the flora with localities for the rarer species, taking account of all previous work and adding considerably to the stock of information about plant distribution in Ireland. The first comprehensive account of the Irish flora was now available to the serious student of botany. A few years previously a descriptive flora had been produced which popularized botany and made identification of plants easier. *An Irish Flora* (1833) is believed to have been written by Katherine Sophia Baily of Newbury, Berkshire, later to become Lady Kane. She is said to have met Robert Kane when he returned the publisher's proofs, which had come to him in error (Cullinane, 1971). Robert Kane became President of the new Queen's College in Cork but his wife steadfastly refused to live there, preferring to remain in Dublin where she is reputed to have had an interesting garden of exotic plants. Many localities in *An Irish Flora* were supplied by John White, gardener at Glasnevin, who also produced an interesting and useful guide to Irish grasses (1808). He expanded the list of Irish names for grasses available to him from published and manuscript sources and his own collection into a comprehensive list of Irish grass names by coining new ones and rearranging them into a binomial system in Irish.

A similar approach was later employed by the Botanical Society of the British Isles in devising a complete list of English names of plants (Dony et al., 1986). Mackay's *Flora Hibernica* included an account of the ferns of the country prepared by Thomas Taylor. The cryptogamic botany (non-flowering plants) had even fewer exponents but significant progress was made with the study of bryophytes (mosses and liverworts) in particular. The Royal Dublin Society assisted by awarding monetary prizes to the discoverers of new plants. Dawson Turner of Yarmouth published in Latin an Irish moss flora in 1804. William Jackson Hooker married Turner's daughter Maria in 1815 and they spent their honeymoon in Ireland, meeting with Taylor and Whitley Stokes in Belfast in July and moving on to Dublin after a month to stay with the Taylors. The friendship that had naturally commenced on the first meeting of Taylor and Hooker now blossomed (Sayre, 1987), and Turner (and later Smith, Hooker and Taylor) named many new mosses and liverworts after their discoverers. Robert Scott, Professor of Botany in Trinity College, had a moss, *Dicranum scottianum*, named in his honour; Stokes, lecturer in Natural History in Trinity College, is commemorated by another moss, *Hypnum stokesii*. Stokes had been a member of the United Irishmen, which did not endear him to the authorities or to the establishment of Trinity College, and he was suspended from his teaching post for three years. However, on reinstatement he became a Senior Fellow and Regius Professor of Physic and founded the College Botanic Gardens in 1806.

Stokes also encouraged the remarkable talents of Ellen Hutchins of Bantry, Co. Cork. As a girl she had been in ill-health; Stokes suggested that she take up an outdoor pursuit and recommended the study of natural history. Hutchins applied herself to the study of the cryptogamic plants of the Bantry area. She corresponded with the English botanists Lewis Dillwyn and Dawson Turner and contributed many of her records and illustrations to their publications. The remarkable achievements of her short life are recorded in the several plants bearing her name, including *Herberta hutchinsiae*, the beautiful hepatic or liverwort, *Jubula hutchinsiae*, the dark companion of the Killarney fern, and *Ulota hutchinsiae*, the amphi-Atlantic moss. The flowering plant genus *Hutchinsia* was named by Robert Brown in her honour after she discovered a plant of this southern European genus growing wild on a cemetery wall in Bantry.

The great flurry of botanical activity in the first third of the nineteenth century had added greatly to the existing knowledge of the Irish flora, giving botanical studies a national framework within which to work. The baseline floras and lists were in place and further work would serve to refine that framework. Botany was now a respectable and legitimate study in its own right while remaining an important component of medical and agricultural studies. At the beginning of the century one of the objectives of the Botanic Gardens at Glasnevin was to advance agriculture and medicine, but as the century progressed a greater emphasis was placed on exotic plant collections for their intrinsic and educational interest and their use in decorative planting.

Just as the increased amount of fieldwork prompted the preparation of Mackay's *Flora Hibernica* in 1836 so did that book point the way to further fieldwork. It highlighted the gaps in the study of the flora and suggested further exploration of those parts of the country that were not well represented among the records. Field workers were thin on the ground, however, and no significant progress was made in the 1840s. Work was still concentrated on the Belfast, Cork and Dublin areas and was a reflection of the distribution of botanists. David Orr had reported some unlikely plants from Colin Glen near Belfast and Powerscourt Waterfall in Wicklow; the reports were charitably ascribed to carelessness by S.A. Stewart in print (1888) but probably not in conversation (Praeger, 1937) and are now believed to have been deliberate fraud. Apart from Orr's impressive list of deceptions Irish botany has not suffered much from frauds or hoaxes, though there are still one or two plants on the current Irish list which might have a flawed pedigree.

Soon the new railways were opening up the country to exploration and making many parts of the west easily accessible. Edward Newman, who had visited Achill Island in the 1830s, described the poverty of the inhabitants and the condition of their dwellings, while noting maidenhair fern and other Achill rarities and describing that incredibly romantic lough, Bunafreeva West, on the western precipice of the Achill coast. He had also been at Torc Waterfall where, with probable exaggeration, he had described the Killarney fern as occurring in such quantity that he had 'stood amid the roar of waters gazing on hundreds of the dark fronds of this fern, as they waved to and fro in the agitated air, and sparkled with myriads of sunlit drops' (Newman, 1839).

The British Association Meeting was held in Cork in 1843. One member, Thomas Power, a lecturer in botany in the Cork School of Medicine, prepared an account of the flora of Cork for the occasion that was published two years later by the Cuvierian Society of Cork (Power, 1845). The list of algae was contributed by Joshua Harvey, Professor of Midwifery at Queen's College, Cork. A more famous algologist was William Henry Harvey, who had returned home from South Africa in 1842 where he had succeeded his brother as Colonial Treasurer (Nelson, 1992). Harvey, who was to become Professor of Botany at the Royal Dublin Society and later in Dublin University, was educated at the celebrated Quaker school at Ballitore, Co. Kildare. He made significant contributions to the study of the South African and North American floras and was the foremost algologist of his day. His *Phytologia Britannica* (1846-51), dealing with British Isles algae or seaweeds, is still much used today.

Agitation for repeal of the Act of Union was the dominant political force at work in the 1840s. A rapidly increasing population of tenant farmers, with each succeeding generation attempting to survive on ever-smaller holdings, became dependent on the potato as a staple food. Corn was grown to pay the rent but the potato was grown for eating. There had been periodic failures of the potato crop, but these were local. In 1845, however, the potato crop was attacked by a new and devastating rot that ravaged the growing plants and the tubers both in the ground and in storage.

At the same time, David Moore was developing the plant collections at Glasnevin for the Royal Dublin Society, and the construction of the curvilinear range of glasshouses, manufactured and built by Richard Turner, was under way. While continuing the developments at Glasnevin, Moore became involved in the investigation of the potato rot. He was quickly converted to the idea that it was caused by a fungus and not, as some suggested, by the dampness of the Irish air or unusual electrical influences. Although he cooperated with various bizarre experiments at the Gardens to try to protect the plants and tubers from rotting he supported a soberly scientific approach to resolving the problem.

The devastation wrought by the Great Famine left its mark on Irish botany, for it caused the death of one of its most respected exponents. Thomas Taylor, who had contributed greatly to the advancement of bryological knowledge, had been variously Physician in Ordinary to Sir Patrick Dun's Hospital, Professor of Natural History and then Secretary at the Cork Institution until its decline in the early 1830s, and then farmer and estate owner at Dunkerron in County Kerry. Taylor was struggling to survive financially by the mid-1840s. He had sought a post at the new Queen's University in Cork but believed that the post would be given to a Catholic. He wrote to William Wilson in February 1845:

But the great drawback to the expectations of either of us, I am sure, is our Protestantism. It is true that the Belfast one is to be Presbyterian but the Galway and Cork ones are understood to be boons to the Catholic Southern and Western parts of Ireland, and to be answers to the cry lately raised and loudly reiterated, that Catholic students receive no encouragement in the University of Dublin. We must take the world as we find it; perhaps it may be in our favour that a Catholic with any pretension at all to Botanical knowledge may not ever be discovered. (Sayre, 1987)

Taylor worked untiringly at medicine in the awful hunger and epidemic fevers that resulted from the potato failure in 1845-7. He was interested in discovering the cause of the potato failure and examined diseased tubers under the microscope as early as 1845 (Sayre, 1987). He was physician to the workhouse at Kenmare and, probably worn out by his exertions, died of fever on 4 February 1848.

The hundreds of thousands who died and the millions who fled the country in the succeeding decade were not likely to be concerned with the gentle and esoteric pursuit of botany. Survival and a search for economic security would have been the chief concern of the masses. Botany was a pursuit for the financially secure if not indeed for the gentlemen and ladies of leisure. The terrible hunger came to an end with a successful harvest in 1848. The country could begin to pick up the pieces. Queen Victoria came to Dublin in 1849 for the opening of the Great Industrial Exhibition organized by the Royal Dublin Society and visited the Botanic Gardens where she admired Turner's beautiful curvilinear glasshouse. David Moore's expansion of the collections at Glasnevin reflected a growing emphasis on exotic plants. However, he did not abandon his interest in the Irish flora and when an energetic and charismatic Englishman, Alexander Goodman More, came to Ireland, he and Moore immediately formed plans to produce a new book on the distribution of Irish plants. *Cybele Hibernica* (1866) was modelled on H.C. Watson's *Cybele Britannica*. It used twelve subdivisions of the Irish provinces as the botanical recording units. The pattern of following the British model had been set by Threlkeld and it would continue with Praeger's 'Irish Topographical Botany' (1901).

More had tasted Irish botany at Castle Taylor on the edge of the Burren during holidays spent there and found it to his liking. He came to spend the summer of 1850 with his schoolfriend Walter Shawe-Taylor. Arriving on 14 June he recorded in his notebook shooting a sparrowhawk, taking a wood white butterfly and finding *Geranium sanguineum*, his first botanical entry and the beginning of an interest in plants that was to become an important part of his life's work. 'It was from gathering specimens of Irish wild flowers to send home to his sister, who took pleasure in drying them, that he was led to begin the study of botany this summer in the west' (Moffat, 1898). The remarkable flora of the Burren was first described in detail in 1862 by Frederick James Foot, a geologist with the Irish Geological Survey. Foot drowned in Lough Key near Boyle in 1867, the first of two such tragedies that deprived Irish botany of two of its more active workers.

A.G. More was Keeper of the Natural History Museum in Dublin from 1881 until he was forced to retire after six years from the ill-health that dogged him in his later years but did not reduce his enthusiasm for botanical organization. He inspired a younger generation of botanists to help with the production of a second edition of the *Cybele Hibernica*, which was dedicated to his memory when it eventually saw the light in 1898, some three years after his death. The second edition was edited by Nathaniel Colgan and Reginald Scully, who were to write classic county floras of Dublin and Kerry respectively. More had entrusted to them the task of completing the second edition of the work he had begun with David Moore a generation earlier.

Richard M. Barrington, estate owner, surveyor, organizer of coastal bird surveys and explorer of islands and mountain ranges, was one of

More's greatest admirers and wrote his obituary. He wrote to Matilda Knowles at the Museum of Science and Art:

I regard him as having been the greatest Irish Botanist of the 19th century – certainly as far as topography & a critical & accurate eye for species is concerned. He originated the idea of a Cybele Hibernica on Watson's lines – & was the initiator of more botanical expeditions in Ireland than any other botanist.

The first edition of *Cybele* had inspired unprecedented exploration of the country. The Belfast Naturalists' Field Club, founded in 1863, provided a perfect focus for studies in Ulster and the Dublin Naturalists' Field Club was formed twenty years later. Henry Chichester Hart, a man of remarkable physique, keen intellect and independent mind, explored the mountains of Ireland, performing many remarkable feats of endurance in the process. He has been criticized for the imprecise nature of his records and the inadequacy of his specimens, but he did not miss much and his investigations of the Irish mountain ranges were of great service to Irish botany. In that heyday of Irish botany when A.G. More was orchestrating the fieldwork for the second edition of *Cybele Hibernica*, 'full advantage was taken of Hart's endurance and skill as a climber and walker, and many of the mountain groups and less accessible areas fell to his share – the Reeks, Galtees, Comeraghs, Twelve Bens, Brandon, Croaghpatrick, Mweelrea, the courses of the Barrow, Suir, Nore, Blackwater, Slaney; and the lonely shore-line of Wexford and Waterford' (Praeger, 1949).

In August 1883 Thomas Hughes Corry, who was still only twenty-three years of age, and his friend Charles Dickson, a young Belfast solicitor, were drowned when their boat overturned in Lough Gill, near Sligo. Corry had received a grant from the Royal Irish Academy to continue his investigation of the flora of the Ben Bulben range. A.G. More put together a paper on the heights of plants there from the notes that Corry had made on a visit the previous year (Corry, 1884). In the introduction to the paper More, lamenting his passing, commented:

Mr Corry's career as a Botanist was only just commencing, but he had already given great promise of distinction as a scientific Naturalist. Himself an Irishman, he took the greatest interest in the Botany of the country. His remarkable zeal and energy, his love for the study of critical plants, together with the position which he held as Curator in the Herbarium at Cambridge, and the trusted friend of Professor Babington, gave him unusual advantages, of which he diligently availed himself; and his early death will be deplored by all who feel an interest in the advance of Botany in Ireland.

A full account of the tragedy is given by S. A. Stewart in his preface to the *Flora of the North-east of Ireland* (1888), of which Corry is credited as co-author. Stewart himself was exploring the shores of Lough Allen in the adjoining county of Leitrim on that fatal day and described the appalling weather (Stewart, 1888). Richard Barrington, writing to Matilda Knowles in December 1906, recalled the grief felt by all of the botanical community at the time: 'Please put enclosed specimens in their places with any letters referring to them attached by pin to sheet. Corry's poem I would like attached to one of his plants. I think I have one somewhere here in herbarium. I well remember seeing the poor chap lying dead in the hotel in Sligo with Charley Dickson by his side also dead.' Stewart completed the work single-handedly and the *Flora* was published in 1888 with financial help from the wealthy Corry family.

Stewart also encouraged the young son of a Dutch linen merchant who lived in Belfast. Robert Lloyd Praeger had been persuaded to join the Belfast Naturalists' Field Club by his father and maternal grandfather: 'I think my earliest contact with a man of science was when my grandfather, Robert Patterson, took me to Cultra on the shores of Belfast Lough to show me the Adder's-tongue' (Praeger, 1949). This early interest in ferns brought Praeger into contact with W.H. Phillips of Holywood, Co. Down, and 'the best of the British fern men', A.M. Jones and E.J. Lowe. Membership of the Field Club brought him to the notice of Stewart, 'whose only fault was his overweening modesty'. While A.G. More and his disciples were working on the second edition of *Cybele Hibernica*, Praeger was already looking beyond it to a greater refinement in plant distribution. The model was again a British one, for H.C. Watson had produced *Topographical Botany* in 1873, with a second edition in 1883, in which plant distribution was given in the newly devised vice-county system. An early attempt was made to devise such a system for Ireland by W.R. McNab, Professor of Botany at the Royal College of Science and Superintendent of the Royal Botanic Gardens at Glasnevin. McNab proposed a division of Ireland into thirty-six vice-counties, each referring to a province based on those in *Cybele Hibernica*, but this resulted in some 'strange alliances', such as South Tipperary being placed in East Munster and North Tipperary being placed in East Shannon (McNab, 1885). The vice-county arrangement was refined by Praeger following suggestions from Hart and others, and almost single-handedly Praeger set about the work of bringing knowledge of Irish plant distribution into line with that of Britain.

Praeger had left Belfast for Dublin in 1893, finding a more specialized approach to the study of natural history in Dublin but 'with a less intimate acquaintance with the animals and plants in relation to their surroundings, and of topographical detail as applied to the fauna and flora' (Praeger, 1949). His post at the National Library gave him ample opportunity for fieldwork, and he used the developing rail network to greatest advantage in surveying those vice-counties which were not already well botanized.

In devising the recording units, in calculating the number of species to be expected within each of the vice-counties and the amount of fieldwork

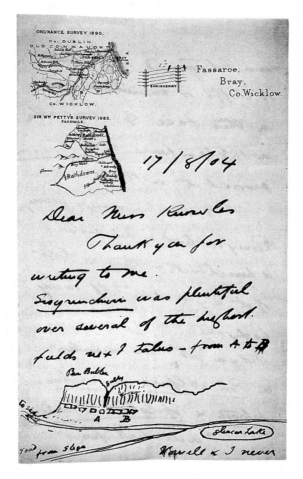

Richard Barrington to Matilda Knowles, 17 August 1904, reporting plentiful Sisyrinchium *on Ben Bulben in Co. Sligo.*

needed to achieve the degree of completeness required for publication of the results, in sticking to his rigorous programme of fieldwork, plant collection, note-taking, and identification of critical specimens, in arranging help for the more critical groups, in editing and selecting material for publication, and in encouraging those correspondents who promised to be useful, Praeger displayed a remarkable ability for organization. His success with the 'Irish Topographical Botany' project, published in 1901, encouraged him to organize the Lambay and Clare Island Surveys for the Royal Irish Academy in later years.

The Twentieth Century

The success of 'Irish Topographical Botany' also established Praeger as the undisputed leader of floristic studies in Ireland. For the next half century Praeger, in the words of G.F. Mitchell (1986), 'bestrode Irish Natural History like a Colossus'. He published a number of additions to the botanical records contained in 'Irish Topographical Botany' in several papers in the *Proceedings of the Royal Irish Academy*. His book on the interesting botanical areas in Ireland, *The Botanist in Ireland* (1934), is still an important stimulus to botanical exploration. However, Praeger's overpowering personal contribution to Irish botany and his assumption of the mantle of botanical controller may have discouraged a generation of botanists from greater effort. The sheer volume of work and the appearance of completeness presented in 'Irish Topographical Botany' may have led to a false sense that all of the fieldwork had been done. Praeger himself may have been of the same opinion. In an article entitled 'Things Left Undone' (1946), he makes no reference to the deficiencies of the vice-county surveys that become apparent to the modern recorder.

Apart from looking to Britain for models for plant recording and the extensive use of the British diagnostic floras for plant identification, Irish botany remained by and large self-sufficient and aloof from developments in Britain. There had been very few Irish members of the Botanical Exchange Club. Allen (1986), noting that this state of affairs was consolidated by Praeger, suggests that this may have been because Praeger did not care for the Club Secretary, G.C. Druce. The success of the *Irish Naturalist*, which Praeger had founded, as a vehicle for publication of botanical records and of more substantial papers such as the 'Flora of Armagh' (Praeger, 1893), contributed to the relative independence of Irish botany.

Local studies continued. Praeger brought out a second edition of the *Flora of the North-east of Ireland* in 1938 aided by Rev. William Megaw, who wrote the bryophyte chapter, which had originally been contributed by Stewart. Megaw was a Presbyterian minister who continued the bryological tradition of Ulster clergymen such as Canon Henry William Lett and Rev. Cosslett Herbert Waddell, who had made a major contribution to the bryology of Ireland. Lett had published a book on British hepatics and a companion volume on mosses to Praeger's 'Irish Topographical Botany'. Waddell had been responsible for setting up the Moss Exchange Club, which was later to become the British Bryological Society. At the end of 1895 he submitted notes to *Science Gossip*, the *Irish Naturalist* and the *Journal of Botany* proposing the establishment of an exchange club for bryophytes and inviting interested botanists to get in touch with him. Twenty-three members enrolled (Foster, 1979) and the future of bryology in Britain and Ireland was secure.

The dependence on British floras for plant identification was partly overcome in 1931 when John Adams, a former lecturer in the Royal College of Science in Dublin who had since retired from his post of Colonial Botanist in Canada, produced *A Student's Illustrated Irish Flora* with keys, descriptions of genera and species and information on ecology, times of flowering and distribution. Although it was packed with information, the book was not an elegant production and did not have a long life. In 1943 *A New Irish Flora* was produced. Published in Dundalk, it was the work of David Webb (*plate 5*), recently returned from Cambridge to Trinity College. Now in its sixth edition, it has been the single most valuable tool for Irish botanical students for fifty years. Since its first edition it has remained a conservative flora. Taxa below the level of species are not included and only outlines of the divisions within the difficult apomictic (non-pollinating) genera, such as *Hieracium*, *Taraxacum* and *Rubus*, are given. The *Flora* may have been partly responsible for the conservative approach of Irish botanists and their reluctance to study critical groups. Reliance on British and to a lesser extent continental botanists for identification of the critical plant groups has been a feature of recent Irish botany. The Rev. H.W. Lett had tackled the bryophytes but also concentrated on *Rubus*, though as Praeger (1949) pointed out, he 'sometimes lacked the caution and patience necessary when dealing with critical plants, thus bringing down on himself the criticism of that prince of caution, S.A. Stewart'. Praeger himself undertook no critical taxonomic work on the Irish flora, though he did tackle the two daunting succulent groups, *Sedum* and *Sempervivum*, for the Royal Horticultural Society. Webb studied the Irish Dactyloid saxifrages and became the acknowledged expert on the group in Europe. R.D. Meikle first came up against the problems of willow identification when working on the flora of Northern Ireland. He continued his interest in the group while at Kew and solved many of the problems associated with British and Irish species.

James Ponsonby Brunker, a leading member of the Dublin Naturalists' Field Club, had worked on the flora of Wicklow since 1918. He was trained in fieldwork by R.W. Scully and in the introduction to his *Flora of the County Wicklow* stresses the importance of that training. Scully undertook the initiation process remembering that A.G. More had done the same for him. Brunker was conscious of that tradition of field workers and spoke of handing on the mantle to a younger generation. Praeger occupied a high place among the people he admired but Scully was spoken of with real affection and gratitude. The notion of an elite group of naturalists probably originated with A.G. More and his recruiting or selecting what he considered suitable or suitably placed people to help with the revision of *Cybele Hibernica*. This idea came to Brunker through Scully. Brunker, who was a member of the Dublin Naturalists' Field Club for more than fifty years, became part of such an elite group within the Field Club. He called it the ASU (for 'active service unit'); membership was by invitation and included such notables as A.W. Stelfox, A. Farrington and G.F. Mitchell. The unit assisted with the flora of County Wicklow and the revision of the Dublin flora but was also interested in geology and ornithology (Mitchell, 1990; Hudson, 1986). The ASU was a strictly male group; the only woman to be allowed on its outings was Mrs R.C. Faris, and then only on one occasion. Some plant localities known to Brunker were not made public and were for selected persons only. Details of the Carlow locality for the Killarney fern were entrusted to Brunker by R.A. Phillips, its first finder. Brunker pre-empted his own intention to pass on this information to the younger male generation when in the late 1960s he made it known for the *The Flora of County Carlow* (1979) being prepared by Evelyn Booth.

The field clubs had always encouraged women to join and participate fully in club organization and activities. Advertisements for the Dublin club had specifically declared that women would be welcome (Bailey, 1986; Doogue, 1986). This distinguished it from the Natural History Society, which excluded women from those meetings at which unsuitable subjects, presumably including references to sexual reproduction, were to be discussed. There seems also to have been a notion that women could not be trusted to keep confidences. A letter from Barrington to Miss Knowles, dated 9 November 1910, implies as much:

I enclose you a private letter from my old friend Colonel Fielden – who is a real veteran in war & science – from the American Rebellion of 1862 to the last Boer War – from Nares Arctic Expedition of 1875 to a recent expedition to Novaya Zemlya. Most of these – (all indeed) he mentions are dead I think – & he wants to see justice done. Tho' a woman you will try to consider the information private in case any Kew entities or non entities pay you a visit. With kind regards & hoping you can help me – to help my old friend I am yrs sincerely, Ricd. M. Barrington. Take care of the letter & remember me to Miss McArdle.

In 1963 the Belfast Naturalists' Field Club celebrated its centenary. The chief guest at the celebrations was Arthur Wilson Stelfox, who had also helped Brunker with his Wicklow flora. Although he worked primarily at entomology and conchology, Stelfox also made important contributions to Irish botany. He retraced much of Hart's mountain routes and began a study of mossy saxifrages that was to be completed by David Webb. Stelfox knew the best routes to the higher mountains and issued precise instructions to anyone who had the good fortune to consult him in advance of a trip to high ground.

The great leap forward, from twelve sub-provinces to forty vice-counties as the basis for biological recording, was to last for over half a century, until the Botanical Society of the British Isles began mapping the flora of the ten-kilometre squares of the National Grid. The key figures in the Irish contribution to this work, begun in the 1950s and completed with the publication of the *Atlas of the British Flora* in 1962, were Webb in the Republic and Patricia Kertland in Northern Ireland. Frequent visits by British-based botanists stimulated an interest in plant recording among Irish botanists and led to the formation of an Irish branch of the Botanical Society of the British Isles. At its first field meeting in the summer of 1963, they made the first Irish record of the Pyrenean species *Minuartia recurva* in the Caha Mountains on the Cork-Kerry border.

Irish botanical studies were being integrated into schemes devised in and for Great Britain. The smaller force of field botanists would find that more and more of their time would be spent on network projects, including recording schemes and recorder-based projects devised for the tight network of vice-county recorders in Great Britain. Unfortunately, the Irish recorder network was overstretched and the benefits of belonging to the British-based society were offset by the demands of that society on the slender resources available. Irish botanists turned their attentions to national needs. By 1977 the Irish Phytogeographical Society had recruited the more active young fieldworkers, including the best of the amateur and professional botanists, and had the support of the older academic botanists. It also provided another outlet for plant and animal records and for publication of preliminary studies, assisting rather than competing with the well-established *Irish Naturalists' Journal* in promoting field botany.

An Foras Forbartha, a semi-state body in the Republic of Ireland set up to advise on planning and development, produced a series of county development reports which included inventories of the best botanical areas. Conservation had come of age and would be the principal consideration behind much of the work of the last quarter of the twentieth century. The National Parks and Wildlife Service of the Department of Arts, Culture and the Gaeltacht continues as the major state watchdog for developments promoting or threatening flora and fauna in the Republic, while the Department of the Environment performs a similar function in Northern Ireland. Co-operation and a desire to conserve and develop what is best informs the work of both. The work of the field botanist – the plant records made often as a recreation, sometimes as a duty, occasionally as an obsession – has now assumed a political importance. Protection of the flora now has a legal basis. Field botany, once regarded as an esoteric pursuit, is now viewed as a practical activity with implications for the kind of environment being planned for the future.

A new generation of regional floras is emerging. The first of these – *The Flora of County Carlow* (Booth, 1979), *Flora of Lough Neagh* (Harron,

1980) and *Flora of Connemara and the Burren* (Webb and Scannell, 1983) – have already stimulated further work in these areas and have been important reference sources for conservation work. A new edition of Stewart and Corry's *Flora of the North-east of Ireland* (Hackney, 1992) contains much new work, and the elegance of its production must improve the image of Irish field botany. It is expected that a revised *Flora of County Dublin* will be published in 1997.

A *Census Catalogue of the Flora of Ireland* (Scannell and Synnott, 1987) and checklists of the floras of several Irish counties have been produced or are being prepared. Although there are still relatively few Irish field botanists, a new heyday of Irish botany has arrived which rivals that begun by Stewart and Corry, More and Barrington, Hart and Praeger, Colgan and Scully, but is in turn dependent, as they were, on the labours of those generations who went before and took the trouble to record their observations and commit them to print.

References

Adams, J. 1931. *A Student's Illustrated Irish Flora*. London: L. Reeve and Co.

Allen, D.E. 1986. *The Botanists: A History of the Botanical Society of the British Isles through a Hundred and Fifty years*. Winchester: St. Paul's Bibliographies.

Bailey, G.W.D. 1986. 'History of the Dublin Naturalists' Field Club,' in *Reflections and Recollections: 100 Years of the Dublin Naturalists' Field Club*. Dublin: Dublin Naturalists' Field Club.

Baily, K.S. 1833. *An Irish Flora*. Dublin.

Barrington, R.M. Letters at National Botanic Gardens, Glasnevin.

Booth, E. 1979. *The Flora of County Carlow*. Dublin: Royal Dublin Society.

Brunker, J.P. 1950. *Flora of the County Wicklow*. Dundalk: Dundalgan Press.

Colgan, N. 1904. *Flora of the County Dublin*. Dublin: Hodges, Figgis and Co. Ltd.

Corry, T.H. 1884. 'On the Heights attained by Plants on Ben Bulben.' *Proceedings of the Royal Irish Academy 2 (4)*: 73-7.

Cullinane, J. 1971. 'Katherine Sophia Baily (Lady Kane), Botanist and Wife of Sir Robert Kane, First President of Queen's College, Cork.' *University College Cork Record 46*: 18-21.

Desmond, R. 1994. *Dictionary of British and Irish Botanists and Horticulturalists*. London: Taylor and Francis and The Natural History Museum.

Dickie, G. 1864. *A Flora of Ulster and Botanist's Guide to the North of Ireland*. Belfast: Aitcheson.

Dony, J.G., S.L. Jury and F. Perring. 1986. *English Names of Wild Flowers: A List Recommended by the Botanical Society of the British Isles*. Reading: Department of Botany, University of Reading.

Doogue, D. 1986. 'Getting Started,' in *Reflections and Recollections: 100 Years of the Dublin Naturalists' Field Club*. Dublin: Dublin Naturalists' Field Club.

Edwards, S. 1992. *Mosses in English Literature. British Bryological Society Special Volume No. 4*. Cardiff: British Bryological Society.

Feehan, J. 1984. *Laois: An Environmental History*. Ballykilcavan Press.

Foster, W.D. 1979. 'The History of the Moss Exchange Club.' *Bulletin of the British Bryological Society 33*: 19-26.

Hackney, P. 1992. *Stewart and Corry's Flora of the North-east of Ireland*. 3rd edn. Belfast: Institute of Irish Studies, Queen's University.

Harron, J. 1980. *Flora of Lough Neagh*. Belfast: Irish Naturalists' Journal; Coleraine: University of Ulster.

Harvey, W.H. 1846-51. *Phytologia Britannia*. London: Reeve Brothers.

Hooker, W.J. and T. Taylor. 1818. *Muscologia Britannica*. London: Longman, Hurst, Rees, Orme and Brown.

Hoppen, K.T. 1970. *The Common Scientist in the Seventeenth Century*. London: Routledge and Kegan Paul.

How, W. 1650. *Phytologia Britannica*. London: O. Pulleyn.

Hudson, H.J. 1986. 'The A.S.U.,' *Reflections and Recollections: 100 years of the Dublin Naturalists' Field Club*. Dublin: Dublin Naturalists' Field Club.

Hudson, W. 1762. *Flora Anglica*. London: J. Nourse and C. Moran.

Knowles, M.C.K. 1929. 'The Lichens of Ireland.' *Proceedings of the Royal Irish Academy 38B*: 179-434.

Lhwyd, E. 1712. 'Some Further Observations relating to the Antiquities and Natural History of Ireland.' *Philosophical Transactions of the Royal Society 27*: 524-6.

Mackay, J.T. 1836. *Flora Hibernica*. Dublin: William Curry Junior and Co.

McNab, W.R. 1885. 'Note on the Botanical Topographical Divisions of Ireland.' *Scientific Proceedings of the Royal Dublin Society (new series) 4*: 197-9.

Mitchell, G.F. 1986. 'For over Fifty Years he Bestrode Irish Natural History like a Colossus.' *Living Heritage: The Voice of An Taisce*. 4: 6-7.

Mitchell, G.F. 1990. *The Way that I Followed: A Naturalist's Journey around Ireland*. Dublin: Country House.

Mitchell, M.E. 1974. 'The Sources of Threlkeld's *Synopsis Stirpium Hibernicarum*.' *Proceedings of the Royal Irish Academy 74B*: 1-6.

Mithcell, M.E. 1975. 'Irish Botany in the Seventeenth Century.' *Proceedings of the Royal Irish Academy 75B*: 275-84.

Moffat, C.B. 1898. *Life and Letters of Alexander Goodman More*. Dublin: Hodges, Figgis.

Moore, D. and A.G. More. 1866. *Contributions towards a Cybele Hibernica*. Dublin: Hodges, Smith and Co.

Nelson, E.C. 1981. 'Sir Arthur Rawdon (1662-1695) of Moira: His Life and Letters, Family and Friends, and his Jamaican Plants.' *Proceedings and Reports of the Belfast Natural History and Philosophical Society 10*: 30-52.

Nelson, E.C. 1988. *The First Irish Flora, Synopsis Stirpium Hibernicarum by Caleb Threlkeld*. [Introduction to facsimile edition.] Kilkenny: Boethius Press.

Nelson, E.C. 1992. 'William Henry Harvey as Colonial Treasurer at the Cape of Good Hope: a Case of Depression and Bowdlerized History.' *Archives for Natural History 19*: 171-80.

Nelson, E.C. 1992a. 'Robert Brown – with Books in Ireland.' *Botanical Society of the British Isles News 62*: 28-30.

Nelson, E.C. 1993. 'Botany and Medicine – Dublin and Leiden.' *Journal of the College of Physicians and Surgeons. 22*: 133-6.

Nelson, E.C., and E. McCracken. 1987. *The Brightest Jewel: A History of the National Botanic Gardens, Glasnevin*. Kilkenny: Boethius Press.

Newman, E. 1839. 'Notes on Irish Natural History.' *Magazine of Natural History 3 (new series)*: 548-51; 569-77.

Newman, E. 1846. *A History of British Ferns*. London: John Van Voorst.

Power, T. 1845. 'The Botanist's Guide for the County of Cork,' in J.R. Harvey, J.O. Humphreys and T. Power, *Contributions towards a Fauna and Flora of the County of Cork*. Cork and London: Cuvierian Society of Cork.

Praeger, R.L. 1893. 'The Flora of County Armagh.' *Irish Naturalist 2*: 11-15, 34-8, 59-62, 91-5, 127-34, 155-9, 182-4, 212-15.

Praeger, R.L. 1901. 'Irish Topographical Botany.' *Proceedings of the Royal Irish Academy 23*: 1-188, 121-410.

Praeger, R.L. 1909. *A Tourist's Flora of the West of Ireland*. Dublin: Hodges, Figgis.

Praeger, R.L. 1934. *The Botanist in Ireland*. Dublin: Hodges, Figgis.

Praeger, R.L. 1937. *The Way that I Went*. Dublin: Hodges, Figgis; London: Methuen.

Praeger, R.L. 1946. 'Things Left Undone.' *Irish Naturalists' Journal 8*: 322-7.

Praeger, R.L. 1949. *Some Irish Naturalists: A Biographical Notebook*. Dundalk: Dundalgan Press.

Praeger, R.L. and W.R. Megaw. 1938. *A Flora of the North-east of Ireland*. 2nd edn. Belfast: The Quota Press.

Ray, J. 1696. *Synopsis Methodica Stirpium Britannicarum*. 2nd edn. London: S. Smith and B. Walford.

Rutty, J. 1772. *An Essay towards a Natural History of the County of Dublin*. Dublin: author.

Sayre, G. 1987. 'Biographical Sketch of Thomas Taylor.' *Journal of Bryology 14*: 415-27.

Scannell, M.J.P. and D.M. Synnott 1987. *Clar de Phlandai na hEireann. Census Catalogue of the Flora of Ireland*. 2nd edn. Dublin: Stationery Office.

Scully, R.W. 1916. *Flora of the County Kerry*. Dublin: Hodges, Figgis.

Smith, C. 1756. *The Antient and Present State of the County of Kerry*. Dublin: author.

Stewart, S.A. and T.H. Corry. 1888. *A Flora of the North-east of Ireland, including the Phanerogamia, the Cryptogamia vascularia, and the Muscineae*. Cambridge: Macmillan and Bowes.

Threlkeld, C. 1726. *Synopsis Stirpium Hibernicarum*. Dublin: S. Powell.

Turner, D. 1804. *Muscologiae Hiberniae Specilegium*. London: J. White; Yarmouth: J. Black.

Wade, W. 1804. 'Plantae Rariores in Hibernia Inventae.' *Transactions of the Royal Dublin Society 4*: i-xiv, 1-214.

Walsh, L. 1978. *Richard Heaton of Ballyskenagh 1601-1666*. Roscrea: Parkmore Press.

Webb, D.A. 1943. *A New Irish Flora*. Dundalk: Dundalgan Press.

Webb, D.A. and M.J.P. Scannell. 1983. *Flora of Connemara and the Burren*. Dublin: Royal Dublin Society; Cambridge: Cambridge University Press.

White, J. 1808. 'An Essay on the Indigenous Grasses of Ireland.' *Bulletin of Ireland*. Dublin.

Bogland: Study and Utilization

PETER FOSS AND CATHERINE O'CONNELL

On 15 June 1919 the first non-stop powered flight across the Atlantic ended nose-down in Derrygimla Bog near Clifden, Co. Galway. The cool, moist westerlies that helped Alcock and Brown to achieve this historic crossing do more than carry intrepid aviators to the western shores of Europe – they also have a very important effect on the climate and vegetation of Ireland. After their 6500-km journey from the eastern seaboard of North America, the westerlies carry enough moisture to produce rain on two out of three days in western Ireland. The Gulf Stream also plays an important role in moderating the Irish climate and ensuring little temperature variation throughout the year. Coupled with a geology of hard, acidic rocks, this has produced landscapes dominated by the vegetational assemblage known as 'peat bog'. The word 'bog' derives from the Irish word *bogach* meaning 'soft ground'.

Today bogs are found on all continents except Antarctica, but are most common in northern latitudes, where retreating glaciers left moist, depressed land with poor drainage. Precipitation is their only water source and as a result they have highly acidic soils, reflected in a pH range between 3.5 and 4.2. If other waters, such as springs, feed into bogs they are then called 'fens' which are alkaline, reflected in a pH range between 7 and 8.

Differences in types of bog reflect differences in climate and terrain. Waterlogging first reduces oxygen levels and slows the decay of dead vegetation, which settles and gradually becomes peat, a precursor of coal. The accumulation of peat is very dramatic in bogs that are dominated by *Sphagnum* mosses. These mosses excrete antibiotics and hydrogen ions, which further raises water acidity, helping to retard decay even more. Many of the postglacial lakes in the centre of Ireland have become in-filled with vegetation and peat; these are called 'raised bogs' (*plate 7*). The other bog type, the 'blanket bogs', spread across poorly drained landscapes, most often in mountainous regions and along the oceanic west coast of Ireland. Here high rainfall causes leaching of the soil and the development of a watertight iron pan layer, making it possible for peat to accumulate directly on the mineral soil (*plate 7*).

The living surface of a bog is made up of a series of well-drained hummocks, flat lawns and damp hollows, with pools present in very wet bogs. In blanket bogs more complex features reflect variations in the peat depth, with ridges and rock outcrops covered with a thin layer of peat. They may contain relatively large lakes, and are drained by swallow holes, streams, and rivers such as the Liffey in Co. Wicklow and the Owenduff in Co. Mayo.

Bog Wildlife

Several different species of bog moss grow in the pools, drains and hummocks of the bog, making up a richly coloured mosaic. *Sphagnum* moss, fully adapted to the hostile environmental conditions of the bog water, abounds. Anaerobic conditions limit the ability of bacteria and fungi to break down dead plants, which means that the essential minerals needed for plant growth are in short supply.

Carnivorous plants such as sundew, bladderwort and butterwort boost the mineral nutrients in their diet, such as nitrogen and phosphorus, by consuming insects. The spoon-shaped leaves of sundew, the most commonly encountered species, are covered with up to two hundred pin-shaped red 'tentacles' (or stalked glands) that respond to touch. Each gland is covered with a mucilaginous secretion that traps and digests prey, including small flies, gnats, beetles and ants, and occasionally, larger prey such as damselflies. On average, a sundew plant traps up to five insects per month.

Evergreen plants conserve nutrients by retaining their leaves each year. In bogland, the most obvious of these are the heathers. In late summer and autumn the colour purple wonderfully transforms the vast expanses of brown bogland. Bogs in the west of Ireland are a gardener's paradise, where mingling with the commoner species of ling heather, cross-leaved heath and bell heather, one also finds rarities such as St Dabeoc's heath, Mackay's heath and a host of hybrid species.

Other plants such as bog cotton, black bog rush, deer sedge, beak sedge and bog asphodel recycle nutrients gathered in their leaves, moving them from the decaying leaves into storage organs. These provide a highly nutritious food source for the small flocks of Greenland white-fronted geese that migrate to Ireland in October to overwinter in remote bogs. Bogs present birds with special problems of survival, as they are almost treeless landscapes. Therefore many bogland birds are ground-nesters, and species such as skylark, golden plover, curlew, red grouse and snipe are beautifully camouflaged for protection from predators such as the fox. The well-known calls and cries of these birds are an evocative part of the atmosphere of the wild boglands.

Bogland pools and lakes are a wildlife haven for frogs, insects and many other invertebrates. The adult frog is an important predator and enjoys a varied diet of insects on the bog. Damselflies and dragonflies, among the most spectacular Irish insects, set up their hunting territories around bog pools. Brilliantly coloured, with glistening wings and their strong purposeful flight, dragonflies are easily identifiable. Other creatures of bog pools include water beetles, midges, water boatmen, freshwater snails, water spiders, water mites, caddis-flies and bloodworms. Even the surface of the pools is inhabited by a variety of specialized animals such as the raft spider (*Dolomedes fimbriatus*), the pond skater and the whirligig beetle, which make use of surface tension to walk on the water and catch prey landing on the surface.

More than Peat Alone

The anaerobic conditions in peat bogs delay the normal processes of decay and give bogs tremendous preservation powers. Through the years, turf cutting has unearthed a fascinating array of ancient gold, bronze, amber, wooden and stone objects preserved by the peat. As the living bog grows, it buries and conserves anything in its path, including the early pine woodland and 'bog oaks' often exposed by turf cutters at the cut-edge of bogs. When the growing bogs encroached upon farmland, the stone walls of fields, houses and tombs of ancient Irish homesteads were swallowed up and deleted from the landscape. Twenty years ago, exploration of peat bog on the north coast of Mayo unearthed the first well-preserved farmsteads, found buried under four metres of peat. These dated back over four thousand years to an era preceding the formation of the bog (Caulfield *et al.*, 1987; Herity, 1971). Perfectly preserved gold and bronze jewellery, weapons and household objects have furnished valuable clues to lifestyles, rituals and warfare in ancient Ireland (Halpin, 1984).

In the Irish midlands, scattered communities grew up on the fertile mineral soils. The growth of some raised bogs gradually prevented easy passage from one community to the next. To maintain contact, local people often built trackways or 'toghers' of wood or stone across the bog, a large number of which have been unearthed, perfectly preserved (Moloney, 1993). For centuries peat bogs were used for storing butter, and 'bog butter' is unearthed occasionally when turf is being cut. Human corpses were sometimes disposed of in bog holes and occasionally these have been found so well preserved that the colour and style of hair and the type of clothing is still evident. By examining the contents of the stomach, archaeologists can sometimes identify what was eaten at the corpse's last meal (O'Floinn, 1988).

Historical Studies of Boglands

The earliest publications on Irish bogs appeared over three hundred years ago: Gerard Boate's *Irelands Naturall History* (1652) and William King's paper to the Royal Society in 1685. In discussing the origin of bogs, Boate asserted that they did not occur 'by any naturall property or primitive constitution, but through the superfluous moysture that in length of time hath been gathered therein', either from springs or from rainwater. He seemed to be in little doubt that the vast area covered by bogs in Ireland could be ascribed to the 'retchlesness of the Irish who let daily more and more of their good land grow boggy through their carelessness'. He was led to this conclusion by the finding, even at this early date, of plough marks and relics of cultivation and habitation on the mineral soil underlying bogs. Boate also described the former presence of trees in bogs, which helped to reinforce his prejudicial view of their origin.

Robert Lloyd Praeger (1949) commented that although Boate, a physician to Cromwell, had not been to Ireland when he wrote his book, 'so slight a drawback was no deterrent to his writing about it, basing his account on reports received from others; and a very interesting and mainly accurate book he made of it'. Boate's account is notable for the first attempted classification of bogs, which he distinguished from heaths. He observed that bogs were of several types, and made an important demarcation between 'red bogs' and 'wet bogs'. Of the former he stated that 'the earth in them for the most part is reddish and overgrown with moss of the same colour: in some parts of vast extent'. These bogs correspond to what we know nowadays as raised bogs. He devoted more attention to the wet bogs, which have 'superfluous moysture', and even sub-divided them into four types: grassy, watery, miry and hassocky (White, 1982).

William King, the Irish divine who became Bishop of Derry and later Archbishop of Dublin, was also a founder member of the Dublin Philosophical Society. His paper to the Royal Society in 1685, 'Of the Bogs and Loughs of Ireland', was largely concerned with the practical problems of land drainage. Although much of his paper was reminiscent of Boate's earlier publication, down to the account of the reason for the extent of the bogs ('no wonder if a country, famous for laziness as Ireland is, abound with them'), his views on the origin of bogs represent the first clear and definite statement of their plant succession.

The next major works on peatlands were the four *Reports of the Commissioners Appointed to Enquire into the Nature and Extent of Several Bogs in Ireland: and the Practicability of Draining and Cultivating them*, published between 1810 and 1814. The second of the four is the most interesting from a vegetational viewpoint. It contains an outstanding series of observations, notably those of 'the ablest land surveyor of his time', Richard Griffith, one of the eight engineers employed on the survey. During the years 1809-13, he surveyed the Bog of Allen, bogs in the valley of the River Suck, the Wicklow Mountains and north of Clew Bay. In total he spent 1300 days on the bog survey and is credited with surveying about 180,000 hectares of bog or 15 per cent of the total in Ireland.

In the *Reports* there are observations and comments on the formation, morphology and vegetation of bogs. Griffith made use of the distinction that had first been made by his contemporary, the chemist Richard Kirwan, between compact or black bogs (fen peat) and fibrous or red bogs (bog peat). Griffith's reports of the raised bogs of the central plain are characterized by meticulous maps and drawings of vertical profiles, and include details of chemical analyses of the various strata which were among the first published on this topic (White, 1982). Although many of the basic concepts of bog ecology were actually established by these engineers long before they were discovered by professional botanists, there are only isolated references to the plant species growing on bogs since the primary object in compiling the *Reports* was to offer advice on bog drainage and exploitation. The engineers put forward many ideas and practical suggestions on this subject, which helped to stimulate landowners' efforts to exploit peatlands.

Bogland received little further study during the remaining years of the nineteenth century, until Ireland's best-known field botanist, Robert Lloyd Praeger, published 'Irish Topographical Botany' in 1901. This paper had a major influence on the knowledge of the geography and ecology of the Irish flora. In 1902 Praeger examined bog vegetation and used the terms 'plant group' and 'plant association' to emphasize the uniqueness and integrity of the plant assemblages of Irish raised bogs, 'one of the few plant associations now to be found which is absolutely uninfluenced by ubiquitous man and his works'. Subsequently, in the introductory section of *The Botanist in Ireland* (1934), he commented on regional variations in peatland flora, bog ecology and the destruction of raised bogs and gave descriptions of specific sites.

Contribution of Ecologists to the Study of Bogs

The next major developments came in 1935 with A.G. Tansley's visit to the Irish midlands, where he studied the vegetation and stratigraphy of raised bogs in the distinguished company of Praeger, Hugo Osvald, Harry Godwin, Knud Jessen and Frank Mitchell. Tansley introduced the term 'bog' into ecological literature in his monumental work *The British Islands and their Vegetation*, which was published in 1939. His account of Irish raised bogs is quite detailed and original and is still the most accessible source of information on Irish vegetation to many foreign botanists, although they will find that many of the fens and raised bogs it describes have since been destroyed (White, 1982).

The 1935 study trip stimulated Godwin (1981), Jessen (1949), Mitchell (1976) and Osvald (1949) to elucidate the stages in the formation of bogs and the vegetation history of Ireland since the Ice Age. Praeger (1937) describes a typical wet visit to Roundstone Bog by this eminent group:

We stood in a ring in that shelterless expanse while discussion raged on the application of the terms soligenous, topogenous and ombrogenous; the rain and wind, like the discussion, waxed in intensity, and under the unusual super-incumbent weight, whether of mere flesh and bone or of intellect, the floating surface of the bog slowly sank till we were all half-way up to our knees in water. The only pause in the flow of argument was when Jessen or Osvald, in an endeavour to solve the question of the origin of the peat, would chew some of the mud brought up by the boring tool from the bottom of the bog, to test the presence or absence of gritty material in the vegetable mass. But out of such occasions does knowledge come, and I think that that aqueous discussion has borne and will bear fruit. For the bogs and what they can teach us of the past history of our country are yet to a great extent a sealed book, though they will not remain so much longer.

True to Praeger's prediction, these workers established in Ireland the tradition of palaeoecological research, the study of ancient plant communities from their fossil remains, and within the last twenty years much important work has been carried out. Michael O'Connell in University College Galway has studied blanket bog formation in detail (1986, 1990). Using fossilized tree trunks of bog oak, John Pilcher and Michael Baillie in Queen's University, Belfast, examined the varying pattern of tree-ring widths from which they established a chronology by cross-matching similar patterns in different trees. With the addition of more early timbers, they have managed now to build a dendrochronology spanning several thousand years, which allows the age of even small pieces of oak to be accurately dated (Pilcher *et al.*, 1977; Pearson *et al.*, 1977). From specific studies on fossil pine and oak stumps, interesting information on the structure of the ancient woodlands that grew on bogs, and reasons for their extinction, have emerged (Pilcher, 1990; McNally and Doyle, 1984, 1984a). This indicates that the 'pine woodland episode' on raised bogs lasted from around 2000–1500 BC. Study of the age structure of these woodlands suggests that their decline was due to a raised water table which inhibited germination of seedlings and eventually led to the extinction of the woodland.

Two German botanists, J. Braun-Blanquet and Reinhold Tüxen, described Irish bog vegetation and categorized it on floristic criteria in 'Irische Planzengesellschaften' (1952). They had a significant influence on several Irish botanists who adopted their scheme, including John J. Moore, who subsequently established the School of Vegetation Science at University College Dublin. Further work refining the earlier classification of Braun-Blanquet and Tüxen was published by Moore in 'A Classification of the Bogs and Wet Heaths of Northern Europe' (1968), and his influence as a teacher at UCD stimulated a steady stream of research on Irish bogs. Another major study in which he played a prime part was the International Biological Programme on Blanket Bogs, undertaken at Glenamoy, Co. Mayo, which ran for twenty years from 1960. Research was undertaken to describe and characterize the vegetation and ecology of virgin blanket bogs (Doyle and Moore, 1980; Doyle, 1982).

In the last decade research on bogs has continued apace, with the emphasis on the relationship between water levels and the growth and regeneration of bogs, in order to develop management plans for conserved areas. Two major studies have been carried out. The first, by the Environmental Science Unit at Trinity College, Dublin, has focused on Mongan Bog in Co. Offaly, near Clonmacnoise (Tubridy, 1984). Ecosystem studies, stimulated by the Royal Irish Academy and undertaken by researchers at UCD and Trinity College, investigated production and decomposition processes (Madden and Doyle, 1990; Doyle and Dowding, 1990). The second study, initiated in 1989 at Clara and Raheenmore Bogs in Co. Offaly, involved Irish and Dutch researchers who examined their geohydrology and ecology with a view to developing suitable management programmes for raised bogs in Ireland.

Paralleling this research into the ecology and formation of bogs has been a growth in interest in wetland archaeology. Many chance archaeological discoveries have been made, usually during turf cutting, and the wide range of artefacts found has been documented by Halpin (1984). However, contemporary archaeological work now places greater emphasis on site research. Seamus Caulfield, who was inspired by his father, has firmly established the importance of bogs as preservers of ancient landscapes. His team's discovery of the Céide Fields in Co. Mayo revealed the largest Stone Age 'monument' yet found in Europe (Caulfield et al., 1987). Recently, the establishment of an Archaeological Wetlands Unit at University College Dublin, directed by Barry Raftery, has been another significant step towards systematic investigations of bog archaeology and has led to significant publications on bog trackways and villages (Raftery, 1990; Moloney, 1993, 1993a).

In conjunction with the archaeological investigations of bogs there has been an emphasis on the importance of preserving the archaeological heritage of peatlands. A national survey co-ordinated by the Office of Public Works is under way to identify and map all the sites and monuments of archaeological importance in bogland, as a first step in ensuring their conservation (Anon., 1992; Condit and Gibbons, 1990).

From Marshland to Peat Production

Hand-won peat has been utilized as a fuel in Ireland throughout recorded history. Traditionally turf was – and in some places still is – cut by hand with a spade known as a *slean*, a Gaelic word anglicized as 'slane'. This is a narrow straight-shafted light steel blade with a wing set at right angles that enables a complete sod to be cut at a single stroke. First a bank is opened up on the bog, and using the *slean*, turves are cut and landed on the top of the bog. The wet sods are spread out to dry using a turf-fork or pike. After one or two weeks, the turves have dried sufficiently to be built into small stacks and then into larger and larger 'turn-foots', 'castles', 'rickles', or 'lumps' to aid drying out. This is called 'footing the turf' and is carried on throughout the summer months. Completely dry turves shrink by an eighth of their original volume and are brick-hard. They are transported home and built into a large pile or 'clamp', often against the house wall, from where they traditionally fuelled heating and cooking. A week's turf cutting would usually provide enough fuel to last one year.

Hand production accelerated in the seventeenth century, following the clearance of most of the native forests, reaching recorded levels of around five million tons per annum. But it was not until the nineteenth century that any serious attempts were made to mechanize the process of peat cutting. In 1844 Charles Wye Williams of Derrylea invented the first turf sod machine, and in 1860 Charles Hodgson perfected a way of milling peat and turning it into 'briquettes'. These pioneering methods were followed by many other attempts at small-scale commercial exploitation of the bogs, most of which failed, although they fostered the notion of turning the vast resource of peat wastelands into an economic resource (Ryan, 1907, 1908).

In 1934 the Irish Free State decided to take a direct role in the development of Irish peat resources and set up the Turf Development Board. The Board purchased a small area of bogland and developed methods of producing milled and sod peat. Development was delayed during World War II but much experience was gained that proved useful for later expansion, and the peat produced during the war made a vital contribution to the nation's fuel supply at a time when imports were severely restricted. Following the war, plans were put in place for a programme to exploit much greater areas of bog.

In line with the proposed expansion, a state peat production company, Bord na Móna, was established in 1946 to develop the country's peat resources on a fully commercial basis. The company eventually acquired a total area of eighty thousand hectares of bogland, making it the largest single owner of peatland in the country today. Peat is harvested mainly from the deep raised bogs of the midlands, with several smaller production centres in the west. In 1990 Bord na Móna's output was eight million tons, and over half of its total output is used for the generation of electricity. Sod peat and peat briquettes are supplied for domestic and industrial consumption, and horticultural peat and fertilized peat products are marketed worldwide, forming an important source of export revenue.

The success of Bord na Móna in exploiting peat and developing the technology to do so stimulated the creation of smaller commercial peat companies throughout the country, all of which have accelerated the depletion of the resource. The rate of peat extraction in the private sector intensified in the 1980s with the introduction of a variety of mechanical turf extractors and the ready availability of grants under the 1981 Turf Development Act. In 1990 nearly one and a half million tons of fuel peat were produced by the private companies.

Bog Reclamation

Irish bogland has many other uses. In addition to peat production, great effort was put into reclaiming bogland for agricultural use by both individual farmers and government committees in the eighteenth and nineteenth centuries. As early as 1716 the government supported the idea of bog reclamation, and by 1729 government duties were imposed on items imported into Ireland to fund bog-reclamation schemes. In 1731 'An Act to Encourage the Improvement of Barren, and Waste Land, and Boggs, and Planting of Timber Trees and Orchards' was passed by Parliament in London. In the same year the Dublin Society was set up, and among its aims was the encouragement of bog reclamation by the awarding of medals to projects with development potential.

With the escalating population in the early nineteenth century, productive land became scarce and bog reclamation became a priority. It was against this background that the government established a commission under Sir Richard Griffith to investigate Irish bogs for reclamation purposes. Bog reclamation continued up to 1848 when famine and evictions forced many of the tenants to abandon their holdings and emigrate. The Land War that followed and the subsequent demise of the landlords effectively halted the major agricultural reclamation of peatlands.

By 1955 Bord na Móna's progress in extracting peat from the bogs led to a renewed discussion of reclamation that continues today (Mollan, 1989). The American aid received through the Marshall Plan after World War II led to the foundation of An Foras Talúntais (Institute of Agricultural Research), now Teagasc. Under the directorship of P.J. O'Hare it undertook every possible experiment on the drainage and cultivation of blanket bog at Glenamoy, Co. Mayo (Moore et al., 1975).

The Forestry Division also established experimental planting on blanket bog at Glenamoy, but concluded that agricultural reclamation of blanket bog was not economically feasible and that planting conifers would only succeed with financial support. However, in 1950 the Food and Agricultural Organization of the United Nations produced the so-called Cameroon Report after a visit to Ireland (Anon., 1951). This recommended that 6 per cent of the land surface of Ireland be devoted to the forestry industry, with half to be planted on blanket bog in the west of Ireland, to try to stimulate economic growth in these areas. There followed an intensive programme of conifer planting on blanket bogs, and between 1974 and 1982 the Forest Service was planting conifers on 5000 hectares per year; some 160,000 hectares of blanket bog are now planted (Ryan and Cross, 1984).

A Change in Attitudes

The cumulative effects of traditional turf-cutting, mechanization of the peat industry and the commencement of tree planting on bogs served to diminish greatly the area of intact peatland in a relatively short period of time. Since conservation was not until recently merited with any economic value, it was not considered important. Tom Barry, an employee of Bord na Móna, was the first to point out to the board that they had an obligation to preserve some bogs. His interest in this issue was stimulated by the case of Pollagh Bog in Co. Offaly, where in 1951 John Moore had discovered the rannoch rush (*Scheuzcheria palustris*) and wintergreen (*Pyrola secunda*). Moore undertook an ecological study of the only Irish station of these rare species, but despite his opposition the site was destroyed for turf development by Bord na Móna (Moore, 1955). This landmark case represented the first time conservation of a bog had been sought primarily due to the presence of rare species, and was the first where conflict arose between development agencies and environmentalists.

A conflict arose between environmentalists and foresters in the early 1950s over Lough Meenameen Fen in Co. Fermanagh. The Northern Ireland Forest Service overruled the conservation of a rare moss, *Homalothecium nitens*, in favour of the planting of a forty-hectare site, and the area was subsequently drained and planted (Parker, 1990). Exploitation of peatlands continued apace until the early 1970s, when the first comprehensive peatland surveys were undertaken by An Foras Talúntais and An Foras Forbartha. Hammond (1979) classified peatlands into major ecological types and mapped intact and man-modified areas. A national survey to identify sites of conservation interest in the Republic of Ireland was undertaken over the period 1968-74 (Anon., 1980).

In response to heightened public consciousness of environmental conservation, stimulated in 1970 with European Conservation Year, the first steps were taken to conserve bogs. An Taisce, Bord na Móna, the Forest and Wildlife Service (Dublin) and the Forest Service in Northern Ireland discussed the value of conserving peatland, and areas were set aside for protection (Barry, 1976; Parker, 1990). However, a period of almost ten years was to follow without any significant results. This forced John Moore to reiterate his concerns for bogland conservation in 1982 when he accepted a European Prize for the Protection of Nature from the Johann Wolfgang Von Goethe-Stiftung Conservation Trust, a German organization. Moore commented in his acceptance speech:

Although I have worked as a member of the Wildlife Advisory Council for four years now, and although we have made recommendations to the Minister to conserve a number of our bogs, nothing concrete has happened, partly due to the unfavourable financial position of the Government Exchequer. However, in recent months, a National Peatland Conservation Committee was set up to promote the conservation of a representative series of our bog types. This very active committee made up mainly of active young workers have drawn up an annotated list of the bog sites they wish to have preserved. They point out that only 6 per cent of the Midland raised bogs remain undrained and their hopes are that, as a result of their efforts, a representative series of bogs, comprising about 4 per cent of the remaining undrained areas, be preserved for posterity. (Anon., 1982)

At this time several other important developments occurred that consolidated the need for a conservation movement relating to peatlands, and in a report on European peatlands to the Council of Europe, the most important Irish sites for peatland conservation were listed (Goodwillie, 1980). In 1981 a Dutch researcher, Matthijs Schouten, came to Ireland to examine the differences in bogs from the east coast to the west coast of Ireland. He was provided with a list of sites to select for study, but found that out of one hundred sites he visited, only twenty-three were sufficiently intact to merit study. Greatly alarmed, Schouten gave a seminar at a bog conservation week held at UCD in 1981, entitled 'Irish Bogs – Who Wants Them?' He pointed out the close similarity between the history of Dutch peatland destruction and the unchecked exploitation of bogs in Ireland. In 1983 Schouten set up the remarkable 'Dutch Foundation for the Conservation of Irish Bogs', which was to raise funds in Holland to purchase bogs in Ireland for conservation purposes (Schouten and Nooren, 1990). In three years the Dutch Foundation raised sufficient funds to purchase three Irish bogs.

In 1982, during 'Bog Conservation Week', a number of experts formed the National Peatland Conservation Committee (known today as the Irish Peatland Conservation Council), which included, apart from Schouten, experts from Irish universities, the Office of Public Works, An Foras Forbartha and An Foras Talúntais (Doyle, 1990). Its priority was to publish a list of the conservation-worthy peatlands in Ireland (O'Connell, 1987). This was considered vital in stimulating government attention and in formulating plans for a programme of site acquisition and conservation. This stimulated the Wildlife Service of the Office of Public Works to undertake a national peatland survey, which was completed in 1992, while in Northern Ireland a peatland survey was co-ordinated by the Countryside and Wildlife Branch of the Department of the Environment (Cross, 1990; Leach and Corbett, 1987; Anon., 1992a).

Conserving the Bogs

Bogs are increasingly under threat from a host of pressures, including development, agriculture and forestry. Although these undoubtedly helped to transform the economies of certain regions of Ireland, the environmental cost of this progress now means that we can point to a date in the very near future when, tragically, the last natural peatlands will have vanished forever from Ireland. On the European mainland it is already too late; all natural peatlands or bogs in the Netherlands have been lost and Switzerland and Germany have only 500 hectares remaining each. In the United Kingdom there has been a 90 per cent loss of blanket bogs with only 125,000 hectares remaining, while 98 per cent of raised bogs are lost and only 1170 hectares remain.

Research by IPCC shows that to date there has been a 92 per cent loss of raised bogs and an 82 per cent loss of blanket bogs in Ireland. At current rates of exploitation IPCC estimates that all unprotected raised bogs and blanket bogs will be extinct early in the new century (Foss and O'Connell, 1996). At present only 30,808 hectares out of a conservation target of 50,000 hectares targeted in 1987 are protected (Treacey, 1990). With only a few years to go before all unprotected raised and blanket bogs become extinct, IPCC has formulated a Peatland Conservation Plan for Ireland (Foss and O'Connell, 1996). The Plan is to be used to draw up a sustainable land policy for peatlands throughout the country, as part of the government's National Conservation Strategy. A similar strategy document exists for Northern Ireland (Anon., 1993).

The Conservation Plan presents a full inventory of peatlands of European Conservation Importance in the Republic and Northern Ireland. Information on some 715 sites (covering an area of nearly 250,000 hectares) is included, as is a strategy to achieve the goal of conserving a representative sample of Irish bogs. Each peatland site of European Conservation Importance is listed in the Conservation Plan as part of a national network of sites representing the full range of peatland habitats in Ireland. These vital land areas are of inestimable value as a key part of the heritage of

Ireland. They must be conserved and protected so that our bogland heritage will be inherited by future generations.

References

Anon. 1731. *An Act to Encourage the Improvement of Barren, and Waste Land, and Boggs, and Planting of Timber Trees and Orchards.* Dublin.

Anon. 1810-14. *Reports of the Commissioners Appointed to Enquire into the Nature and Extent of the Several Bogs in Ireland; and the Practicability of Draining and Cultivating them. 1-4.* House of Commons.

Anon. 1951. *Report on the Forestry Mission to Ireland by the Food and Agricultural Organisation of the United Nations.* Dublin: Government Publications.

Anon. 1980. *Peatland Sites of Scientific Interest in Ireland.* Dublin: An Foras Forbartha.

Anon. 1982. *Verleihung des Europa-Preises Für Landespflege an Professor John J. Moore S.J., D.Sc., Dublin/Irland, und der Peter Joseph Lenné-Medaille in gold an Herrn Byron Anthony Antipas, Athen/Griechenland.* Johann Wolfgang Von Goethe-Stiftung zu Basel.

Anon. 1992a. *Peatland Conservation Strategy.* Belfast: Council for Nature Conservation and the Countryside.

Anon. 1993. *Conserving Peatland in Northern Ireland: A Statement of Policy.* Belfast: Environment Service.

Barry, T.A. 1976. 'Environmental Protection and the Bogs of Ireland.' *Proceedings of the 5th International Peat Congress, Foznan:* 17-35.

Boate, Gerard. 1652. *Irelands Naturall History. Being a true Description of its Situation, Greatness, Shape and Nature.* London: Samuel Hartlib.

Braun-Blanquet, J. and R. Tüxen. 1952. 'Irische Pflanzengesellschaften.' *Veroff. Geobot. Inst. Zurich* 25: 224-415.

Caulfield, S., A. Lynch and B. Raftery. 1987. 'The Archaeology of Peatlands,' in C. O'Connell (ed.), *The IPCC Guide to Irish Peatlands.* Dublin: Irish Peatland Conservation Council.

Condit, T. and M. Gibbons. 1990. 'The Bird's Eye View of Our Past.' *Technology Ireland 22 (5):* 50-4.

Cross, J.R. 1990. 'Survey and Selection of Peatland Sites for Conservation in the Republic of Ireland,' in G.J. Doyle (ed.), *Ecology and Conservation of Irish Peatlands.* Dublin: Royal Irish Academy.

Doyle, G.J. 1982. 'The Vegetation, Ecology and Productivity of Atlantic Blanket Bog in Mayo and Galway, Western Ireland.' *Journal of Life Sciences of the Royal Dublin Society 3:* 147-64.

Doyle, G.J. 1990. 'Bog Conservation in Ireland,' in M.G.C. Schouten and M.J. Nooren (eds), *Peatlands, Economy and Conservation.* The Netherlands: SPB Academic Publishing.

Doyle, G.J. and J.J. Moore. 1980. 'Western Blanket Bog *(Pleurozio purpureae – Ericetum tetralicis)* in Ireland and Great Britain.' *Colloques phytosociologiques 7:* 213-23.

Doyle, T. and P. Dowding. 1990. 'Decomposition and Aspects of the Physical Environment in the Surface Layers of Mongan Bog,' in G. J. Doyle (ed.), *Ecology and Conservation of Irish Peatlands.* Dublin: Royal Irish Academy.

Foss, P.J. and C.A. O'Connell. 1996. *Irish Peatland Conservation Plan 2000.* Dublin: Irish Peatland Conservation Council.

Godwin, H. 1981. *The Archives of the Peat Bogs.* Cambridge: Cambridge University Press.

Goodwillie, R. 1980. *European Peatlands.* Strasbourg: Council of Europe, Nature and Environment Series 19.

Halpin, A. 1984. *A Preliminary Survey of Archaeological Material Recovered from Peatlands in the Republic of Ireland.* Dublin: Office of Public Works.

Hammond, R.F. 1979. *The Peatlands of Ireland.* Dublin: An Foras Taluntais Soil Survey Bulletin 35.

Herity, M. 1971. 'Prehistoric Fields in Ireland.' *Irish University Review 1*: 258-65.

Jessen, K. 1949. 'Studies in Late Quaternary Deposits and Flora History of Ireland.' *Proceedings of the Royal Irish Academy 52B*: 88-279.

King, William. 1685. 'Of the bogs and loughs of Ireland.' *Philosophical Transactions of the Royal Society 15*: 948-60.

Leach, S.J. and P. McM. Corbett 1987. 'A Preliminary Survey of Raised Bogs in Northern Ireland.' *Glasra 10*: 57-73.

Madden, B. and G.J. Doyle. 1990. 'Primary Production on Mongan Bog,' in G J. Doyle, (ed.), *Ecology and Conservation of Irish Peatlands*. Dublin: Royal Irish Academy.

McNally, A. and G.J. Doyle. 1984. 'A Study of Subfossil Pine Layers in a Raised Bog Complex in the Irish Midlands. I. Palaeowoodland Extent and Dynamics.' *Proceedings of the Royal Irish Academy 84B*: 57-70.

McNally, A. and G.J. Doyle. 1984a. 'A Study of Subfossil Pine Layers in a Raised Bog Complex in the Irish Midlands. II. Serial Relationships and Floristics.' *Proceedings of the Royal Irish Academy 84B*: 71-81.

Mitchell, F. 1976. *The Irish Landscape*. Glasgow: Collins & Son.

Mollan, C. 1989. *The Utilisation of Irish Midland Peatlands*. Dublin: Royal Dublin Society.

Moloney, A. 1993. 'Survey of the Raised Bogs of County Longford.' *Transactions of the Irish Archaeological Wetland Unit 1*: 1-120.

Moloney, A. 1993a. 'Excavations at Clonfinlough, County Offaly.' *Transactions of the Irish Archaeological Wetland Unit 2*: 1-131.

Moore, J.J. 1955. 'The Distribution and Ecology of *Scheuchzeria palustris* on a Raised Bog in Co. Offaly.' *Irish Naturalists' Journal 11*: 1-7.

Moore, J.J. 1968. 'A Classification of the Bogs and Wet Heaths of Northern Europe.' *Ber. Int. Symp. Pflanzensoz., Stolzenau/Weser 1964*: 306-20.

Moore, J.J., P. Dowding and B. Healy. 1975. 'Glenamoy, Ireland,' in T. Rosswall and O.W. Heal (eds), *Structure and Function of Tundra Ecosystems*. Stockholm: Ecological Bulletin 20.

O'Connell, C.A. 1987. *The IPCC Guide to Irish Peatlands*. Dublin: Irish Peatland Conservation Council.

O'Connell, M. 1986. 'Reconstruction of Local Landscape Development in the Post-Atlantic based on Palaeoecological Investigations at Carrownaglogh Field System, County Mayo, Ireland.' *Review of Palaeobotany and Palynology 49*: 117-76.

O'Connell, M. 1990. 'Origins of Irish Lowland Blanket Bog,' in G.J. Doyle (ed.), *Ecology and Conservation of Irish Peatlands*. Dublin: Royal Irish Academy.

O'Floinn, R. 1988. 'Irish Bog Bodies.' *Archeology Ireland 2*: 94-7.

Osvald, H. 1949. 'Notes on the Vegetation of British and Irish Mosses.' *Acta phytogeographica Suecica 26*: 1-62.

Parker, R. 1990. 'Peatland Conservation in Northern Ireland,' in G.J. Doyle (ed.), *Ecology and Conservation of Irish Peatlands*. Dublin: Royal Irish Academy.

Pearson, G.W., J.R. Pilcher, M.G.L. Baillie and J. Hillam. 1977. 'Absolute Radiocarbon Dating using a Low Altitude European Tree-ring Calibration.' *Nature 270*: 25-8.

Pilcher, J.R. 1990. 'The Ecology of Sub-fossil Oakwoods,' in G.J. Doyle (ed.), *Ecology and Conservation of Irish Peatlands*. Dublin: Royal Irish Academy.

Pilcher, J.R., J. Hillam, M.G.L. Baillie and G.W. Pearson 1977. 'A Long Subfossil Oak Tree-ring Chronology from the North of Ireland.' *New Phytologist 79*: 713-29.

Praeger, R.L. 1901. 'Irish Topographical Botany.' *Proceedings of the Royal Irish Academy. 3rd Ser. 7* i-clxxxviii, 1-410

Praeger, R.L. 1934. *The Botanist in Ireland*. Dublin: Hodges Figgis & Company.

Praeger, R.L. 1937. *The Way That I Went*. Dublin: Hodges Figgis & Company.

Praeger, R.L. 1949. *Some Irish Naturalists: A Biographical Note Book*. Dundalk: Dundalgan Press.

Raftery, B. 1990. *Trackways through Time*. Dublin: Headline Publishing.

Ryan, H. 1907/8. 'Report upon the Irish Peatland Industries. Parts 1 and 2.' *Economic Proceedings of the Royal Dublin Society 1*: 371-420; 465-546.

Ryan, J.B. and J.R. Cross. 1984. 'Conservation of Peatlands in Ireland.' *Proceedings of the 5th International Peat Congress*, Dublin.

Schouten, M.G.C. and M.J. Nooren. 1990. *Peatlands, Economy & Conservation*. The Hague: SPB Academic Publishing.

Tansley, A.G. 1939. *The British Islands and their Vegetation*. Cambridge: Cambridge University Press.

Treacey, N. 1990. 'Closing address at the "Peatlands in Perspective" Conference 1987,' in M.G.C. Schouten and M.J. Nooren (eds), *Peatlands, Economy and Conservation*. The Hague: SPB Academic Publishing.

Tubridy, M. 1984. *Creation and Management of a Heritage Zone at Clonmacnoise, Co. Offaly, Ireland*. Dublin: Trinity College Environmental Sciences Unit.

White, J. 1982. 'A History of Irish Vegetation Studies.' *Journal of Life Sciences of the Royal Dublin Society 3*: 15-24.

Paper Landscapes:
Mapping Ireland's Physical Geography

J.H. ANDREWS

Tudor Cartography

Ireland is too small to have developed a native map-making tradition. The first maps to show any close knowledge of the interior were those commissioned by the English government between the 1520s and the 1600s. It was a late start by the best continental European standards, but when they did appear such maps were surprisingly numerous, and also surprisingly varied in both form and content. Paradoxically this fortunate state of affairs owed much to official incompetence. The Tudors had no regular map-producing department, they made no provision for the safeguard of cartographic images by printing, and they kept no properly organized archive of manuscript maps. Most of their surveyors and draughtsmen in Ireland were recruited from a military background, usually on short-term *ad hoc* engagements. Some had already acquired professional expertise as geometers or engineers and became well known in this capacity to their contemporaries and to future historians. Others were obscure and nameless amateurs. But despite its wide range of merit, style and subject-matter their work shows a number of common features.

The areas assigned to Anglo-Irish surveyors at this period were seldom larger than a province and often much smaller. Map scales usually ranged between about seven miles and two miles to an inch. The cartographer's objectives were strictly practical. Most of his interest was in human geography, particularly the location of towns, forts, castles and other defensible sites. Special attention was also given to the names and approximate boundaries of political divisions. In this outsider's view of Ireland, nature played a largely tactical role as an obstacle to movement and as a refuge for the government's enemies. Its main components were mountain, forest and water – or land that was mixed with water such as bogs and foreshores – and it was these kinds of negative terrain that cartographers chose to emphasize by colour or line-work, ordinary arable or pasture land generally being left blank.

Water was usually shown either by a blue wash (a convention imported to north-European cartography from the Mediterranean) or by more plausible if less attractive colours such as grey. Waves or currents were often simulated by pen strokes and could be made to look frighteningly turbulent. Drawings of ships served as guides to navigability as well as for decoration. Woods were masses of trees in profile, usually forming a continuous canopy and sometimes shaded in dark green. Not all colour conventions were equally appropriate. In John Browne's 1585 map of Mayo green was used for 'bogges and wast groundes' (MPF 92), and a greenish blue remained common for bogs until gradually superseded by a more realistic brown around the turn of the century. Bog, already recognized as the most characteristic of Ireland's terrain types, could also be given prominence by short conventional pen-strokes, horizontal for water and vertical for plants, sometimes further conventionalized to produce a woven or plaited effect (MPF 38-64). The only unvegetated surfaces distinguished at this period were those on which ships might run aground, rocks being shown by crosses, sands by a close stipple.

The surface of Ireland is fascinatingly irregular, but the landforms of modern geography-teaching – scarps, plateaux, spurs etc. – had no place in Elizabethan cartography. The only relief features recognizable on contemporary maps were hills, depicted in side view and at first, like bogs, coloured green as often as brown. Some profile drawings denoted particular summits, others were simply components in an assemblage of symbols collectively signifying an upland and individually signifying nothing. This second, aggregative function of hill symbolism, though intellectually more sophisticated, was for most draughtsmen the easier option. In theory a hill could be varied in size, smoothness and gradient as well as in colour to imitate reality, but few observers had either the time or the artistic ability for such refinements, and without their names very few of the hill profiles drawn by sixteenth-century cartographers could be identified individually on the ground. Fortunately, hill names are quite common on these maps, and often more vividly descriptive than the corresponding symbols. Verbal language could also hint at different orders of relief feature, as when Robert Lythe's 'Petworth' map of 1571 reported that within broad upland regions such as Slew Grott and Slew Goe in Munster every individual hill had 'his particular name'.

The difference between realism and convention in the portrayal of hill features may be illustrated by two characteristically Irish relief types for which special provision was made in Elizabethan cartography. In a well known but anonymous regional map of c. 1563 covering the recently pacified countries of Leix and Offaly, numerous esker ridges appear in their correct positions as snake-like features each composed of two closely spaced parallel lines with a brown filling, perhaps the first use of planiform methods in the history of Irish relief representation (Hardiman Maps, 9) and a great improvement on the chain of separate hills used for one of these eskers in the earliest known town plan of Maryborough (MPF 277). A contrasting example was provided a few years later by the most successful of all Elizabethan surveyors in Ireland, Robert Lythe (MPF 73). For the rocky surfaces of north Co. Clare Lythe chose an array of purely conventional profiles (*plate 8*). His small and tightly packed Burren hills, though quite unrealistic, are at least immediately distinguishable from all the other uplands on his maps and in areal extent they closely match the 'karstic [i.e. limestone] plateaux' of a modern geomorphological cartographer (Haughton, 1979). Neither of these techniques was imitated by later artists.

Symbolism and representationalism in early physical cartography are interesting mainly as a means of separating professional map-makers from amateurs. Sometimes, however, a symbol may hint at contemporary scientific or pseudo-scientific beliefs. A good example is the tendency for uplands to be mapped as long narrow strings regardless of their true shapes. This fashion probably derived from the Greek geographer Ptolemy and reflected the actual form of hill masses around the Mediterranean basin. Other errors can be explained without recourse to foreign models. One long-standing cartographer's habit was to make rivers rise in lakes. Another, not exactly conventional but similar in its dependence on extrapolation, was to draw a river flowing simultaneously downhill and uphill to different outlets, a practice first exemplified in Ireland by the River Shannon as shown on a famous medieval map. Here the double-mouthed Shannon was doubtless inspired by the hydrographic theories of Giraldus Cambrensis (the map in question occurs in a copy of his *Topographia Hiberniae*) and there was also authority in the Book of Genesis for interconnected river systems unknown to modern physical geography (Wright, 1965). However, on many later maps such backward-running rivers simply betrayed a copyist's misinterpretation of a territorial boundary.

Since maps are not read serially like a passage of prose, their irrelevances are less irritating than those of a literary text: cartographers are correspondingly less afraid of being deflected from their main purpose, especially as most of them regard blank paper as a discreditable admission of ignorance. Animals have been favourite space-fillers since medieval times. They also illustrate the nearest approach in cartographic language to a negative judgment. Empty space on a map may be simply a gesture of agnosticism, but it may also constitute a statement about the world. In the same way, by depicting 'elephants for want of towns' a cartographer can indirectly assert that towns do not exist. This is the function of the fox, wolf, deer and rabbits seen in an Elizabethan map of north Antrim, and it is revealing in the same map to find wild Irishmen peeping from behind the rocks or sand dunes as one more element in the natural scene (MPF 88).

The most common channel for supplementary information on maps of the Tudor period, however, was ordinary verbal language, either written *in situ* or linked with its correlative location by some equivalent of the asterisk. Written captions economize on artistic ability and inventiveness. They also carry a meta-linguistic message. A map's blank spaces, as noted above, can sometimes be legitimately read as statements of non-existence: by switching to a purely verbal medium a cartographer may hope to avoid any impression of promising equivalent data for the rest of his survey area.

In fact, inscriptions other than names are not as numerous on Elizabethan Irish maps as one could wish, but several modern natural sciences are represented in them. Thus geology: 'whyt stones pointed lyke diamonds', near Tralee (MPF 73). Geomorphology: 'a claye ground wher ye lande wasteth', on the Wexford coast near Rosslare (Petworth map). Ecology: 'thys wodde ys greate okes and moche small woodes as crabbtre thorne hasell wth such lykes' (Petworth map). Hydrography: 'the poynte of Arkelowe wher is four tymes full sea in a 24 howrer' (Petworth map). Zoology: 'the high Hills of Benbolbin where yearlie limbereth a Falcon esteemed the Hardiest in Ireland' (MPF 37). Limnology: 'A[nn]o [15]98. O'Donnell camped by this logh where his men did see 2 waterhorses of a huge bigness', the lake in question being Glencar Lough on the borders of Co. Sligo and Co. Leitrim (Dartmouth Maps, 7). Perhaps psychology is the best scientific affiliation for another note on the same map recording that 'In this bog ... there is every whott [hot?] summer strange fighting of battles, sometimes at foot sometimes wt horse, sometimes castles seen on a sudden, sometimes great store of cows driving & fighting for them'.

The Seventeenth and Eighteenth Centuries

A new factor in late sixteenth-century European cartography was the growing number and influence of maps printed from engraved copper plates. In Ireland this trend had two consequences. Manuscript maps on small and medium scales gradually began to resemble their printed counterparts, a trend that becomes noticeable around 1580; and eventually politico-military regional maps ceased for a considerable period to be preserved in manuscript. This last development owed much to the Irish section of John Speed's *Theatre of the Empire of Great Britaine* (1612), for these were the first published maps of Ireland accepted as reliable by contemporaries who knew or thought they knew the country at first hand. It was not until late in the eighteenth century that regional military mapping reappeared in Ireland as a manuscript genre, and by that time its style and content were quite different.

Engraving made maps more professional and more international. Symbols for buildings, hills and other minor features became smaller, neater and more standardized, though individually less informative. Colour, which still had to be added by hand, became a way of emphasizing rather than conveying information; on many maps it was reduced to narrow transparent strips alongside printed political or administrative boundaries. At the same time the cartographer's subject-matter shrank to a low common denominator comprising coasts, rivers, hills, woods, settlements and territorial divisions, leaving only placenames like Hawks Rocks or Seal Island to preserve some element of animation in the landscape. For nearly a hundred and fifty years the one extensive and permanent addition to this repertoire was main roads, which were not shown regularly on maps of Ireland until nearly the end of the seventeenth century but which then became almost universal. Professional cartographers now accepted that verbal sentences and clauses do not blend easily into a graphic medium, and inscriptions of the here-be-dragons type went out of favour. (A rare late example was the phenomenon on the Donegal coast known as McSwine's Gun, described on William Petty's county map of 1685 as 'a place where the water howls'.) The new ideal was for maps and text to be complementary but separate, and from Petty's time onwards there were many dual publishing projects designed to embody this relationship. For some psychological reason the task proved remarkably difficult: in most cases, the better the map, the less effective the accompanying memoir and vice versa. Only in comparatively recent times has an Irish map-maker, Tim Robinson, achieved equal success with both forms, adding for good measure a poetic appreciation of landscape all too rare among geographical communicators in any country.

Progress in seventeenth-century cartography took several paths. One was the development of specialized map types. Among the categories that established themselves in Ireland during this period were the fort plan, the plantation map and the estate map. Common to all three were a large scale and a restricted consumer demand, making manuscript a more appropriate medium than print at least until the introduction of lithography in the nineteenth century. Fort plans were naturally confined to very small areas; it was not until the late eighteenth century that Irish military map-makers returned to the surveying of extensive landscapes, and then they chose a style that quickly spread to civil cartography on comparable scales. Plantation and early estate surveys dealt mainly with actual and potential property boundaries, typically on scales of forty Irish perches to an inch (1:10,080) or more. Since many such boundaries followed coasts and waterways these maps can often be instructively compared with the modern Ordnance Survey to demonstrate the progress of erosion or aggradation (natural or artificial) along the shoreline and of both planned and unplanned realignments of

rivers in their flood plains. Such comparisons show the deliberate alteration
of watercourses to be perhaps the commonest kind of mapped landscape
change in eighteenth- and nineteenth-century Ireland. Surface character was
less effectively depicted on early property maps. Often the only reference to
it was a distinction between profitable and unprofitable land, but this makes
it possible for the margins of at least some bogs and unreclaimed mountains
to be traced before the great increase of rural population that preceded the
Famine. Compared with the Ordnance Survey, the old maps show cultiva-
tion-limits being pushed up many Irish hillsides, between the 1650s and the
1830s, from about five hundred feet to about eight hundred feet above sea
level.

Meanwhile, maps of more extensive areas were still being printed for
travellers, administrators and businessmen, a popular format from c. 1750
onwards being the survey of a single county published in two, four or six
sheets at a scale of one or two inches to an Irish mile. All-Ireland maps at
smaller scales were improved by incorporating the results of these new county surveys in simplified form. Once road networks had become normal cartographic fare there was little change in the content of such 'topographical'
maps. Improvement consisted of recording a limited range of everyday topics more comprehensively and with directions and distances that were more
nearly correct. This trend was continued when the government decided to
establish its own map-making department in the shape of the Ordnance
Survey and to publish its own national one-inch map. More accurate travellers' maps constituted scientific progress to the extent that geography and
the related disciplines of topography and chorography (as anciently defined
by Ptolemy) were sciences, but not in any other sense. Indeed one of the
most striking features of post-medieval map history is that the great intellectual efflorescence of the late seventeenth century had virtually no cartographic expression. It was not that maps themselves were unnoticed or
unappreciated by the scientific community. Techniques and instruments had
been perfected for the determination of latitudes, longitudes and azimuths,
and the advantages of triangulation and precise base-line measurement were
generally understood. Yet very little was actually done at this high level of
accuracy (Andrews, 1980).

The same was true of what eventually became known as distribution
maps or thematic maps. The possibility of mapping spatial patterns for their
own sake was noted (though without applying any particular name to this
process) by several scientific authors in the late seventeenth century. At
some time in or before 1697, for instance, Thomas Molyneux plotted traces
of the former presence of the giant Irish deer on a map of Ireland.
Cartographically this would have been in no way innovative: it would simply call for some variant of the kind of symbol that had long since been

devised for churches, towns, forts etc. A more interesting proposal was put to the Royal Society of London in 1684 by the English naturalist Martin Lister. 'It were advisable', he wrote,

that a soil or mineral map, as I may call it, were devised .... It might be distinguished into countries, with the river[s] and some of the noted towns put in. The soil might either be coloured, by variety of lines, or etchings; but the great care must be, very exactly to note upon the map, where such and such soils are bounded .... Now if it were noted, how far these extended, and the limits of each soil appeared upon a map, something more might be comprehended from the whole, and from every part, than I can possibly foresee, which would make such a labour very well worth the pains. For I am of the opinion, such upper soils, if natural, infallibly produce such under minerals, and for the most part in such order. (Mendyk, 1989)

Here Lister refers by implication to two essential features of a thematic map. One is the distinction between foreground (in this case soils) and background (counties, rivers and 'noted' towns). The other was more important. In a general or non-thematic map, individual occurrences of a phenomenon may be omitted if they are judged unhelpful to a majority of readers or if there is insufficient room for them. On the other hand a thematic map within its narrow limits is a complete record, of the author's knowledge if not of reality. As such it can facilitate the inductive method of reasoning commended to scientists by Francis Bacon, as Lister showed by suggesting an inductive generalization (linking soils and subjacent rock minerals) that his own proposal might help to verify.

Lister's programme was more demanding than Molyneux's since it called for positive judgments on a whole territory and not just a selection of points. But cartographically it was no more original, having been anticipated in numerous maps distinguishing political divisions by different colours. In fact, the only cartographic application of the new natural philosophy that had not already appeared in standard atlases was the isopleth or line of constant numerical value (Robinson, A.H. et al., 1985). This was first used in a scientific context by Edmond Halley in 1701 to show the variation of the magnetic compass in the Atlantic Ocean (Thrower, 1978). Several kinds of intellectual breakthrough were involved in the precise numerical mapping of an invisible gradient by the controlled extrapolation of discrete line symbols, but Halley's 'curves' found few imitators until over a hundred years later. This may have been because most contemporaries regarded them as an unusual form of meridian line rather than as a revolutionary technique applicable to all kinds of geographical continuum.

One obvious cause of the scientists' failure to make more progress with either thematic or non-thematic cartography in the late seventeenth and early eighteenth centuries is that for purely logistical reasons conception had outrun execution among would-be researchers. Certainly there were still insufficient field data to make one of Lister's 'wholes'. But this theory cannot encompass the socio-economic sphere, where (as modern historical geographers have found) much mappable statistical information already existed for whole kingdoms and their subdivisions without any cartographer having made use of it. There is a mystery here that historians have hardly begun to solve, but at least it seems clear that in the story of thematic maps, traditional explanations of Irish backwardness – war, poverty, excessive spirituality – are not particularly relevant.

The Representation of Relief

There was one major exception to the somewhat uninspiring picture drawn in the foregoing paragraphs. In the representation of surface relief on maps, the eighteenth century witnessed important changes. The first was a shift from profile to planiform methods. For a hundred years before c. 1750 the hills on European maps were becoming gradually smaller and less realistic, until some cartographers seemed to forget that they were meant to look like natural forms. A later and more promising fashion was for hachures (a French term not recorded in English until the mid-nineteenth century), which were lines or brush strokes following the direction of steepest slope, their thickness or darkness roughly proportional to the gradient. Although in cartographic literature profile and planiform hills are sharply contrasted, they can also be seen as limits to a perceptual continuum in which the observer's angle of vision is gradually increased from nought to ninety degrees. Intermediate forms, in which the hills are viewed obliquely, became common in military maps during the seventeenth century and can be quite effective where there is little competing detail to be portrayed. These transitional styles are well shown in Richard Bartlett's surveys of Ulster, with something very like a true hachured hill occurring in his map of the Blackwater valley, Co. Armagh, as early as 1602 (Hayes-McCoy, 1965). The original reason for improving on profile symbols was to help the tactician in his placement of soldiers and artillery. But whatever their purpose, hachures had the advantages of embracing a greater variety of relief features than did profiles and of being easier to reconcile with other planiform detail such as stream and road networks.

Every form of relief representation works best within a certain range of horizontal scales, and the advantages of hachuring were most evident on the county maps of half an inch or more to a mile that became common in the eighteenth century. During the 1750s vertical hachures were introduced by the Anglo-French cartographer John Rocque to published Irish county and town maps as well as to manuscript estate surveys. Twenty years later they were featuring prominently in the manuscript military surveys of Colonel

Charles Vallancey. From 1792 onwards they began to appear in privately published general maps of Ireland, of which the most effectively hachured was Aaron Arrowsmith's of 1811, which drew from unpublished surveys by Vallancey (Andrews, 1966). The British one-inch Ordnance Survey maps were elaborately hachured from the beginning and when the Survey went to Ireland a similar map was produced there, though it took from 1855 to 1895 to publish its 205 sheets.

Apart from its success with broad and massive uplands developed on resistant rocks, careful hachuring at the one-inch scale could pick up smaller and more localized features such as gorges, gullies, hillside terraces, dunes and bog islands. It could also show the results of glacial erosion and deposition, including corries, kettle-holes and eskers. In this respect the Ordnance Survey's hill artists can stand comparison with modern geomorphologists. The moraines mapped by T.W. Freeman near Castlemaine Harbour in 1950 are plainly identifiable on the Victorian one-inch map, for example; so are all the drumlins shown by the same author in the vicinity of Castleblayney, Co. Monaghan.

Hachuring was widely admired and respected as the most 'artistic' of all eighteenth- and nineteenth-century cartographic processes. This may help to explain why little was done, in the English-speaking world, to make it more scientific by incorporating exact measurements of altitude and slope. In practice the technique depended throughout its history on a field sketcher's subjective assessment of land form, and the only way to give precision to a normal hachured map was by the addition of numbers showing the altitudes of selected points, usually hilltops. For all the graphic effectiveness of hachures they were hardly ever used in the study of landforms by non-military scientists. It was not until 1873 that the Geological Survey decided to show the relation of rocks to relief by printing future sheets of its Irish one-inch geological map on a hachured base. By that time an even more effective system of hill representation was well established.

Contour lines, generally called contours for short, are isopleths joining points judged to be the same vertical distance above or below some specified datum, usually sea level. In areas of complex relief, contours are harder to apprehend at a glance than hachuring. But unlike hachures they yield heights and (for readers willing to measure and calculate) gradients that are strictly numerical. Contours began as a way of depicting submarine relief, which could be measured at 'spot depths' with a weighted cord but not sketched from direct observation. Like hachures, they were first used on land maps by military cartographers in France. Depending as they did on accurate measurements by level or theodolite, contours also presupposed a horizontally accurate base map, which meant that in Ireland they had to wait for the advent of the Ordnance Survey, though even then their introduction was delayed by the department's traditional adherence to hachures.

A leading advocate of contours in the Ordnance Survey was the head of its Dublin office in the 1830s, Captain Thomas Larcom. The main basis for his enthusiasm was not military (this motive had grown weaker in the cartography of post-Napoleonic Ireland) or scientific in any academic sense. His intended readership was the civil engineering profession, for whom contours would be useful in the laying out of roads, railways and drainage channels while also assisting agricultural development through their portrayal of height, slope, aspect and by implication local climate. Other economic factors conditioned the Survey's choice of a vertical contour interval which was closer on low ground than on the less valuable uplands, creating at first glance the cartographic illusion that many Irish hill slopes flatten out towards their summits. Contours were first added to the Survey's six-inch map of Donegal in 1839 and were first published seven years later. Their apotheosis was in a national half-inch map of 1912-18, which belatedly introduced a constant interval of one hundred feet from sea level to the tops of the highest hills (Andrews, 1975). Unlike hachures, contours have been extensively used by Irish geomorphologists as an indication of relief.

Geology and Soils

Martin Lister in 1684 had left the construction of a geological map to 'the industry of future times'. His phrase was well chosen in more than one sense. Only an industrial revolution could generate enough wealth to support the nationwide data-gathering services that most kinds of thematic cartography require, even if that wealth had to pass through government departments or state-supported institutions rather than coming directly from private sources. Apart from this general dependence of cartography upon economics the British industrial revolution provoked a special curiosity about the subterranean world by increasing the demand for coal and iron, so it is not surprising that geology was quick to benefit from the increased resources now available for map-making. Ireland was inevitably drawn into this new pattern of events. Its geology seemed both scientifically interesting and economically promising. Its intellectual and professional communities had always been receptive to British thought, and with the political union of the two kingdoms in 1801 cross-channel relations became even closer.

Before the Union the only Irishmen known to have attempted geological mapping were Charles Smith in Cork and William Hamilton in Antrim. Smith in 1750 had been content with writing 'L.V.' (limestone vale) at appropriate places in a county map. Forty years later Hamilton, inspired like many artists and writers by the wonders of the Giant's Causeway, had taken several steps forward by drawing a line to show the limits of Ireland's north-eastern basaltic plateau. But both achievements were overshadowed when the Dublin Society for Improving Husbandry, Manufactures and other Useful Arts and Sciences provided Irish geology with its first effective institutional sponsor. In 1800 this body recruited a number of authors, mainly country gentlemen, to undertake 'statistical surveys' of the Irish counties, with soils and minerals among the topics chosen for inclusion. Four of the surveys included some kind of geological map, the best being that of Kilkenny by William Tighe (*plate 9*). None of these proto-geologists pursued their studies outside their own county, but a broader view emerged when the Society began to work with natural rather than administrative units.

One kind of natural unit to claim attention at an early stage was bogland. In 1809, under the stimulus of wartime agricultural prices, the government appointed a commission to survey and take levels of all Irish bogs occupying more than five hundred acres and to report on the practicability of reclaiming and cultivating them, with suggestions for new roads and navigable canals as well as drainage channels. The work was completed in 1813. It was performed by some of Ireland's most gifted civil engineers, of whom several – most notably Richard Griffith, Alexander Nimmo and William Bald – were to win fame within their own profession and outside. Their talents included the making of new topographical surveys where previous maps were inadequate, as was often the case, and the writing of reports not just on technical questions of drainage and road construction but on a wide range of attendant agricultural and social problems. The scale of the original bogs commission surveys was four inches to a mile, reduced by half for engraving. The work was organized by river basins and the irregularity of the resulting sheet layout did not make for easy reference (*Coimisiun na gCanalach*, 1923). Nor did these surveys combine to make a single large map of the whole country. (It was not until 1920 that every bog in Ireland appeared on one thematic sheet at the smaller scale of ten miles to an inch [Hellyer, 1992]). Their value lay rather in contributing information to later maps and in helping to inspire and educate the authors' Irish colleagues. But no engineer could control the course of international trade. With the postwar fall in corn prices, marginal land lost much of its value and Ireland's bogs remained unproductive except as a diminishing store of turf.

A more lastingly fashionable source of fuel in the early nineteenth century was coal. In the end Ireland turned out to be poorly endowed in this respect, but each province had at least one small area with rocks of coalbearing age. In 1809 the Dublin Society commissioned a survey of the Leinster (Castlecomer) coalfield from Richard Griffith, who apart from his expertise in civil engineering was the nearest thing to a trained geologist that Ireland could then produce and who had already shown his mettle by including some information about solid geology in two of his maps for the bogs commission. In 1812 Griffith acquired a permanent position as the Dublin Society's mining engineer and a year later he began to map the country's remaining coalfields. It was at some time during this period, probably in 1811, that he decided to put the whole island on the geological map.

In England and Wales the recent work of G.B. Greenough had shown that quasi-academic motives need no longer be a handicap in the mapping of rocks and rock structures. Griffith's early geological interests, like Greenough's, were not so much practical as scientific, and this may explain why in Ireland he managed to anticipate the government's more utilitarian efforts. In the end, however, his success depended not only on scientific ability but also on a happy knack of finding official positions in which geology could legitimately be pursued as a sideline. In the 1820s this combination was spectacularly exemplified by Griffith's appointment as head of the official Irish boundary survey and the general valuation of rateable property. The second of these tasks, begun in 1827, was to prove especially rewarding, for the assessment of land values required a knowledge of soils, subsoils and minerals, and in the valuation office Griffith controlled a large staff whom he could train in methods of geological surveying. He was in fact running 'a rudimentary and quite unofficial geological survey of Ireland' (Herries Davies, 1983).

From all these surveys Griffith finally produced a geologically coloured copy of Arrowsmith's *Ireland* which he exhibited to the British Association for the Advancement of Science in 1835. Its main weakness was the base map, but here Griffith had a further stroke of luck when he joined a new government commission charged with recommending lines of railway for Ireland. The railway commissioners entertained high hopes of geology both for the light it could throw on future economic development and for its particular relevance to the problem of selecting and developing suitable routes. Accordingly they arranged for the reconstruction of Griffith's map. In 1839 his geological findings, much revised, were shown in print on a superior base compiled with great skill at the Ordnance Survey office in Dublin from the best materials then available, including the Survey's own triangulation and its own six-inch maps of the northern counties (*plate 10*). The 'railway map' was also sold with considerable success as a separate publication. Its practical value is well illustrated in the commission's report:

The geological map of Ireland will serve as a valuable guide in determining the best lines for improved internal communication, whether by ordinary roads, by railways, or canals: for every variation from the blue colour on the map indicates not only a change in the character and composition of the rock, but also the commencement of a hilly or mountainous tract, through which no internal communication can be made without encountering steep ascents or descents, and other engineering difficulties; in

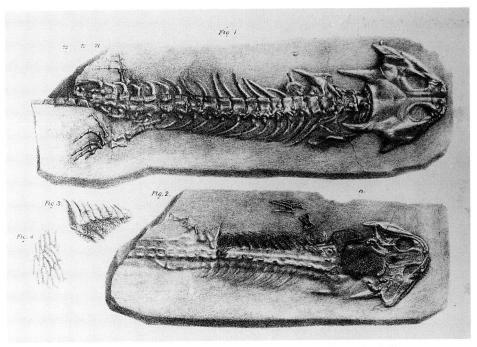

Keraterpeton Galvani, an amphibian fossil found in the Jarrow colliery, Co. Kilkenny.

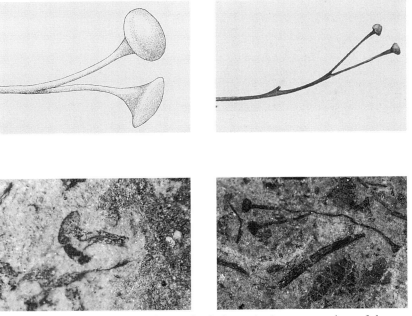

Cooksonia, the world's earliest known land plants: (*top*) reconstructions of the fertile axes; (*bottom*) the fossils themselves.

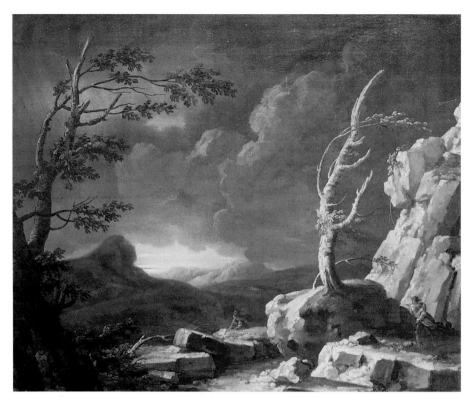

George Barret, *A Stormy Landscape* (1760).

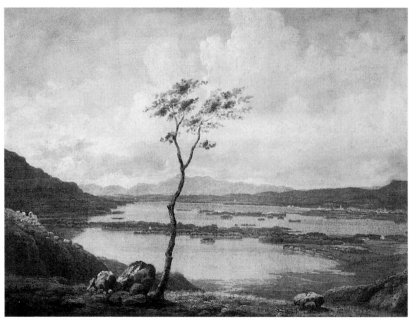

Jonathan Fisher, *A View of the Lower Lake, Killarney* (1797).

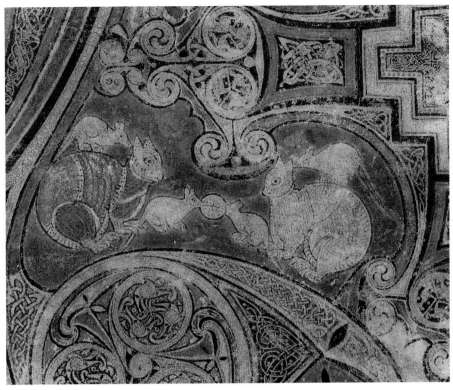

Cats and rats from the Book of Kells. This is the earliest
suggestion of the presence of the ship rat in Ireland.

Wolf with devil's tail from the Book of Kells, depicting
the association of the animal with evil.

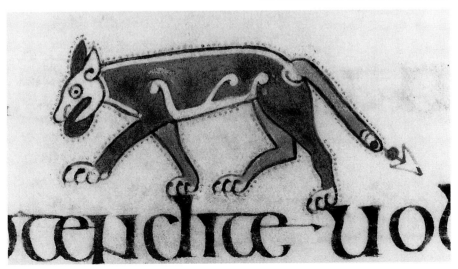

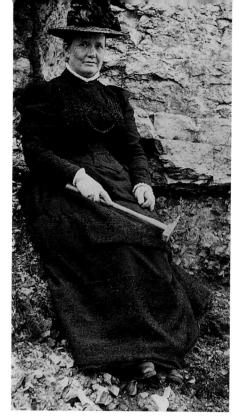

Sydney Mary Thompson (Madam Christen), 1847-1923, artist and geologist, at junction of chalk/greensand and New Red Sandstone, Murlough Bay, Co. Antrim, 1898.

Below: St John's eagle – actually an osprey – from the Book of Armagh.

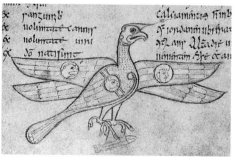

Edwin Sandys, *A True Prospect of the Giants Cawsway* (1696), one of the earliest graphic representations of the Giant's Causeway, commissioned by Thomas Molyneux. Later geologists ridiculed the presence of trees and houses on the basalt.

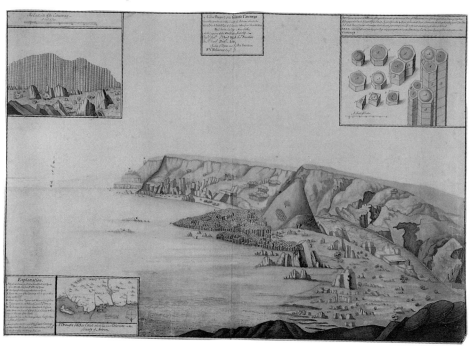

Reginald W. Scully, author of *Flora of the County Kerry*, 1916, and co-editor of the second edition of *Cybele Hibernica*, 1898.

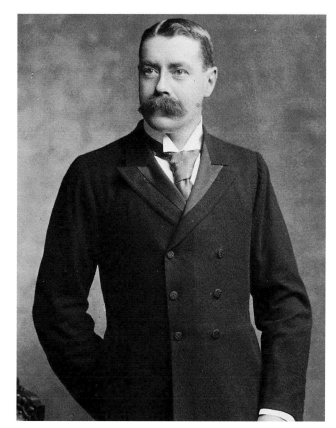

Below: D.A. Webb of Trinity College, Dublin, author of *A New Irish Flora*, 1943, which remains the standard work.

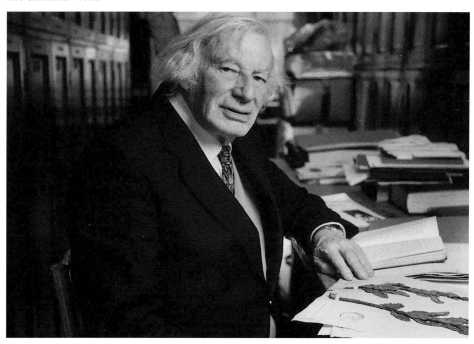

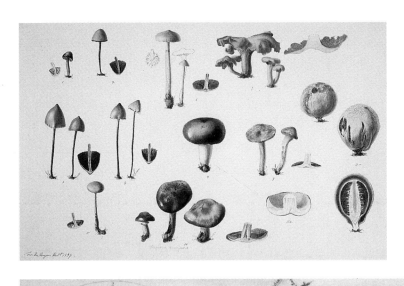

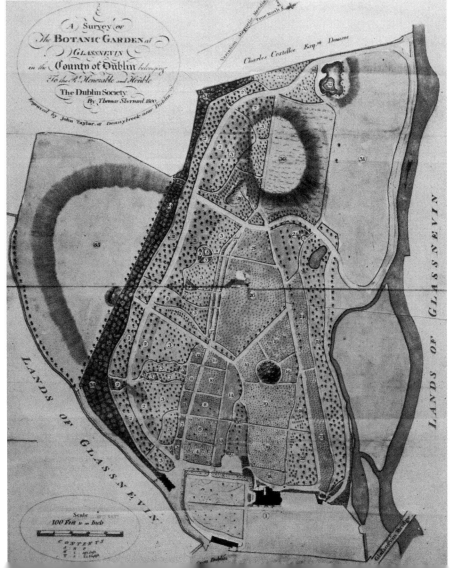

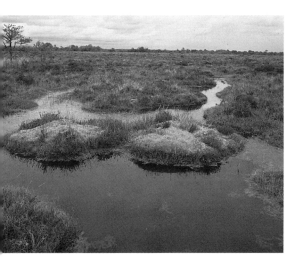

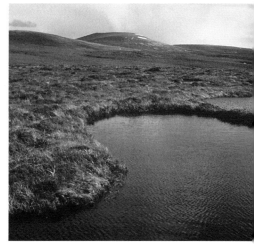

Above, left: Raised bog at Garriskill,
Co. Westmeath.

Facing, above: Watercolour illustration of Irish
fungi by George Victor Du Noyer, 1839.

Above, right: Blanket bog at Sally Gap,
Co. Wicklow.

Facing, below: Map of the Botanic Gardens,
Glasnevin, by Thomas Sherard, 1800.

Below: Bank of hand-cut turf on a raised bog
in Co. Clare.

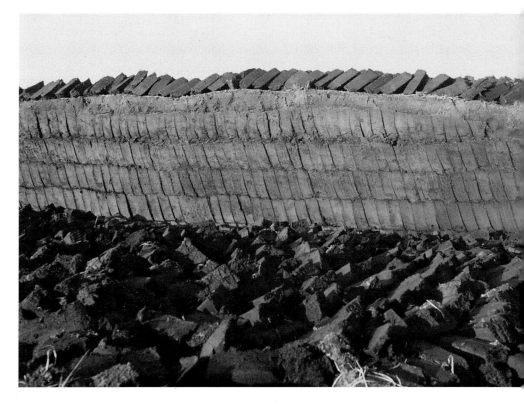

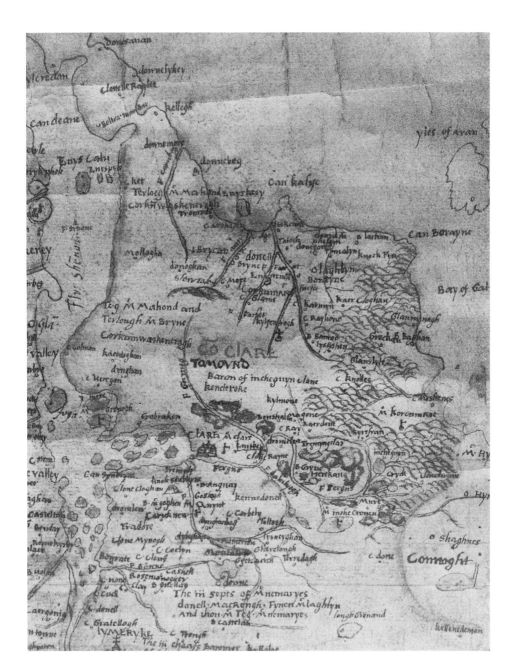

The Burren of Co. Clare from Robert Lythe's 'A Single Draght of Mounster', 1571.
North is to the right.

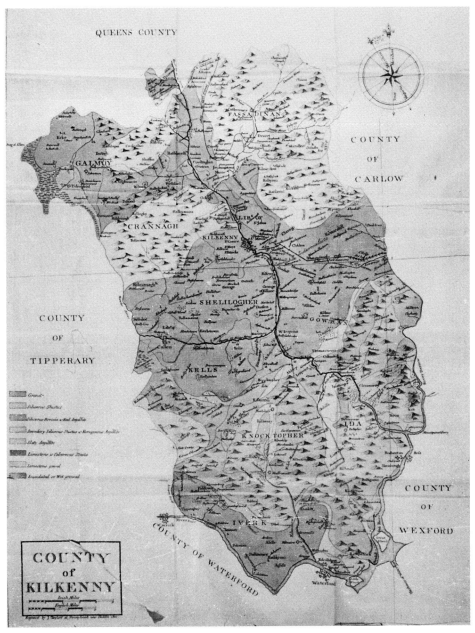

The geology of Co. Kilkenny, from William Tighe's *Statistical Observations relative to the County of Kilkenny* (Dublin 1802).

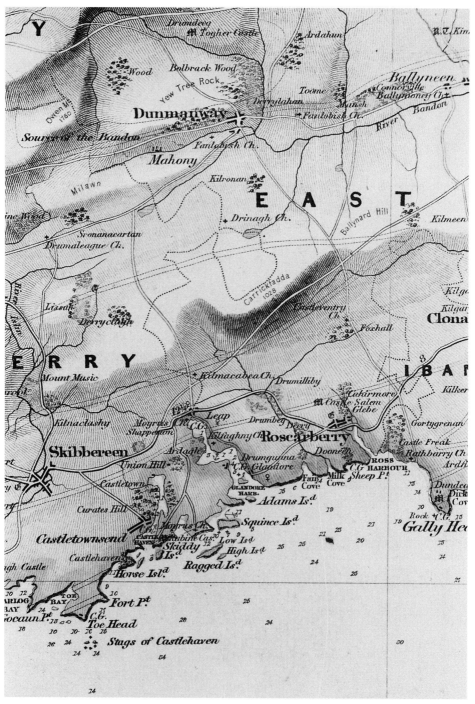

West Cork detail from *A General Map of Ireland to accompany the Report of the Railway Commissioners* (Dublin 1839). Geological boundaries are dotted. The closely spaced parallel lines represent the Carboniferous yellow sandstone separating the Old Red Sandstone of the Carrickfadda region from the Carboniferous slate.

Facing: Frontispiece of the Clare Island Survey from *Transactions of the Royal Irish Academy*. The photograph by R.J. Welch shows Croaghmore from the north-east.

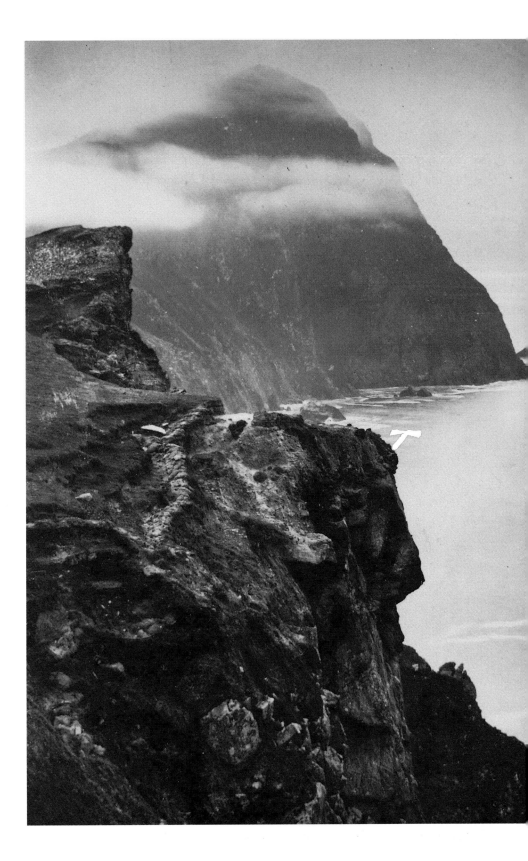

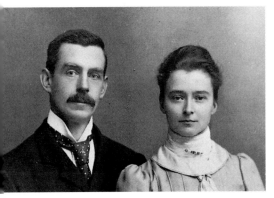

Wedding photograph of the Praegers, 1901, the year in which 'Irish Topographical Botany' was published.

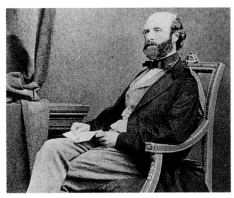

Alexander Henry Haliday of Holywood, Co. Down, one of the leading European entomologists of the nineteenth century.

Ninth Party visit to Clare Island during the Survey, June 1910. Posing on a pucaun beside the pier at Kinacorra are (*front, l. to r.*) Thomas Greer (entomologist), W.F. de Vismes Kane (entomologist), R.J. Ussher (ornithologist), P. Kuckuck (phycologist), H. Wallis Kew (zoologist); (*back, l. to r.*) N.H. Foster (*inset*), R.L. Praeger, Carl Lindner (ornithologist), A.D. Cotton (phycologist), W.J. Lyons (meteorologist), and R.J. Welch.

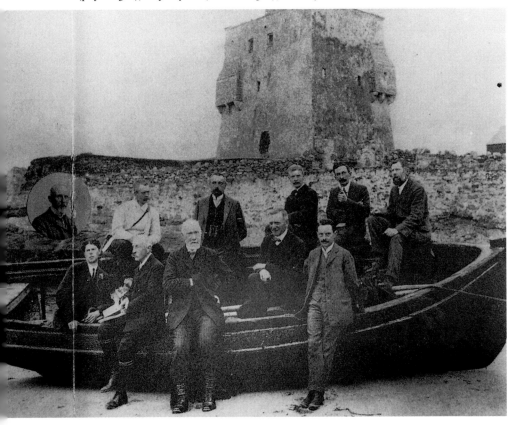

addition to which it may be observed that the whole of the populous towns of the interior of Ireland are situated in the limestone country, and nearly the whole of the rich arable and pasture lands are confined within its limits. It is true that this valuable district is encumbered by vast tracts of bog, at present in a state of nature, and nearly inaccessible; but no doubt these bogs, as well as the flooded lands on the banks of the rivers, will hereafter be drained and improved, and become valuable appendages to the adjoining uplands.

Like so many good maps, Griffith's was becoming obsolete by the time he managed to publish it. Before 1839 the government had already begun work on an official geological survey of England and Wales at four times the Irish railway commissioners' scale. Sooner or later Ireland would have to follow suit. At one inch to a mile geology was no longer a sideline. It needed its own organization, a need that gradually became clearer during the period 1825-45 when the Ordnance Survey (ignoring Griffith) tried to map the geology and topography of Ireland as a single enterprise. The combination produced one masterpiece in Captain J.E. Portlock's *Report on the Geology of the County of Londonderry*, which included a coloured half-inch geological map. Otherwise the Ordnance Survey had little success as a corporate geologist, and in 1845 the government admitted as much by transferring the whole subject to a separate department, responsible for both Britain and Ireland. This arrangement remained in force until 1905.

Although geological knowledge made great progress in the nineteenth century, the fundamental nature of a geological map was established at least as early as Tighe's *Statistical Observations* in 1802. Its essence was that every part of the mapped area should be classified and that no part could belong to more than one class. Categories were based on either the lithology or the age of the rock immediately below the land surface. It was a lucky accident that a scientific classification could be accommodated by a familiar cartographic technique and that the limits of each formation could be mapped in much the same way as any other kind of boundary. Nor was there anything unusual about the symbols chosen by early geologists for localized rock occurrences where data were as yet insufficient for the interpolation of boundaries. Such symbols remained in vogue for special cases like the sites of economically useful minerals. But the best way to characterize the formations themselves was by colour, which having become inessential on ordinary topographical maps by the late eighteenth century could now be applied exclusively to the third dimension.

Colours suited the logic of geological classification by being spatially incompatible, and the principles governing their use were easily understood. As the Scottish mineralogist Robert Jameson had pointed out, they should be transparent enough to show the underlying topographical map detail; and they should 'agree as nearly as possible with nature, that is, they must correspond with the most common colour of the rock, or at least differ from it as little as possible'. For a time colour was almost indissolubly associated in the minds of cartographers with geology: in England for instance the government's advisers spoke not of making a geoiogical survey but of affixing geological colours to a topographical map. The advantages of chromaticism were ample recompense for the necessity of painting each individual impression of the map by hand, a practice applied to all 205 sheets of Ireland's official geological map before it was eventually superseded by colour printing.

All this prompts the question whether geological or at any rate lithological maps can rightly be considered thematic at all, or whether they simply extended the concept of a topographical map by treating the landscape as a solid mass rather than a surface. (Maps showing only one formation, like those of the Irish bogs commission, are unaffected by this argument and may be accepted as thematic.) The second view gains support from the ease with which many of the rock types recognized by geologists can be identified by laymen without instrumental aids. What should or should not count as thematic may strike non-cartographers as an excessively abstract question, but the concept of three-dimensionality does carry one or two practical implications. For instance, a map of sub-surface conditions should be able to distinguish the vertical relationships of different rock layers. In England William Smith did this in 1815 by using darker tones of colour near the base of a formation, though other cartographers failed to follow suit, perhaps because this practice required too much artistic skill from the colourist. It is also arguable that if the land surface is represented without colour, geological deposits nearer the top of the stratigraphic column should be shown in lighter tints. This would justify the Irish Geological Survey in representing glacial drift, from 1856 onwards, by an inconspicuous open stipple (Herries Davies, 1983). It might also explain the Survey's choice of pale yellow for peat bogs instead of the traditional brown.

Another, more general question related to the issue of thematic versus non-thematic was whether or not geology required a special base map. Here opinions differed, as the Dublin Society's *Statistical Surveys* made clear. Tighe's answer in Kilkenny was affirmative, all roads being omitted from his map for the sake of clarity, whereas in Cork Horatio Townsend began with a 'single all-purpose representation of the county' (Herries Davies, 1983) before switching to a simpler base map in the second edition of his book. Of course a skeleton base made the rocks harder to find in the field and also missed the chance of showing how geology was related to other geographical variables; and eventually it was accepted that even a complex map could take a coating of colour without its black and white content having to be simplified. For the Geological Survey the problem solved itself, because the only base accurate enough to accommodate its findings was the ordnance map. In England the one-inch sheets were used for this purpose from the beginning; in Ireland geology was published first on the Ordnance Survey's county indexes to its six-inch maps (from 1848 to 1851) but thereafter at one inch to one mile, the entire country being geologically covered on this scale between 1856 and 1890. A redesigned one-inch base map would have been intolerably expensive, but it was relatively cheap to engrave the geological boundaries on duplicate printing-plates of the standard Ordnance Survey sheets already completed, especially as from the 1840s such duplicates could be electrotyped without recourse to further engraving. In the twentieth century the drawing and photolithographic printing of more specialized geological maps have become a commonplace of scientific publication in innumerable monographs and journals. Cartographically the most recent innovation in this area has been the use of isopleths in the mapping of gravitational anomalies (Haughton, 1979).

Combining geology and topography in the same map was never easy. The zone of greatest discordance between the two spheres lay immediately beneath the surface of the ground among the roots of Ireland's natural and artificial vegetation. Soils were the favourite medium of a pioneer agricultural chemist, Sir Robert Kane, director of the Museum of Irish Industry in Dublin from 1845 (Simington and Wheeler, 1947). Three years after his appointment Kane announced a scheme for preparing two sets of maps based on the same county indexes as were currently being used by the geologists. One was a set of choropleth maps (as they would be called in the twentieth century), in which each townland would be shaded or coloured according to its Griffith valuation. The other maps were to be 'agrological', showing soils and contour lines. Griffith's valuators had been instructed to study soils but Kane intended to depend on samples collected by the officers of the Geological Survey. Two or three counties were mapped according to this programme, but unfortunately the maps appear to have been lost and Kane's system is known only by description. His main soil types were calcareous and non-calcareous (to be shown in red and blue respectively), both categories being subdivided into clay, clay loam, loam, 'sandy' and 'peaty'. This was an idea before its time. In practice the collection of soils proved impossible to harmonize with the Geological Survey's other activities and in 1852 the whole arrangement came to an end. One underlying reason for the collapse of Kane's scheme was the gradual abandonment of tillage by Irish farmers in response to post-famine economic conditions. Soil science revived only after an independent government began to encourage arable farming, and in 1959 the Republic of Ireland finally created its own official soil survey. But since soil types are harder to recognize than rock types the subject and its maps have never developed much appeal for the layman.

Climate and Vegetation

After the lithosphere, the atmosphere. With climate, as with geology, it was only in the nineteenth century that data became sufficiently abundant to attract much attention from cartographers. Ireland's climate is better known to the world at large than any other aspect of its physical geography, but the subject has played little part in Irish map history. Geologically and physiographically the country is highly complex; so too are its local climates as determined by altitude, aspect, shelter and the physical properties of soil and vegetation. But the island is too small to generate the broad horizontal differences of climate that have stimulated cartographic interest in other countries, and there has been little attempt to delimit its climatic regions.

Climatic statistics can be mapped as 'raw' numbers placed *in situ*, by proportional shading (especially favoured for precipitation) or by proportional symbols, a good example of the last method being a 'hyetographic' or rainfall map of the British Isles in 1851 that included ten stations in Ireland (Robinson, A.H., 1982). But the dominant technique has always been the isopleth, first applied to climate with Alexander von Humboldt's isotherms or lines of equal temperature devised in 1816. By the mid-nineteenth century isopleths were also being used for barometric pressure and precipitation. These applications had been made widely known through Heinrich Berghaus's *Physikalisher Atlas* (1845) and in the English-speaking world through its derivative, the *Physical Atlas* published by the Edinburgh firm of W. and A.K. Johnston. It was only a matter of time before climatic isopleth maps would be produced for individual countries. Air moves freely across coastlines as well as political boundaries so it was natural to treat the British Isles as a unit, especially as western Ireland provided British weather forecasters with an essential lookout post towards a meteorological future that generally came to them from the Atlantic Ocean.

In 1851 Humphrey Lloyd of Trinity College, Dublin, drew June, December and mean annual isotherms for Ireland at intervals of one degree Fahrenheit based on observations at sixteen stations. They were all straight lines, and were perhaps conceived as lines of latitude (the 'climates' of ancient geography) that had been deflected by influences from continental Europe. Seven years later a more modern-looking mean annual temperature map of the British Isles was published by Henry Hennessy of the Catholic University of Ireland. This time there were twenty-three stations and the curves for Ireland gave realistic expression to the island's own 'continentality'. Hennessy saw a promising future for the isopleth technique, but the systematic separate mapping of climatic elements in Ireland had to wait for the appearance of advanced geographical textbooks beginning with T.W. Freeman's *Ireland* in 1950.

The scientific mapping of vegetation has taken two forms. Philosophically the simpler process is to map the locations of individual species (an idea obviously applicable to fauna as well as flora) by the same techniques used for mineral occurrences in geology, a method pioneered for botanic mapping by Hermann Hoffmann in 1860. As observations and symbols multiply, such maps may become excessively complicated. An obvious though rather subjective simplification is to replace the individual dots by a generalized regional boundary that encloses all of them, thus defining the outer limit of a species. Ireland's pioneer in regional botanic cartography was Frederick James Foot, who mapped the Burren of Co. Clare at three miles to an inch in 1862, using dots for some plants and boundaries for others (Nelson, 1993). Foot was evidently inspired by the field techniques of the Geological Survey (in which he served for many years) and by incorporating a true geological boundary as well as botanical boundaries his map brought out the relation between limestone soils and vegetation. In 1866 the same method was applied to the whole of Ireland by David Moore and A.G. More. On a national scale climate rather than geology was the dominant influence, and Moore and More's map acknowledged this by combining floral boundaries with isotherms derived from Hennessy. The most famous biogeographical limits in Ireland are those of American and Lusitanian flora in the west and south-west, thought to be of pre-glacial origin and relevant to geological theories of former land bridges.

A more objective way of generalizing plant distribution maps – by describing areas rather than individual points – is related to the choropleth technique. In theory this might be achieved by shading counties or other administrative divisions as is often done in socio-economic geography, but of course such territories have no biogeographic significance. An attempt to devise more suitable unit areas was published by the Ordnance Survey of Ireland in 1949 (Hellyer, 1992), but maps based on arbitrary grid squares of uniform size are now generally considered more scientific, and since the Survey's map sheets began to carry the Irish National Grid in the 1950s the ten-kilometre square has become the standard method of mapping both botanical and zoological distributions. Equally standard is the use of uniform dots to indicate the presence of a species within a given square, though sometimes additional information has been given by varying the size or colour of the dots. An early use of this technique for Ireland was F.H. Perring and S.M. Walters's misleadingly titled *Atlas of the British Flora*, first published in 1962. Since then both floral and faunal grid-square distribution maps have proliferated, both for Ireland individually and for the British Isles, and the subject now needs its own cartobibliography.

A more comprehensive form of botanic map-making is the large-scale survey of vegetation types. Cartographically this resembles geological mapping but conceptually it is more complex, imposing stronger demands on the scientist's powers of classification. Though at first sight the large-scale vegetation survey represents an evolution from the land-use divisions seen on early plantation and estate maps, in fact its categories are formed by aggregating individual species rather than by simply forming general impressions of the vegetated surface. Here the model was G.H. Pethybridge and R.L. Praeger's survey of upland and coastal vegetation in Co. Dublin. Of course scope for such studies is limited in Ireland by the dominance of agricultural land. Further progress requires the classification and mapping of improved grasslands, a task first attempted on a rudimentary all-Ireland map by Austin O'Sullivan in 1979 (Haughton, 1979).

The mapping of flora and fauna raises a more general issue. Most scientific maps are analytical and seemingly objective. They reduce the world to individual elements, each abstracted from reality and recorded in isolation, or at best in company with a few other variables. This can hardly be described as mapping 'nature'. Within individual sciences there can be some degree of synthesis, as in maps of landform types or vegetation types. The idea of a single grand synthesis is more elusive. It has had a certain currency among geographers, for instance with Andrew Herbertson's idea of natural regions, which was actually expressed in map form, and with S.W. Wooldridge's concept of 'sites', which was not. Such ideas have usually been formulated in regions of rare geographical simplicity like south-east England. Ireland's landscapes are not simple.

References

Andrews, J.H. 1966. 'Charles Vallancey and the Map of Ireland.' *Geographical Journal 132*: 48-61.

Andrews, J.H. 1975. *A Paper Landscape: the Ordnance Survey in Nineteenth Century Ireland.* Oxford: Oxford University Press.

Andrews, J.H. 1980. 'Science and Cartography in the Ireland of William and Samuel Molyneux.' *Proceedings of the Royal Irish Academy 80* C: 231-50.

Coimisiun na gCanalach agus na mBothar Uisce Intire, Report: July 1923, (IPP 1923, III, 607 (250 11.23)) Map 2: 'Districts Selected by the Commissioners Appointed to Inquire into their Nature & Extent and the Practicability of Draining and Cultivating Them' 1810.

Dartmouth maps of Ireland, National Maritime Museum, Greenwich, MS P.49.

Foot, F.J. 1862. 'On the Distribution of Plants in Burren, County of Clare.' *Transactions of the Royal Irish Academy 24 Science*: 143-60.

Freeman, T.W. 1950. *Ireland: Its Physical, Historical, Social and Economic Geography.* London and New York: Methuen.

Giraldus Cambrensis (trans. J.J. O'Meara). 1951. *The First Version of the Topography of Ireland by Giraldus Cambrensis.* Dundalk: Dundalgan Press.

Hamilton, W. 1790. *Letters Concerning the Northern Coast of the County of Antrim.* Dublin.

Hardiman maps. Early maps of Ireland catalogued by James Hardiman in the Library of Trinity College, Dublin (MS 1209).

Haughton, J.P. (ed.). 1979. *Atlas of Ireland.* Dublin: Royal Irish Academy.

Hayes-McCoy, G.A. 1965. *Ulster and Other Irish Maps, c.1600.* Dublin: Irish Manuscripts Commission.

Hellyer, R. 1992. *The 'Ten-Mile' Maps of the Ordnance Surveys.* London: The Charles Close Society.

Hennessy, H. 1858. 'On the Distribution of Heat over Islands, and especially over the British Isles.' *London, Edinburgh and Dublin Philosophical Magazine and Journal of Science 16.* New Series: 241-67.

Herbertson, A. 1905. 'The Major Natural Regions: an Essay in Systematic Geography.' *Geographical Journal 25:* 300-12.

Herries Davies, G.L. 1983. *Sheets of Many Colours: the Mapping of Ireland's Rocks 1750-1890.* Dublin: Royal Dublin Society.

Jameson, R. 1808. 'On Colouring Geological Maps.' *Memoirs of the Wernerian Natural History Society 1:* 149-60.

Lloyd, H. 1855. 'Notes on the Meteorology of Ireland, Deduced from the Observations Made in the Year 1851, under the Direction of the Royal Irish Academy.' *Transactions of the Royal Irish Academy 22:* 411-98.

Mendyk, S.A.E. 1989. *'Speculum Britanniae': Regional Study, Antiquarianism, and Science in Britain to 1700.* Toronto: University of Toronto Press.

Moore, D., and A.G. More. 1866. *Contributions towards a Cybele Hibernica, being an Outline of the Geographical Distribution of Plants in Ireland.* Dublin: Hodges, Smith & Co.

Moore, D., and A.G. More. 1867. 'On the Climate, Flora, and Crops of Ireland.' *Report of the Proceedings of the International Horticultural Exhibition and Botanical Congress Held in London, May 1866.* London: Truscott, Son & Simmons: 165-76.

MPF. Maps and plans in the Public Record Office, London.

Nelson, E.C. 1993. 'Mapping Plant Distribution Patterns: Two Pioneering Examples from Ireland Published in the 1860s.' *Archives of Natural History 20:* 391-403.

Perring, F.H. and S.M. Walters. 1962. *Atlas of the British Flora.* Wakefield: E.P. Publishing Ltd.

Pethybridge, G.H. and R.L. Praeger. 1905. 'The Vegetation of the District Lying South of Dublin.' *Proceedings of the Royal Irish Academy 25 B:* 124-80.

Petty, W. 1685. *Hiberniae Delineatio.* London: William Petty.

Petworth map. Map of Central and Southern Ireland by Robert Lythe, 1571. West Sussex Record Office, Chichester, PHA 9581.

Portlock, J.E. 1843. *Report on the Geology of the County of Londonderry, and of Parts of Tyrone and Fermanagh.* Dublin: Andrew Milliken; Hodges and Smith; London: Longman, Brown, Green and Longmans.

Railway Commission. 1838. *Second Report of the Irish Railway Commission.* House of Commons Papers, 1837-8: xxxv.

Robinson, A.H. 1982. *Early Thematic Mapping in the History of Cartography.* Chicago and London: University of Chicago Press.

Robinson, A.H., R.D. Sale, J.L. Morrison and P.C. Muehrcke. 1985. *Elements of Cartography.* 5th ed., New York: John Wiley and Sons.

Robinson, T. 1976. *Oileáin Árann, The Aran Islands, Co. Galway: A Map and Guide.* Roundstone: Folding Landscapes.

Robinson, T. 1977. *The Burren: A Map of the Uplands of North-West Clare.* Roundstone: Folding Landscapes.

Robinson, Tim. 1990. *Connemara: Part One, Introduction and Gazetteer; Part Two, A One-Inch Map.* Roundstone: Folding Landscapes.

Simington, R.C. and T.S. Wheeler. 1947. 'Sir Robert Kane's Lost Maps.' *Department of Agriculture Journal 44:* 2-20.

Smith, C. 1750. *The Antient and Present State of the County and City of Cork.* Dublin.

Thrower, N.J.W. 1978. 'Edmond Halley and Thematic Geo-cartography,' in N.J.W. Thrower (ed.), *The Compleat Plattmaker: Essays on Chart, Map, and Globe Making in England in the Seventeenth and Eighteenth Centuries.* Los Angeles: University of California Press: 195-228.

Tighe, W. 1802. *Statistical Observations Relative to the County of Kilkenny, Made in the Years 1800 and 1801.* Dublin: Dublin Society.

Townsend, H. 1810. *Statistical Survey of the County of Cork, with Observations on the Means of Improvement*. Dublin: Dublin Society.

White, J. 1982. 'A History of Irish Vegetation Studies.' *Journal of Life Sciences, Royal Dublin Society* *3*: 5, 22.

Wooldridge, S.W. 1945. *The Land of Britain. The Report of the Land Utilisation Survey of Britain* (ed. L. Dudley Stamp), Part 51, *Yorkshire (North Riding)*. London: Geographical Publications.

Wright, J.K. 1965. *The Geographical Lore of the Time of the Crusades*. New York: Dover Publications.

Acknowledgments

Thanks are due to Dr Gordon Herries Davies and Dr Arnold Horner for their helpful comments on a draft of this chapter; also to Dr Karen Cook and to Dr E. Charles Nelson for much valuable assistance with the history of geological mapping and vegetation mapping respectively.

Insects and Entomology

JAMES P. O'CONNOR

Man and Insects

Since ancient times man and insects have been linked in many ways. Insects are present in every nook and cranny, field and garden and even in the most remote and unlikely places. We share our lives with them in many obvious and other less obvious ways, in relationships that are sometimes 'nurturing', sometimes 'competitive', and of which we are often unaware. One of our earliest links with insects arose through the cultivation of honey bees, an art developed in many civilizations. Bee cultivation was in practice in Ireland in the early Celtic period, although it probably dates from even earlier (Stelfox, 1927). Some Irish placenames reflect ancient links with bee culture: Mellifont, where an early abbey existed, means 'place of honey'. Honey formed an easily stored, long lasting and healthy supplement to often meagre and boring diets and has been a highly valued food throughout Irish history. In 1800 the Dublin Society, one of whose goals was the pursuit of excellence in agriculture, offered assistance towards improvements in beekeeping: 'A premium of 10 shillings will be given for every stock of bees preserved by any person through the succeeding winter over and above 10 stocks – such claimants to return the best method in their opinion for feeding bees in winter. N.B. the society recommend the removal of the hives to a northern aspect at the beginning of winter and in the spring to bring them to a warm situation' (Anon., 1800).

Bees form part of the imagined bliss of a rural retreat in one of the best known and most evocative poems of W.B. Yeats:

> I will arise and go now, and go to Inisfree,
> And a small cabin build there with clay and wattles made,
> Nine bean rows will I have there, and a hive for the honey bee,
> And live alone in the bee-loud glade.

In Ireland knowledge of insects always had close links with medicine, folklore and agriculture. A plentiful supply of insects is essential for the successful fruiting of many crops, but as might be expected, many of the first insect records concern pests. Through the centuries farmers had to contend with the ravages of turnip flies, wireworms and caterpillars on crops, and timber beetles, which caused much damage to both standing and building timber. We find a report of an outbreak of cockchafers in Co. Galway as early as 1688, a detailed description of an infestation, evidently of a small ermine moth, in Co. Monaghan in 1737-40, and a discussion of the wheat midge as a pest in 1802. Biological controls were introduced, such as turkeys to destroy larvae of cockchafers (Ball, 1856). Eradication of these pests required knowledge of insects, not only of the adults but of all the different stages in their metamorphoses, and their food and life habits. Thus the need for the collection and study of insects: in short, for entomology.

The use of insects in medicinal treatments, charms and cures forms another ancient link between insect and man in Ireland. Among the animals listed in John K'Eogh's 'animal herbal', *Zoologica Medicinalis Hibernica*, published in 1739, were ant, bee, beetle, butterfly, cricket, earwig, flea, fly, gadfly, grasshopper, glow-worm, locust, louse, maggot, moth and silkworm, with recommendations for the preparation methods and application procedures of each:

A MOTH, Hib. Leone, Lat. Tinea. It is reported, that if a live moth be laid on the navel till it dies, it will cure jaundice: Moths being pulverised, mixt with wine, honey, and the juice of an onion cure deafness, and the pain of the ears being applied to them. The oil extracted from them cures the said disorders, also warts: They draw thorns and splinters out of the body, being applied to it. Garments are defended from them by lavender, flowers, rosemary, mints, wormwood, stoechas, and water germander, also by the oil of spike.

Although today these medicines would be more likely to make us feel ill than to cure us, in the days before the widespread use of antibiotics and vaccines everything that might be useful was experimented with. It is interesting that today many Chinese herbal and animal medicines are given increasing credence by Western medicine. Nevertheless it is evident that close observation and collection of certain insects, and the recognition and eradication of others, was part of everyday life in Ireland many centuries ago and continues to this day.

The relationship between insects and man was, and is, often benign. According to old Irish superstitions, crickets singing in the hearth were considered lucky and to kill them was unlucky. Ladybirds have always been known as the gardener's ally and treated with great respect. (Although more than thirty species occur in Great Britain only fourteen are found in Ireland, the most common being the familiar seven-spot and ten-spot ladybirds.)

Flying insects are, of course, valued by farmers as pollinators of crops, particularly fruit trees and bushes, which depend on insect activity early in the season to produce good harvests. Fly fishermen form another large fraternity who are totally dependent on the presence of suitable flying prey and who therefore need insects, whose accurate representations they must fabricate to 'fool the fishes'. A caddisfly (*Apatania auricula*) that is confined to south-west Ireland in the British Isles, is so plentiful in the lakes of Co. Kerry that local anglers have imitated the adults with an artificial fly called the plain rail, which lake trout take in season. Harris's famous book *An Angler's Entomology* (1950) remains an extremely useful work providing a wonderful source of information on the aquatic insect life of Ireland, relating to a sport that brings large numbers of anglers from both Ireland and abroad on fishing holidays. The book forms a bridge between scientific entomology and the 'rule of thumb' field methods of anglers who produce imitations such as the watery dun, the green drake and the grey flag to lure their prey. Harris includes descriptions of flies tied by one Corny Gorman – who dressed flies for Inchiquin and other lakes in Co. Clare in the 1790s – that must rank as some of the oldest trout flies known to fishermen in these islands. Not surprisingly the non-biting midges or chironomids, a group of aquatic insects highly valued by anglers, have been extensively studied in Ireland, especially at University College Dublin, with now more than 360 species recognized on the island. Among other insects welcomed particularly for their beauty of form and colour, but also for their usefulness as pollinators are, of course, the butterflies, which along with the hum of bees add delightfully to fine summer days.

Ireland's Insects

Inhabiting an island on the western margins of Europe, the insect fauna of Ireland is smaller than that of Great Britain and much smaller than that of mainland Europe, but it is nevertheless a surprisingly rich one, containing about sixteen thousand species. A comparison between the British and Irish faunas shows that about three quarters of the British freshwater insects and about half of the terrestrial insect fauna are found in Ireland. It is fascinating to consider what particular characteristics of climate, ecology and environment in Ireland, combined with opportunism and accident, have influenced the content of our recorded insect fauna. For example, only 40 per cent of ant species and 70 per cent of syrphid fly species found in Britain occur in Ireland. Certainly, like human beings, sun-loving insects are affected by the notoriously variable Irish climate. Frequent cloud cover means that the country receives only about 30 per cent of the bright sunshine possible throughout the year and the number of days on which rain falls in an average year is exceedingly high, with August being the wettest month throughout central and eastern Ireland (Orme, 1970).

The last Ice Age, which began drawing to a close some thirteen to fourteen thousand years ago, must have had a profound effect on Ireland's insect fauna. It is fascinating to visualize the conditions that then prevailed in the island, with vast areas of frozen tundra pitted with scattered pools and ponds, icy temperatures, and scarcely any visible tree or plant cover. Amazingly, although conditions have changed so much, we still have some interesting species that have probably survived here since the glacial period. These include the small alpine caddisfly (*Tinodes dives*) discovered in 1983 near the summit of Ben Bulben, Co. Sligo (O'Connor and Good, 1984). It is still unknown elsewhere in Ireland and I was delighted to have the opportunity of observing this species in its more usual habitat in a stream high up in the French Alps, where it was the dominant aquatic insect.

In the Killarney lakes of Co. Kerry, chironomid midges that are also glacial relicts have been discovered, while in the nearby Devil's Punch Bowl, high in the mountains, a short-winged stonefly (*Capnia atra*) has also been found. Its adaptation of short wings has helped to prevent its being blown away in the high mountain habitat. Terrestrial relict species also occur, such as the rare alpine rove beetle (*Stenus glacialis*) found living at 630 metres on the summit of Muckish Mountain in west Donegal and on Slievemore on Achill Island, Co. Mayo (Anderson, 1979).

Although Ireland as an island has not been isolated from mainland Europe long enough for any recognizably endemic insect species to evolve, Irish subspecies and varieties of various insects have arisen. The most noticeable occur in some species of Irish moths and butterflies in which consistent colour and/or pattern variation identifies them as distinct subspecies, such as the Irish forms of the orange tip and marsh fritillary butterflies. The Burren green (*Calamia tridens*) is a moth with an Irish subspecies (*occidentalis*) discovered in 1949. This unusual green moth proved to be a species previously unknown in the British Isles. Its capture caused considerable excitement among British entomologists, many of whom invaded the Burren to collect specimens. Unexpectedly, as a result of their forays, numerous other insects were recorded for the first time in the area. Soon, entomologists with their nets and light traps became a common sight there. The Burren is famed as a haven for butterfly collectors, but few will compete with the sartorial elegance of 'The Butterfly Collector of Corofin', who in that poem by Paul Durcan

> Is himself a butterfly: in a red cardigan
> And skintight pants striped bluegreen
> And white cravat stippled with yellow
> He flutters about the back-garden
> Completely at home amongst the 'speckled woods' and the 'red admirals'.

It is known that faunas, especially of islands, are never static in terms of numbers of species present or population sizes, so that Ireland's insect fauna continuously fluctuates, with new insects arriving and others decreasing or disappearing from time to time. Most species would have been able to colonize the island unaided by man, a process that continues today. However, it is possible that many of the new arrivals will not be recognized due to the thin spread of entomologists working here. Noticeable immigrants are often quickly recorded, such as a large desert locust that arrived at Cobh, Co. Cork, in November 1979, blown here with red sand dust from Africa. Fortunately the locust was in its 'solitary phase' and apparently originated in Western Mauritania, indicating that its journey would have been entirely over the sea once the African coast was crossed (Bond and Blackith, 1987).

Most people will be familiar with some of the attractive migrant butterflies and moths which regularly visit our shores, the most common being red admirals and painted ladies. Other spectacular and obvious migrants are hummingbird hawkmoths, deathshead hawkmoths and monarch butterflies. Less well known are several migratory dragonflies that also visit here, one of the most beautiful being the red-veined sympetrum (*Sympetrum fonscolombei*) whose European distribution is principally Mediterranean but whose migrations sporadically take it northwards. Migratory and unusual insects arouse such interest that 'Annual Reports on Migrant Insects' are published in the *Irish Naturalists' Journal*.

Another class of 'foreign imports' could be called the 'immigrant hitchhikers', the many species that have hitched a ride on colonizing vertebrates. Thus a whole range of fleas, biting and sucking lice and other parasites have arrived in Ireland on their vertebrate hosts. One such visitor was the lethal oriental rat flea (*Xenopsylla cheopis*), which carried bubonic plague to Ireland on several occasions in previous centuries. Some of these hitchhikers only survive for a short time, such as a minute flightless water bug (*Microvelia pygmaea*) first discovered in Ireland in the 1970s. It was probably carried here on the plumage of migrating wildfowl and managed to establish itself for some years on several lakes in Co. Cork. Scarcity of shorebirds in Ireland permits this bug to occupy the open water on lake margins where enormous uncontrolled populations of it arise and soon exhaust the food supply, resulting in extinction (Walton, 1985).

Previously unrecorded species are added continually to our faunal lists, and even in well-studied groups exciting additions to the Irish fauna are discovered, as in 1981 when a strange damselfly found in Co. Sligo proved unknown in the British Isles and was named the Irish damselfly (*Coenagrion lunulatum*) (Cotton, 1982). Although most of the Irish species of insects originated in Northern Europe, some arrive from even further afield. An

American hoverfly (*Platycheirus amplus*) that was 'swept', or netted, from fen meadow in Co. Kildare constituted the first European record of this insect, and it has proved to be one of several species now known to occur in both Europe and North America whose presence in Europe was previously unsuspected (Speight and Vockeroth, 1988). Therefore, Ireland's position as the last outpost of Europe and the first landfall from North American continues to provide entomologists with both the unusual and the unexpected.

Irish Entomology: The Early Days

The Dublin Society was responsible for the first record of a collection of insects in Ireland when in 1792 it made a purchase, funded by a grant from the Irish Parliament of some £1350, which was to be of inestimable value to Irish natural history. Through the negotiations of the chemist and mineralogist Richard Kirwan (c. 1733-1821), who has close links with his German counterparts, it acquired the magnificent 'natural history museum' of Nathaniel Gottfried Leske (1752-86). Among the 'subjects of natural history' was a collection of insects from Europe and farther afield, which amounted to some 2500 species in 1813 when the entomological part was catalogued by Bernard O'Reilly (O'Connor, 1985). A comparison of O'Reilly's catalogue with the original sale catalogue – *Museum Leskeanum. Pars entomologica ad systema entomologiae. CL. Fabreicii ordinata etc.* – shows that the insect collection had not been greatly augmented in the twenty years since its purchase.

However, the basis of entomological collections in Ireland had been formed. By 1820 the collections in the Dublin Society Museum contained some eleven thousand insects, having been supplemented mainly by Irish material which the Society was intent on acquiring as part of its plan to have specimens to illustrate all of Ireland's natural history. In 1826 it dispatched Sir Charles Giesecke, its Professor of Mineralogy and Curator of the Museum, to undertake a tour in Co. Donegal to collect specimens and 'to direct his attention to the subject of native entomology and ornithology, and to collect, if opportunity occurs, any specimens in these departments he may conceive likely to be useful in completing these classes in the Museum' (White, 1911). The Leskean collection appears to have greatly stimulated interest among naturalists, because by 1843 William Thompson wrote that several collections of insects existed in the city, some in various other institutions and others in private collections. He noted: 'In Dublin there are of public collections, the Ordnance Museum, Phoenix Park, good in various departments of Vertebrata and Invertebrata; ... Trinity College containing the late Mr Tardy's fine collection of insects, added to by Dr Coulter; ... Royal Dublin Society, Vertebrata and Invertebrata: of private collections in the metropolis ... Miss M. Ball's, Insects chiefly, and Shells; ... Mr Egan's, in Insects; ...' (Thompson, 1843).

Of these, the Ordnance Collections were handed to the newly opened Museum of Irish Industry in 1847, and following the disbandment of that museum in 1867 the zoological collections were given to the Royal Dublin Society's Natural History Museum, which is now part of the National Museum of Ireland's collections. A Mr Egan of Dublin was a member of Council of the Dublin Natural History Society and in 1838 presented 'a large glazed case of rare Lepidoptera including several rare Sphingidae' to the Society's collections (Anon., 1844).

James Tardy (c. 1773-1835), whose Huguenot parents had settled in Dublin around 1760, was described by a contemporary as 'the most active of the few entomologists in Dublin' (Good and Linnie, 1990). He did not publish anything, but his collection contained about ten thousand specimens of Irish insects when purchased in 1843 by Trinity College, along with another collection of British insects made by John Curtis, the English entomologist, and a collection of eighteen thousand foreign shells made by Hugh Cuming which were 'unequalled in Ireland' (Coulter, 1843). In 1825 John Curtis named a beetle *Cossonus tardii* after Tardy and commented:

I have great pleasure in adopting the specific name proposed by Mr Vigors in honour of his friend James Tardy, Esq., of Dublin, to whom I have to acknowledge my obligations for specimens of this fine *Cossonus* taken by himself and Mr Vigors in July 1822, near Powerscourt waterfall, county of Wicklow, Ireland, under the bark of decayed hollies: it appears, like all other wood-feeding insects, to be extremely local; for Mr Tardy in a letter says, 'I have in vain sought for it in places abounding as much in holly and in similar situations in the same county.'

Tardy was therefore not merely an avid amasser of specimens but a careful and accurate observer of insects and their habits, and he illustrates what was taking place (see also Good and Linnie, 1990). This was the development of collecting into the full-blown scientific study of nature.

In the eighteenth and nineteenth centuries, contributions to Irish entomology came mainly from the leisured, wealthy members of the Anglo-Irish population, who had time and money to pursue the study of insects and whose numbers were supplemented occasionally by visiting English entomological acquaintances. The study and collection of specimens had become a fashionable recreation for the gentry, being a thoroughly respectable, intellectual and constructive pursuit. In addition, there was always the possibility of the added excitement of the personal recognition that might come from finding an unexpected rarity or making a new discovery, which stimulated collecting efforts in wild and remote places or unusual habitats.

The important early collections of the Dublin Society became the basis of the National Museum collections, which expanded greatly over the following hundred years. Other Irish societies became involved in the fashion for the study of all branches of natural history, including entomology. Of these, the Belfast Reading Society (founded 1788), which had a 'natural history cabinet' that included insects, and the Belfast Natural History Society, which accrued collections from its foundation in 1821, are outstanding examples. Following the impetus given by the doyen of Irish natural history, John Templeton, many developments took place and the Belfast naturalists diligently assembled collections and books and provided the requisite intellectual setting as an encouragement for others (Ross and Nash, 1985). Notable naturalists of this era in the north included George Crawford Hyndman, Robert Templeton and Robert Patterson. Hyndman's collection, consisting entirely of British Isles insects, the majority of them Irish, was classified and pinned out in his cabinets according to the system introduced by the French naturalist Fabricius, which was superseded by the more popular Linnaean system. It now forms part of the entomological collections in the Ulster Museum, Belfast.

Robert Templeton, the son of John Templeton, devoted much of his youth in Ireland to the pursuits of entomology and arachnology. He qualified in medicine and joined the Royal Artillery. In 1836 he published *Thysanurae Hibernicae* (Irish bristletails and springtails), the first work in English on these primitive insects, in which he described two new genera and a dozen new species. Later, outside his medical commitments, he was to make a significant contribution to the entomology of Ceylon and altogether published some twenty-five zoological papers between 1833 and 1858 (Nash and Ross, 1980). His close friend Patterson collected widely and contributed much to early knowledge of the Irish insect fauna, especially beetles. A less serious entomologist, Patterson wrote several important works on zoology and was responsible for giving the study of insects a cultural aspect by publishing what is probably the only book of its kind, *Letters on the Natural History of the Insects Mentioned in Shakespeare's Plays with Incidental Notes on the Insects of Ireland* (1838; see p. 492).

Alexander Henry Haliday commenced work on insects in the 1820s and became one of Europe's greatest entomologists, but remains virtually unknown in Ireland (*plate* . He was born in 1806 in Holywood, Co. Down. He was the son of one of Belfast's best-known physicians, who was a man of literary taste, a Whig and a founding subscriber of the school that his son was to attend, the Belfast Academy. His grandfather, the Rev. Samuel Haliday, 'was a very learned man who had studied under some of the great theologians at Leyden and had served as chaplain to Colonel Anstruther's Regiment of Cameronians throughout Marlborough's campaigns' (Stewart, 1985). Coming from this cultured and learned background, the youthful Haliday decided to study law at Trinity College, Dublin but was never to practise his profession. He returned north around 1826 to run the family's estates in Co. Down, but his natural-history interests had already been ignited by his coterie of friends, most of whom were already in the 'throes of the bug'. The following year, after meeting John Curtis, his interest became focused on the insects that had been neglected by previous entomologists. He possessed, according to Nash (1983), 'decided gifts as an entomologist. His rare capacity for observation, his descriptive powers and extraordinary ability to recognize relationships combined to foster his precocious talent. Furthermore his attention was largely directed to the obscure in the insect world – the minute Hymenoptera, the Diptera and the Thysanoptera [parasitic wasps, two-winged flies and thrips]'.

In addition, Haliday became an adept linguist and his influence on many other continental entomologists, particularly the German Hermann Loew and the Italian Camillo Rondani, and the leading English entomologists – Francis Walker, J.C. Dale, John Stephens and John Curtis – was considerable. He was the first to suggest that the type specimens from which the species descriptions had been made should be deposited in museums. This is now standard scientific practice worldwide. He published seventy-five entomological papers, including descriptions of numerous species new to science, and contributed substantial amounts of information to Curtis's *British Entomology* (published in sections between 1827 and 1840) and *Guide to the Arrangement of British Insects* (1837) and Walker's *Insecta Brittanica Diptera* (1851-6). Of Haliday, the notable English entomologist Joseph Westwood wrote: 'Nothing has ever exceeded the clearness and precision of his general views, as well as his minute and elaborate details. He was our foremost entomologist' (1870). The German entomologist Baron Osten Sacken mentioned his 'desire for completeness and perfection, which was quite disinterested, because shy of publicity; he had an intense desire of being useful, by imparting useful knowledge to others, unmindful of the amount of work it involved' (1903). In line with this wish to promote his subject and natural history as a whole, he became one of five Irish editors of the widely read *Natural History Review* in the 1850s.

In 1861 ill-health forced Haliday to leave Ireland to live in Lucca, Italy, where he helped to found the Italian Entomological Society. Edward Percival Wright, Professor of Zoology at Trinity College, his closest personal friend, joined him on an exhausting entomological tour of Sicily in 1870, from which Haliday never fully recovered, dying soon afterwards. Today his main insect collection and manuscripts are preserved in the Natural History Museum, Dublin, the remaining part of his library is in the Royal Irish Academy, and a manuscript list of Irish insects is in the Ulster Museum, Belfast. These are a continuing source of information to entomologists throughout the world.

Collections and Museums

The extraordinary outburst of work beginning in the 1860s after the founding of the Belfast, Cork, Dublin and Limerick Field Clubs provided great
encouragement for a new wave of naturalists. Field work and collecting were
no longer solitary activities; now they were carried out in groups, or even
'droves' on the clubs' well-organized outings. The correct identification of
the collected specimens completely depended on published checklists, keys
and field notes and on the availability and accessibility of reference material for comparison. Therefore, from the early nineteenth century to the present day, the academic institutions and museums devoted to natural history
accumulated entomological libraries and collections of insects. A catalogue of
the entomological works in Belfast Museum Library in 1847 reveals that
both 'fashionable' and 'foreign' publications were acquired, with the latter
probably finding a place there due to Haliday, whose linguistic ability gave
him wide access to continental literature. *Dialogues on Entomology* (1819),
Insect Architecture (1830) and *Insect Transformations* (1831) stood alongside
Latreille's *Cours d'Entomologie* (1831), *Atlas d'Entomologie* (1831) and the
Annals de la Societe Entomologique (1832-45) and the personal publications of
Haliday and Patterson.

Likewise in Dublin, the Royal Irish Academy and the Royal Dublin
Society would have acquired most of the relevant publications then available. Important reference journals publishing information on Irish insects
have been the *Natural History Review*, *The Entomologist's Monthly Magazine*,
The Entomologist's Record and *The Entomologist's Gazette*. The invaluable
Irish Naturalist and its successor the *Irish Naturalists' Journal* served the
field clubs as the publishing outlet for their collected information and com-
plemented the more academic and formal *Proceedings of the Royal Irish
Academy*. The more recent *Bulletin of the Irish Biogeographical Society*
reflects the growth in interest beyond the identification and naming of specimens to an interest in the range and distribution of our flora and fauna.
Much of the published literature on Irish insects consists of papers reporting additions to the fauna and checklists for various groups, which are listed in *A Bibliography of Irish Entomology* (Ryan, O'Connor and Beirne, 1984).

The various institutions and societies also set about acquiring and
building up their collections. The insect collections in the Belfast Museum
expanded quickly following its opening in 1831 so that by 1833 it had eleven
cases of foreign insects, including specimens from Rio de Janeiro, North
America, the West Indies and China. The thirteen cases of native insects
contained principally Irish specimens, supplemented with some English
specimens donated by, for example, William Curtis and Joseph Westwood.

In 1855 Haliday listed the numbers of named specimens in the collections as 929 beetles (Coleoptera), 243 alder and lacewing flies (Neuroptera), 645 butterflies and moths (Lepidoptera), 1247 bees and their allies (Hymenoptera), 1130 true flies (Diptera) and 246 bugs (Hemiptera), making a taxonomic collection totalling some 4500 specimens, with many more awaiting naming by specialists. In the Dublin Museum at this time, a similar picture emerges of an increasing interest in the acquisition of a comprehensive and scientific national collection illustrating the insect world. The collection of British Lepidoptera benefited from valuable additions from Rev. Joseph Greene and Richard Shield, and the Coleoptera were augmented with collections of several hundred British specimens from Percival Wright and Edward Newman and more than 250 species of European beetles from the Museum Societé Philomatique at Verdun. The Duke of Leinster donated two cases of insects from China to the foreign collections from, for example, Australia, Burma, the East Indies, Hong Kong, India, Russia, St Helena and Trinidad.

Many notable Irish entomological collections have subsequently been presented to or purchased by the National Museums in Belfast and Dublin. These have been greatly enriched by the professional entomologists employed by the institutions, among whom have been G.H. Carpenter, J.N. Halbert, A.W. Stelfox and E. O'Mahony, all of the National Museum, Dublin. The contributions of George Carpenter, who later became Professor of Zoology in the Royal College of Science, were mainly in the important field of economic entomology, which had wide implications in the vital agricultural field. For thirty years his valuable contributions were published annually in *Reports on Insect Pests*. In a key piece of work he successfully tackled the problems caused by attacks of the highly injurious warble flies, which then plagued cattle and reduced the value of hides. Carpenter was succeeded in Dublin by James Nathaniel Halbert, who devoted his time to producing valuable checklists of many Irish insect groups including caddisflies, lacewings, book lice, damselflies, dragonflies, stoneflies, mayflies, true bugs and (with W.F. Johnson) beetles. Halbert's interests extended beyond insects to other arthropods, and he identified and described many new species of marine and freshwater mites and compiled the Irish checklist.

In 1920 Halbert was joined in the Museum by Arthur Wilson Stelfox of Belfast, an architect by training who had an exceptional interest in natural history. Stelfox also benefited by training from Carpenter, and was put to work on Irish Hymenoptera and became a world authority on this insect order, which includes the familiar bees, wasps and ants. This group also contains the parasitic wasps so beloved by Haliday, and like him, Stelfox excelled in the study of these insects, continuing Haliday's work and revising parts of his collection which had been acquired by the Museum.

In 1922 Eugene O'Mahony joined the staff as a technical assistant. He was assigned to work on insects, thus strengthening the Museum's team of entomologists. However, this happy situation did not last since outside the Museum, momentous events were taking place. The War of Independence resulted in a new administration taking over in southern Ireland in 1922. Although all three remained productive entomologists, Halbert soon took early retirement and Stelfox and O'Mahony subsequently became disillusioned with the regime in the Museum following partition, though both continued to research Irish insects and amass their own collections (Beirne, 1985). Stelfox retired at sixty-five in 1948 and moved back to Northern Ireland, where he continued his wide-ranging researches for many more years. Although he had been promoted from Assistant to Deputy Keeper in 1931, he remained embittered about the new administation and the treatment of the Natural History Museum and its staff. As a result his magnificent collection of Irish parasitic Hymenoptera was presented to the Smithsonian Institution in Washington, D.C., meaning that scarcely any of his specimens in these groups were available in Dublin for others to study. After O'Mahony's death in 1951, Stelfox had arranged for his insect collection to be presented to the Hope Entomological Collections in Oxford University. Fortunately, in the 1980s, the O'Mahony Collection and voucher specimens from the Stelfox Collection from both museums were subsequently returned to the Natural History Museum, Dublin. The repatriation of these most valuable entomological collections has enabled a succeeding generation to advance the researches of these two great entomologists. After Stelfox's retirement, twenty-seven years were to elapse before another entomologist was appointed to the National Museum to resume the tradition of entomological research. The Ulster Museum acquired its first full-time entomologist in 1970.

Unlike entomologists in the early nineteenth century, the succeeding generation belonged to a diverse range of professions. Indeed, one of the great attractions of entomology as a hobby rather than as a profession stems from the size and diversity of the subject, which make it possible to become an authority on virtually any group. Colonel Niall MacNeill (1899-1969) is a good example of such an amateur. An officer in the Irish Army and also Assistant Director of the Ordnance Survey, in middle age he became interested in the dragonflies and damselflies. Encouraged by Cynthia Longfield, he was the first to discover morphological details of the nymphs and wrote some fascinating accounts of their larval stages and life-histories. On a wider scale he pioneered the National Grid System on Irish maps: the mapping of the distribution of plants and animals by 10-km or 100-km squares.

The work of the relatively small number of Irish entomologists has been supplemented by others, particularly from Great Britain, who have made significant contributions to our knowledge of the Irish fauna. Examples include the work of Peter Chandler on two-winged flies, Ted Pelham Clinton and others on micromoths, Marcus de Vere Graham on parasitic wasps, Raymond Haynes on macromoths, Mike Morris on weevils, Courtenay Smithers on psocids and Phil Withers on moth-flies. Bryan P. Beirne, who started working on entomology under Halbert's tutelage, became a prolific researcher on the Irish insects. Although he emigrated to Canada in 1949 to pursue his career he never lost his interest in Irish entomology, eventually contributing to *A Bibliography of Irish Entomology* (Ryan *et al.*, 1984). His 1985 paper, 'Irish Entomology: The First Hundred Years', vividly describes the developments and those involved. Of one of those, E.F. Bullock, Beirne wrote that he 'remained obviously English. He had a strong Dorsetshire accent and an Edwardian appearance with spiked moustache, tiny-rimmed spectacles, curly-brimmed hat, high collar, expansive waistcoat with heavy watch and chain, narrow trousers and massive out-turned boots. He was a genial, kindly and beaming man of rather endearing simplicity and sincerity and with a sense of humour' (Beirne, 1985).

The recent introduction of novel and imaginative collecting techniques has enabled many significant discoveries to be made. These include the rearing of larvae and pupae from previously overlooked habitats such as rot holes in trees and the use of new equipment like Malaise traps, light-traps, d-vacs (large vacuum cleaners) and 'pyrethrum fogging' (which involves the rapid 'knockdown' or temporary paralysis of insects from the usually inaccessible tree canopy). More recently, faunal studies on Irish insects have produced new perspectives on the interrelationships of various insect groups with their environment. A fine example is the recently completed research on the two-winged flies, or Diptera, of the Murrough, Co. Wicklow. This has yielded records of more than 650 species of which one fifth were breeding there, and as it includes a bibliography of relevant faunistic and taxonomic literature it provides an excellent model for future studies (Blackith *et al.*, 1991). In another interesting study, the conservation value of the rich Clonmacnoise Heritage Zone in Co. Offaly was assessed using its butterfly and moth fauna. Surprisingly this site was home to about 20 per cent of the currently known Irish Lepidoptera fauna (Bond, 1989). Other aspects of insect life in Ireland that have received recent attention include insect behaviour, the biogeography and ecology of individual species, insect diets and the parasites of various Irish vertebrates.

The Contribution of Women

Although relatively few Irish women have been interested in studying insects, some have made significant contributions – yet even today, despite encouragement, their numbers remain small. The collection of insects, rather than the detailed study of them, was for long one of the areas of natural history favoured by women. Robert Ball (1802-57) made mention of a lady of his acquaintance who formed a collection of over two hundred species of insects taken 'from the windows of her drawing-room'! It is unlikely that he was referring to either of his sisters, who were naturalists, not of the 'closet' variety, but rather exceptional field naturalists.

Mary Ball (1812-98) became one of Ireland's first female entomologists and also contributed to conchology, the study of shells (Ross, 1985). She was born in Cobh, Co. Cork, and later lived with her sister, Anne Elizabeth, in Youghal and Dublin. She communicated her accurate observations to Haliday and others, including Baron de Selys-Longchamps, the Belgian naturalist and authority on dragonflies who visited Ireland and examined her collection of these attractive insects. Around 1840, Mary Ball was the first person to identify the sounds produced by Water Boatmen (Corixids) as a mating call, known as 'stridulation' (Hutchinson, 1982). Although today it may appear extraordinary to us, her discoveries were normally published under her brother Robert's name, or passed to others, such as Haliday, for inclusion in their work, since even as late as the 1850s it was unusual for women to publish their own papers in scientific journals. She made several interesting finds, including that of the first migratory locust to be recorded in Ireland. This specimen of *Locusta christii* was taken on 1 August 1836 at Ardmore, Co. Waterford, and is recorded in John Curtis's famous work, *British Entomology*.

Mary Ward (1827-69) was born Mary King in Ferbane, Co. Offaly, and was the cousin of William, 3rd Earl of Rosse, the renowned Irish astronomer, and a frequent visitor to his home and observatory at Birr Castle. An exceptionally fine artist and painter, she drew many accurate and delightful illustrations of insects. One of her books (co-authored with her sister Lady Mahon) had the unusual title *Entomology in Sport* (1853). She became well known as a naturalist, astronomer, microscopist and artist and was the first woman to write and have published a book on the microscope and its uses in 1858 (under the name of 'the Hon. Mrs W.'). This was reprinted at least eight times between 1858 and 1880 (Harry, 1984, 1985).

The collection of another entomologist, Mrs Battersby of Rathowen, Westmeath, which was given to the Belfast Museum, illustrates the special appeal that butterflies and moths held for women. In about 1850 she joined a growing band of enthusiasts in Ireland and England who collected, bred and exchanged, not just dried specimens of Lepidoptera, but also their pupae, through a sort of 'Pupal Exchange Club'. She had exchanged specimens in her collection with James Tardy, a Mrs Hutchinson, a Mr Corbin and a Mr Doubleday, among others. About 1843, the English entomologists

Henry Doubleday and his brother Edward had invented the 'treacling pan' as a method of attracting and capturing nocturnal moths, 'in no time at all effecting a veritable revolution in the range of species represented in the average collector's cabinet' (Allen, 1976). Their interest in curiosities and rarities is evident, for the collection contained many specimens of sub-species, varieties and forms. Not surprisingly, these curiosity-hunters, with their keen notion of the unusual, also contributed the first Irish records of several moths and butterflies.

One of the most remarkable entomologists of recent times was another Irish woman, Cynthia Longfield (1896-1991), who represented a last flow-ering of the Victorian tradition, having a passionate interest in natural his-tory and ample private means. Although born in London, her family came from Cloyne, Co. Cork, and she always considered herself to be Irish. She became a world authority on the dragonflies and damselflies (Odonata) of Europe and Africa and wrote what was, until recently, the standard work on the group in the British Isles (Longfield, 1937). Longfield collected and studied Odonata in many parts of the world, taking part in the St George Scientific Expedition to the Pacific in 1924 and subsequently travelling fear-lessly in many parts of Africa and South America between 1927 and 1937 (Hayter-Hames, 1991; Scannell, 1992). In the last twenty years the appeal of entomology has widened for women, as a glance at current publications shows.

Arrivals: Friends or Foes?

Man has not only studied insects in Ireland, but has also played his part in importing them into the island, either accidentally or on purpose. While the honey bee and the large copper butterfly were deliberately introduced, most introductions have been unintentional. The discovery of the cellar beetle (*Blaps lethifera*) at the Viking site at Wood Quay, Dublin, dating from around the mid-eleventh century, provides early evidence of an accidental introduction since the specimens were probably imported in produce from abroad (O'Connor, 1979). Despite the benign relationship man has often had with insects, some insect introductions may pose a serious economic threat if they are not quickly identified, and they may also have devastating effects on the landscape. The most obvious instance arose with the bark beetles responsible for spreading the fungus that causes Dutch elm disease, the wilt-ing and death of elm trees brought about when the fungus blocks the tree's vital water-conducting tubes. The large elm bark beetle (*Scolytus scolytus*) was first discovered here in 1943 and might easily have been eradicated. However, by 1982 the small elm bark beetle (*Scolytus multistriatus*) had also reached Ireland. It was found in the Phoenix Park in Dublin by the use of special pheromone traps which are sexually attractive to the beetles. The extensive tracts of our countryside now planted with a restricted range of conifer species therefore risk extensive damage should some foreign species of bark beetles become established. Several potentially serious pest species have already been detected during inspections of imported timber in Irish ports. These include the spruce bark beetle (*Ips typographus*), the most aggressive scolytid known in Europe, particularly in Germany where it has devastated large numbers of spruce trees, and the spruce beetle (*Dendroctonus rufipennis*), now considered a chronic pest in North America where it attacks standing trees in addition to freshly cut or windfelled ones (O'Connor *et al.*, 1991).

There is ample evidence of some recently imported species that have managed to establish themselves in Ireland at considerable risk to public health. Cockroaches have for centuries been among the most detested 'domestic' insects. In the last twenty years the brown-banded cockroach (*Supella supellectilium*), originally from tropical Africa, has increasingly been recorded here in buildings, including hospitals. It can infest premises and is not solely confined to kitchens and eating areas. How it has been introduced is not known, but it may have been in the personal luggage of foreign visitors or with imported fruit. A fruit fly (*Drosophila repleta*) is another recently detected pest which, in Ireland, seems to have a taste for public houses (O'Connor and Ashe, 1992).

It often comes as a surprise to people to discover that mosquitoes are found in Ireland and even more of a surprise that altogether eighteen species have been recorded here, but malaria is not now present. Before 1844, malaria was still unknown in Ireland but subsequently, year after year, it increased, particularly in Cork, and a plague occurred in 1857. The Crimean War was a possible contributory factor because of the large numbers of infective soldiers returning home with regiments stationed in Ireland. Malaria may be re-introduced in future from other parts of the world if evidence from an outbreak in England is significant. In 1983, residents living close to Gatwick Airport near London, who had not themselves travelled to any malarious country, contracted malignant tertian malaria. Its transmission was attributed to infective tropical mosquitoes escaping from intercontinental aircraft, and now over twenty cases of 'airport malaria' have been reported close to other European airports.

In the economically important horticultural field, several serious pests have recently been introduced. One of our most alarming introductions is the western flower thrips (*Frankliniella occidentalis*), a North American species now spreading throughout north-western Europe. In Ireland this notorious greenhouse pest was first found on imported sweet peppers and is a virus vector on chrysanthemums, lettuce and many other plants, resulting in heavy financial losses to the industry (Dunne and O'Connor, 1989). The South American leafminer (*Liriomyza huidobrensis*) – a highly polyphagous species which can feed on plants of at least nine different families – has also been accidentally imported here recently (Hume *et al.*, 1990). Fortunately prompt action quickly eradicated it, although continuous vigilance will be necessary to prevent its re-introduction.

It is not every day that one comes across pests that impose grave economic damage by causing pigs to catch colds! Yet this is precisely the problem caused by the lesser mealworm beetle and the broad-horned flour beetle. In 1983 the Natural History Museum received a plea for help from an intensive pig farm in Co. Cavan, along with a sample of polystyrene insulation riddled with large and small holes. The flour beetle damage had totally impaired its insulating properties, making many pigs ill in the cold and draughty conditions (O'Connor, 1987).

Insect Conservation

However, there is another story to tell, this time of human destruction of harmless or beneficial insects. We often fail to realize the profound influence on the associated fauna of the progressive destruction of almost all the native Irish forests, dating from soon after the first arrival of man and continuing until the early nineteenth century. Obviously the insect fauna of the forests would have been greatly affected; many woodland species were unable to survive in the almost treeless landscape. Some species did manage to survive and these demonstrate a typical relict distribution pattern exhibited by 'old-forest insects' which today remain in only a few localities in the small total area of remaining native woodland. An example is the red-brown lycid beetle (*Pyropterus nigroruber*), still found in Kerry, whose future is not secure, as it requires dead wood in which its larvae can develop and is therefore extremely vulnerable to any 'tidying up' of the woodland which could eradicate both habitat and beetle (Speight, 1990). It also appears that the Scots pine (*Pinus sylvestris*) became extinct in Ireland along with its associated insect fauna. Amazingly, present-day insects have been found feeding on the thousand-year-old wood of the long-dead pines excavated from Irish bogs during the course of peat extraction (Speight, 1985)

Untold numbers of Irish insects are now under threat mainly due to habitat destruction from afforestation, drainage and land reclamation. In recent years many locations have been destroyed or badly damaged in the name of 'improvement'. These include a delightful section of the Royal Canal at Luttrellstown, Co. Dublin, which was cleaned by dredging. An official faunal survey was belatedly carried out *after* the dredging, when it was impossible to know what effects the destruction of this habitat had caused!

In the Republic in the past, the general population often had little sympathy for, or understanding of, insects. Part of the reason may be traced to the removal of rural science or nature study from the primary school curriculum in the Irish Free State in the 1930s to make more time available for the teaching of the Irish language. As a result, complete ignorance of the natural world is often evident, especially in urban environments.

Amazingly, even those responsible for making decisions affecting our natural environment frequently display a lack of concern for it. A preoccupation with 'tidiness' results in the widespread practice of spraying verges, hedgerows and areas around trees, which in a short time may seriously reduce the insect diversity in an area. A poignant example concerns a very rare soldier fly (*Oxycera fallenii*). Haliday had noted that James Tardy had collected two specimens of this beautiful little black and yellow insect in the vicinity of Enniskerry, Co. Wicklow, but for a century no further individuals were seen. A European authority dismissed the original record as erroneous, noting that the species closely resembled others and had never been found in Great Britain. There the matter rested until the 1930s, when the fly was rediscovered in Glen of the Downs, not far from Enniskerry. Subsequently, both sites were eradicated by building works. In 1980, in an intensive collecting effort, a small population was located at a rather undistinguished roadside marsh, midway between Enniskerry and Glen of the Downs. Therefore the past and present known range of this fly in Ireland roughly encompasses about five square miles. This pretty little fly is unrecorded in Great Britain; geographically the closest populations of it to Ireland are now in Denmark and Switzerland. Although it is of singular zoogeographic interest, the small area it inhabits in Ireland has neither been designated nor acquired for conservation purposes and the colony is further threatened by a road-widening scheme made possible with funding from the European Community. The Irish Government is a signatory of the Berne Convention of the European Community which legislates for the protection of species and their habitats and it is to be hoped that the protection of important habitats will be easier in the future.

The situation is beginning to change and public awareness of the environment is increasing slowly. This has been helped greatly by natural history programmes on television and radio, resulting in a dramatic increase in interest in the work of institutions such as the two national museums, in Dublin and Belfast. Although *The Irish Times* publishes occasional entomological articles, the press in general has done little to promote an understanding of insects and the natural environment even though these creatures constitute a large, noticeable, and often commercially important part of our fauna. The Wildlife Service of the Office of Public Works in the Republic has conducted some exceptional public-relations work for insect conservation and the Conservation Branch of the Department of the Environment in Northern Ireland has financed surveys and reports on endangered species and their habitats. Apart from these moves there are positive indications of a fundamental advance in public awareness. Recently, a more enlightened approach by some county councils and in the Republic by organizations such as the Electricity Supply Board, has resulted in the preservation of a number of important sites.

'Insect gardens' have become fashionable. Henry Heal of Belfast was one of the pioneers in designing insect-friendly gardens. In 1964 he created Europe's first butterfly garden at Drum Manor in Co. Tyrone, and in later years he was to see hundreds of butterfly gardeners at work all over Britain and Ireland (Heal, 1986). A few years ago, having been invited to talk about insects and wildlife gardening to a local gardening club, I prepared with some trepidation, for the slides unfortunately showed large areas of my garden filled with stinging nettles and other 'weeds'. To my surprise, the lecture was very well received by these gardening enthusiasts and aroused the interest of other gardening groups. Incidentally, my garden wild patch has been very good for insects and to date has produced eight species new to Ireland and the first Irish record of a strepsipteran (a two-winged parasitic insect) for 150 years.

Although so many aspects of our lives are interdependent on our insect fauna, it is difficult to foresee a bright future for the study of insects in Ireland. In most universities here and across the water, the teaching of systematic zoology and nomenclature, or taxonomy, has almost disappeared from the syllabus. Taxonomists have been replaced by, among others, biochemists, behaviourists and physiologists, meaning that there is little encouragement to undergraduates to consider entomology as a career, a situation that has not been helped by the dearth of jobs. While posts have multiplied in many disciplines, the number of entomologists employed has effectively declined. A review of the state of taxonomy in Ireland (O'Connor et al., 1988), produced for the National Committee for Biology of the Royal Irish Academy, published a list of recommendations to alleviate some of the problems bedevilling Irish taxonomic studies but these have not yet been implemented. We must therefore conclude that knowledge of insects and their ways is not at the moment considered to have any economic importance. This is despite the fact that investigations such as the now-fashionable Environmental Impact Assessments are meaningless unless the collected specimens are correctly named, since most of them rely on the total number of species collected, or on species diversity, in assessing the environmental value of sites to counteract or prevent unwelcome commercial developments in vulnerable areas.

With the increasing trade with the European Union and elsewhere, entomologists will be needed also to identify the many insects that will be imported accidentally into Ireland. Potentially serious economic pests will need to be detected quickly and speedily eradicated or they may become established here. Given our ageing population of professional specialists and declining numbers of amateurs, it is also certain that without encouragement to the younger generation to take an interest in entomology either as a career or as a worthwhile hobby, there will be very few people capable of accurately identifying insects, the dominant group of animals in Irish freshwater and terrestrial habitats.

However, we must hope that increasing public interest in nature conservation, coupled with the new awareness of the importance of maintaining plant and animal biodiversity, may help to recruit young entomologists. From a cultural point of view, our way of life requires an enormous interchange in people and goods between countries. It is therefore essential that knowledge and appreciation of the diversity of the Irish insect fauna, which is both a key element in many food chains and also of economic importance in industry, agriculture and forestry, is widely available and accessible. The challenge is a great one, for Ireland's insects have been an important part of our lives since man first stepped on to these shores and these fascinating creatures are too important to ignore or neglect. As William Peck, the first American entomologist and a contemporary of George Hyndman, aptly wrote of insects in 1819: 'In the execution of the task assigned them, they often frustrate the designs and subvert the arrangements of man, thus constraining him to attend to objects which are generally deemed beneath his notice, and obliging him to feel how effective is the smallest instrument in the hand of Omnipotence.'

References

Allen, D.E. 1976. *The Naturalist in Britain*. London: Allen Lane.

Anderson, R. 1979. '*Stenus glacialis* Heer (Col., Staphylinidae) in West Donegal.' *Entomologist's Monthly Magazine 114*: 20.

Anon. 1800. *Premiums of the Dublin Society*. Dublin: Dublin Society.

Anon. 1844. *Report of the Dublin Society – Acquisitions for the Museum*. Dublin: Dublin Society.

Ball, R. 1856. 'Proceedings of Societies: Dublin University Zoological Association.' *Natural History Review 3*: 1-9.

Beirne, B.P. 1985. 'Irish Entomology: the First Hundred Years.' *Irish Naturalists' Journal*: Special Entomological Supplement 1-40.

Blackith, R.E., R.M. Blackith, M.C.D. Speight and M. de Courcy Williams. 1991. 'A First List of Diptera from the Murrough, Co. Wicklow, Ireland, including 663 Species and 140 Breeding Records.' *Bulletin of the Irish Biogeographical Society 14*: 185-253.

Bond, K.G.M. 1989. 'Clonmacnoise Heritage Zone, Co. Offaly, Ireland: Assessment of Conservation Value based on Lepidoptera Recorded from 1983 to 1987.' *Bulletin of the Irish Biogeographical Society 12*: 6:3-89.

Bond, K.G.M. and R.E. Blackith. 1987. 'A Desert Locust of the Solitary Phase in Ireland.' *Irish Naturalists' Journal 22*: 356-8.

Carpenter, G.H. 1902-16. 'Reports on Injurious Insects and other Animals.' *Economic Proceedings of the Royal Dublin Society*. Dublin.

Cotton, D.C.F. 1982. '*Coenagrion lunulatum* (Charpentier) (Odonata: Coenagrionidae) New to the British Isles.' *Entomologist's Gazette 33*: 213-14.

Coulter, T. 1843. Letter to McDonnell, Bursar of Trinity College, 11 January.

Curtis, J. 1824-40. *British Entomology – being Illustrations and Descriptions of the Genera of Insects found in Great Britain and Ireland Containing Coloured Figures from Nature of the most Beautiful Species, etc*. 7 vols. London: author.

Curtis, J. 1837. *A Guide to the Arrangement of British Insects*. 2 vols. London: author.

Dunne, R., and J.P. O'Connor. 1989. 'Some Insects (Thysanoptera: Diptera) of Economic Importance, New to Ireland.' *Irish Naturalists' Journal 23*: 63-5.

Good, J.A., and M. Linnie. 1990. 'The History of the Early Nineteenth Century Coleoptera Collection of James Tardy at Trinity College, Dublin, and the Validity of Records based on his Collection.' *Irish Naturalists' Journal 23*: 298-305.

Harris, W. 1950. *An Angler's Entomology*. London: Collins.

Harry, O.G. 1984. 'The Hon. Mrs Ward (1827-1869) Artist, Naturalist, Astronomer and Ireland's First Lady of the Microscope.' *Irish Naturalists' Journal 21*: 193-200.

Harry, O.G. 1985. 'Mary Ward – Microscopist, Astronomer, Naturalist, Artist,' in C. Mollan, W. Davis and B. Finucane (eds), *Some People and Places in Irish Science and Technology*. Dublin: Royal Irish Academy.

Hayter-Hames, J. 1991. *Madam Dragonfly: The Life and Times of Cynthia Longfield*. Edinburgh, Cambridge and Durham: The Pentland Press.

Heal, H. 1986. 'Drum Manor Butterfly Garden.' *Irish Naturalists' Journal 22*: 131-2.

Hume, H., R. Dunne and J.P. O'Connor 1990. '*Liriomyza huidobrensis* (Blanchard) (Diptera: Agromyzidae), an Imported Pest New to Ireland.' *Irish Naturalists' Journal 23*: 325-6.

Hutchinson, G.E. 1982. 'The harp that once ... a Note on the Discovery of Stridulation in the Corixid Water Bugs.' *Irish Naturalists' Journal 20*: 457-66.

Longfield, C. 1937. *The Dragonflies of the British Isles*. London: Warne.

Nash, R. 1975. 'The Butterflies of Ireland.' *Proceedings of the British Entomological and Natural History Society 7*: 69-73.

Nash, R. 1983. 'A Brief Summary of the Development of Entomology in Ireland during the Years 1790-1870.' *Irish Naturalists' Journal 21*: 145-50.

Nash, R. and H.C.G. Ross. 1980. *Dr Robert Templeton Roy. Art. (1802-1892)*. Belfast: Ulster Museum.

O'Connor, J.P. 1979. '*Blaps lethifera* Marsham (Coleoptera: Tenebrionidae), a Beetle New to Ireland from Viking Dublin.' *Entomologists' Gazette 30*: 295-7.

O'Connor, J.P. 1985. 'Bernard O'Reilly – Genius or Rogue?' *Irish Naturalists' Journal 21*: 379-84.

O'Connor, J.P. 1987. '*Alphitobius diaperinus* (Panzer) (Col, Tenebrionidae) Damaging Polystyrene Insulation in an Irish Piggery.' *Entomologist's Monthly Magazine 123*: 50.

O'Connor, J.P. and P. Ashe. 1992. '*Drosophila repleta* Wollaston (Dipt., Drosophilidae), an Unsavory Find in a Dublin Pub.' *Entomologist's Monthly Magazine 128*: 146.

O'Connor, J.P. and J.A. Good. 1984. '*Tinodes dives* (Pictet): A Caddisfly New to Ireland from Ben Bulben, Co. Sligo.' *Entomologist's Record and Journal of Variation 96*: 108-9.

O'Connor, J.P., M.J.P. Scannell and M.C.D. Speight. 1988. 'The State of Taxonomy in Ireland,' in C. Moriarty (ed.), *Taxonomy, Putting Plants and Animals in their Place*. Dublin: Royal Irish Academy.

O'Connor, J.P., T.G. Winter and J.A. Good. 1991. 'A Review of the Irish Scolytidae (Insecta: Coleoptera).' *Irish Naturalists' Journal 23*: 403-9.

Orme, A.R. 1970. *The World's Landscapes 4. Ireland*. London: Longman.

Osten-Sacken, C.R. 1903-4. *Record of my Life Work in Entomology*. 3 vols. Cambridge, Mass. (1-2), Heidelberg (3): author.

Patterson, R. 1838. *Letters on the Natural History of Insects Mentioned in Shakespeare's Plays, with Incidental Notes on the Insects of Ireland*. London: W. S. Orr and Co.

Ross, H.C.G. 1985. 'Mary Ball – Naturalist,' in C. Mollan, W. Davis and B. Finucane (eds), *Some People and Places in Irish Science and Technology*. Dublin, Royal Irish Academy.

Ross, H.C.G. and R. Nash. 1985. 'The Development of Natural History in early Nineteenth Century Ireland,' in *From Linnaeus to Darwin: Commentaries on the History of Biology and Geology*. London: Society for the History of Natural History.

Ryan, J.G., J.P. O'Connor and B.P. Beirne. 1984. *A Bibliography of Irish Entomology*. Dublin: Flyleaf Press.

Scannell, M.J.P. 1992. 'Cynthia Evelyn Longfield (1896-1991) – a Tribute.' *Botanical Society of the British Isles Newsletter 60*: 25-6.

Speight, M.C.D. 1985. 'Present-day Use of Prehistoric Pine Timber ('bog-deal') by Woodboring Insects and its Faunal Implications.' *Irish Naturalists' Journal 21*: 448-9.

Speight, M.C.D. 1990. '*Pyropterus nigroruber* (Degeer) in Ireland (Coleoptera: Lycidae), with a Key to Distinguish this Beetle from Related European Species.' *Bulletin of the Irish Biogeographical Society 13*: 166-72.

Speight, M.C.D. and J.R. Vockeroth. 1988. '*Platycheirus amplus*: an Insect New to Ireland not Previously Recorded from Europe (Diptera: Syrphidae).' *Irish Naturalists' Journal 22*: 518-21.

Stelfox, A.W. 1927. 'A List of the Hymenoptera Aculeata (sensu lato) of Ireland.' *Proceedings of the Royal Irish Academy 37B*: 201-355.

Stewart, A.T.Q. 1985. *Belfast Royal Academy – The First Century 1785-1885*. Antrim: Greystone Press.

Templeton, R. 1836. 'Thysanurae Hibernicae, or Descriptions of such Species of Spring-tailed Insects (Podura and Lepisma Linn.) as have been Observed in Ireland.' *Transactions of the Entomological Society of London 1*: 89-98.

Thompson, W. 1843. 'Report on the Fauna of Ireland: Div Invertebrata. Drawn up at the request of the British Association.' *Reports of the British Association 1843*: 245-91.

Walker, F. 1851-6. *Insecta Brittanica Diptera*. 3 vols. London: Reeve and Benham (1), Lovell and Reeve (2-3).

Ward, Hon. Mrs M. and Lady M. 1856. *Entomology in Sport*. London: Paul Jerrard & Son.

Walton, G.A. 1985. '*Microvelia pygmaea* (Dufour) (Hemiptera: Veliidae) in Ireland.' *Irish Naturalists' Journal 21*: 493-5.

Westwood, J.O. 1870. 'Alexander Henry Haliday – Obituary.' *Transactions of the Entomological Society of London 47*: 113.

White, H.B. 1911. 'History of the Science and Art Institutions, Dublin.' *Museum Bulletin of the National Museum of Science and Art 1.4*: 7-34.

Mammals and Mammalogy

PATRICK SLEEMAN

Quis enim, verbi gratia, lupos, cervos et sylvaticos porcos, et vulpes, taxones et lepusculos et sequivolos in Hiberniam deveheret?

– Augustin, seventh century

Origins of Ireland's Mammal Fauna

The origins of Ireland's present fauna have long been the subject of speculation and controversy among scientists. Our native mammal fauna was present after the last Ice Age, about thirteen to fourteen thousand years ago. It is believed that reindeer, hare, stoat, pygmy shrew and otter, all of which can live in Arctic conditions, survived the extreme cold. It is probable that Arctic foxes and lemmings, characteristic species of the cold, survived only to go extinct when the warmer conditions returned, but as yet we have no evidence for this. Hares, stoats and otters have changed sufficiently to become recognizable native Irish subspecies (*Table 1*) and can therefore be distinguished from those from other countries. For example, the Irish stoat can be told apart from the British stoat by the irregular back/belly line and by its darker colouring. How did the other native wild mammals, which could not have survived the cold, get here?

In Ireland there are about half the mammal species found in Britain. Weasels, voles and moles, as well as polecats, brown hares, beavers and roe deer, never made it to Ireland. Today we have twenty-one species of terrestrial wild mammal in Ireland (*Table 1*), compared with thirty-eight species in Britain. This indicates that considerable obstacles must have existed to their colonization. There has been much intriguing speculation about the origin of Irish mammals in general, and about certain species in particular. This latter phenomenon has been labelled the 'pygmy shrew syndrome' (named for an unexpected and much speculated-about mammal in the Irish

*Table 1: Wild terrestrial mammals of Ireland and their probable status
(*species extinct in Ireland)*

ASSUMED NATIVE

Giant Irish deer*	*Megaceros giganteus*
Reindeer*	*Rangifer tarandus*
Brown bear*	*Ursus arctos*
Wild boar*	*Sus scofa*
Wolf*	*Canis lupus*
Wild cat*	*Felis sylvestris*
Red squirrel*	*Sciurius vulgaris*
Red deer	*Cervus elaphus*
Pygmy shrew	*Sorex minutus*
Fox	*Vulpes vulpes*
Badger	*Meles meles*
Pine marten	*Martes martes*
Irish (Mountain) hare	*Lepus timidus hibernicus*
Irish stoat	*Mustela erminea hibernica*
Irish otter	*Lutra lutra roensis*
Wood mouse	*Apodemus sylvaticus*

INTRODUCED

Hedgehog	*Erinaceus europaeus*
Rabbit	*Oryctolagus cuniculus*
Brown hare	*Lepus europaeus*
Red squirrel*	*Sciurius vulgaris*
Grey squirrel	*Sciurius carolinensis*
Bank vole	*Clethrionomys glareolus*
Ship (Black) rat	*Rattus rattus*
Common (Brown) rat	*Rattus norvegicus*
House mouse	*Mus domesticus*
Mink	*Mustela vison*
Fallow deer	*Dama dama*
Sika deer	*Cervus nippon*
Muskrat*	*Ondata zibethicus*
Roe deer*	*Capreolus capreolus*
Wild pig (Greyhound pig)*	*Sus domestica*
Goat (Feral)	*Capra hircus*

fauna) and leads people to use a limited amount of anomalous data to explain island colonization (Sleeman *et al.*, 1986).

One theory about the origin of the Irish flora and fauna concerns a number of species that occur both in Ireland and the Iberian peninsula, which are referred to as the 'Lusitanian' elements of our fauna, since Lusitania was the name used by the Romans for their province in Portugal and part of Spain. Lusitanian animals and plants have been used in speculations about the survival of life in unglaciated regions, or 'refuges', during the last glaciation, or to postulate the existence of land bridges between Ireland and Iberia. The Lusitanian element of the Irish flora and fauna held great fascination for Robert Francis Scharff, of whom more later. However, Lusitanian animals represent less than 1 per cent of Ireland's total fauna (Speight, 1986) and are of small size and thus easily transported. It would appear, therefore, that they were introduced accidentally from time to time.

Thirty-one wild terrestrial mammals and six species of bats have lived in Ireland since the last glaciation (*Table 1*), although at least sixteen of these have been introduced by man. Originally only a single representative of each genus of mammals was present in Ireland and only through introductions were other representatives of the same group added to the fauna. For example in the deer genus *Cervus*, red deer (*Cervus elaphus*) are native, but sika deer (*Cervus nippon*) are introduced; in the genus Sciurus, red squirrels are native but became extinct and were re-introduced, while grey squirrels are introduced; and in the genus Rattus, both ship and common rats are introduced, but at different times.

Are the introductions to be considered as Irish? Seven of the fifteen species assumed to be native became extinct; to further complicate matters, three introduced species are also now extinct in Ireland. All introduced wild mammals are now considered to be Irish, and therefore it is mainly due to the successive waves of colonization since humans first arrived at these shores that we owe much of the present-day mammalian fauna of Ireland. As the monk Augustin wisely observed in the seventh century: 'Who indeed would have brought wolves, deer, wild swine, foxes, badgers, little hares and squirrels to Ireland?' Some have suggested that many, if not all, Irish mammals were introduced by people in boats. Spectacular evidence in support of this view is the skeleton of a Barbary ape, *Maca sylvans*, with a chain around its neck, which was found at a Bronze Age site at Emain Macha, Co. Armagh. This captive animal must have been brought to Ireland by boat (Woodman, 1986).

Is it possible that other wild mammals, especially fierce carnivores such as bears, wolves, badgers and foxes, were brought by boat to Ireland? Since these predatory mammals range widely in search of food it seems more likely that some crossed over ice bridges or land bridges that may have remained after the glaciers departed. Others may have taken to the water and swum the relatively short distance from Scotland. Wolves are known to cross water on ice floes and have been seen on drifting ice off North America (Banfield, 1954). Sea-level changes must be considered as well; the consensus of opinion is that during glaciation the sea level would have been about fifty fathoms below present levels (Savage, 1966), which would allow for a number of possible land bridges in the north of the island or, as Mitchell (1963) has argued, between Wicklow and the Lleyn Peninsula and between Louth, the Isle of Man and Cumbria.

Without doubt, people did bring in domestic dogs, pigs, cattle, sheep, goats and horses at different times, and perhaps like the Barbary ape, some carnivores were brought as captives, or even with a view to exploiting their fur. John Millington Synge, in his book *The Aran Islands* (1907), gives a graphic description of the islanders moving cattle and horses by boat at the turn of this century, providing a glimpse of how this might have been done.

Human Impact on the Mammals

Human beings, then, especially as hunters and fishermen, have had enormous impact on Irish mammal life from early times. Ireland was one of the last areas of Europe to be colonized by Mesolithic people. These hunter-fishers settled here around 7000 BC, and at their camp sites archaeologists have found traces of the animals they used, including wild boar, wolf, brown bear, hare and red deer (Woodman, 1981). Reindeer, wild boar and brown bear appear to have become extinct during the following prehistoric times, as they fail to turn up in later archaeological sites (Stuart and Wijngaarden-Bakker, 1985). It was once considered unlikely that primitive peoples could cause extinctions of large animals; however, this is now accepted to have occurred frequently, particularly on islands with their limited animal populations. The extinction of giant birds, such as the moa on the islands of New Zealand and others on Madagascar and Hawaii, are now believed to have been due to primitive hunters (Diamond, 1991). Likewise in Ireland, the extinction of reindeer, boar and bear, and possibly other animals such as large bird species, was probably due to overhunting by early colonizers. The wild pigs encountered in later historic times were smaller and are thought to have been escaped descendants of domestic pigs, called greyhound pigs, that had bred in the wild or become 'feral' (Harting, 1880). Other domestic animals that became feral in Ireland were goats and, arguably, horses.

These early hunters had to know and understand the habits of wild mammals. By Early Christian times hunters were using ingenious methods such as wooden traps, which caught deer by the leg, a device beautifully illustrated in a panel on Banagher High Cross, dating from around AD 800.

The wolf survived in Ireland long after it had disappeared from Britain; its presence resulted in the name 'Wolf-Land' being used for Ireland (Harting, 1880). Exactly when the last Irish wolf was killed is a matter of great debate, but it appears to have been about two hundred years ago (Fairley, 1975). Evidence suggests that the Irish wild cat was also hunted to extinction.

The wolf, incidentally, is an example of a wild mammal that has left its mark not only on our landscape but also on our culture. Contrary to popular myth, wolves rarely attack humans, unless rabid; they do, however, pose a grave threat to domestic animals. Their predation on cattle, sheep, goats and even dogs, as well as the terror of rabid wolves, led to the association of wolves with evil – hence the demonic wolf, with devil's tail, illustrated in the ninth-century Book of Kells (*plate 3*). In order to protect their stock the early Irish farmers drove them into secure areas at night. This resulted in the building of thousands of ring forts which dot the Irish countryside (Fairley, 1975), and probably also the lake island habitations called 'crannógs'. The practice of housing and protecting domestic animals was still commonplace in seventeenth-century Ireland (MacLysaght, 1979) and survives in areas such as Spain, where the wolf is still found (Grande, 1984). Echoes of wolves remain not only on our landscape, but in our language. 'Wolf words' sprinkle our every day speech: to 'cry wolf'; to 'keep the wolf from the door'; to 'wolf down' one's food; a 'wolf in sheep's clothing'.

The forced extinction or extermination of wild mammals is sometimes both wise and necessary. The muskrat was originally introduced to Ireland from America in 1929 for fur-farming, but some escaped and became feral and these destructive rodents were finally exterminated in 1935 (Fairley, 1982). Roe deer were imported into some estates in the west of Ireland in the last century for sport, but had disappeared completely by the 1930s, probably due to overhunting (Barclay, 1932). People have caused declines in wild mammals not only by hunting but also by accidental and intentional habitat destruction. Since the impenetrable woods provided refuge for Irish rebels, priests and outlaws, as well as for wolves, their destruction, under the pretext of civilizing the country, made economic and political sense from the government's and colonist's point of view. The decline of formerly widespread species, such as red deer and pine marten, which now have a very restricted distribution (Harrington, 1980; O'Sullivan, 1983), was initiated with the devastation of vast areas of Irish woodland. Roughly between 1580 and 1750, landowners made huge profits from Irish hardwoods, selling them not just for industry and shipbuilding, but even for pit props, barrel staves and charcoal burning (McCracken, 1971).

As deer grew scarce and hare-hunting was increasingly impeded by enclosures, other animals were hunted, particularly foxes. By the eighteenth century hunting had become so popular that a specialist book on hunting in Ireland appeared: *The Experienced Huntsman* (1714) by Arthur Stringer, huntsman at the Earl of Conway's estate at Portmore, Co. Antrim. Fox-hunting had originally been regarded as socially inferior to deer-hunting, but it gained popularity around this time as deer became scarcer (Thomas, 1983). Today Ireland, still famous for hunting, has many packs of fox and hare hounds and even a few packs of deer hounds. One example is the Duhallow Hunt in Co. Cork, believed to be one of Ireland's oldest fox hunts, having been formed in 1745.

The pine marten was also in decline at this time, causing complaints in 1638 from the Lord Deputy, who was experiencing difficulty in obtaining marten fur for his garments (MacLysaght, 1979). Curiously, the growth of fox-hunting encouraged measures to protect foxes for the chase; these may have helped martens also, since the 'fox coverts' of planted woods would also have provided suitable habitat for martens. According to Charles Moffat (1927), if martens were 'caught at mischief' (i.e. in the hen run) they might be mistaken for young foxes, which they superficially resemble, and released. The planting of trees, including fox coverts, by landlords provided important habitats for Ireland's remaining woodland animals in an otherwise tree-less landscape. During the seventeenth century these plantations were main-ly coniferous, as they are today, with hardwoods being reserved for orna-mental planting in parklands (MacLysaght, 1979). However, although the scarcity of hardwoods has deleterious effects on some wildlife, it also has interesting side-effects. From the late sixteenth century red deer, normally forest-dwellers, became associated in Ireland with the open hills, the only habitat left to them after the disappearance of the woods. Grey squirrels, originally from North America, were introduced into Ireland in 1911. They prefer hardwood habitats to conifers, and the shortage of such hardwoods here is presumed to have caused the grey squirrel to spread less rapidly than in England (Ní Lamhna and Goodwillie, 1979).

With the woods all but gone by 1700, people increasingly turned to bogs for fuel, initiating the destruction of bogland which continues to this day. Turf-digging unearthed numerous remains of a giant deer, the so-called 'Irish Elk', *Megaceros giganteus*. The Giant Irish deer will forever be associ-ated with Ireland but appears to have become extinct here around 8000 BC before the arrival of the first Mesolithic people. The males of this large deer had enormous antlers up to three metres across and thirty-five kilograms in weight. The skulls of females are poorly represented in collections, but they did not have antlers and their skulls may be mistaken for those of horses (Stuart, 1982). The American evolutionary biologist Stephen Jay Gould (1977) has explained that the name 'Irish elk' is a double misnomer since, although most common in Ireland, they were not exclusively Irish, their remains having been found elsewhere in Europe. Neither is it an elk but rather a member of the deer family Cervidae. On account of its enormous antlers the Giant Irish deer gained a central role in debates about evolution, as has been skilfully described by Gould. This species was first brought to the attention of scientists by Thomas Molyneux (1697) who, making an understandable error, declared it to be an American moose. Despite all of these misconceptions the Giant Irish deer has become a key icon for Ireland's natural history, and its impressive antlers may still be seen decorating many Irish and British stately homes and museums.

The fox, red squirrel and marten may originally have been introduced to Ireland to supply fur (Fairley, 1983). Wild foxes are still hunted for their fur in Ireland and Britain. When fox fur prices soared in the 1978-80 period (responding to a fashion for fox fur), unprecedented numbers of foxes were killed (Macdonald and Carr, 1981). Several thousands were killed in Ireland each winter (only winter coats are of value), leading to incorrect assertions that Irish foxes were threatened (e.g., Rochford, 1980). In fact the fox is a versatile survivor and is still very common in the countryside and even in suburban areas. The predatory American mink was introduced to Ireland by fur farmers in the 1950s and, like the muskrat, it escaped to the wild and is now widespread across the country. There is no evidence of lasting damage to our fauna by mink, despite widespread hysteria about their presence, although they have been a threat to some colonies of seabirds, reared gamebirds and domestic poultry (Smal, 1991). The introduction of mink and muskrat, and the killing of thousands of foxes, are alarming examples of how human culture, in this case the fashion for fur, can have a huge impact on our wild mammals.

Some introduced mammals also brought harmful diseases and parasites with them. Ship rats carried fleas and bubonic plague, which ravaged cities and towns in medieval Ireland. More recently, the highly infectious rabbit disease myxomatosis, carried by rabbit fleas, was deliberately introduced in 1954 to control the huge numbers of rabbits. Similarly, red deer introduced to Donegal carried deer warbleflies, and nasal bot-flies which live as larvae in the nasal passages of deer (Sleeman, 1979).

Another relatively recent introduction is a reclusive rodent, the bank vole, which was discovered in 1964 near the River Shannon by a Dutch student, Andreas Claassens (Claassens and O'Gorman, 1965). Although Claassens was mistakenly thought to have imported the voles himself from Holland, the true story was even more interesting. In a subsequent study of the spread of the voles, Smal and Fairley (1984) estimated that they arrived in the Shannon area around the 1940s or 1950s. Between July 1925 and October 1929 Siemens-Schuckert of Berlin had carried out construction on the massive Shannon Hydroelectric Scheme. Contemporary film shows huge earth-moving machines and trains transported from Germany for the task, and it is remotely possible that bank voles were accidentally imported in these machines. However, this would date the arrival of the voles at about two decades before Smal and Fairley's estimate. Genetic analysis, coupled with the rate of spread, has already confirmed that the voles were introduced (Byrne et al., 1990) and may eventually establish their provenance.

In modern times, some mammals such as the badger and the pipistelle bat have increased. Badgers in Ireland feed mainly on earthworms and therefore rely on pastures to provide their principal food (Kruuk, 1989). Since the end of the Great Famine in 1849, the acreage of pasture has increased – extending earthworm habitats – and rural human population densities have decreased. These two factors, coupled with recent legal protection, appear to have given Ireland one of the largest badger populations of any European country, with the current estimate numbering between 210,000-250,000 (Griffiths, 1991; Smal, 1995). The prevalence of the badger, reflected in its placing in the road casualty list of mammals (fifth behind rat, rabbit, cat and hedgehog), may also account for lower numbers of hedgehogs in Ireland. Both G.H. Pentland, a bird-watching landowner from Drogheda, Co. Louth, and Charles Moffat, suggested that badgers reduced the numbers of hedgehogs (Pentland, 1917; Moffat, 1938). Recent results from an English study showed that of thirty hedgehogs released, seven had been killed by badgers within two months (Doncaster, 1992).

Old buildings such as castles and fortified towers often provide roosts for certain bats. Thoor Ballylee, Co. Galway, the restored fifteenth-century tower house formerly inhabited by W.B. Yeats, is today a summer roost for lesser horseshoes, one of our rarer bats. Pipistrelles often roost in recently built houses, and the increasing numbers of new buildings have allowed them to breed successfully, making them now one of our most common bats (Moffat, 1922; Fairley, 1975). While pipistrelles and perhaps other bats gained from the increased numbers of buildings, woodland mammals declined as their habitats became smaller, or disappeared.

The small number of Irish terrestrial mammal species is in sharp contrast to the large number of species of marine mammals – whales, dolphins, porpoises and seals – that spend time in Irish waters. Since early times their presence brought whalers and whaling to the seas of Ireland. A medieval Arab geographer writing in Spain referred to people, perhaps Vikings, hunting whales 'near an island in the north Atlantic' some time between AD 450 and 1058 (Fairley, 1981). The existence of whales off our coasts was almost certainly known to the Spanish Moors, and probably also to the Basque whalers of northern Spain. Evidence for this comes from the work of a Canadian researcher, Selma Barkham. In the 1970s she discovered some references in sixteenth-century Spanish archives to Basques whaling off North

America. Acting on this information, divers discovered a sixteenth-century Basque whaling port at Red Bay in Labrador, complete with sunken ships and whale remains (Barkham and Grenier, 1979). This startling evidence that the Basques crossed the Atlantic in pursuit of whales shows the ability and determination of these early seafarers. Given that Ireland is much nearer than America, the possibility of a Basque whaling presence here must be considered. If evidence for such a presence, including perhaps shore-based whaling ports, is ever found, it would constitute one explanation for our Lusitanian fauna.

The slaughter of whales continued rather sporadically until the advent of modern whaling in the last century, which in Ireland, as elsewhere, led to a greatly increased killing efficiency and soon to a severe reduction in numbers of the great whales. Today, worldwide attitudes to whales have changed, due in part to a change in our perception of them as more than merely a source of meat and oil. The realization that some species of whales are on the verge of extinction, or are indeed extinct, has led to a renewed interest in their biology and behaviour. Ever-popular dolphins 'make good television' and have become an international icon for conservation. A bottle-nosed dolphin named Fungi, living off Dingle, Co. Kerry, has won many hearts and minds and features in several books. Ireland now has an active Whale and Dolphin Conservation Group, formed in March 1991 and in the same year Irish waters became the first official Whale Sanctuary in Europe.

Two species of seal live around Ireland's coasts: the grey seal, which is relatively common, and the common (or harbour) seal which is scarce in Ireland. Seals, with their large eyes and endearing appearance, provoke a strong emotional reaction in people and this may account for the numerous Irish myths about seal-people interactions. Seals are particularly vulnerable when they come on land to breed and have long been hunted. Seal meat and skin were highly valued and seal skin was used in Early Christian footwear (Barber, 1981). Tomás Ó Crohan in *The Islandman* (1934) graphically describes a seal hunt on the island of Inishvickillaun off Co. Kerry. The islanders hunted the seals by candle-light in a dark, dangerous sea cave, and after the hunt had great difficulty in getting the seals, now dead, out of the cave. In the end, however, the results were worthwhile: 'Our big boat was loaded down to the gunwale with four seal cows, two bulls and two two-year-olds – one for each member of the crew. Every one of the men had a barrelfull of seal meat, we reckoned in those days that every barrel of seal meat was worth a barrel of pork.'

Today there is considerable concern about seal predation among fishermen, who claim that seals greatly damage commercial fisheries. Prior to the Wildlife Act (1976, Republic of Ireland) which now protects them, bounties were paid out for dead seals and more than 450 seals were killed between 1972 and 1976 (Summers et al., 1980). In autumn 1981, one of the largest Irish colonies of breeding grey seals on the island of Inishkea North, Co. Mayo, was brutally and illegally attacked, with hundreds of seals being killed. The attack and subsequent plans to have an official cull provoked considerable public outcry and the killing of seals became a major issue, another illustration of the changing attitudes to wild mammals in Ireland. In the late 1980s, the arrival of a viral disease of seals, which had swept across from the North Sea, killed large numbers of seals and again caused great public concern.

Otters, inhabitants of both the sea coast and freshwater, have a recent history similar to that of seals. Although in the past persecuted for alleged damage to fisheries and also killed for their pelts, Irish otters, hunting records and a national survey show, have not recently declined, unlike the situation in most of the rest of Europe (Channin and Jefferies, 1978; Chapman and Chapman, 1982). The otter now enjoys full legal protection and otter-hunting with hounds is no longer licenced in the Republic. Changed attitudes are, once again, evident. However, other dangers, such as pesticide use, appear to be much graver and more insidious threats to our otter populations. These aquatic predators are at the top of the food chain and vulnerable to poisoning from certain pesticides and other chemicals, which have already caused their decline in Britain. Recently, high pesticide concentrations have been found in some otters, and incidentally mink, in Co. Cork (Mason and O'Sullivan, 1992).

Invasions, diseases, wars, civil unrest and famines all have had their effects on wild mammals. The invading Vikings in the ninth and tenth centuries probably hunted whales for food. In the twelfth century, Norman invaders introduced fallow deer and probably rabbits. Initially both were kept in captivity – the deer in parks or so-called 'deer forests', the rabbits in enclosed 'warrens' – from which both escaped from time to time. The Vikings and Normans established the earliest towns, with the latter also being responsible for some of the magnificent stone castles that are still to be seen here. The crowded buildings of towns would have provided ideal habitats for another introduction, the ship rat. This rat, also called the black rat, is now known to have been present in Roman Britain (Armitage et al., 1984), and the first suggestion of its presence in Ireland is in a drawing (*Plate 3*) in the Book of Kells (Shrewsbury, 1971). Although the animals in the illustration have been described as 'cats and kittens', the four smaller animals with the cats have long tails, pointed snouts and big ears and are clearly rodents. They are too big to be mice and have the characteristics of ship rats. They are not common rats, which only invaded Europe from Asia in the eighteenth century. The ship rat's presence was very bad news for the colonists, as through its fleas it is a victim and a vector of bubonic plague. Plague periodically struck the inhabitants of Irish towns for about three hundred years, between 1348 and 1650. Away from ships, ship rats are most at home in cities and towns, and because of this the rural Irish were less affected than those in the towns. The lack of success of campaigns to subdue the rural Irish clans during the period was due in part to plague among the colonists. It also played a role in many sieges, with often the besieged town falling to the effects of plague.

The clustered nature of the monastic settlements of this time ensured that they too were severely affected. Because monks were often the only educated people in the district, such settlements were then of great religious, economic, and cultural significance. Therefore plague had important effects in many areas of life. The effects of diseases on human history often have been overlooked, as historians have tended to concentrate on more glamorous affairs, such as wars (McNeill, 1976).

The many wars fought in Ireland produced marked effects on some of the island's wild mammals. For example, during the brutal Cromwellian campaign, wolves were said to have increased due to the general state of disorganization, even becoming common in the outskirts of Dublin, where a wolf-hunt was organized at Castleknock in December 1652 (MacLysaght, 1979). In the same year Cromwell himself prohibited the export of Irish wolfhounds, in order that wolves might be controlled.

Arthur Stringer (1714) claimed that during the Jacobite War of 1688 most of the deer parks were 'broke and the deer beat out into the country'. In the more recent Anglo-Irish Troubles (1919-21), red deer in the Glenveagh Estate in Co. Donegal were released when the 'forest' fence was breached; feral populations were soon established which survived and spread (Whitehead, 1964). During the two world wars, many of the famous fallow deer herd of the Phoenix Park in Dublin were removed, with the population becoming the lowest on record there during World War II (Hayden et al., 1992). In Ulster during that war the remaining herds of park deer were devastated, in at least one instance by American troops (Kilpatrick, 1987).

Charles Moffat noted in his 'Mammals of Ireland' (1938) that from correspondence with people all over the country he formed the impression that rabbits, hares, foxes and badgers had increased during World War I, but hedgehogs had decreased due, he suggested, to the increase in badgers. Another effect of World War I was that whaling halted on the west coast, although it resumed following the war and continued until 1922 (Fairley, 1981). We may well owe the survival of some of the great whale species off our coasts to the interruption of that war. The 'Troubles' have had other local effects on mammal populations, such as during the Anglo-Irish war, when many bridges in Co. Cork were blown up. Colonies of Daubenton's bat had roosted underneath many of the arches and their local distribution has been affected to this day (Smiddy, 1990, 1991).

More beneficial effects of World War II were not altogether predictable. One British soldier stationed in Northern Ireland, Michael
Blackmore, was also a leading British bat researcher and his wartime observations formed a valuable core of early knowledge of bats in that area.
Subsequently he returned to Ireland to pass on some of his knowledge and
expertise to local bat workers (Skillen, 1959), and as a result the post-war
Irish distribution maps tend, like many other distribution maps, to have
clusters of bat records in particular areas, such as around Armagh, reflecting the distribution of bat workers rather than of bats.

Sadly the troubles continue, and resulted in the omission, in the most
recent National Otter Survey (Chapman and Chapman, 1982), of certain
border areas, due to the dangers of bombs around bridges (Peter Chapman,
pers. comm.). Similarly, the latest National Badger Survey also avoided border areas. One recent positive side-effect of these troubles occurred in 1977,
when British troops were able to assist in the study of one of the most celebrated of Ireland's whales, a killer whale that strayed into the River Foyle
in Derry city. They enabled researchers from the University of Ulster to
study the whale's behaviour from one of the Royal Marine landing craft
(Wilson and Pitcher, 1979). The visit of that whale, dubbed 'Dopey Dick',
lives on in Derry's cultural life, celebrated in song and story.

Famine has also affected Ireland's wild mammals. During the Great
Famine (1845-9) the last remaining native Irish red deer, in the Erris area
of Co. Mayo, were slaughtered for food (Ussher, 1882) and, according to
local tradition, whales were used for food in west Cork (Sleeman, 1988).
This was not the first time whales had provided food during famines in
Ireland. It is recorded that in medieval Dublin a famine was relieved when
some whales became stranded, an event mentioned by James Joyce in *Ulysses*
(Somerville-Large, 1979). To this day many Irish people disdain 'wild
foods', such as rabbit, nettle and edible seaweed, because they are regarded
as 'famine foods' whose consumption is still a bitter reminder of famine.

Developments in Irish Mammalogy

It is to the seventh-century monk Augustin that we owe the first accounts of
Irish mammals. He is sometimes given the title of 'Ireland's First Naturalist'
(Scharff, 1921). Giraldus Cambrensis, the twelfth-century ecclesiastic, wrote
a wide-ranging description of Ireland, *Topographia Hiberniae*, though in
places his text is often more travellers' tales than fact. Giraldus, a Norman
Welshman, annoyed the Irish with his biased and frequently fanciful text.
His portrait of the Irish was the subject of several refutations, two of the
best known being by the poet Geoffrey Keating (c. 1580-c. 1650) in Irish
and the scholar John Lynch (c. 1599-c. 1673) in Latin.

Giraldus, Keating and Lynch were topographical and hitorical writers, and their accounts are a blend of fact, fiction and political comment. A pioneer of more factual topography was Charles Smith. His books on counties Waterford (1746), Cork (1750) and Kerry (1756) mention deer, rabbits, hares, seals and whales. There were few others who wrote about mammals in the eighteenth century; one was Arthur Stringer, whom we have already met, another John Rutty, whom we will meet later.

In more recent times, those who have made a scientific study of Ireland's wild mammals can be divided into two distinct groups, namely those who specialized in mammals and those whose main interest was in some other group of animals, usually birds. An example from the second group is William Thompson. The mammal section of his *Natural History of Ireland* (1849-56), a book which covers many fields of natural history and avifauna in greatest detail, forms, in the words of James Fairley, 'the basis of modern mammalogy in Ireland' (Fairley, 1975). Other naturalists who were predominantly ornithologists but who took an interest in mammals were Robert Patterson (1802-72) of Belfast and his son Robert Lloyd Patterson (1836-1906), and Robert Warren of Sligo (1829-1915), all of whom published useful notes on mammals. This tradition is followed by today's leading Irish ornithologist, Robin Ruttledge. Although today there is a growing interest in Irish birds, only a few ornithologists take more than a passing interest in mammals, though with some important exceptions. Pat Smiddy of Cork, as we have seen, has contributed some important work on bats and fleas, as well as recording whale-strandings and road casualties. Ornithologists at Cape Clear Island Bird Observatory record whale sightings and contribute notes on other mammals on the island. Peter Robertson, who studied wild and released pheasant, has examined the role of the fox as pheasant predator (Robertson and Whelan, 1987). There are only four species of small mammal in Ireland – wood mouse, house mouse, pygmy shrew and bank vole – compared with fourteen in Britain. The diet of owls consists largely of small mammals. The diets of Irish owls are therefore of considerable interest. Although most studies have been done by mammalogists, significant studies of owl diet have been carried out by ornithologists such as Paul Walsh (1984, 1988).

Photographers have also contributed to the understanding of Ireland's wild mammals, from the first days of still cameras. The Belfastman Robert J. Welch, a famous photographer, contributed some interesting observations on mammals, including an account of the last native red deer in Donegal (Welch, 1905). Today the Corkmen Richard T. Mills and Sean Ryan have added to our knowledge and appreciation of wild mammals, not only by their photographs but also by their stunning illustrated lectures. Fr Paudie Doolan, another talented photographer, writes and illustrates popular natural history articles (under the pen-name Francis Field) in *The Sacred Heart Messenger* magazine, and his work has appeared elsewhere, as in Carolyn King's *Weasels and Stoats* (1989). Many television programmes feature wild Irish mammals, the most notable being those of Eamon de Buitléar and the late Gerrit van Gelderen, which have helped to inform people and influence attitudes to local wildlife. However, television has drawbacks as a medium for natural history: by presenting the products of many hours' patient filming in a matter of minutes, nature films give a rather misleading impression of the patience and skill necessary to observe and record wild animals.

Among the entomologists who have contributed to studies of Irish mammals are the Irish-Canadian Bryan P. Beirne, who has speculated on the origins of the fauna of Britain and Ireland (Beirne, 1952). However, the major overlap between entomology and mammalogy arises in studies of insect parasites and insects in the diets of mammals. Fleas in particular have attracted attention, from Nathan Charles Rothschild's first published note in 1899, through to the fascinating observation that Irish hedgehogs appear to harbour fewer fleas than hedgehogs in Britain and elsewhere (Mulcahy, 1987). On the other hand, mammalogists often have to study insects as constituents of mammal diets. For example, since bats and shrews eat insects, work on their diets involves the identification of insect remains in their guts or droppings.

There have long been established links between medicine and the study of natural history. One such was the work of Thomas Molyneux (1661-1733), Professor of Medicine at Dublin University, who wrote the first description of the Giant Irish deer. In 1772, another medical doctor, John Rutty, contributed a useful account of the mammals of the Dublin area, while Nathaniel Alcock, also a doctor, produced an early account of Ireland's bats in 1899. A medical man who took a special interest in whales was Alexander McAlister of the Royal College of Surgeons, who took part in the dissection of a minke whale (Carte and McAlister, 1868). Fergus O'Rourke, Professor of Zoology at University College Cork, was also a medical doctor and wrote *The Fauna of Ireland* (1970). Today Jim Barry, another Cork doctor, continues the tradition, his interests being mainly in the area of animal welfare and badgers.

Mammal specialists first started publishing around the latter half of the nineteenth century. Although Charles Moffat was also interested in birds, his contribution to the study of bats, and indeed of all Irish mammals, is such that he must be considered a mammalogist. His important review 'The Mammals of Ireland' (1938), and his observations on bats still form the basis of our knowledge of some species today. He was a notable journalist and also played a role in promoting bird-protection legislation. Another noted mammalogist who also made contributions to ornithology was Richard Barrington.

He detailed the re-introductions of red squirrels to Ireland (1880) and was justifiably concerned about the survival of the pine marten. In a note on the measurements of dead martens (1910), Barrington made a point of urging naturalists to discourage killing of martens. A generous man, he also personally financed research on whales (Fairley, 1981).

Lester Jameson was interested in bats; however, his most important contribution was a study of sandy-coloured mice on Bull Island, Dublin. These, he speculated, were products of natural selection by bird predation (Jameson, 1898). In the 1890s, when Darwin's theory of evolution was still relatively new, these observations attracted considerable attention. Although his theory is not accepted today, the Bull Island mice, along with the Giant Irish deer and Irish stoat, form an unlikely but significant selection of Irish examples in the story of evolutionary theory.

Gerald Barrett-Hamilton was primarily interested in mammals and published a large number of papers and notes, under both his own name and his pen name, 'Lepus hibernicus', and as this suggests, his attention focussed on endemic Irish mammals. Owing to his death, *The History of British Mammals* (Barrett-Hamilton and Hinton, 1910-21) remained unfinished but is still widely used today. He played a part in describing the Irish stoat as a distinct form or subspecies (Thomas and Barrett-Hamilton, 1895). He and others considered it to be an intermediate form between the British stoat and the weasel, because of the black-tipped tail, a characteristic of stoats, and its possession of a wiggly back-belly line that is a characteristic of British weasels. This idea was taken up later by ecologists, who speculated that in the absence of the weasel, the Irish stoat had evolved to fill both weasel and stoat roles (Hutchinson, 1959). However, there appears to be little evidence for this (Sleeman, 1989).

Robert Francis Scharff (1858-1934), Keeper of Natural History in the National Museum, Dublin, was an 'all-rounder' who made contributions to the study of Irish mammals. A pioneering biogeographer, he became caught up in rather confused efforts to explain postglacial colonization of Ireland and was one of those who promoted the idea of the Lusitanian element of Ireland's flora and fauna.

In more recent times Irish mammalogy has been well served by many workers, the most important of whom is James Fairley, Professor of Zoology at University College Galway. His initial studies were on wood mice and foxes but he has continued to work on a number of other Irish mammals at Galway. He has published three important books, *Irish Wild Mammals: A Guide to the Literature* (1972), *An Irish Beast Book* (1975) and *Irish Whales and Whaling* (1981). Fairley has also produced a steady flow of papers, with various co-authors, on mammals such as bank voles, pygmy shrews and bats. His work has given much impetus to our understanding of mammals and his book on whales created increased interest in recording these animals around our coasts. *The Irish Naturalists' Journal* quickly responded with a section of 'Cetacean Notes' to record Irish whale and dolphin strandings and sightings. Several years on, it is clear that this has been a success, with contributions from people from all walks of life.

Modern technology has also contributed to our understanding of Ireland's wild mammals and dramatically changed methods used to study them. Radio-carbon dating, genetics and computerized data analysis have revolutionized our understanding of mammals and their origins. Particular developments in electronics have led to bat detectors and, more significantly, radio-tracking.

In radio-tracking, a small radio transmitter is attached to an animal allowing it to be located and identified as it moves around its range (Kenward, 1987). Red squirrels, common rats, wood mice, martens, badgers and stoats have been radio-tracked successfully. For example, stoats, like most small carnivores, are notoriously difficult to trap; in the 1970s a study of stoats in Co. Kerry produced few results, because only six stoats were captured over about a year (Thompson and Fairley, 1978). Although in the 1980s the same number of stoats was trapped in a year's field work in Co. Cork, radio-tracking provided additional information on the stoat's habits (Sleeman, 1989). This work showed that stoats frequently climb and inspect trees for suitable prey. Since birds and bats use holes in trees for roosting and nesting, they would be among the most vulnerable prey. However, the rather limited area of woodland in Ireland means that predation by stoats might have an impact on any potential users of trees. This may partly explain why Ireland has fewer bat species than Britain (seven in Ireland to twelve in Britain) and similarly why birds that nest in tree-holes, such as woodpeckers, redstarts and flycatchers, are absent from Ireland (Sleeman, 1993).

As noted, badgers are common in Ireland and bovine tuberculosis is endemic in the badger population. The possible role of badgers in the spread of tuberculosis to cattle is a matter of great controversy (O'Connor and O'Malley, 1989). Badgers are perhaps the classic example of a wild mammal towards which attitudes have changed; today there is a conflict between a perceived need to cull them to control tuberculosis and their protected status. Research has been conducted on badgers, through the use of radio-tracking, to study their interaction with cattle, which they usually try to avoid. This has challenged the idea that badgers are sedentary and confine themselves to a particular social-group territory (thereby giving rise to localized tuberculosis) by the discovery that they often move long distances (Sleeman, 1992). Quotes from field notes give the 'atmosphere' of radio-tracking and an idea of the results of such work. Badgers did not emerge from their setts (holes) if cattle were present at the entrances. A note taken in July 1989 read:

Radio-tagged badger in sett C had not emerged by 22:10, despite the fact that badgers elsewhere in the area were emerging much earlier. At 22:10 there was one cow 'hanging around' the sett entrances. By 22:15 three cows were present, one grazing and eventually a total of five cows turned up. During this time the signal from the badger varied, becoming weaker, and then stronger, indicating that she (a female No 14) was active. Finally at 22:40 the cattle moved away and the badger emerged and stayed in the undergrowth around the sett until 23:30. She then headed off in the direction of a damp foraging area.

Curious cattle often moved close and on one occasion actually chased a badger:

Badger No 14 emerges from sett C at 20:10 and immediately moves off through undergrowth. She emerges at a field edge where many cattle are spread out. As she moves along broken hedges nearby cattle become active and are seen to pursue the badger. The badger moves rapidly and tracker has to run to keep up. She eventually gets to a foraging area, a woodland stream edge well away from the cattle at 21:30 and remains there until 01:45.

Today, then, the study of Ireland's mammals uses the latest data-collection techniques to build up a picture of their behaviour and biology. Unfortunately, the latest results are not always reported in new books about British and Irish mammals. For example, the recent *Handbook of British Mammals* (Corbet and Harris, 1990), though excellent on British mammals, gives inaccurate distribution maps and species lists for some Irish mammals. As Fairley (1992) commented, 'the tendency of some mammalogists to think less critically where Ireland is concerned has not quite vanished'. It is to be hoped that it soon will.

With such a small Irish list of wild mammals it is not surprising that their study was somewhat neglected in the past. But now, happily, attitudes to wild mammals in Ireland are changing. This increased interest and curiosity about our wild mammals is perhaps unexpected, for many are, by their nature, shy and nocturnal and therefore elusive and unseen. Those people who become interested in natural history are often attracted to more visible animals such as birds or insects, which by their sheer numbers make up for what they lack in size. Mammals constitute a tiny proportion of the Irish fauna when compared with even one group of insects, such as the rove beetles (*Staphylinidae*), which has nearly 570 Irish species (Good, 1990). In earlier times mammals were trapped or hunted as pests, food, or quarry, and only since the middle of this century have perceptions of their value altered. For example bats, once regarded as feared spirits of the night, are now actively conserved and fully protected. Publicity about environmental issues has focused greater attention on our fauna. Events such as the European Conservation Year (1970) and new organizations such as the Irish Wildlife Federation and Ulster Wildlife Trust have fostered new attitudes towards our native wildlife. This has resulted in the legal protection of most mammals and in the setting up of specialist organizations such as Badgerwatch, Regional Bat Groups, various Deer Societies, the Whale and Dolphin Group and even the Irish Hedgehog Preservation Society.

Human beings have exerted considerable and often harmful influence upon wild mammals; in turn, we have today a responsibility to ensure that they survive in our landscape. An increased awareness of wild mammals and their role in the ecology of Ireland's flora and fauna will enable us better to understand and cherish them.

References

Alcock, N.H. 1899. 'The Natural History of Irish Bats.' *Irish Naturalist 8*: 29-36, 53-7, 169-74.

Armitage, P., B. West and K. Steedman. 1984. 'New Evidence of the Black Rat in Roman London.' *The London Archaeologist 4*: 375-83.

Banfield, A.W.F. 1954. 'The Role of Ice in the Distribution of Mammals.' *Journal of Mammalogy 35*: 104-7.

Barber, J.W. 1981. 'Some Observations on Early Christian Footwear.' *Journal of Cork Historical and Archaeological Society 94*: 103-6.

Barclay, E.N. 1932. 'The Introduction and Extermination of Roe Deer in Ireland.' *Natural History Magazine 3*: 265-7.

Barkham, S. and R. Grenier. 1979. 'Divers Find Sunken Basque Galleon in Labrador.' *Canadian Geographical Journal 97*: 60-3.

Barrett-Hamilton, G.E.H and M.A.C. Hinton. 1910-21. *A History of British Mammals*. London: Gurney and Jackson.

Barrington, R.M. 1880. 'On the Introduction of the Squirrel into Ireland.' *Scientific Proceedings of the Royal Dublin Society 2*: 615-31.

Barrington, R.M. 1910. 'Measurements of Martens.' *Irish Naturalist 19*: 104.

Beirne, B.P. 1952. *The Origin and History of the British Fauna*. London: Methuen.

Byrne, J.M., E.J. Duke and J.S. Fairley. 1990. 'Some Mitochondrial DNA Polymorphism in Irish Wood Mice (Apodemus sylvaticus) and Bank Voles (Clethrionomys glareolus).' *Journal of Zoology 221*: 299-302.

Carte, A. and A. McAlister 1868. 'On the Anatomy of Balaenoptera rostrata.' *Philosophical Transactions of the Royal Society 158*: 201-61.

Channin, P.R.F and D.J. Jefferies. 1978. 'The Decline of the Otter *Lutra lutra* L. in Britain: an Analysis of Hunting Records and Discussion of Causes.' *Biological Journal of the Linnean Society 10*: 305-28.

Chapman, P.J. and L.L. Chapman. 1982. *Otter Survey of Ireland*. London: The Vincent Wildlife Trust.

Claassens, A.J.M. and F. O'Gorman. 1965. 'The Bank Vole Clethrionomys glareolus Schreber: a Mammal New to Ireland.' *Nature 205*: 923-4.

Corbet, G.B. and S. Harris (eds). 1990. *The Handbook of British Mammals*. 3rd edn. Oxford: Blackwells.

Diamond, J. 1991. *The Rise and Fall of the Third Chimpanzee*. London: Vintage Books.

Doncaster, C.P. 1992. 'Testing the Role of Intraguild Predation in Regulating Hedgehog

Populations.' *Proceedings of the Royal Society of London B 249*: 113-17.

Fairley, J.S. 1972. *Irish Wild Mammals: A Guide to the Literature*. Galway: privately published.

Fairley, J.S. 1975. *An Irish Beast Book*. Belfast: Blackstaff Press. 2nd edn 1984.

Fairley, J.S. 1981. *Irish Whales and Whaling*. Belfast: Blackstaff Press.

Fairley, J.S. 1982. 'The Muskrat in Ireland.' *Irish Naturalists' Journal 20*: 405-11.

Fairley, J S. 1983. 'Exports of Wild Mammal Skins from Ireland in the Eighteenth Century.' *Irish Naturalists' Journal 21*: 75-9.

Fairley, J.S. 1992. Review of *The Handbook of British Mammals*, 3rd edn. *Mammal Review 22*: 54-5.

Giraldus Cambrensis. [c. 1188] 1982.. *Topographia Hiberniae*. Trans. John J. O'Meara as *The History and Topography of Ireland*. Portlaoise: Dolmen Press.

Good, J.A. 1990. 'Megarthrus hemipterus (Illiger) (Coleoptera: Staphylinidae) to be Deleted from the Irish list.' *Irish Naturalist's Journal 23*: 283.

Gould, S.J. 1977. 'The Misnamed, Mistreated and Misunderstood Irish Elk,' in *Ever Since Darwin: Reflections on Natural History*. New York: Norton.

Grande, R. 1984. 'El lobo ibérico.' *Biologia y mitologia*. Madrid: Hermann Blume.

Griffiths, H. 1991. *On Hunting Badgers*. Glanmorgan: Piglet Press.

Harrington, R. 1980. 'Exotic Deer in Ireland,' in R.P. Kernan, O.V. Mooney & A.E.J. Went (eds), *The Introduction of Exotic Species Advantages and Problems*. Dublin: Royal Irish Academy.

Harting, J.E. 1880. *British Animals Extinct within Historic Times*. London: Trüber and Co.

Hayden, T.J., N.A. Moore and P.F. Kelly. 1992. 'The Fallow Deer of the Phoenix Park: An Evolving Management Plan,' in O. J. Bullock and C.R. Goldspink (eds), *Management, Welfare and Conservation of Park Deer*. Potter's Bar, Herts: Universities Federation for Animal Welfare.

Hutchinson, G.E. 1959. 'Homage to Santa Rosalia or Why are there so Many Kinds of Animals?' *American Naturalist 870*: 145-59.

Jameson, H.L. 1898. 'On a Probable Case of Protective Colouration in the House Mouse (*Mus musculus*').' *Journal of the Linnean Society 26*: 456-73.

Keating, G. [c. 1634] 1991. *Foras Feasa Ar Éirinn* (*A Basis of Knowledge about Ireland*), in S. Deane (ed.), *The Field Day Anthology of Irish Writing*, vol. I. Derry: Field Day.

Kenward, R. 1987. *Wildlife Radio Tagging*. London: Academic Press.

Kilpatrick, C. 1987. 'Deer in Ulster–IV: The Twentieth Century.' *Deer: Journal of the British Deer Society 7*: 87-91.

King, C. 1989. *Weasels and Stoats*. Bromley: Helm.

Kruuk, H. 1989. *The Social Badger*. London: Oxford University Press.

Lynch, J. [1662] 1991. *Cambrensis Eversus ... (Or Refutation of the Authority of Giraldis Cambrensis on the History of Ireland)*, in S. Deane (ed.), *The Field Day Anthology of Irish Writing*, vol. 1. Derry: Field Day.

Macdonald, D. and G. Carr. 1981. 'Foxes Beware: You are Back in Fashion.' *New Scientist* January: 9-11.

MacLysaght, E. 1979. *Irish Life in the Seventeenth Century*. Dublin: Irish Academic Press.

Mason, C.F. and W.M. O'Sullivan. 1992. 'Organochlorine Pesticide Residues, PCBs and Heavy Metal in Irish Mink and Pine Marten.' *Irish Naturalists' Journal 24*: 153-5.

McCracken, E. 1971. *Irish Woods Since Tudor Times*. Newton Abbot: David and Charles.

McNeill, W.H. 1976. *Plagues and Peoples*. Oxford: Blackwell.

Moffat, C.B. 1922. 'What Bats are Common?' *Irish Naturalist 31*: 12.

Moffat, C.B. 1927. 'The Pine Marten.' *Irish Naturalists' Journal 1*: 170-1.

Moffat, C.B. 1938. 'The Mammals of Ireland.' *Proceedings of the Royal Irish Academy 44B*: 61-128.

Molyneux, T. 1697. 'A Discourse Concerning the Large Horns Frequently Found Underground in Ireland, Concluding from them that the Great American Deer, Call'd a Moose, was Formerly Common in Ireland: with Remarks on Other Things Natural to that Country.' *Philosophical Transactions of the Royal Society 19*: 509-12.

Morris, P.A. 1987. 'Changing Attitudes towards British Mammals.' *Biological Journal of the Linnean Society 32*: 225-33.

Mulcahy, R.M. 1987. 'Fleas from Hedgehogs in Ireland.' *Irish Naturalists' Journal 22*: 346-7.

Ní Lamhna, E. and R. Goodwillie. 1979. 'Distribution of Mammals in Ireland (1979).' *Irish Journal of Environmental Science 8*: 1-82.

O'Connor, R. and E. O'Malley. 1989. *Badgers and Bovine Tuberculosis.* Dublin: Eradication of Animal Diseases Board.

Ó Crohan, T. (1934) 1951. *The Islandman.* Trans. from Irish by R. Flower. Oxford: University Press.

O'Riordan, C. E. 1972. 'Provisional List of Cetacea and Turtles Stranded or Captured on the Irish Coast.' *Proceedings of the Royal Irish Academy 72B*: 253-74.

O'Rourke, F. J. 1970. *The Fauna of Ireland.* Cork: Mercier Press.

O'Sullivan, P. 1983. 'The Distribution of the Pine Marten (*Martes martes*) in the Republic of Ireland.' *Mammal Review 13*: 39-44.

Pentland, G. H. 1917. 'Badgers and Hedgehogs.' *Irish Naturalist 26*: 20.

Robertson, P.A. and J. Whelan. 1987. 'The Food of Red Fox (*Vulpes vulpes*) in Co. Kildare, Ireland.' *Journal of Zoology 213*: 740-3.

Rochford, J. 1980. 'Fox in a Fix.' *The Badger: Newsletter of the Irish Wildlife Federation 2*: 3-5.

Rothschild, N. C. 1899. 'Irish Fleas.' *Irish Naturalist 8*: 266.

Rutty, J. 1772. *An Essay towards a Natural History of the County of Dublin.* Dublin: Sleator.

Savage, R.J.G. 1966. 'Irish Pleistocene Mammals.' *Irish Naturalists' Journal 15*: 117-30.

Scharff, R. F. 1921. 'The Earliest Irish Zoologist.' *Irish Naturalist 30*: 128-32.

Shrewsbury, J.F.D. 1971. *A History of Bubonic Plague in the British Isles.* Cambridge: Cambridge University Press.

Skillen, S. 1959. 'Irish Bats.' *Irish Naturalists' Journal 13*: 66-9.

Sleeman, D.P. 1979. 'Larvae of Cephenomyia auribarbis (Meigen) and Hypoderma diana (Brauer) (Diptera: Oestridae) from a Red Deer in Co. Donegal.' *Irish Naturalists' Journal 19*: 441-2.

Sleeman, D.P. 1988. 'Some Whale Arches in Co. Cork.' *Irish Naturalists' Journal 22*: 539.

Sleeman, D.P. 1989. *Stoats and Weasels, Polecats & Martens.* London: Whittet Books.

Sleeman, D.P. 1992. 'Long-distance Movements in an Irish Badger Population,' in I.G. Priede and S.M. Swift (eds), *Wildlife Telemetry.* London: Ellis Harwood.

Sleeman, D.P. 1993. 'Habitats of the Irish Stoat.' *Irish Naturalist's Journal 24*: 318-21.

Sleeman, D.P. R.J. Devoy and P.C. Woodman (eds). 1986. *Proceedings of the Postglacial Colonisation Conference.* Occasional Publication of the Irish Biogeographical Society No. 1.

Sleeman, D.P., P. Smiddy and P.G. Sweeney. 1985. 'Irish Mammal Road Casualties.' *Irish Naturalists' Journal 21*: 544.

Smal, C.M. 1991. *Feral Mink in Ireland.* Dublin: Office of Public Works.

Smal, C.M. 1995. *The Badger and Habitat Survey of Ireland.* Dublin: Government Publications.

Smal, C.M. and J.S. Fairley. 1984. 'The Spread of the Bank Vole *Clethrionomys glareolus* in Ireland.' *Mammal Review 4*: 71-8.

Smiddy, P. 1990. 'A Survey of Bats and Bridges.' *The Natterer: Newsletter of the Dublin Bat Group 1*: 6.

Smiddy, P. 1991. 'Bats and Bridges.' *Irish Naturalists' Journal 23*: 425-6.

Smith, C. 1746. *The Antient and Present State of the County and City of Waterford.* Dublin: author.

Smith, C. 1750. *The Antient and Present State of the County and City of Cork.* Dublin: author.

Smith, C. 1756. *The Antient and Present State of the County and City of Kerry.* Dublin: author.

Somerville-Large, P. 1979. *Dublin.* London: Hamish Hamilton.

Speight, M.C.D. 1986. 'Use of Invertebrates, as Exemplified by Certain Insect Groups, in Considering Hypotheses about the History of the Irish Postglacial Fauna,' in D.P. Sleeman, R.J. Devoy and P.C. Woodman (eds), *Proceedings of the Postglacial Colonisation Conference.* Occasional Publication of the Irish Biogeographical Society 1: 60-6.

Stringer, A. [1714] 1977. *The Experienced Huntsman.* Ed. J.S. Fairley. Belfast: Blackstaff Press.

Stuart, A.J. 1982. *Pleistocene Vertebrates in the British Isles.* London: Longmans.

Stuart, A.J. and L.H van Wijngaarden-Bakker. 1985. 'Quaternary Vertebrates,' in K.J. Edwards and W.P. Warren (eds), *The Quaternary History of Ireland.* London: Academic Press.

Summers, C.F., P.J. Warner, R.G.W. Nairn, M.G. Curry and J. Flynn. 1980. 'An Assessment of the Status of the Common Seal Phoca vitulina in Ireland.' *Biological Conservation 17*: 115-25.

Synge, J.M. 1907. *The Aran Islands.* London: Oxford University Press.

Thomas, K. 1983. *Man and the Natural World.* London: Penguin.

Thomas, O. and G.E.H. Barrett-Hamilton. 1895. 'The Irish Stoat Distinct from the British Species.' *Zoologist 19*: 124-9.

Thompson, E.H. and J.S. Fairley. 1978. 'Notes on the Irish Stoat in the Bourn-Vincent Memorial Park, Killarney.' *Irish Naturalists' Journal 19*: 158-9.

Thompson, W. 1849-56. *The Natural History of Ireland.* 4 vols. London: Bohn.

Ussher, R.J. 1882. 'Notes on Irish Red Deer.' *Zoologist 6*: 81-4.

Walsh, P.M. 1984. 'Diet of Barn Owl at an Urban Waterford Roost.' *Irish Birds 2*: 437-44.

Walsh, P.M. 1988. 'Black Rats *Rattus rattus* (L.) as Prey of Short-eared Owls *Asio flammeus* (Pontopiddan) on Lambay Island, Co. Dublin.' *Irish Naturalists' Journal 22*: 536-7.

Welch, R.J. 1905. 'The Last Red Deer, Co. Donegal.' *Irish Naturalist 14*: 120.

Whitehead, G.K. 1964. *The Deer of Great Britain and Ireland: An Account of their History, Status and Distribution.* London: Routledge and Kegan Paul.

Wijngaarden-Bakker, L.H. van. 1974. 'The Animal Remains from a Braker Settlement in Newgrange, Co. Meath: first report.' *Proceedings of the Royal Irish Academy 74C*: 313-83.

Wilson, J.P.F. and A.J. Pitcher. 1979. 'Feeding and Behaviour of a Killer Whale *Orcinus orca* L. in the Foyle Estuary.' *Irish Naturalists' Journal 19*: 352-5.

Woodman, P.C. 1981. 'A Mesolithic Camp in Ireland.' *Scientific American 245*: 120-32.

Woodman, P.C. 1986. 'Man's First Appearance in Ireland and his Importance in the Colonisation Process,' in D.P. Sleeman, R.J. Devoy and P.C. Woodman (eds), *Proceedings of the Postglacial Colonisation Conference.* Occasional Publication of the Irish Biogeographical Society 1: 34-7.

Bird Study in Ireland

CLIVE HUTCHINSON

Introduction

Robert Lloyd Praeger put it well in his *Natural History of Ireland* (1950) when he pointed out that the relative prominence of the science of ornithology was due to the large number of people who saw it as a hobby. This has been the case in Ireland as elsewhere since the early nineteenth century, but Praeger's slightly envious attitude to birdwatchers has been replaced by an attitude among many zoological professionals that ornithology is more of a pastime than a science. Yet one of the strengths of the study of Irish birds has been the body of informed amateurs: the few scientists have been able to correspond with and use the enthusiasm of far greater numbers of active participants than have the leaders of any other branch of natural science. Birds satisfy the collecting instinct more readily than most organisms. They are quite easy to identify, there are not too many species to learn, and they are prone to wander so that the thrill of vagrants is always a possibility.

Indeed Praeger himself, in his autobiographical *A Populous Solitude*, published in 1941, described how his own interest in natural history was stimulated by an early interest in birds and their nests. Like so many children of the time he collected eggs, but he 'soon realized the futility and undesirability' of this activity and commenced observing the nests. Writing fifty-seven years later, he was able to tabulate for 282 nests recorded in 1884 the number of each species recorded, the success rate of each and the principal reasons for failure. His scientific bent was obviously present at an early age, as indeed was his thorough approach to note-taking.

Neither his rigorous attitude to recording what he saw nor his disapproval of egg-collecting was representative of the traditional Irish attitude to birds. Birds have normally been seen in rural Ireland as objects of utility. Some, such as pheasants and mallard, are of value as sporting targets; others, such as hooded crows and woodpigeons, are pests to be exterminated.

Most farmers own shotguns for 'vermin destruction' and many rural dwellers (though probably not mainly farmers) shoot game. Among the urban working class, goldfinches and linnets have been valued as songbirds, and have been seen as suitable for capture and putting in cages. Until very recent years and the influence of television, birds have not been seen by the general public as animals worthy of admiration or study in their own right. Those of us who watched birds in the countryside twenty-five years ago remember the curiosity with which we were viewed. What were we looking at and why? Nowadays, a person walking along a path or roadside with a pair of binoculars is assumed to be looking for birds and curiosity is directed more at whatever rare species may be about than at the birdwatcher. Yet it remains true that a common response to an unusual and colourful bird is to shoot it; two of the three American belted kingfishers known to have visited Ireland in the 1980s were shot.*

The Irish avifauna is quite distinctive and markedly different from that of the island of Britain. The smaller size of the island, its more limited climatic and altitudinal ranges and the resultant smaller number of habitats are the principal reasons why the number of species recorded in Ireland is only two-thirds the number recorded in Britain, and why a similar proportion applies to the numbers of breeding species. Yet Ireland has a long and indented coastline with high cliffs providing nest sites for seabirds and shallow bays with ice-free inter-tidal mudflats where wintering wildfowl and waders come from northern Canada, Greenland, Iceland, Siberia and Scandinavia to feed in great flocks. In addition, the location of the island on the western periphery of the European land mass, projecting into the Atlantic, makes it an ideal location for studying the migration of passing seabirds and for sighting vagrant stragglers from North America.

Most of those who have provided the baseline material for our knowledge of Irish birds have been gifted amateurs. The earliest published account of Irish birds is that of Giraldus Cambrensis, who visited Ireland on three occasions between 1185 and 1204 and wrote an outline of *The History and Topography of Ireland* (*Topographia Hiberniae*) setting out, among many other items, an account of the birds. Game birds are referred to in several seventeenth- and eighteenth-century accounts of Irish life and in game preservation legislation, but the first lists of birds were very brief ones published in the early county histories of the eighteenth century. Real ornithology, being the sytematic and scientific study of birds, began in the nineteenth century.

---

*In *Birds of Ireland* (1900), R.J. Ussher observed that the indigenous kingfishers in Ireland 'are unmercifully shot' (ed.).

William Thompson

A look at the acknowledgments to the standard texts on Irish birds of the end of the nineteenth century (Ussher and Warren's *Birds of Ireland*, 1900) and the mid-twentieth century (Kennedy, Ruttledge and Scroope's *Birds of Ireland*, 1954) provides interesting sociological insights into the backgrounds of the contributors. A total of 106 people are credited in the earlier book with providing material. Of these, eleven were clergy, six were doctors, five were army officers and four were baronets. Only three were women. Clearly, many of those involved in the study of birds in the late nineteenth century were professional men. Some fifty years later, not much had changed, except that more women were contributing information. Of the 137 contributors listed in the introduction to the 1954 book, five were doctors (probably academics in the main rather than general practitioners), five were army officers, four were clergy; but for an activity still dominated by men, it is remarkable that ten were women. Indeed, the occupations of the authors of the later book are a pointer to the background of so many of those who provided the material for them. None was a trained scientist: Ruttledge and Scroope were both retired army officers and Kennedy was a Jesuit priest.

The pioneering work on Irish birds was William Thompson's *The Natural History of Ireland*, published in the mid-nineteenth century. Unfortunately, he did not list his contributors at the beginning of each of the three volumes that dealt with the birds, but a perusal of the accounts of the bird species shows that the bulk of his information came from a small number of correspondents scattered around the country. As in the later books, many of them were doctors, clergy and members of the professional class. Dr Burkitt of Waterford, Dr Harvey of Cork, Rev. Joseph Stopford of Cork and Mr Watters of Dublin were representative of Thompson's sources. These were the hobbyists Praeger referred to. They were the informed, well-educated and curious. They formed the backbone of the archaeological and antiquarian societies as well as the field clubs, philosophical societies and, later, the ornithological clubs that were the predecessors of our modern conservation bodies. They read widely. William Yarrell's *History of British Birds* went through several editions and sold well in the nineteenth century. Copies can be found in many old private libraries in Ireland. Books like this provided the detailed descriptions of plumage, behaviour and nesting habits that the isolated pioneers needed to identify the birds they saw.

Sight records were not enough on their own in the late nineteenth and early twentieth centuries. Eggs were collected and unusual birds shot so that identification was certain. The taking of specimens was not restricted to bird study; botanists, entomologists, geologists and others based their studies on the same technique. But many more people were engaged in game shooting in habitats where rare ducks and waders occurred (and were therefore in a position to kill an unusual bird) than were capable of recognizing a rare plant. Taxidermists were much in demand at this time as sportsmen sought to have their finest specimens mounted for the drawing-room. The taxidermist firm of the Williams family in Dame Street in Dublin became an extraordinarily important source of records of Irish birds. William Williams (who died in 1901) and his sons Edward and W.J. Williams carried on business for more than seventy years and contributed many notes to the *Irish Naturalist* and the *Irish Naturalists' Journal* on the specimens they received. Dealing daily with so many birds, they were quick to notice an unusual plumage and to research the identity of the species by comparing the skins with the text in books like Yarrell's. The work of the Williams family is often seen in auction rooms and is well represented in the Natural History Museum in Dublin. The best examples of their taxidermy were mounted against a carefully painted backdrop of the site where the birds were taken. The Williams family, though the best known, were far from being the only taxidermists in the country; the Sheals family of Belfast and the Rohu firm in Cork were both responsible for fine work and also produced records of unusual birds.

Although many of those who sent unusual specimens to the Williams family may not have known what it was they had shot, some sportsmen were remarkably knowledgeable about birds. Sir Ralph Payne-Gallwey, whom Praeger did not deign worthy of mention in his book of potted biographies of Irish naturalists (*Some Irish Naturalists*, 1949), was a unique figure as an Irish wildfowl shooter who recorded his observations. Some might say that it is perhaps just as well for the Irish avifauna that he was unique, for he described in his book *The Fowler in Ireland* (1882) how he shot fifteen hundred duck in the winter of 1880/81, eight hundred of which were killed in one month. Yet his book is a wonderful combination of technical advice on guns, punts and shooting technique with accounts of the distribution and behaviour of all the common wildfowl and wading species. The rarer species are dealt with briefly but always with authority. Many contemporary conservationists decry the activity of wildfowlers, and there are accounts in Payne-Gallwey's book of large bags which repel modern sensibilities, but he was representative of many sportsmen who provided the raw material for much of our knowledge of Irish birds in the nineteenth century.

These therefore were the people who generated the data for the development of bird study in Ireland: the professional and monied middle classes who had time to travel and indulge their hobbies. But they needed leadership, a focal point for their interest, which was provided in part by learned societies but to a much greater extent by the enthusiasm of a small number of gifted amateurs. The earliest lists of Irish birds were produced in the eighteenth century in the county histories, in Dr John Rutty's *An Essay towards a Natural History of the County of Dublin* (1772), and in Dr Patrick Browne's 'A Catalogue of the Birds of Ireland ...' (1774); but these were modest works. William Thompson's *Natural History* (1849-56) was a much more formidable book. The three volumes on birds that were completed during his lifetime comprise over twelve hundred pages based on an extensive correspondence with a network of letter-writers all over Ireland. The fourth volume, published posthumously, includes memoirs of his life that serve to place in context the importance of his work and the central position he held in the second quarter of the nineteenth century.

Thompson was born in Belfast in 1805, the son of a wealthy linen merchant. His school years were not particularly distinguished and at the age of sixteen he was apprenticed to a firm in the linen trade. Like many young men of his class he was an enthusiastic shot and his interest in birds developed when he had difficulty in identifying some of the species he brought home. In the autumn, apparently, he spent the early morning shooting on the shores of Belfast Lough before going to work. In 1826, when he was twenty-one years old, his apprenticeship was complete. Two significant events occurred in that year. He undertook a tour of the Continent, which he documented in detail in his journals, and he joined the Natural History Society of Belfast. Shortly after he returned from his four months abroad he set up in business on his own account, but was apparently not successful and abandoned his career about 1831 to become a full-time student of natural science. How he supported himself in this work is not clear, but it seems likely that he was able to rely on family resources.

Thompson read his first paper to the Natural History Society in Belfast in 1827 when he was still very much an amateur; in 1834, by which time he was devoting all his time to research on the fauna of Ireland, he had his first papers published in the *Proceedings of the Zoological Society of London* and the *London and Edinburgh Philosophical Journal*. Thereafter he published regularly in the journals of the London learned societies and was an annual visitor to their meetings, frequently bringing specimens which he had difficulty in determining and obviously revelling in the discussions he had with others who shared his enthusiasm.

As the acknowledged natural-history expert in Belfast he was brought news of all the unusual specimens that were found in the area. In time he became known throughout the country as an expert who was assembling data for a book on the fauna of Ireland. He had the essential attribute of anyone who seeks to write a book on Irish birds: he was a painstaking correspondent. All records were investigated thoroughly and, in many cases, specimens were examined before the occurrence was considered acceptable for publication. He published regularly, and was careful to acknowledge fully the sources of his material. This conscientious attitude must have encouraged his correspondents to keep him informed.

Thompson had no university education or institutional connection. Like many other amateur scientists of his time, he attended the annual meetings of the British Association for the Advancement of Science and, when it met in Glasgow in 1840, he produced a report on the vertebrate fauna of Ireland, which included the birds. The first volume of his *Natural History* appeared in 1849, the second in 1850 and the third in 1851, but sadly he died early in 1852, having only completed the sections on birds.

He was obviously an important leader in two respects. Firstly, he seems to have dominated the intellectual life of Belfast zoology for nearly twenty years. He was President of the Natural History Society in 1843 and was re-elected annually until his death; he was a conduit for the publication of observations by many people which would otherwise have been completely lost; and he provided a bridge between the natural historians of Belfast and London. But more importantly for the future of the study of Irish birds, he set rigorous standards in the first significant account of the status of Irish birds. He was an original in Ireland in this respect, but he was greatly influenced by the standards of acceptance of records of unusual species that were employed by the editors of the London journals and the authors of the books on British birds that were appearing.

Barrington and Ussher

Thompson was an amateur – as were all the figures who provided the route to publication that was so important if the hobbyists were to continue to feel it worthwhile to communicate their observations. He was also very much a representative of the thrusting Belfast merchant class that had produced the Belfast Natural History Society and later the Belfast Naturalists' Field Club. But the leadership the widely distributed Irish bird enthusiasts needed did not come again from Belfast, perhaps because in the late nineteenth century, as the demand for Home Rule grew throughout the country, the middle classes centred their scientific interests more and more on Ulster and looked less to the remainder of the island of Ireland.

Richard Ussher, the principal author of the next major textbook on Irish birds, *Birds of Ireland* (1900), lived in Waterford and spent much of his life in full-time egg-collecting and research on birds. Major R.F. Ruttledge, one of the authors of the 1954 book *Birds of Ireland* and the sole author of the 1966 *Ireland's Birds*, was invalided out of the Indian Cavalry in 1942 and spent most of his time after that on the study of Irish bird distribution, living in Mayo and Wicklow. Ussher and Ruttledge shared with

Thompson the essential characteristic of being exceptional correspondents, and like Thompson they drew the bulk of their material from the professional classes. One man, however, himself also a remarkable correspondent, tapped a completely new vein of material for the study of Irish bird distribution: Richard M. Barrington, who perceived the value of collecting data from Irish lightkeepers.

Barrington was born at Fassaroe, near Bray in Co. Wicklow, and published his first note on birds in 1866 at the age of seventeen. He graduated from Trinity College, Dublin, and was called to the Bar but earned his living mainly from his large farm. Like many other naturalists of the time he was greatly stimulated by A.G. More, an English botanist and ornithologist who came to Dublin to take up a post in the Natural History Museum in 1867. More was one of the few students of Irish birds prior to the 1960s who could in any sense be considered to have an employment related to his research interest. He published relatively little on Irish birds but a major paper in *The Ibis* on the distribution of British birds, using the counties as units, was a precursor of the modern bird atlases. He was also a great letter-writer and he encouraged the young Barrington to produce botanical reports. The scientific training was influential for Barrington's massive survey of the birds that occurred at Irish lighthouses.

This work had as its principal objective the study of bird migration. It had become well known that large numbers of migrant birds were attracted to the beams of the lighthouses that had recently been constructed around the coasts of Britain and Ireland. Following a meeting at Heligoland with Heinrich Gatke, who had been studying bird migration there since 1843, John Cordeaux and J.A. Harvie-Brown, ornithologists from England and Scotland respectively, decided in 1879 to circularize lightkeepers with printed schedules requesting the date, number of birds seen, time when seen, weather conditions and the number of birds striking the light. To their surprise, almost two-thirds were returned completed. This success stimulated them to seek sponsorship for a systematic survey of the lighthouses and lightships around all of the coasts of Britain and Ireland. The organization they turned to for support, the British Association, set up a Committee on Migration to which More and Barrington were appointed. Schedules were sent out to lightkeepers around the shores of both islands from 1881 to 1887 and an enormous volume of material was collected and summarized annually by the British Association. In 1888 the BA decided that sufficient data had been collected for analysis and William Eagle Clarke, the youngest member of the committee, was given the task of preparing a digest of the survey's findings. Barrington, however, was unhappy with the short time-span of the survey. He believed that observations should be continued over many more years so that uncorroborated records could be confirmed by subsequent occurrences, and that more specimens should be collected. As a result, he personally financed the survey in Ireland until 1897 and, with the help of C.B. Moffat, analyzed the results for the years 1881-97 in an enormous tome published in a tiny edition of only 350 copies in 1900. In the introduction to *The Migration of Birds as Observed at Irish Lighthouses and Lightships* he wrote that 'few, perhaps, can realize what the collection of statistics, the preparation, the printing and the publication, of this work have cost in time and money .... Birds are a very attractive subject, but even if all the copies were sold, the expenses would not nearly be defrayed.'

His book remained the standard work on Irish bird migration up to the early 1950s when the first bird observatories opened. His assessment of the returns of lightkeepers was thorough. Besides sending out schedules, Barrington also sent out labels for specimens and envelopes for the legs and wings of species that could not be identified. Among the two thousand specimens he collected from lightkeepers were several records of birds never before seen in Ireland, and indeed not recorded again until the 1950s. Lapland bunting, short-toed lark, lesser whitethroat, yellow-browed warbler, red-breasted flycatcher and woodchat shrike, all species now known to be regular migrants on the coast, were added to the Irish list by Barrington as a result of his correspondence with lightkeepers. Some were found dead at the light but others were shot, obviously by very knowledgable lightkeepers, and the specimens forwarded to Fassaroe.

Barrington's circularization of lightkeepers was repeated at intervals in subsequent years by J.S. Barrington, his son, by George Humphreys and by Major R.F. Ruttledge, but none carried out the work so comprehensively as Richard Barrington had done.

Barrington had an interest in travel and climbed in Switzerland and Canada. He visited Rockall in 1896 with Praeger, Harvie-Brown and others on an expedition partly financed by the Royal Irish Academy and partly by Barrington and Harvie-Brown. Even though they travelled in June, the seas were far too rough to land on the rock so they had to content themselves with observations of the birds and with shooting a number of specimens, which were recovered by dinghy. Obviously, Barrington was a formidable man in the field. Praeger related in *The Way that I Went* (1937) that Barrington and H.C. Hart, a prominent contemporary botanist, visited Powerscourt one wet day in search of singing wood warblers and scarce plants. The weather was appalling, but Hart showed his contempt for the conditions by walking through the longest grass and the briars close to the edge of the stream. Barrington, not to be outdone, reacted by stepping into the stream, sitting down on a submerged stone and eating his lunch. Without a word, Hart joined him there. All rivalry, we are told, ceased forthwith.

The dominant ornithologists of the last quarter of the nineteenth century were Barrington, A.G. More (who died in 1895), Richard Ussher of Waterford, Robert Warren of Sligo and C.B. Moffat. The first four of these decided in 1890 that the time was right for a new book on Irish birds to replace and update Thompson's volumes. Barrington was heavily involved in his migration reports, More was in poor health and Warren wrote sections on only six species, so the bulk of the book was prepared by Ussher. Both Ussher and Warren were amateurs. Robert Warren was born in Cork but spent most of his life on the estuary of the River Moy with easy access to Killala Bay and Bartragh Island. Here he spent fifty years noting the birds of a part of the west of Ireland that was almost unknown to ornithologists, and if *Birds of Ireland* has few pages actually written by Robert Warren, the text of the entire book benefited from his knowledge.

Richard Ussher, like Barrington and Thompson before him, was an indefatigable correspondent. He was born in 1841 and spent much of his early life abroad before settling down after marriage in the family home at Cappagh, Co. Waterford, where he was occupied as a landowner and magistrate. His great passion was the collection of eggs and he was particularly fascinated by the breeding birds of coastal cliffs. His discovery on his own property at Cappagh of a cave containing remains of man as well as the Irish elk attracted him to palaeontology, and he spent a great deal of time and money in later years digging caves in Cork, Waterford, Clare and Sligo. His collection of seven thousand eggs was acquired by the National Museum and his notes were bequeathed to the Royal Irish Academy where they remain an important source for students of Irish birds. As recently as 1982, the organizer of a survey of breeding choughs around the Irish coastline was able to compare his results with the researches of Ussher and found that choughs continued to nest in the same sites as those where Ussher had found them a century earlier. The egg collection is of less contemporary interest in these changed times, though Praeger wrote approvingly (1949) that in later years 'he atoned by relinquishing the collection of eggs, by helping energetically the work of the Irish Society for the Protection of Birds, and by widespread explorations of the west coast and the bogs and lakes of the midlands to determine the breeding-range in Ireland of rarer species'.

Ussher was apparently a rather shy man, but his determination in seeking out nests and in exploring caves was legendary. He needed this quality when he commenced the ten years of work that preceded the publication of *Birds of Ireland*. His correspondence and research were extensive and the resulting book remains a wonderful read – perhaps the most interesting, because of its detail, of all the Irish bird books to dip into. It remained the standard textbook for over fifty years. I have found his account of the distribution of quail particularly interesting because the species is now known only as a spasmodic summer visitor:

The extensive growth of wheat, leaving stubbles full of weeds, in the early part of the century, and the multiplication of potato-gardens up to the time of the famine (1846-48), were facts in favour of this bird at that period, and bevies of Quails used to be met with commonly through the winter months in every cultivated district; this species was then considered more numerous than the Partridge, and appeared to be resident from its abundance at all seasons .... The birds often frequented rough elevated ground full of furze but were particularly attached to the small holdings of the peasantry, where they could feed on the seeds of various weeds and lurk in the headlands and straggling fences. In such situations, Quails were to be met with on the edges of bogs, but did not resort to the latter .... After the famine, much of the tilled lands were turned into pasture or reverted into moor; and about 1850-53 I heard an old sportsman remark that Quails were then much less frequently met with in co. Waterford than they had been, while the Rev. C. Irvine dated their decrease in co. Tyrone from 1848. Still they continued common up to about 1860, and I can remember their frequent calls during August 1858; but in the 'sixties' there was a steady decrease, which advanced during the 'seventies', when the occurrence of a Quail became a fact to be noted ...

Later in the text, Ussher suggests that the decrease of the quail was not only due to the conversion of tillage into pasture but also to the wholesale netting of the birds on spring migration in the Mediterranean.

Émigrés and Popularizers

Within a very short period the outstanding figures of late Victorian Irish ornithology passed away. More died in 1895, Ussher in 1913 and both Barrington and Warren in 1915. Moffat remained as a focal point in Dublin, interesting himself in the work of the Irish Society for the Protection of Birds, of which he was Secretary for more than twenty years prior to his death in 1945, and individuals like George Humphreys in Dublin, R.F. Ruttledge in Mayo and Lance Turtle in Belfast kept the interest in bird distribution alive, until a new generation came along in the late 1950s and 1960s.

As well, of course, as the leading synthesizers of work on Irish bird distribution, there were also popularizers. The books on birds produced by Thompson, Barrington and Ussher were substantial doorstops and aimed at a relatively small market. John Watters saw the need for a small handbook on Irish birds and, borrowing heavily from Thompson, produced a *Natural History of the Birds of Ireland* in 1853. Unashamedly aiming the little book at the general reader for whom Thompson's volumes would be too expensive, he combined rather unsystematic accounts of each species with poetic quotes and classical allusions. The book seems to have sold well: certainly it is frequently to be found in the lists of antiquarian booksellers, but, alas, Watters was much less critical than his contemporaries and successors. A different sort of book was the attractive and unpretentious little *Our Irish Song Birds* by Rev. Charles Benson, headmaster of Rathmines School, which first appeared in 1886 and sold out in little more than three months. This success stimulated Benson to produce a second edition in 1901 which, while brought up to date, did not have the exquisite colour plates of the first issue. Benson admitted that his book was not a scientific one but he hoped to pass on to the reader something of his love of birds and their song, and he succeeded, for his obvious admiration for them still charms the reader.

There was clearly a market for popular books on Irish birds, but it remained untapped again for many decades. Rev. P.G. Kennedy SJ, some forty years later, broadcast on Radio Éireann about the birds of the North Bull Island, Dublin Bay. He wrote articles on the birds of the area in *Studies* and the *Irish Naturalists' Journal* and, finally, published a little book in 1953 entitled *An Irish Sanctuary – Birds of the North Bull*. The book appears to have sold fairly well, but was still widely available in Dublin in the late 1960s. Unlike most modern books and papers about birds, it is a readable and highly personalized account not just of the birds but of the experiences of the author and his friends watching them on the Bull.

Some important Irish ornithologists went abroad and published their best work outside Ireland. Professor C.J. Patten, for example, was born in Dublin and graduated from Trinity College, Dublin, in medicine. He specialized in anatomy, and while in Ireland and later in England (where he became Professor of Anatomy at the University of Sheffield), he spent his spare time studying the birds of the lakes, rivers and coast. He was a keen ornithologist and advised birdwatchers to use binoculars and to dress in a manner in which they would harmonize with their natural surroundings. Although he shot wildfowl he was opposed to unnecessary killing and, in particular, to the shooting of seabirds for the millinery trade. His *The Aquatic Birds of Great Britain and Ireland* (1906) was not just a book about the distribution of the birds, though he did cover that aspect, but a thorough account for its time of the plumage, behaviour, nest, food, voice, flight and measurements of the wildfowl, waders and seabirds occurring around the coasts and on the lakes, rivers and marshes of both Britain and Ireland. Although published in England and dealing with the birds of Britain as well as Ireland, the Irish influence on the book is obvious. Richard Ussher read the proofs, Edward Williams was particularly acknowledged for the help he provided from his Dublin taxidermists, and the texts were heavily dependent on material from the *Irish Naturalist*. Patten noted in his introduction that the book was based on fieldwork on the Irish coast over more than twenty years, as well as on more recent investigations in Britain. The book was illustrated with a mixture of drawings, monochrome paintings and photographs. The drawings are strangely uncredited but include some exquisite line drawings by George Lodge and reproductions of paintings by Archibald Thorburn. There are several photographs of nests and eggs but they are mostly of mounted specimens and very unlifelike.

While Patten published a number of papers in addition to his large book, he was nowhere near as prolific as the most notable of all the émigrés, the Rev. E.A. Armstrong. Although remembered in Ireland for his book on Northern Ireland, *Birds of the Grey Wind* (1940), his interest was primarily in the behaviour of birds and far less in their distribution. The fascination of Thompson, Ussher and Barrington for documenting the occurrences of species was something he did not share. His book on Northern Ireland is an evocation of the birds, flowers, legends and folklore of the area. Although he had a heightened aesthetic sense of birds, Armstrong wrote a number of scholarly books about behaviour, including *Bird Display: an Introduction to the Study of Bird Psychology* (1942), *A Study of Bird Song* (1963) and two books in the Collins New Naturalist series: *The Wren* (1955) and *The Folklore of Birds* (1958). These were all erudite works that were distinguished by an easy writing style and a sense of wonder at the natural world. His book on folklore includes an extensive account of the Irish wren boys and the origins of the St Stephen's Day (26 December) custom. This ritual involves groups of boys, carrying a wren, dressed in fancy garb and often with faces blackened, going from house to house, singing a song and collecting coins. Armstrong showed that this was not just an Irish custom but was also known from Britain and France. He suggested that the ritual came to Ireland from the Mediterranean during the Bronze Age and was a New Year ceremonial having as its purpose the defeat of the dark earth-powers and identification with the hoped-for triumph of light and life. He trained in Queen's University, Belfast, but he spent the remainder of his life outside Ireland, working as an Anglican clergyman in parishes as varied as Kowloon, Leeds and St Mark's, Cambridge. What he achieved in terms of original ornithological research and extraordinarily wide reading, all in the limited spare time of a clergyman, was quite remarkable.

Those ornithologists who found the behaviour of birds much more fascinating than their distribution have always been in a small minority. The pages of the *Irish Naturalist* and the *Irish Naturalists' Journal* included many notes on birds, but very few major publications appeared. C.B. Moffat's paper on 'The Spring Rivalry of Birds', published in the *Irish Naturalist* in 1903, was an exception. Moffat concluded that the chief purpose of bird song is to advertise the presence in an area of an unvanquished cock bird, who claims the area as his and will allow no other cock to enter it without a battle. This was an original contribution at a time when birds were widely believed to sing purely for enjoyment.

J.P. Burkitt

The most original of all the ornithologists of the first half of the twentieth century, however, was a man little known to the public and so little known to the naturalists of his time that Praeger did not mention him in his book *Some Irish Naturalists*. This was J.P. Burkitt, who was born in 1870, trained as a civil engineer and spent the years between 1900 and 1940 as County Surveyor for Fermanagh. He placed different patterns of metal bands on the legs of robins in his garden – not coloured rings because he was colour-blind – and thus made possible for the first time the study in the field of individual birds. He discovered new information about territorial behaviour and song, including female song; he observed robin display and realized that this was a threat display aimed at intimidating other robins and not (as had hitherto been thought) part of courtship; and he was the first to use ringing returns to estimate average age. He assumed that the number of new robins produced each year must be balanced by a similar number of deaths among the existing population and, after estimating the replacement rate, he calculated the average age of a robin at about two years and ten months, an age which seemed shockingly short at the time. In fact, subsequent research has shown that this figure is too high. He told David Lack, the author of a monograph on the robin, that he did not look at a bird until he was thirty-seven, at which time he had no ornithological friends. He published a pioneering paper in *British Birds* entitled 'A Study of the Robin by Means of Marked Birds' and a few short papers in the *Irish Naturalists' Journal*. He told Lack in 1944 that he had pricks of conscience when studying the robin, in case he might be more interested in the created than in the Creator. He was deeply religious and extremely humble. His later years were spent reading the Bible and working in his garden.

Developments at Mid-century

Mainstream work on Irish birds from the First World War to the early 1950s was limited in scope and clearly suffered from a lack of stimulating leadership. A number of moves in the early 1950s changed all this. Firstly, Saltee Bird Observatory was formed in 1950; then a new book, *Birds of Ireland*, and a booklet on the birds of Northern Ireland were published in 1954; and finally, and probably most importantly, the *Irish Bird Report* was started.

Saltee was founded in the flush of enthusiasm that had followed the formation of a bird observatory at Fair Isle, and its success was assured when it was discovered that interesting migrants could be found that would enable Barrington's lighthouse work of more than fifty years earlier to be updated. Major R.F. Ruttledge was a central figure in starting the first Irish bird observatory; he was also one of the authors of the new book on Irish birds and the first editor of the *Irish Bird Report*.

Ruttledge, who has been known to generations of birdwatchers as 'the Major', was born in Carlow in 1899 but moved at an early age to Mayo where he concentrated on studies of the distribution of birds in the west of Ireland. His particular interests were seabirds breeding on the islands off the west coast and the geese that wintered on the midland and western bogs. A significant paper on the birds of Galway and Mayo (1950) was the first modern county avifauna produced in Ireland, and his paper on the numbers and distribution of geese with Mrs Hall Watt (1958) was the summary of many years watching geese. His work on seabirds and his search for Leach's petrels nesting in Ireland led him to spend a night on every island off the coasts of Galway and Mayo, including memorable stays in 1946 and 1947 on the Stags of Broadhaven, four rocky pinnacles off the north Mayo coast, where his tent was blown away in a storm on the second visit. Despite the discomfort Ruttledge saw and heard Leach's petrels on both occasions, but failed to prove breeding. This had to wait until 1982 when a team of bird ringers caught Leach's petrels and found nests and eggs.

The new book on Irish birds was written by a triumvirate of Rev. P.G. Kennedy (who had written so evocatively of the North Bull), Lt-Col. C.F. Scroope (another ex-Army officer) and Ruttledge, with assistance from George Humphreys. It was in many respects an update of Ussher and Warren's work of fifty years earlier and nowadays is of particular interest in showing how little progress had been made. What was to prove much more important in the long run was the formation of the *Irish Bird Report* by the Dublin-based Irish Ornithologists' Club, with Ruttledge as its editor. It sought to publish all the interesting records of Irish birds each year and immediately generated a new interest in documenting bird records. As so often in the past, the success of the venture was heavily dependent on the letter-writing ability of its editor, and those of us who contributed to it in its earlier years remember the closely written and searching requests for further documentation that we received by return of post when we sent in records. The new report generated so much information in a short time that Ruttledge was able to produce a completely new book on Irish birds within twelve years, *Ireland's Birds*. Only after its appearance in 1966 did Ruttledge feel that the systematic list of species could be somewhat curtailed and short papers included. So in due course the simple report of the 1950s evolved into an ornithological journal, *Irish Birds*, in the 1970s.

The authors of *Birds of Ireland* were relative loners in Irish ornithology. Organization was provided in the first half of this century by the Dublin Naturalists' Field Club. Founded in 1886, it had ornithologists among its members from an early stage (Moriarty 1986, 1988). Barrington was its first treasurer, Ussher an early president and Patten and Moffat were among the lecturers. There were occasional ornithological excursions by the Club but the study of birds was peripheral to the main interests of the members and it was not until 1939 that a Bird Group was formed and more attention paid to ornithology. Regular visits were made to the North Bull and censuses of heronries were carried out. The heyday of the DNFC's leadership was from the late 1930s to the early 1950s, though the population to be led was very small.

In 1950 the Irish Ornithologists' Club was formed as an offshoot of the Irish Society for the Protection of Birds. Alec Mason, M.J. Rowan and Ivan Goodbody were the founder members and George Humphreys joined shortly afterwards. Goodbody had been studying the autumn movement of skylarks in Wexford and the others had been involved in wildfowl counts in Dublin. They got together and decided to form a new club. It was intended for serious ornithologists and its principal rule was that there were to be no rules and no minutes. Wildfowl counts and other useful studies were contemplated but it was felt that junior birdwatchers were adequately catered for by the Dublin Naturalists' Field Club. The IOC remained alive and active until the late 1960s when it merged with other bodies to form the Irish Wildbird Conservancy. Meetings were held at The Brazen Head bar and women were excluded from membership for much of the life of the organization. There were forty-five members in 1960 and about ten people attended outings, but membership rose to over 140 by 1968. It was very much a Dublin organization and its membership held aloof from general birdwatching. Yet it was responsible for the foundation of the *Irish Bird Report.*

In Northern Ireland leadership was provided by a few individuals. Arnold Benington was a very influential figure and one of the founders of the Copeland Bird Observatory. C. Douglas Deane, universally known as Jimmy Deane, was the author of the Ulster Museum's *Handbook of the Birds of Northern Ireland* in 1954 and a prolific correspondent in the press. The Northern Ireland Ornithologists' Club was formed in the mid-1960s and the Ulster Society for the Protection of Birds was absorbed into the Royal Society for the Protection of Birds in 1965. This heralded a significant advance for bird conservation in Northern Ireland as the RSPB had substantial expertise and financial resources.

The issue that most intrigued ornithologists in the 1950s and early 1960s was the study of bird migration. Saltee Bird Observatory was founded in 1950 but closed in 1964. Copeland Bird Observatory and Cape Clear Bird Observatory, both still thriving, were founded in 1954 and 1959 respectively. Observatories also existed briefly at Tory Island (1958-65) and Malin Head (1961-5). A great deal was learned in a few years at these sites about patterns of bird migration, but perhaps the greatest long-term value of the

observatory network was the cross-fertilization fostered by the mix of relatively experienced British and novice Irish birdwatchers, and the opportunities provided for Irish birdwatchers to learn the techniques of bird-ringing
and the use of mist-nets to catch birds. Ken Williamson, former warden of
Fair Isle Bird Observatory, was one of those instrumental in setting up
Saltee, and Tim Sharrock, currently editor of *British Birds* magazine, was
the principal moving force behind Cape Clear in 1959.

The late 1960s were exciting years for ornithologists. Increasing urbanization, changes in land use, land drainage, pollution and the effect of pesticides all appeared as major threats to birds. The voluntary conservation
movement developed rapidly in response; government in both Northern
Ireland and the Republic committed more resources to wildlife conservation;
the general public showed a heightened awareness of wildlife; and close-up
views of birds and their behaviour on television proved to be popular early-
evening entertainment. No longer was the study of birds an isolated activity.
Attitudes seemed to be changing very rapidly.

In Northern Ireland the Royal Society for the Protection of Birds established its presence with professional organization. In the Republic the various organizations concerned with birdwatching and conservation that had
developed over the years came together in 1968 to form the Irish Wildbird
Conservancy, now named Birdwatch Ireland. The new organizations both
saw co-operative field ornithology as a means of providing essential baseline
conservation material on the distribution of Irish birds and as a popular outlet for the enthusiasm of active members. Four principal surveys were promoted from the beginning: wildfowl counts, breeding-seabird counts, the
survey of breeding birds on the basis of the ten-kilometre squares of the
National Grid, and the breeding peregrine census.

Wildfowl counts had first been carried out in Ireland in the late 1940s
and early 1950s under the auspices of the Severn Wildfowl Trust and were
concentrated on locations close to Dublin and Belfast. Then, in 1964-5, the
Northern Ireland Ornithologists' Club commenced a survey of the wildfowl
of the Lough Neagh basin which showed for the first time the immensity of
the numbers of duck wintering in the area. From 1967 onwards, country-
wide counts of geese and wildfowl were organized as part of international
census efforts.

The carrying out of wildfowl counts was spurred initially by a growing
consciousness of the threat to the habitat of ducks, geese and swans posed
by increasing drainage and the obvious lack of information on the numbers
and distribution of these birds in Ireland. An additional motivation to these
surveys was the international interest in wildfowl and their habitats. When
the Seabird Group, a mainly British organization of workers interested in
seabirds, proposed a census of all the breeding seabirds around the coastlines

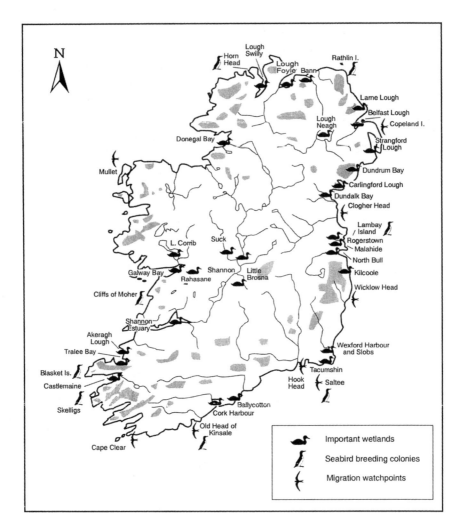

Birdwatching sites in Ireland (courtesy Clive Hutchinson).

of Britain and Ireland in 1969 and 1970, the Irish reaction was as enthusi-astic as the response to wildfowl counts. The habitat on which these birds spend so much of their lives, the inshore waters around our coast, was seen as threatened by oil pollution and by concentrations of poly-chlorinated biphenyls or PCBs. As with the wildfowl, virtually nothing was known about the numbers of birds breeding around our shores.

The two-year census, known as 'Operation Seafarer', generated enor-mous enthusiasm among the growing body of amateur ornithologists and, although the survey's techniques have been much criticized in recent years on the grounds that census methodology was inadequately standardized, it did pinpoint all the major seabird colonies and, for some species, provided valuable baseline data.

The third survey promoted by the Irish Wildbird Conservancy in its early years was the plan to map the breeding birds of Britain and Ireland on a ten-kilometre square grid over the five years from 1969 to 1973. The Ordnance Surveys of Ireland and Northern Ireland construct most of their maps on the basis of the ten-kilometre grid, dividing the country into 1010 squares, all of which were to be visited for this survey. There was no obvious conservation motive behind this survey, unlike the wildfowl and seabird counts. But there was a sense that if the British and Northern Irish were going to do it – it was the idea of the British Trust for Ornithology – then the Republic should join in. Very little consideration was given to the difficulty involved or indeed to who would organize the survey, but there was great enthusiasm from the amateur ornithologists. The project had a scientific value in that it mapped with unprecedented accuracy all the records of confirmed, probable or possible breeding over the five-year period. It also propagated the idea of field ornithology as an activity of interest in itself, and many Irish amateur birdwatchers were introduced to rigorous recording techniques. At the end of the *Atlas* period many called for a new survey to keep them occupied in useful activity, but the replacement survey on important bird habitats which was adopted in Britain proved too complex and too demanding of most Irish observers and was not a success in Ireland. Indeed, it would probably not have been a success in Britain without substantial professional input.

Finally, in reponse to the declining population of the peregrine, the IWC promoted annual censuses of the species in the Republic. This survey was organized by John Temple Lang, a Dublin-based lawyer who had been one of those responsible for uniting the various bodies into the Irish Wildbird Conservancy. Like the wildfowl counts and the seabird censuses, the peregrine survey marked a reaction to conservation problems and the threat to a species. Peregrines had been found in the early 1960s to have declined sharply in Britain as a result of the effects of pesticide contamination. The Irish censuses found a similar decline and formed the basis for lobbying to restrict the availability of certain pesticides. The end result has been a revival in the population of the species to a stage where numbers now are probably as high as they have ever been. The species has even bred on a gasometer in the centre of Dublin.

Each of these surveys reflected the interest of Irish ornithologists in numbers and distribution of birds. The wildfowl counts developed in due course into an enquiry into both wildfowl and wading birds of coastal and inland wetlands. A great deal of material on the seasonal distribution and numbers of most Irish wildfowl and waders in the early 1970s was amassed and published in my own *Ireland's Wetlands and their Birds* (1979). The survey was repeated in the 1980s, but there was no spin-off into studies of why the birds feed on particular estuaries, where they moult, or how many of them actually utilize individual sites. These were the problems that increasingly interested British and continental ornithologists from the mid-1970s on, but apart from a small amount of wader and wildfowl ringing and a handful of other studies there was no research on ducks, geese or waders. There was little improvement in the 1980s despite all the protests about threats to waterfowl, though a state-funded research programme commenced on white-fronted geese and a couple of postgraduate projects took place.

One is drawn inexorably to the conclusion that while amateur ornithology flourished in Ireland in the nineteenth century, it parted company from British and continental movements in the early years of this century. As both amateur and professional research developed abroad, Irish ornithologists focused on bird distribution and on adding as many species as possible to their life lists. It could be argued that such a strong statement is not fair to bird ringers, but Irish ringing has been notable for the dearth of publications from its proponents. The British Trust for Ornithology provided essential assistance in both Northern Ireland and the Republic in the late 1960s and early 1970s by providing intensive ringing courses, and there are now approximately a hundred ringers in the country, but only a handful of serious research projects have been started and very few papers relying mainly on ringing results have been published. One would hardly think that this is the country of J.P. Burkitt, the father of the marking of individual birds.

Ornithology Today

In the foregoing I have dealt very largely with Irish amateur ornithology. The reason for this emphasis is the scarcity of professional opportunities for ornithologists in Ireland. There is no university with an interest in ornithology to rival Oxford, Aberdeen or Durham in Great Britain, though there are indications that this may be changing. At each of the colleges of the National University in Cork, Dublin and Galway there is now at least one member of staff prepared to encourage students to work on birds. Secondly, there has been an increase in the number of professional ornithologists working in the civil service since the mid-1970s. It would not be true to say that there is a plethora of opportunities in the state service but there does seem to be an increase in the number of ornithologists earning a living from research either as employees of or under contract to government departments. In particular, the Department of the Environment for Northern Ireland has commissioned a substantial amount of work from the Royal Society for the Protection of Birds in the last five years. Surveys of breeding peregrines, breeding common scoters and breeding waders have provided contract work for ornithologists in Northern Ireland. In the Republic the National Parks and Wildlife Service has commissioned research into seabird breeding ecology, white-fronted goose feeding ecology, the effect of cormorants on fisheries and the effect of drainage of a river system on the birds of the area. Thirdly, there are signs of a few amateurs carrying out first-rate ornithological research and being prepared to contemplate publishing it. One of the aims of the journal *Irish Birds*, which was founded in 1977, was to encourage both amateur and professional ornithologists to publish original work on Irish birds and, while the emphasis of the majority of papers has been on bird distribution, there have been important contributions on other topics. The journal, an annual periodical, has been a remarkable success, stimulating a flow of publications over the first twenty years of its life that has no parallel in the past.

Public attitudes to birds have changed significantly in the 1980s and 1990s, with continuing pressure on the environment and a growing view that animals and birds have 'rights' of a sort – though it is still worth pointing out that far more people shoot game than are members of all the bird conservation and ornithological bodies in the country. In Ireland, north and south, there are over 160,000 shotgun licences; the number of members of bird conservation organizations is less than 10,000. The gun club movement is strong enough to have supported several shooting magazines over the years. The ornithological and the nature conservation public in Ireland has never been considered large enough by any Irish publisher to support a commercial magazine, though a number of British magazines are sold into this market. However, a handful of books on Irish birds, in particular Gordon D'Arcy's beautifully illustrated *The Guide to the Birds of Ireland* (1981), have found commercial success and several enterprising pioneers have made a living from organizing courses on field studies and wildlife-related topics.

Today there are clear signs of change in approach to bird study. Where the amateur had been dominant for over a century in contributing new information there are now indications that serious bird study is being taken over by professionals. The necessity for statistical analysis in a modern scientific paper deters amateurs. Most are frightened off by p values and chi-square tests. A recent (1996) issue of the journal *Irish Birds*, for example, contains no paper by an amateur ornithologist. There remains, however, a large body of enquiring and energetic birdwatchers whose energies are ready to be harnessed in co-operative surveys. It would be a shame if the tradition that produced Barrington's twenty-year survey of birds at light-stations and the recent bird atlases were allowed to die. What is required is imaginative leadership. After all, most PhD studies cover a very short three-year period; amateurs are prepared to carry on research for much longer.

References

Armstrong, E.A. 1940. *Birds of the Grey Wind*. London: Oxford University Press.

Armstrong, E.A. 1942. *Bird Display: an Introduction to the Study of Bird Psychology*. Cambridge: Cambridge University Press.

Armstrong, E.A. 1955. *The Wren*. London: Collins.

Armstrong, E.A. 1958. *The Folklore of Birds*. London: Collins.

Armstrong, E.A. 1963. *A Study of Bird Song*. London: Oxford University Press.

Barrington, R.M. 1900. *The Migration of Birds as Observed at Irish Lighthouses and Lightships*. London and Dublin: R.H. Porter and Edward Ponsonby.

Benson, Rev. C.W.. 1886. *Our Irish Song Birds*. Dublin: Hodges Figgis and Co.

Browne, P. 1774. 'A Catalogue of the Birds of Ireland, whether Natives, Casual Visitors or Birds of Passage, Taken from Observation; Classed and Disposed According to Linnaeus.' *The Gentleman's and London Magazine: or, Monthly Chronologer*. Dublin: Exshaw.

Burkitt, J.P. 1924-6. 'A Study of the Robin by Means of Marked Birds.' *Brit. Birds 17*: 294-303; *18*: 97-103; *19*: 120-4; *20*: 91-101.

Cramp, S., W.R.P. Bourne and D. Saunders. 1974. *The Seabirds of Britain and Ireland*. London: Collins.

D'Arcy, G. 1981. *The Guide to the Birds of Ireland*. Dublin: Irish Wildlife Publications.

Deane, C.D. 1954. *Handbook of the Birds of Northern Ireland*. Bulletin of the Belfast Museum and Art Gallery 1: 6.

Giraldus Cambrensis (Gerald of Wales). Trans. John J. O'Meara, 1982. *The History and Topography of Ireland*. London: Penguin Books.

Hutchinson, C.D. 1979. *Ireland's Wetlands and their Birds*. Dublin: Irish Wildbird Conservancy.

Hutchinson, C.D. 1989. *Birds in Ireland*. Calton: T & A.D. Poyser.

Kennedy, Rev. P.G. 1953. *An Irish Sanctuary – Birds of the North Bull*. Dublin: At the Sign of the Three Candles.

Kennedy, Rev. P.G., R.F. Ruttledge, and C.F. Scroope. 1954. *The Birds of Ireland*. London and Edinburgh: Oliver & Boyd.

Moffat, C.B. 1903. 'The Spring Rivalry of Birds.' *Irish Nat. 33*: 25-9.

Moriarty, C. 1986. 'Of Bird Groups and Birding,' in *Reflections and Recollections: 100 Years of the Dublin Naturalists' Field Club*. Dublin: DNFC.

Moriarty, C. 1988. 'Birds and Bird People,' in *In the Field of the Naturalists: Proceedings of the D.N.F.C. Centenary Seminar*. Dublin: DNFC.

Patten, C.F. 1906. *The Aquatic Birds of Great Britain and Ireland*. London: R.H. Porter.

Payne-Gallwey, Sir R. [1882] 1985. *The Fowler in Ireland*. London: John van Voorst. Rpt. Shedfield, Hampshire: Ashford.

Praeger, R.L. 1931. *The Way that I Went*. Dublin: Hodges Figgis.

Praeger, R.L. 1941. *A Populous Solitude*. Dublin: Hodges Figgis.

Praeger, R.L. 1949. *Some Irish Naturalists: A Biographical Notebook*. Dundalk: Dundalgan Press.

Praeger, Robert Lloyd. 1950. *Natural History of Ireland*. London: Collins.

Ruttledge, R.F. 1950. 'A List of the Birds of the Counties Galway and Mayo, Showing their Status and Distribution.' *Proc. Roy. Ir. Acad. 52 B*: 315-81.

Ruttledge, R.F. and R. Hall Watt. 1958. 'The Distribution and Status of Wild Geese in Ireland.' *Bird Study 5*: 22-33.

Rutty, J. 1772. *An Essay towards a Natural History of the County of Dublin*. 2 vols. Dublin: W. Sleator.

Sharrock, J.T.R. 1976. *The Atlas of Breeding Birds in Britain and Ireland*. Berkhamsted: T & AD Poyser.

Thompson, W. 1849-56. *The Natural History of Ireland*. 4 vols. London: Reeve, Benham and Reeve.

Ussher, R.J. and R. Warren. 1900. *Birds of Ireland*. London: Gurney and Jackson.

Watters, J.J. 1853. *The Natural History of the Birds of Ireland*. Dublin: James McGlashan.

Yarrell, W. 1871-85. *A History of British Birds*. 4th ed. (revised and enlarged by Alfred Newton and Howard Saunders). 4 vols. London: John van Voorst.

Fish and Fisheries

CHRISTOPHER MORIARTY

Fish and Fishing in Antiquity

The earliest inhabitants of Ireland known to archaeology were the Mesolithic hunter-gatherers whose encampments have been found in a number of places beside rivers and at the seaside. They arrived about nine thousand years ago. One of the major sites is Mount Sandel on the River Bann, excavated by Peter Woodman (1985). The significance of Edmund Spenser's 'fruitful fishy Bann' is that it remains to this day the most productive source of eels in the country. Eels are highly exploitable and can be caught from the river-bank using simple equipment. In April or May the young elvers, newly arrived from the ocean, enter freshwater in enormous numbers. At waterfalls, they actually leave the water to wriggle over damp stones where they can be easily caught by hand. In unobstructed streams, the greatest numbers swim close to the bank where hand-nets can reach them. Growing eels, after the elver stage, can often be caught by turning over the stones where they lie hidden. Where the river bed is muddy, eels can be speared throughout the winter as well as in the warmer months. The characteristic stone artefact of the Mesolithic people is the 'microlith', a small flint point believed to be part of a wooden fishing spear. In autumn, fully grown eels migrate seawards and they are still caught on the Bann using walls of wattle – woven rods of hazel. The construction of such walls would have been well within the capabilities of a Mesolithic community. The Bann also provided salmon, trout, sea-bass and flounder and probably other species.

It is possible that Fionn Mac Cumhail and his tradition may have survived from the time of the hunter-gatherers. Whatever his date in history, one of the best-loved of the stories about him has an important place in the relationship between fish and Irishman. This relates that nine hazels of wisdom grow beside the well that lies hidden near the source of the River

Boyne. Once in seven years their nuts fall into the water and are eaten by a salmon, which thus inherits wisdom. He who first eats this salmon will attain to all knowledge. Fionn went to the Boyne to learn the art of poetry from Finegas, who had waited there for seven long years to capture the salmon. To cut a long and delightful tale short, Fionn accidentally tasted the salmon and deprived Finegas of his prize.

Salmon seldom, if ever, eat hazel nuts, and scientists might question the plausibility of this means of transmitting learning. But the story may point to something more. The Neolithic farmers suffered from severe scarcity of food in winter, as did Irish farming communities for thousands of years after them. Preservation and storage of food were never easy. However, large salmon in the peak of condition enter the Boyne soon after mid-winter and make their way upstream towards the tributaries where they spawn. The salmon run continues at least until the month of May and enabled communities living by the Boyne to enjoy abundant food all through the season, when the majority of people subsisted only with difficulty. It may be no coincidence that the greatest Neolithic civilization known to Ireland was centred in Newgrange in the Boyne valley. This culture's wisdom, great engineering skills and considerable knowledge of astronomy command respect to this day; it is not surprising that the region came to be looked on as an abode of gods. The Boyne people's diet of salmon would have been well known to those who lived in less favoured regions, and a simple deduction on their part would have suggested that the salmon was the fountain of their knowledge.

Fionn Mac Cumhail and his followers (the Fianna) feasted on salmon and eel from the River Shannon, and over and over again they praised the salmon in their poetry. The saga of Fionn includes a very early reference to catching salmon with rod and line in which a companion of Diarmuid Ó Duibhne went into a wood on the banks of the River Laune and 'picked in it a straight long rod from a rowan tree and put a hair and a hook upon the rod, and put a berry upon the hook and went on the stream, and took a fish that cast. He put up the second berry and killed the second fish and he put up the third berry and killed the third fish' (Gregory, 1904). Not only does the tale place the technique far back in history, but it gives a very respectable antiquity to the ability of the honest angler to embroider his prowess.

The absence from Ireland of purely freshwater fish was noticed as early as the twelfth century by Giraldus Cambrensis in his *Topographia Hiberniae* (O'Meara, 1951). Arthur Went, in the course of his studies of the history of Irish fisheries (1946), traced records of the earliest mention or introduction of a number of species. The first reference to the pike in Ireland just makes the sixteenth century – Spenser mentioned it in *Epithalamion* (1595):

Ye Nymphes of Mulla, which with carefull heed,
The silver scaly trouts doo tend full well,
The greedy pikes which use therein to feed,
(Those trouts and fishes all others doo excell)
And ye likewise which keepe the rushy lake,
Where none doo fishes take.

The reference to the rushy lake is very interesting. Unless they had been introduced by man, there would be no trout in an isolated lake, nor any other freshwater fish. Carp and tench were first brought to Ireland early in the seventeenth century by the first Earl of Cork. Species such as perch, bream, gudgeon, minnow, rudd and loach appeared between then and the eighteenth century, but Went failed to trace specific references to their arrival. Roach and dace escaped from two cans of live bait into the Munster Blackwater in 1889. The introduced species subsequently spread throughout many river systems.

Early references to sea-fish are very few: they are mentioned in passing in the diet of the Fianna, and Giraldus stated that the sea coasts 'abounded sufficiently' with them. In Viking Dublin, cod and ling bones have been found, to say nothing of abundant cockles and mussels and smaller numbers of other molluscs, including oysters and scallops (Mitchell, 1987).

The greatest Irish achievement in fisheries in medieval times was the discovery of a technique of mussel culture. In 1235 an Irish merchant seaman named Walton survived shipwreck near La Rochelle on the Bay of Biscay. He settled on the shore of the Bay of Aiguillon where he used a large net attached to poles to catch the wading birds as they flew low over the mud. Enormous numbers of mussels settled on the poles. Walton is credited with the idea of setting up an array of stakes, with interlacing branches to provide additional anchorages for the mussels (Wilkins, 1989). The system has remained in use to this day, but history does not relate whether it was tried in Ireland before the twentieth century.

References to fishing rights are virtually absent from Fergus Kelly's *Early Irish Law* (1988), which deals with the Brehon laws from the seventh century. The sole reference is to the right of a landowner to erect a fishing weir on or adjacent to his neighbour's land. It is significant that this issue was sufficiently important to merit a place in the law. Fishing weirs exist in rivers in most parts of the world and always indicate a considerable degree of knowledge of the migratory habits of certain species: in Ireland of the salmon and the eel. The weir has one or more gaps or 'eyes' in which nets are placed and for salmon the opening faces downstream as the mature salmon journeys in from the sea. For eels the opposite arrangement is made as the adult eel migrates towards the ocean.

Legal ownership of fishing rights, for salmon above all others, has been traced in many rivers and set down in detail in many papers, including one on the Liffey (Went, 1953). Whether the Irish enforced such rights prior to the Norman Conquest is uncertain. Went quotes a great many records of fishery ownership and disputes from the twelfth century onwards. The purpose of the restrictions is far from clear: there seems to be no mention of knowledge of the need to conserve sufficient stock for spawning; the exercise of ownership may simply have been to hoard a valuable property. However, concern over salmon did lead to water pollution legislation. The Corporation of Dublin, a major owner of fishing rights, ordered in 1466 'that no tanner, glover nor any person use limed ware or leather work in the River Liffey on account of the destruction of the salmon. Penalty 3/4d for each offence, one half to be paid to the detector and 1/2d to the court.'

Sea-fisheries from the Fourteenth to Sixteenth Centuries

Timothy O'Neill, in his study of medieval Irish trade (1987), makes it clear that major fisheries were in progress in Irish coastal waters. Herring were caught in the Irish Sea and off the west and south-west coasts throughout the fourteenth, fifteenth and sixteenth centuries and a fishery developed to the north-west towards the end of the sixteenth. Cod, ling, hake and haddock also appear regularly in official papers for both domestic trade and export. Salmon and eel naturally continued to be of major importance, though eel apparently were used mainly for local consumption and records of their export are few.

The most interesting account of the history of Irish fisheries is that published in 1902 by William Spotswood Green who, we will see, was himself the most influential individual in that history. Until the seventeenth century, a large share of the fishery was taken by foreign vessels, usually on payment of substantial sums of money to the Crown or to major warlords. Ireland did little compared with its European neighbours to develop an indigenous fishing industry. One reason, Green suggested, was that the Irish were largely pastoralists who enjoyed a rich, if ill-balanced, diet largely of fresh meat: 'With such a complete menu, varied in some places by an abundance of salmon, sea-fishing was an unnecessary employment, and could not have been attractive to a population mainly pastoral.'

The reports on the trade indicate little more than an awareness of the existence of the inshore sea fish and an ability to capture them in large numbers. Scientific observation on the fish had to wait for the work of Roderic O'Flaherty in the seventeenth century. He lists fifteen marine finfish and nine freshwater species together with shrimp, lobster, crab, goose barnacle and the freshwater pearl mussel and five marine molluscs. The sea, in addition, 'now and then casts ashore great whales, gramps, porcupisses, thunies'. His observations are systematic and set out in descriptions of the lakes, rivers and bays of western Connaught. The sea-fish named are those which can be caught inshore from small boats. Herring and pilchard require nets but the others can be taken on baited lines.

Two of O'Flaherty's tales are particularly interesting. The first has the air of a fish story, but sounds as if the exaggeration is only of the size of the eel in question and of its burden:

From hence [Cong] an eele carryed a purse of 13s 4d sterling, and a knife, for about sixteen miles through Lough Orbsen, till it was catched on the river of Galway; which thus happened. One William McGhoill, a fisherman at Cong, lighted on a good eel; and being busie about catching more, thrust his girdle through its guill, which had the purse and knife on it; the eel by chance slides into the river with the purse and knife.

It must have been a very good eel. But the recapture of an eel at Galway is entirely plausible since all the migrants from Cong must go to sea in Galway through the River Corrib.

The second O'Flaherty story is a remarkable description of a true research project, perhaps the first experiment in animal behaviour to be recorded in Ireland. It deals with the Ballinahinch River in Galway, still a renowned salmon fishery:

This river springs from Balynahinsy lake, two miles from the sea. It is shallow and full of wares and stones, from the lake down, for a mile, to Wine Island; on which island is a salmon fishing, worth £30 a year. On this island experience was made how the salmon hath still recourse from the sea to its first offspring; for here, eighteen salmon were marked, with a finn cut of each of them at their going to the sea, and seavneteen [sic] of them were taken next season, in the same place, coming back.

The recovery of seventeen out of eighteen sounds too good to be true, and it seems likely that somebody adjusted the actual results. However, there is no good reason to doubt that the experiment did take place and the conclusion, establishing the very strong homing instinct of salmon, has been tested and confirmed over and over again.

The Dublin Society and Eighteenth-Century Developments

Fifty years or more were to pass before there is further evidence of a scientific approach to fisheries. The Dublin Society was founded in 1731 and incorporated by Royal Charter in 1820 to encourage the application of scientific principles to many fields of development. Went (1981) has given an outline of its work in fisheries. On 1 November 1733, a paper on the destruction of fisheries by trawling was read and 'recommended to those of the Society, who are members of Parliament'. Objections to trawling were to continue to be made through the Royal Dublin Society and through other channels until well into the nineteenth century. These stemmed mainly from the perfectly reasonable but generally false belief that the marine fish spawned on the bottom as trout and salmon were known to do.

Until the end of the eighteenth century the Dublin Society spent considerable sums of money by way of 'premiums' to encourage the development of the fishing industry. Attention was paid in particular to the provision of salt, the only effective preservative available on a large scale, and to improving the distribution of fish both for home consumption and for export. Funds for much of this work were provided by Parliament, with the Society acting to a great extent as an agency of the government, though strictly preserving its own identity.

The eighteenth century saw three more significant steps taken by the Society: distribution of charts of the coast, provision of marker buoys and the building of quays, and the translation and publication of continental treatises on fishing. Four of these were published in 1800: one on fishing for herring, cod and salmon, a Dutch essay on the herring fishery, and two works on salmon and trout.

Fisheries in the Nineteenth Century

Studies of fish and fisheries followed three parallel paths through the nineteenth century. Commercial fishing in the sea received attention in varying degrees. The artificial culture of fish and molluscs developed in a remarkable way. And naturalists, beginning with John Templeton and reaching their most distinguished in William Thompson, set to work in systematic ichthyology, the scientific classification of fish species.

The liberal distribution of premiums, according to Green, was not altogether beneficial. It did indeed lead to a spectacular increase in the numbers of Irish vessels and, of course, in men employed and communities fed. By 1829 the number of men engaged in the Irish fisheries had reached 64,771. But the industry was so dependent on government bounties that, when these ceased in the same year, there was a rapid collapse.

By this time the population of Ireland was approaching its peak of over eight million. Then came the failure of the potato crop beginning in 1845 and the consequent disastrous population decline. The seagoing fleet was already reduced and, even if fish had been available on the market, the subsistence farming communities would have had no money to buy them. There are some indications, however, that the coastal populations fared a little better than those dwelling inland. Quaker-organized famine relief work made an important contribution to the local fishing industries (Johnson and Goodbody, 1996).

A curious side issue was the pursuit of the sunfish, or basking shark. The most recent of many authors who have been inspired by the glamour of the fishery was Kenneth McNally, whose excellent book *The Sun-fish Hunt* was published in 1976. These enormous but peaceable fishes swim inshore in spring and early summer. Thanks to their habit of lying close to the surface and their lack of fear of man or boat, they are easily harpooned. The fact that a large shark was about the same size as the curragh used in the hunt introduced a considerable element of danger to the fishermen. The prize was the liver of the shark, which yields on average 250 kilograms of valuable oil. This was used for lamp-lighting and other purposes in the nineteenth century and, more recently, for specialized purposes including the tempering of steel and the lubrication of delicate machinery. The fishery declined in the latter half of the nineteenth century, but was revived on Achill Island in 1947 to enjoy a further thirty years of profitable existence for a small number of fishermen and shore-based workers.

Estuarine and freshwater fisheries in the nineteenth century were concentrated mainly on salmon and eel. Both species were exploited by stake nets, box cribs and other permanent structures described in law as 'fixed engines'. Salmon were also captured by net, and in some of the larger estuaries there were 'sprat weirs' which caught a great variety of small fish (Went, 1959). Unrestricted use of fixed engines for salmon led to something approaching warfare between fishermen, prompting the establishment of stringent conditions to reduce the numbers and effectiveness of the traps. Commercial fishing in fresh water for other species was limited, the major exception being the pollan of Lough Neagh which were caught in large quantities. William Thompson (1856) mentions the capture of more than seventeen thousand at one time in 1734, the greatest catch ever remembered by the fishermen: 'They altogether filled five one-horse carts.' Pollan were sold locally and transported to Belfast and sometimes exported to England. Char, however, were captured for pig feed where they were abundant, as were elvers.

In 1820 the Dublin Society received its first Royal Charter and came to be known as the Royal Dublin Society. Its interest in fish continued through the nineteenth century. An influential figure in natural-history studies in Ireland over a considerable part of the century was William Andrews. Born in England in 1802, he spent most of his life in Dublin and was a founder member in 1838 of the Natural History Society of Dublin. Between 1861 and 1877 he published nine papers in fishery science in the *Journal of the Royal Dublin Society* (Mollan, 1987). His papers described the cod, ling, herring and salmon fisheries of Ireland and also dealt with the subject of the fishing industry. At the same time Andrews was an enthusiastic collector of marine organisms and published important species lists from the south coast. These studies added considerably to the basic understanding of the requirements of fisheries and dispelled many misconceptions. Their importance, however, lay more in the way of maintaining a tradition within the Society of an appreciation of the need to develop the fishing industry and to approach this on a scientific basis.

Aquaculture

Noel Wilkins (1989) gives a comprehensive account of the remarkable development of aquaculture in Victorian times in his book *Ponds, Passes and Parcs*. The greatest successes were achieved in the extensive culture of salmon and of oysters. Wilkins gives pride of place to the work of the astronomer Edward Joshua Cooper (1798-1863), owner of Markree Castle and Observatory in Co. Sligo. 'Of all the Irish aquaculture ventures in the nineteenth century, that at Ballisodare, Co. Sligo, was the very first, the most successful and the most enduring. It reflects the skilled management and innovative approach of three generations of the Cooper family who continue to this day to own and manage the fishery which is synonymous with their name.'

The splendid waterfall that flows into the estuary at Ballisodare is too high for salmon to ascend and therefore they were absent from the river system above it. After some years of artificially stocking the waters upstream, Cooper in 1852 and 1853 built salmon ladders to take the adults past the falls and in 1856 built the first hatchery. The venture was a complete success and the annual catch of salmon numbered in thousands. The 1850s also saw salmon hatchery schemes in the Corrib and other river systems. There was one attempt to rear salmon at sea in a cage: artificially reared smolts were released into a tidal tank in Kingstown (Dun Laoghaire) Harbour, but the experiment failed, largely because the supply of food was inadequate. More than a hundred years were to pass before this technique would meet with success.

Oyster culture came a little later than salmon rearing, although the licensing of oyster beds had begun in 1846. There were continuous problems in enforcing ownership of the licensed beds. Indiscriminate capture of young oysters can deplete a bed very quickly, but carefully controlled fishing, including the replacement of all small specimens, is usually very successful. From 1864 onwards the Commissioners of Fisheries encouraged oyster culture, initially publishing guidebooks based on foreign publications. In 1868 a commission of four members was set up and instructed to visit oyster culture installations on the British and French coasts and also to inspect the Irish oyster fisheries. They published a report in 1870 which advised measures such as the re-laying of small oysters but did not encourage the collection of the newly settled 'spat' (i.e. spawn). One reason for this was the irregularity of oyster breeding on the Irish coast, where in some years the water is not warm enough for success. Sadly, although the principles of oyster farming were clearly understood and widely known, the practice met with little success in the absence of effective policing and the industry declined in the final decades of the century.

Fauna Studies

While William Andrews studied fisheries, William Thompson was studying the fishes. Born in 1805 into a relatively affluent family, Thompson while working in the family linen business spent much of his leisure time hunting and walking in the country. By 1832 he had retired from the linen business and devoted himself to the study of the fauna of Ireland, systematically collecting material and corresponding with observers in all parts of the country. His aim was to write a monumental work dealing with the entire fauna. His early death in 1852 prevented any such achievement. He had published extensively in the major natural history journals and completed three volumes on Irish birds. He left also a large collection of manuscript notes on the remaining vertebrates and invertebrates, and his will requested that his friends Robert Patterson and James Garrett 'undertake the duties of superintending editors of same, in order that the whole may be carefully edited'. This they did faithfully, and the final volume of *Natural History of Ireland* runs to 548 pages, of which 199 deal with the fishes and nearly two hundred more cover the invertebrates.

Thompson described a number of species new to science, of which one, the pearlfish, has survived all attempts to unite it with others. His friend Dr James L. Drummond had picked up a dead specimen on the shore at Carnlough, Co. Antrim, and Thompson named it *Echiodon drummondii* in his honour in 1837. To this day it remains a little-known species that is believed to live parasitically within the bodies of sea cucumbers.

The pollan of Lough Neagh, at the time a very popular market fish in Belfast, Thompson named *Coregonus pollan* in 1838, but with characteristic modesty suggested that it might not be a new species – 'being fully aware that the same species is often very differently described by different authors, and under the impression that it may eventually prove identical with some of the continental Coregoni, with which I have not had an opportunity of comparing it ...'. He regarded the much rarer Lough Erne pollan as belonging to the same species, but proposed a different name for the even scarcer Lough Derg pollan. At present all three are considered to be vendace, described by Linnaeus in 1758 as *Coregonus albula*, but that may be far from the end of the story and Thompson's view may yet return to favour.

Thompson gives a good list of localities for the char which includes a number of important nineteenth-century populations, such as those of Lough Neagh in the north *(plate 19)* and Lough Owel in Co. Westmeath, that are now extinct. Like the pollan, the char is a survivor from early post-glacial times and is relatively rare, with a discontinuous distribution, as present populations are isolated from each other and have no obvious link between them, genetic or otherwise. Thompson had noticed the variation in appearance between separate populations and considered that this was a result of habitat differences rather than an indication of separate species.

The Research Cruises of the 1890s

The Royal Irish Academy's initiative in deep-sea faunal studies in 1885 was followed very quickly by a decision of the Royal Dublin Society to develop scientific investigation of the sea fisheries. The headquarters of the Royal Irish Academy and the Royal Dublin Society were but a short walk away from each other, and there was a considerable overlap in membership. In 1887 the Royal Dublin Society Council appointed a fisheries committee, which in turn commissioned W.S. Green to collect information on the fisheries of the south-west and suggest how the industry in Ireland could best be promoted. Between 1887 and 1889 he made an extensive investigation of the situation in Ireland and a valuable comparative study on the North American Atlantic coast.

One important economic outcome of the transatlantic visit was to establish a major export trade in salt mackerel from Ireland to the United States. There was in the U.S. a considerable demand for the commodity because of a regulation that alcoholic drink could be served only as part of a meal. A piece of salt mackerel legally constituted the required repast. As it happened, indeed perhaps as a consequence of the regulation, mackerel had become scarce on the American coast. Green was able to learn the accepted way of smoking and introduced the technique to Ireland. The industry developed quickly and continued to thrive – apart from a break in the 1914-18 war years – until the 1930s and the imposition of a salt duty.

However, Green's work was to have much farther-reaching results than this. The government in 1890 appointed him as one of three Inspectors of Irish Fisheries. At the same time, in 1890-91 the Royal Dublin Society, with the assistance of a government subvention, conducted surveys of fishing potential around the entire coast of Ireland.

Green not only planned the cruises, but chartered the vessels and skip-

pered for part of the time. In April 1890, in his first task of actually finding and hiring a suitable vessel, he chartered the 158-ton steam yacht
Fingal. In early May they left Cobh, Co. Cork, heading south-westwards,
and then travelled north as far as Killybegs, Co. Donegal, where the
exploratory trip ended in August. Alfred Cort Haddon, 'Naturalist to the
Survey', Professor of Zoology in the Royal College of Science in Ireland
and a pioneer in marine biology, was responsible for recruiting the scientific personnel. He later moved to Cambridge and transformed his interests
from marine fauna to people, attaining equal distinction as a founder of
modern anthropology.

A number of eminent scientists took part in the *Fingal* cruise: ornithologists, entomologists and even an anatomist. The team also included scientists besides Green who were primarily interested in fisheries matters, in
particular Ernest W.L. Holt, T.H. Poole and C.H.T. Beamish. The following year Green chartered the steam yacht *Harlequin* and with Holt again
made the trip from Cobh to Killybegs. They were joined on the way by
Haddon. From Killybegs they headed north to Lough Foyle on the north
coast, then down the east coast, ending in Kingstown, Co. Dublin.

The research work undertaken on the voyages ranged widely. Poole and
Beamish made the first extensive oceanographic records in Irish waters,
recording temperatures and salinities. Various fishing gears were investigated and detailed measurements of the quantities and sizes of the specimens
in the catch were recorded. The first descriptions of eggs and larvae of a
number of fish species were published in the scientific literature. This was
mainly the work of Holt, the 'Assistant Naturalist', who in the course of the
next few years published a series of detailed papers on the fishes and crustacea, including much descriptive work on species then little known to science. These papers are illustrated with his beautiful drawings, all the more
remarkable for having been executed on shipboard.

Green always took the opportunity to visit fishermen and local enthusiasts when the yachts arrived in port. Voluminous reports on all aspects of
the cruises were published and to this day provide valuable source material
on both the Irish marine fauna and the potential for fishery development.
The study also had a dramatic effect on the local economy, as Green wrote
in 1902: 'At the time of the survey there were practically no fisheries of
importance on the west coast, and the great development which has since
taken place may be attributed in large measure to the information which was
obtained by the survey.'

The next great step was to be taken in 1898, and Green may be quoted once more. A modest man, he makes no reference to his own considerable influence in the establishment of Ireland's first marine laboratory: 'In
1898 the Royal Dublin Society once more entered the field of fisheries

research, and, having obtained from Her Majesty's Treasury a grant of money equal to half the proposed cost, proceeded to establish a Marine Laboratory for the purpose of studying, for a period of five years, the various problems affecting the mackerel fishery and the proceedings of salmon in the sea. The Laboratory commenced work in February 1899.'

Mobility of the laboratory was considered to be essential, so the approach already adopted by the Danish government was followed. The 220-ton brigantine *Saturn* was converted to a floating laboratory with spacious and comfortable accommodation. She was berthed on the Mayo/Galway coast in Ballynakill Harbour in winter and off Inishbofin in summer, towed to her place of work and anchored there while a number of smaller vessels were employed in providing the fish for study. The sites were selected because of their proximity to Cleggan, then the headquarters of one of the principal mackerel fisheries.

The Establishment of Fisheries Research

In 1900 a permanent fishery research body, based in Dublin, was set up by the Department of Agriculture and Technical Instruction for Ireland; Green, now promoted to Chief Inspector, was placed in charge of it. The research team grew in the early years of the century, reaching a peak with eight scientists in 1905. These were the permanent staff, but there were additional 'temporary' workers not recorded in the published lists of 'officers'. Among the latter was Anne L. Massy, who became a leading international expert on a number of groups of molluscs, particularly squids, collected on the Irish expeditions and on international research cruises. She published important monographs on various groups from 1901 until her death thirty years later – a temporary employee to the end.

Also in 1900 the steam cruiser *Helga* was partly transferred from fishery-protection duties to research-cruise duties and was used in a programme to study the life history of the food fishes. Much of the ship's time was devoted to taking part in internationally planned cruises studying fish eggs, plankton and hydrography under the auspices of the International Council for the Exploration of the Sea. The council had been established in 1902 to co-ordinate research in the waters shared by the countries of northern and western Europe. The first international scientific body in the world, its Irish members have continued to play a major part in its work.

Green served as Chief Inspector until his retirement in 1915 and was succeeded by Ernest Holt, who died in office in 1922. Two of their junior officers were George P. Farran and Rowland W. Southern. Between them these four were responsible for some of the most important basic accounts of Irish fisheries science. The first decade of the century saw the publication of no fewer than seventy-seven scientific papers. Holt, in the Department's Annual Report for 1906, laid down the principles underlying the scientific investigations:

For the most part these [Atlantic waters], previous to the inception of the Department's work, were aquae incognitae, and in consequence we have to deal with a vast number of organisms, the presence of which on or near our coast was unsuspected or at least unrecorded, while many of them are new to human observation. Before proceeding to an orderly survey of the distributional relationships of these forms as elements of the whole fauna and to speculations as to their influence upon the present or probable future objects of commercial fisheries it is essential to obtain a knowledge of them individually. Their treatment, therefore, on a strictly zoological basis is to be regarded not as a diversion of the energies of fishery officials into the realms of what is called pure science, but as a preliminary to the necessary collation of all the factors which may affect the commercial fish supply.

Fisheries after 1918

The war years tragically saw a great reduction in research effort, and the death in action of A.C. Hillas, one of the younger members of the biological team. Although the government of the newly independent Irish Free State had a Minister for Fisheries for a while, the importance of research was not fully appreciated and staff numbers remained low until 1959, though Farran and Southern continued to carry out important work. Wartime food shortages had led them to begin studies of freshwater fish and their habitats in 1917. In 1920 a Limnological Laboratory was established, again a vessel at anchor, in Lough Derg on the River Shannon, and observations on freshwater plankton and on the food and growth of trout were published. Southern's samples of trout were small, as specimens were collected by rod and line after the day's work in the laboratory – an idyllic but inefficient technique. The Limnological Laboratory was closed in 1923 and Southern returned to Dublin where he made further close studies of trout and salmon. He was the anonymous author of an authoritative *Angler's Guide* in 1924. Its publication marked the beginning of serious consideration of the sport-fishing sector, which has developed to become today the most important element in inland fisheries, attracting many thousands of Irish, British and continental fishermen each season.

Two young English scientists were appointed to the Free State's fishery research team – Winifred E. Frost in 1928 and Arthur E.J. Went in 1936. This was perhaps remarkable at a time of vigorous nationalism. Two factors must have played a part: Frost and Went were both exceptionally talented scientists, and very little biology and practically no field studies were taught in Ireland at the time. The two English scientists added to Southern's ecological studies of trout and young salmon in Ireland, working mainly in the River Liffey, where because of the geological substrate they had the opportunity to compare fish and invertebrate populations in acid upstream and lime-rich downstream portions of the same river.

In 1939 Frost left to take up a post at the new laboratory of the Freshwater Biological Association on Lake Windermere in England. Went remained in Dublin where he specialized in the growth and migration of salmon, his work providing the essential baseline material on the species. Even though Green in 1900 had accepted that the salmon was the most valuable fish in the Irish economy, salmonid research at the beginning of the century was limited to straightforward marking experiments. Green may have felt that it was more important to concentrate on the less valuable species.

Went, in addition to his overriding interest in salmon, was an enthusiastic recorder of unusual fish and an amateur historian of formidable energy. He devoted much of his spare time to research on the history of Irish fisheries, giving particular attention to records of ownership of salmon-fishing rights, many of which have been well documented from the twelfth century onwards. In a review paper on 'The Pursuit of Salmon in Ireland' (1964) he set out the early records of rod-fishing in Ireland, beginning with the tale of the mythical Diarmuid Ó Duibhne, after whose time there is little recorded until 1593 or later. A reference in the State Papers tells that 'Tirone and his young lady lie at Castleroe for a time. They are salmon fishing on the Bann.' This is far from being a clear reference to the use of the rod but there is no doubt about a record of the Blake family in 1633 as owners of a salmon fishery near the town of Galway in which they had the right to 'one-fourth part of every salmon and trout taken by angling'. The Liffey is mentioned in connection with angling in 1706, and in 1791 comes the first reference to 'salmon flies'.

In 1958, after the lean period from the 1920s to the 1950s, expansion and modernization in the Irish Republic began when the Minister for Lands, Erskine Childers, accepted the view of the scientists that the research sector needed to be greatly expanded. Five biologists were appointed in 1959, doubling the size of the team. Around the same time an Inland Fisheries Trust funded by the State was established and the Sea Fisheries Board was greatly strengthened. This period also marked a considerable change in the scientific approach from largely direct observation to present-day mathematical modelling of the stocks. In the north, following partition, fisheries were in the control of the Department of Agriculture and Fisheries and the 1960s saw the establishment of their first Fisheries Research Laboratory at Coleraine, Co. Derry. All the university zoology departments became actively engaged in freshwater and marine biology.

Conclusion

Fishing has fed or entertained the people of Ireland for nine thousand years. Some aspects of its recorded history are surprising: above all, the apparent lack of interest in fish and fishing by the majority of the population throughout the ages of written history. Green may very well have put his finger on the explanation by suggesting that the people of medieval Ireland had easy access to flesh of many kinds. Throughout this period, salmon and eel remained popular, being readily obtainable without the trouble or expense of going to sea, or even setting out on a lake. Furthermore, it is easy to forget that, while salmon retain a good flavour some days after death and eels can be transported alive, most fish deteriorate rapidly after capture. Unless heavily salted, they could not be moved far from the coast until the railways came. This may be the reason that fish from monastic times until recently was considered a penitential food.

The development of inland fisheries in the eighteenth and nineteenth centuries may well have been a response to an increasing population that was no longer able to find as much meat as they wanted and willing to eat more fish. The success of the expansion of both inland and marine fisheries from the last decade of the nineteenth century owes much to the inspiration and researches of the naturalists. In their current guise as fishery scientists their work continues to be the essential factor in the survival of the fishery and its future developments.

References

Green, W.S. 1902. 'The Sea Fisheries of Ireland,' in W.P. Coyne (ed.), *Ireland Industrial and Agricultural*. Dublin: Browne and Nolan.

Gregory, A. 1904. *Gods and Fighting Men: The Story of the Tuatha de Danaan and the Fianna of Ireland*. London: John Murray

Johnson, J. and R. Goodbody (eds). 1996. *Transactions of the Central Relief Committee of the Society of Friends during the Famine in Ireland in 1846 and 1847*. Dublin: Edmund Burke Publisher.

Kelly, F. 1988. *A Guide to Early Irish Law*. Dublin: Institute for Advanced Studies.

McNally, K. 1976. *The Sun-fish Hunt*. Belfast: Blackstaff Press.

Mitchell, G.F. 1987. *Archaeology and Environment in Early Dublin*. Dublin: Royal Irish Academy.

Mollan, C.B. 1987. *Nostri Plena Laboris: An Author Index to the RDS Scientific Journals – 1800 to 1985*. Dublin: Royal Dublin Society.

O'Flaherty, R. 1978 (1684, 1846). *The Territory of West or H-Iar Connaught*. Ed. J. Hardiman, rpt. with Introduction by W.J. Hogan. Galway: Kenny's Bookshop.

O'Meara, J.J. 1951. *The First Version of the Topography of Ireland by Giraldus Cambrensis*. Dundalk: Dundalgan Press.

O'Neill, T. 1987. *Merchants and Mariners in Medieval Ireland*. Dublin: Irish Academic Press.

Thompson, W. 1849-56. *The Natural History of Ireland*, vol. 4. London: Henry G. Bohn.

Went, A.E.J. 1946. 'Irish Freshwater Fish – Some Notes on their Distribution.' *Salmon and Trout Magazine 118*: 1-9.

Went, A.E.J. 1953. 'Fisheries of the River Liffey.' *Journal of the Royal Society of Antiquaries of Ireland 83*: 163-73.

Went, A.E.J. 1959. 'Sprat or White-fish Weirs in Waterford Harbour.' *Journal of the Royal Society of Antiquaries of Ireland 89*: 91-3.

Went, A.E.J. 1964. 'The Pursuit of Salmon in Ireland.' *Proceedings of the Royal Irish Academy 63* C: 191-244.

Went, A.E.J. 1981. 'Fisheries,' in J. Meenan and D. Clarke (eds), *The Royal Dublin Society 1731-1981*. Dublin: Gill and Macmillan.

Wilkins, N.P. 1989. *Ponds, Passes and Parcs: Aquaculture in Victorian Ireland*. Dublin: Glendale.

Woodman, P.C. 1985. *Excavations at Mount Sandel 1973-77*. Belfast: HMSO.

No Stone Unturned:
Robert Lloyd Praeger and the Major Surveys

MICHAEL D. GUIRY

Background

A remarkable phenomenon of late nineteenth- and early twentieth-century natural history in Ireland was the concentration of the talents of amateur and professional biologists on large-scale projects. Field-trips, forays, dredging parties and localized surveys grew increasingly extensive and well organized, and eventually culminated in what became the best-known of all such ventures, the Clare Island Survey. These endeavours constituted the last hurrah of the Victorian naturalist in Ireland, marking a transition between the sometimes fanatical collecting and list-making of the nineteenth-century amateurs and the ecological approach that has been the hallmark of late twentieth-century biology.

Non-professional interest in biological matters was a phenomenon born out of the new-found leisure of the merchant classes, nurtured initially by the advent of the penny post and later by the increasing availability of rapid and efficient transport systems. After T.H. Huxley, J.D. Hooker and others had wrested natural science from the stultifying influence of the Established Church in England (Desmond and Moore, 1991) and made a separate profession of it, the field and microscopical clubs in Britain and Ireland blossomed to encourage all things amateur, and with them flowered the talented naturalist.

The Clare Island Survey was a magnificent example of the systematic and exhaustive cataloguing of a relatively small area and is a milestone in Irish and, indeed, European biology. Between 1909 and 1911, more than a hundred persons, both amateur and professional, took an active part in the field-work for the Survey. The Royal Irish Academy contributed enormously by its encouragement of the endeavour and by undertaking publication of the results, and is thus intimately connected with the Clare Island Survey in the minds of most Irish biologists and antiquarians. The Survey Committee, chaired by R.F. Scharff, then Keeper of Natural History in the National Museum, with R.L. Praeger as Secretary, first met in the National Library in April 1908. The committee was to consider the possibility of organizing a survey similar to that of Lambay for a western island.

Lambay, off the Dublin coast, was purchased in 1903 by Cecil Baring, a wealthy merchant banker, later third Baron Revelstoke. He and his wife called to the National Library looking for advice and were easily persuaded by Praeger to agree to a systematic investigation of the fauna and flora of Lambay, gleefully referred to in *The Way that I Went* (Praeger, 1937) as a ransacking of the island. This study was carried out between 1905 and 1906 under the direction of Praeger, and the results were published in the *Irish Naturalist* (Praeger, 1907). Some ninety organisms were added to the Irish list and seventeen species previously unrecorded in the British Isles were found.

Praeger's organizational talents stemmed in large measure from his apprenticeship from 1890 to 1893 as Hon. Secretary of the Belfast Naturalists' Field Club, in which post he was responsible for planning the various summer outings. Collins (1993) tells of Praeger 'dragooning the mixed crowd of naturalists from one place to another, dragging along the stragglers and moving on the serious collectors whose intense application to particular problems endangered the timetable'. Praeger apparently used a whistle freely to keep things on schedule.

On his move from Belfast to Dublin in 1893, he joined the Dublin Naturalists' Field Club and quickly became Hon. Secretary. Additionally, he was asked to be part of a committee whose brief was to report 'on the present state of our knowledge of the fauna and flora of Ireland, and as to what is needed to bring this up to date' (Collins, 1993). This committee subsequently became the Fauna and Flora Committee of the Royal Irish Academy, which thrives to this day, having appropriately changed its name in 1955 to the Praeger Committee. It is partly funded by a bequest from the Praeger estate.

Irish Field Club Union conferences, with the aim of improving knowledge of the national biological heritage, were held at three-yearly intervals at various locations starting with Galway in July 1895, of which a detailed account is given by Collins (1993). Again, Praeger was primarily responsible for the organization of what were essentially field trips, and he doubtless made many friends and contacts that would serve him well in later endeavours. Although the naturalists' field clubs and similar societies were somewhat facetiously known as 'Field and Flirtation Societies' (Allen, 1988), their activities were scientifically beyond reproach and clearly they provided a solid foundation for the later detailed studies of Lambay and Clare Island. It is abundantly clear that Praeger was the cornerstone of these activities.

Robert Lloyd Praeger

Robert Lloyd Praeger (1865-1953) was born in Belfast, the son of Willem Emil Praeger from the Netherlands and Maria Patterson, daughter of Robert Patterson. Maria Patterson was a member of a remarkable family of Belfast naturalists, from whom Praeger claimed in *Some Irish Naturalists* (1949) to have inherited his passion for natural history. Praeger was named for his maternal uncle Sir Robert Lloyd Patterson, with whom he struck up a particularly firm friendship in later life. Surprisingly, for one who confessed to having written his first nature poem at the age of five (Collins, 1985) and who joined the Belfast Naturalists' Field Club at the tender age of eleven, Praeger's primary degrees from Queen's College, Belfast (now Queen's University) were in Arts and Engineering. His lack of interest in a formal training in natural history seems to have stemmed from his aversion to the way in which the subject was taught at the universities of the time. He bluntly states his dislike of examinations in *A Populous Solitude* (1941): 'The whole system by which young people stuff themselves full of facts and theories, which with luck, will help them to answer a few of an examiner's questions, following which most of them will serve no further purpose throughout life, was always distasteful to me, and the harvest that examiners glean must often I think make them ready to weep ... '

These are sentiments with which many a contemporary examiner and student would now agree. Scraping through his examinations after much 'matutinal cramming', he graduated from Queen's with a B.A. in 1885 and a B.E. in 1886. Praeger then reluctantly took employment in civil engineering and became deeply involved in the activities of the Belfast Naturalists' Field Club. At this time the Club was a very active mixture of professionals and amateurs, many of whom were extraordinarily gifted. It is significant, in the light of later events, to note that Praeger immediately assumed a diligent role in the organization of the Club's field activities and excursions.

Praeger was exceedingly well connected: in 1888 he was invited to take part in a dredging party aboard the *Flying Falcon* off the south and west coasts of Ireland in the august company of Charles Ball (of the talented and well-known Ball family of Youghal in Co. Cork), William Spotswood Green (zoologist and Chief Inspector of Fisheries, also of Youghal), William Francis de Vismes Kane (zoologist and entomologist), Joseph Wright (amateur geologist and protozoologist), and others. To be dredging in such princely company at the age of twenty-three is testimony indeed to the great regard in which Praeger was held, even as a neophyte. From 1888 to 1891 he found irregular and seemingly unsatisfactory employment as a civil engineer while privately trying to indulge his interests in Quaternary geology and in the botany of the north-east of Ireland. He was elected to the Royal Irish Academy in 1891 at the age of twenty-six, beginning what became a life-long association.

In 1892 he and George Carpenter, then an assistant in the National Museum in Dublin, founded the *Irish Naturalist*. Under their joint editor-ship the journal appeared virtually every month for the next thirty-three years and flourished for much of this time. The *Irish Naturalist* was ideally suited as a forum for the many naturalists, natural history societies and field clubs that graced Ireland during this uniquely peaceful period of its histo-ry. That these were also stable times economically is testified to by the fact that the cover price of the *Irish Naturalist*, 6d. (six old pence), did not change in the first twenty-eight years of its life. Its demise was hastened, perhaps prophetically, by the aftermath of the 1916 Easter Rising during which fire destroyed the presses used for printing and the stock of five years' back numbers (Collins, 1985).* The place of the *Irish Naturalist* was taken by the *Irish Naturalists' Journal*, which continues publication to this day and admirably fulfils the function of its illustrious predecessor.

Moving to Dublin in 1893, in a truly remarkable career volte-face, Praeger obtained a post as Librarian in the National Library in which he remained until his retirement in 1923. Though a successful librarian, Praeger was first and foremost a dedicated and gifted field botanist. After five years of the most gruelling investigations, during which he spent two hundred days on fieldwork in thirty-three of the forty biological subdivisions of Ireland, mostly on a part-time basis, he published *Irish Topographical Botany* (1901), an astonishing compilation of knowledge relating to the vascular flora of Ireland. Praeger's travels during the course of this study and later are enchantingly described in *The Way that I Went* – a book that, even today, the zealous tourist in Ireland cannot be without – and *A Populous Solitude*, a mellifluous account of his country and his life. The now rather dated *Natural History of Ireland* (1950) was a valuable work of reference in its time and certainly has not been replaced by any comparable single volume useful to professional and amateur alike. Praeger was clearly very proud of his orga-nizational ability as regards both fieldwork and surveys, as he stresses this in the account he wrote of himself in *Some Irish Naturalists*, a book that oth-erwise suffers somewhat from fading memories. His research output was Herculean: starting in 1885 he is credited with 789 publications (Collins, 1985); furthermore, one can say without fear of contradiction that the result-ing pile of grain was higher than that of the chaff.

---

*These fires may, by an interesting coincidence, have been started by inept shelling from the *Helga II*, a requisitioned fishery protection vessel also used for dredging during the Clare Island Survey. Clearly a case of 'The Lord giveth ...'.

Heaped with honours in later life – all three of the then Irish universities conferred honorary Doctorates in Science upon him – he was elected Hon. Librarian (1905-31) and President (1931-4) of the Royal Irish Academy, and was first President of the National Trust for Ireland (*An Taisce*) when it was founded in 1947. This latter honour is indeed an interesting link between our Victorian naturalist past and our environmentally correct present. It would not be excessive to claim that Praeger was the last of the great Irish naturalists. A detailed account of the life and times of this most industrious of naturalists is given by Collins in his *Floreat Hibernia* (1985). Suitable eponymous honour was done with the dedication by Rowland Southern of *Praegeria*, a polychaete worm discovered during the Clare Island Survey, though now relegated to synonymy with *Pisione*.

The Clare Island Survey

Although Praeger was clearly the rudder that guided the Clare Island Survey, there were stalwart oarsmen of whom mention must be made. Robert Francis Scharff (1858-1934), Chairman of the Survey Committee, was born in Leeds of German parentage. Appointed to the Museum of Science and Art (now the National Museum) in 1887 as Assistant in the Natural History Division, he became Keeper in 1890. Scharff had been trained as a zoologist in Britain and in mainland Europe, and his great biological passion was the geographical distribution of animals. In addition to Praeger and Scharff, the National Museum meeting in April 1908 was attended by Richard Manliffe Barrington, Nathaniel Colgan, Rev. Canon Henry William Lett and Professor Grenville A. J. Cole. Some of these were amateurs and others professionals, but all were very experienced in field studies. Barrington was an ornithologist; Colgan was a botanist, best known for his *Flora of the County Dublin* (1904); Lett was a bryologist (a student of mosses); and Cole was Professor of Geology at the Royal College for Science in Ireland and Director of the Irish Geological Survey.

The discussions on a suitable survey site ranged from Aran Island in Co. Donegal through the Aran Islands in Galway Bay to the Great Blasket Island and Valencia in Co. Kerry. Clare Island was chosen largely because of its central location in relation to the west coast, its unusual elevation (Croaghmore [*plate 11*] reaches a height of 1520 feet and has some interesting alpine plants and unusual habitats), its proximity to the mainland (for ease of access), and, seemingly paradoxically, its distance from the mainland (sufficiently far so that questions about natural colonization, a particular interest of Praeger's, could be raised). Additionally, the natives may have been regarded as being relatively friendly as the Irish language had largely died out, which was unusual for an offshore western island. For ease of operations, there was a ferry and a modest hotel, and the Congested Districts Board was willing to provide a shed, which could be fitted out as a laboratory (Praeger, 1915). In one way the choice of Clare Island was unfortunate in that the island, which is in Co. Mayo, is sometimes – mainly outside Ireland – confused with Co. Clare, and some latter-day scientific works erroneously cite plants or animals found in the Clare Island Survey as, for example, 'occurring north to Co. Clare'. Similarly, it is frequently not appreciated, even within Ireland, that the Survey was, as is clearly stated in the published title, of 'Clare Island and the adjoining district'; results of the Survey occasionally are cited as if they were exclusively from Clare Island itself.

Clare Island lies at the mouth of Clew Bay, about three miles from the mainland on the eastern side. In the public eye, it is perhaps best known as the island fortress of Grainuile Ó Máille (Grace O'Malley, c. 1530-1600), rather romantically celebrated as an Elizabethan pirate queen. Her tower house survives in good condition, protecting the entrance to the harbour at Kinacorra. The dominating feature of Clare Island is a ridge running from east to west and forming precipitous sea cliffs along the northern shore. These cliffs are listed as an area of international scientific importance because of their rare Arctic alpine plants and breeding seabird colonies. The area of the Survey was roughly bounded by Achill Island to the north and Killary Harbour in the south and inland to Castlebar, so that some limestone terrain could be included (Praeger, 1915a). This is actually a much larger area than is generally appreciated, and in some of the published papers it is occasionally unclear whether a particular entity was found on Clare Island or on the mainland. Collins (1993) goes so far as to suggest that, if one were pedantic, the survey should be known as the 'West Mayo Survey'.

The Committee met several times in 1908 (Scharff, 1915), and it quickly became apparent that this was to be the most comprehensive of all the surveys carried out in Ireland up to that time. Besides plants and animals, the archaeology, history, place and family names, Irish plant and animal names, and climate were to be examined. The Committee obtained funding from the Royal Irish Academy, the Royal Dublin Society, the British Association for the Advancement of Science and the Royal Society in addition to the co-operation of the many workers and their institutions, most dipping into their own pockets to fund the work. In all over two hundred specialists played some part (Collins, 1993), although about half of these did not visit the region but examined material referred to them by other workers. Owing to the Dublin meeting of the British Association for the Advancement of Science in 1908, fieldwork did not begin until 1909; it continued to 1911 with parties of workers from six to sixteen in number visiting the island at approximately monthly intervals. Dredging got under way using the *Helga II*, under the supervision of Rowland Southern, a zoologist with the Fisheries Branch of the Department of Agriculture and Technical Instruction in Dublin.

Over the next three years parties of experts and various collectors continued to visit the island and the nearby mainland (Praeger, 1915), and in 1911 the first results began to appear in the *Proceedings of the Royal Irish Academy* as Volume 31, edited by Praeger. Parts 2-7, although largely dealing with non-biological matters, established the historical, cultural and geological background to the Survey. (Part 8, planned to be 'Peat Deposits' by F.J. Lewis, was never published.) The other sixty parts were exclusively biological except for an informative summary and history of the survey written by Praeger as parts 1 and 68 (Praeger, 1915, 1915a). The General Introduction is significantly concentrated on the nature of island faunas and floras and how these might have come into being, and the General Summary attempts to account for the results. Collins (1993) recounts how Praeger made several attempts to calculate from what height seeds would have to be released so that they would reach Clare Island; these experiments involved, at various times, the main mast of the *Helga II* while moored at Roonagh Quay, and the staircase of the Royal College of Science in Dublin (now refurbished as Government Buildings).

Postscript

While the Lambay study and similar surveys of Valencia (1895-6) and other areas were painstakingly carried out, the Clare Island Survey seems to have marked the end of such ventures, as no similar investigation of any size was subsequently undertaken. World War I, the Easter Rising, the War of Independence and the Civil War were partially responsible, but later the fledgling Saorstát (Free State) had little money for such pursuits. By 1915 Praeger was fifty years of age and although he was to do some fine taxonomic work on the cultivated stonecrops (Praeger, 1921) and on the *Sempervivum* or Houseleek group (Praeger, 1932), he never attempted to organize fieldwork on such an heroic scale again.

There is no doubt, however, that the Clare Island Survey is a jewel in the crown of Irish natural history. It was certainly one of the most comprehensive biological surveys of a single area carried out up to that time. Many of the marine papers, particularly those of Rowland Southern and A.D. Cotton (Kew Gardens, London), included the emergent science of ecology with extensive descriptions of communities and associations. The statistics are indeed impressive: nearly nine thousand organisms (3219 plants and 5629 animals) were found during the survey, of which 585 plants and 1253 animals were new to Ireland, and 55 and 343, respectively, were new to the British Isles. Eleven plant species and 109 animals new to science were discovered. It is significant to note, however, that none of the new species of plants were from the terrestrial groups and, in the marine algae, only one of the three described species from the Survey was to stand the test of time; a similar situation may pertain to the other groups. A re-survey of the marine algae in 1990, which concentrated on the subtidal, resulted in the discovery of thirty-five species not previously reported from the island, including one new to science (Maggs *et al.*, 1991) and one new to the British Isles (Guiry *et al.*, 1991). These results do not reflect badly on the original survey but serve rather to underline the utility of today's SCUBA diving versus the dredging of yesteryear and the ability of new eyes to see new things. Similarly, re-investigations of the flowering plants have resulted in redis- covery of an acceptable majority of the species noted by Praeger (Doyle and Foss, 1986; Brodie, 1991).

In 1988, the Praeger Committee of the Royal Irish Academy agreed to recommend to the Council of the Academy that a re-survey of Clare Island was desirable. A grant for a feasibility study was obtained from the National Heritage Council and a multidisciplinary Clare Island Study Committee was established. Preliminary fieldwork carried out in 1990 suggested that a new survey would be worthwhile. Comparative data could be obtained that would chart the changes that have taken place in the intervening eighty years. It is particularly encouraging that indigenous expertise is now available for prac- tically every group, which was not the entirely the case with the original sur- vey. Contemporary investigations (Doyle and Foss, 1986) had shown that profound changes had taken place in the terrestrial vegetation, largely as a result, as elsewhere in the west of Ireland, of overgrazing by sheep. Studies of the archaeology of the island resulted in the conclusion that the island was far richer than formerly thought; the discovery of a megalithic court tomb and other artefacts indicated settlement by at least 3500 BC (Gosling, 1990). A critical factor in the Academy's decision to sanction a re-survey was the support of the local community expressed via the Centre for Island Studies. Although the population of the island has declined from about 700 in 1891 to some 140 souls today, community spirit has probably never been stronger and the islanders are dedicated to rural renewal via community development and self-help.

The re-survey of Clare Island is still proceeding. Some projects are scheduled to be complete by April 1998, notably the archaeology, vegeta- tional studies and intertidal ecology.

References

Allen, D.E. 1988. 'The Role of the Amateur,' in P.S. Wyse Jackson, C. Moriarty and J.R. Akeroyd (eds), *In the Field of the Naturalists: Proceedings of a Seminar ... Held on 27 September 1986 in Celebration of 100 Years of the Dublin Naturalists' Field Club*. Dublin: Dublin Naturalists' Field Club.

Brodie, J. 1991. 'Some Observations on the Flora of Clare Island, Western Ireland.' *Irish Naturalists'*
Journal 23: 376-7.

Colgan, N. 1904. *Flora of the County of Dublin. Flowering Plants, Higher Cryptogams, and Characeae.*
Dublin: Hodges Figgis.

Collins, T. 1985. *Floreat Hibernia: A Bio-bibliography of Robert Lloyd Praeger 1865-1953.* Dublin:
Royal Dublin Society.

Collins, T. 1993. 'Praeger in the West: Naturalists and Antiquarians in Connemara and the Islands
1884-1914.' *Journal of the Galway Archaeological and Historical Society 45*: 124-54.

Desmond, A., and J. Moore. 1991. *Darwin.* London: Michael Joseph.

Doyle, G.J. and P.J. Foss 1986. 'A Resurvey of the Clare Island flora.' *Irish Naturalists' Journal 22*:
85-9.

Gosling, P. 1990. 'The Archaeology of Clare Island.' *Archaeology, Ireland 4(1)*: 7-12.

Guiry, M.D., C.A. Maggs and C. Adair. 1991. '*Antithamnion densum* (Suhr) Howe from Clare
Island, Ireland: A Marine Red Alga New to the British Isles.' *Cryptogamie: Algologie 12*: 189-94.

Maggs, C.A., M.D. Guiry and J. Rueness. 1991. '*Aglaothamnion priceanum* sp. nov. (Ceramiaceae,
Rhodophyta) from the North-eastern Atlantic: Morphology and Life History of Parasporangial
Plants.' *British Phycological Journal 26*: 343-52.

Praeger, R.L. 1901. 'Irish Topographical Botany.' *Proceedings of the Royal Irish Academy 7 (ser.3)*:
1-140.

Praeger, R.L. (ed.) 1907. 'Contributions to the Natural History of Lambay, Co. Dublin.' *Irish
Naturalist 16*: 1-112.

Praeger, R.L. 1915. 'General Introduction and Narrative.' *Proceedings of the Royal Irish Academy
31(1)*: 1-12, 9 pls.

Praeger, R.L. 1915a. 'General Summary.' *Proceedings of the Royal Irish Academy 31(68)*: 1-15.

Praeger, R.L. 1921. 'An Account of the Genus *Sedum* as Found in Cultivation.' *Journal of the Royal
Horticultural Society 46*: 1-314.

Praeger, R.L. 1932. *An Account of the* Sempervivum *Group.* London: Royal Horticultural Society.

Praeger, R.L. 1934. *The Botanist in Ireland.* Dublin: Hodges Figgis.

Praeger, R.L. 1937. *The Way that I Went: an Irishman in Ireland.* Dublin: Hodges Figgis; London:
Methuen.

Praeger, R.L. 1941. *A Populous Solitude.* Dublin: Hodges Figgis; London: Methuen.

Praeger, R.L. 1949. *Some Irish Naturalists: a Biographical Notebook.* Dundalk: Dundalgan Press.

Praeger, R.L. 1950. *Natural History of Ireland: a Sketch of its Flora and Fauna.* London: Collins.

Scharff, R.F. 1915. 'The Clare Island Survey.' *Irish Naturalist 24*: 177-87.

Out of Ireland:
Naturalists Abroad

JOHN WILSON FOSTER

'Out of Ireland we have come'
– W.B. Yeats

Introduction

This chapter presents brief lives of seven men of Irish origin who made their contributions to natural history mainly, notably, or exclusively outside Ireland. These are Sir Francis Beaufort, Sir Edward Sabine, Francis Rawdon Chesney, Sir Leopold McClintock, Robert Templeton, John Macoun and Henry Chichester Hart. They are an almost random selection from among the lives available, and represent varying degrees of attachment to their island of birth, but there is in each case an instructive significance beyond the uniqueness of the life. All exhibit the centrifugal energy of a small island on the edges of an ocean and a continent. In the study of nature this energy has taken the forms of exploration, emigration, exile or excursion, and has been fruitful for natural history in doing so.

The Voyages of Mythology

Throughout their history the inhabitants of Ireland have ventured abroad for one reason or another, often recording the marvellous and the quotidian they met with in nature. Indeed, the story of travel and exile, of expatriation and expedition, begins with the mythology. Of the races recorded in *The Book of Invasions* (revised until the end of the twelfth century), the Nemedians (who succeeded Partholon, who succeeded the Fomorians) were the first distinguishable inhabitants of Ireland to go overseas, leaving for lands in northern Europe. They weren't the first Irish to do so, if by 'Irish' we mean Gaels, who it is said came after the Tuatha de Danann, Firbolgs and Milesians. Once defeated by the latter invaders, the Tuatha de Danann (the

People of the Goddess Dana) fled to Tír-na-nÓg, the Land of Youth. In the Irish mythological tales of pre-Christian Ireland, the routed gods became the elusive sidhe (or fairies), making their home inside hills, on faraway islands, or beneath the waves. In the Ossianic or Fenian Cycle of tales (said by early historians to depict life in the third century AD), the adventures of the Fianna, the young warriors who followed Fionn Mac Cumhail, included voyages to the Isles of the Blessed that lay to the west of Ireland (Knott, 1966; Foster, 1977).

Early voyage-tales are called *Immrama*, and the earliest known (from an eighth-century text) is *Immram Brain* (*The Voyage of Bran*), a mythological tale in which the hero is seduced by a woman's poetic catalogue of the charms of the Otherworld, a paradise of islands ('thrice fifty distant isles/In the ocean to the west of us'), and journeys there (Joyce, 1879; Seymour, 1930). Under magical influence, Bran sees the ocean as a flowery plain or an orchard and the fish as calves or gambolling lambs. When he returns he discovers, like Oisín (hero of the Ossianic Cycle), that he has passed into legend and cannot live in the real Ireland; all he can do is embark on a renewed and different exile. Despite its supernaturalism, this tale might provide evidence of the Gaels' involvement with the sea and possible voyages of exploration (Ranelagh, 1983).

By the ninth century the *Immrama* had been Christianized, and one such voyage-tale is *Immram Maíle Dúin* (*The Voyage of Maelduin*), dated variably from the eight to the tenth centuries. The hero sets out over the western sea to avenge his slain father, an Aran Islander. But he violates a druid's interdiction and he and his comrades are blown off course and make a strange voyage (as though in punishment) among many islands, the curious inventories of which – early island surveys of natural history, one might say – constitute the bulk of the tale. While some of the islands are paradisal, the tale is particularly fond of the grotesque. There are monstrous ants, 'each of them as large as a foal', a horse-shaped, dog-legged, blue-clawed monster, invisible giant race-horses, and this curious fellow:

When they came near the shore, an animal of vast size, with a thick, rough skin, started up inside the wall, and ran round the island with the swiftness of the wind. When he had ended his race, he went to a high point, and standing on a large, flat stone, began to exercise himself according to his daily custom, in the following manner. He kept turning himself completely round and round in his skin, the bones and flesh moving, while the skin remained at rest. When he was tired of this exercise, he rested a little; and he then began turning his skin continually round his body, down at one side and up at the other like a mill-wheel; but the bones and flesh did not move. (Joyce, 1879)

In the deceptive appearances and illusory splendour Maelduin encounters, one senses an Early Christian distrust of the blandishments of the natural

world. St John Seymour (1930) has even detected 'a certain infernal significance' in such elements as a burning river and an island with red-hot animals. Such significance is more obvious in *Immram Uí Corra* (*The Voyage
of the Sons of O'Corra*, possibly eleventh-century) where Nature is of spiritual meaning: everywhere, for example, are tortured souls in the shapes of
birds, a figure in medieval Irish literature.

Some late ninth-, early tenth-century Irish Latinist modelled his
Navigatio Brendani (*The Voyage of Brendan*) on *Immram Maíle Dúin*. *The
Voyage of Brendan* was translated into various European languages and had
great impact on European medieval literature and thought (Knott, 1966).
Like many of these tales, it is a hybrid of truth and fiction. In fact Brendan
in the sixth century visited Iona and western Scotland and perhaps Brittany;
in legend he survived the perils of sea monsters, voracious birds, sea-fogs,
demons and thirst while voyaging among marvellous islands west of Ireland,
including a beautiful Land of Promise which held sheep bigger than cows,
chanting birds, and great bounties of fruit. The effect of Brendan's story is
said to have been real, inasmuch as it inspired voyages that culminated in
the discovery of that actual Land of Promise, America (Knott, 1966).

Of course, both trade and warfare induced the Irish across the water in
reality early in their history. By the fourth century AD the Celts were raid-
ing Roman settlements in mainland Britain, from which they returned with
coins and other treasures. In 470 Fergus Mac Erc, prince of Dalriada in
north Antrim, crossed the water and founded the kingdom of Argyll, or
Scottish Dalriada (to which St Columba travelled in 563), and so began the
long history of Gaelic Scotland (Curtis, 1950). It seems that the Irish established kingdoms in Wales during the fifth century, while during the same
period east-Cork Irish (the Uí Liatháin) settled themselves in Cornwall
(Doherty, 1991). Warfare was a way of life to the Celtic aristocracy, and
Celtic mercenaries were employed in the Balkans and Greece early in the
first millennium (Chadwick, 1970). Although it is hard to document archae-
ologically, it appears that there was Celtic trade with the classical world,
which would have involved sailors and messengers, agents of some early
variety, travelling overseas (Chadwick, 1970).

The Scholar Exiles

According to Seymour, certain incidents in the Christianized *Immrama*
derive 'from the customs of Irish monks seeking out lonely islands ... that
they might lead a solitary life of undisturbed contemplation and prayer'
(Seymour, 1930). This practice, known as anchoritism, is an ascetic feature
of early Irish (pre-centralized Roman) Christianity. However, apparently the
Irish scribe, in the words of Chadwick (1970), 'knew well how to season his

learning with the lighter side of life, in particular with a close and humorous watch on animals and wild things of all kinds. The Leinster St Moling had in his solitude both a fox and a wren, and "a little fly that used to buzz to him when he came in from Matins".'

Anchoritism was one species of the Irish Christian's love of wandering, *peregrinatio*; another was travel to Christian communities overseas (Italy, France, Spain, Germany, and central Europe) to seek asylum or to teach (Ranelagh, 1983). Yet another was the founding of monasteries abroad (like those founded by St Columbanus in Annegray, Luxeuil and Bobbio between 590 and 615) and, from the seventh to the ninth centuries, missionary work throughout Europe where the Irish holy men were known for their 'nomadic instinct or impulse', specimens of *Hibernicus exul*, and sometimes regarded by Anglo-Saxon monks as heretical (Zimmer, 1891). They were 'scholar exiles' (in Robin Flower's phrase) and kept alive Latin culture. Curtis remarks that 'The map of Europe before the year 900 shows the footprints of many such men' (Curtis, 1950). The ninth century particularly saw Irish scholars thronging to the cathedral and palace schools of Europe, partly in response to Viking attacks on their homeland (Doherty, 1991). One wonders if these men perceived the European animals and landscape with the affectionate glances that their homebound fellows turned in their verses into deft impressionism or whether their exile led them to indulge a lingering gaze of homesickness for Irish nature.

It would be difficult to associate a pious and poetic impressionism of Nature and her creatures with the name of the greatest of these scholar exiles. Johannes Scottus (c. 810–c. 877) called himself Eriugena ('Born in Ireland'); he joined a number of Irishmen at the court of Charles the Bald at Laon. He has been described by Charles Doherty (1991) as the only original thinker between Boethius (c. 470–c. 525) and St Anselm (1033-1109). His *magnum opus*, a work in five books entitled *De Divisione Naturae*, is a philosophical taxonomy of 'Nature', by which Eriugena means 'God and His creation', Nature being capable of a fourfold division: Nature that creates and is not created; Nature that is created and creates; Nature that is created and does not create; and Nature that is neither created nor creates. The Christian philosophical originality of the work notwithstanding, such theological systematics militated against an objective attention to the structural and organic nature of the earth and the plant and animal kingdoms it supported.

In the seventh century Isidore, Bishop of Seville, wrote *De Natura Rerum*, which produced a Eurocentric geographical world view. This portrays three continents separated not just by the Mediterranean but also by two rivers: the Don divides Europe from Asia while the Nile flows between Africa and Europe (America was unsuspected at this time). Irish scholars were among the first to use Isidore's work, initially to help with scriptural problems, then to enlarge the concepts of world geography; the Irish abbot of Iona, Adamnán, in his *De Locis Sanctis*, written about AD 680, saw Jerusalem as the centre of the lands. The contribution of Irish scholars was highly influential at monasteries in Verona, Salzburg and St Gallen in Switzerland, where an important school involved with geographical subjects was conducted by Virgilius (Feargal). New interpretations of world geography were offered in *Liber De Mensura Orbis Terrae* (*On Measuring the Lands of the Earth*); though this book drew on works by Pliny, Sedulius and Priscian as well as Isidore, its author consulted these sources at first hand. Dícuil, an Irishman who flourished between 760 and 825, finished this work in the latter year, probably at the palace school of Louis the Pious at Aix-la-Chapelle (Doherty, 1991). (It seems Dícuil had lived on the Hebrides and the Orkneys and perhaps Iona before going to the Continent.) Dícuil was the author of an earlier book on astronomy, *Liber de Astronomia*. The influence of the so-called T-O maps (maps of the earth) was 'transmitted to virtually every place in which there were books during the early Middle Ages' and coloured conceptions of world geography for centuries (O'Loughlin, 1993).

Seventeenth-Century Exiles

At home, the successive incursions of the Danes, Normans and Old English (between the ninth and fifteenth centuries) depleted the strength of the Gaels, and in 1601 the Battle of Kinsale spelled the end of the Gaelic order in Ireland. Hugh O'Neill and the rebel earls submitted to Elizabeth, then James, and in 1607 left with their subordinates for continental exile. Towards the end of the century, the Flight of the Earls was echoed by the wingbeats of the Wild Geese – the Irish Catholic military survivors of the successful Williamite campaign who then and in the following century fought in European armies in a variety of causes and in a semi-permanent state of armed exile. An estimated 120,000 Wild Geese left Ireland between 1690 and 1730. (Ranelagh, 1983); a soldierly tradition of expatriation and mobility sprang up, in the New World as well as the Old (for instance, in Chile and Peru), an early and sparse diaspora of some civilian impact over the succeeding generations.

Although Irish continued to be written in the seventeenth century, and Latin widely used, the Penal Laws prevented Roman Catholics and Dissenters (non-subscribing Protestants) from enrolling at Trinity College, Dublin, Oxford or Cambridge; as a result, those disqualified in such fashion but ambitious and with the means travelled to universities in Scotland and the continent for their education or to teach. Some were involved in the founding or staffing of Irish colleges on the Continent. Some were editors and collectors of rare works of scholarship. Most of those who published their learning did so as theologians, either as historians or hagiographers. Some combined polemics with scholarship; for example, John Lynch, Bishop of Killala, exiled in France by the spillover into Ireland of the English civil war, wrote a rebuttal of the anti-Irish portions of Giraldus Cambrensis's *Topographia Hiberniae* in 1662.

In *The Irish Writers of the Seventeenth Century* (1857) Thomas D'Arcy McGee has colourful pages on the mostly Catholic expatriates of the pen ('extern lights', he calls them) but also on the Protestant founder of the Dublin Philosophical Society, William Molyneux, whom McGee sees as 'doomed to be the connecting character between the disappearing Catholic nationalists, and their, as yet, invisible Protestant successors'. Molyneux was Surveyor-General of the King's Works and M.P. for Dublin University, but later the author of *The Case of Ireland Stated* (1698). In 1685 he travelled in Europe, surveying fortresses in Flanders for the government, then went on to Holland and France and joined his brother Thomas in Leyden. The city and college of Leyden had a long and distinguished tradition in medicine and many journeyed there to acquire their education (Innes-Smith, 1932). One of these, Patrick Browne (1720-90) of Co. Galway, came into contact with Linnaeus, a fellow student and enthusiastic traveller. Although Browne later naturalized in Ireland and produced the first scientific catalogue of Irish birds and fishes, his talents were directed towards the natural history of the West Indies, in particular Jamaica, where his medical work took him (Nelson, 1994). For his part, the versatile Thomas Molyneux (1661-1733) returned to Ireland in 1687 where he wrote numerous papers, including observations on the Irish wolfhound and Irish elk, on the remains of an elephant found on the Monaghan-Cavan border, and on Irish flowers (he discovered *Saxifraga umbrosa* in 1697). He also visited Roderic O'Flaherty near Galway Bay ('I never saw so strangely stony and wild a country') where, according to McGee, 'The ganet and the sea-eagle dwelt in its cliffs' (McGee, 1857).

The Ulster Scots and the New World

Many descendants of the Scots who were planted in Ulster after the Battle of Kinsale left Ireland in the eighteenth century, mainly for colonial America. Indeed, as early as 1636, 140 passengers sailed from Carrickfergus to found a colony on the Merrimack river; the enterprise was abandoned and not revived until 1719 when 'the Londonderry settlement' spread the Presbyterian settlers through New Hampshire and Vermont. As late as the 1730s, the Irish in Boston were chiefly Protestant. (Of course, we find the Irish much earlier in America: for instance, a Darbie Glaven and Denice Carroll turn up on the second voyage to Virginia, in 1585 [Hakluyt, 1907], and an Irish boy and one Nugent on the fourth voyage of 1587 [Burrage, 1906].) Emigration from Ulster accelerated after 1720; in the 1760s, it is estimated, twenty thousand sailed from the Ulster ports, and thirty thousand between 1770 and 1774. We are told that two-fifths of the total of American immigrants in the colonial period came from Ulster (Foster, 1989).

There was competition for land in Ulster, which motivated some of these emigrants to leave, while economic discrimination and anti-Presbyterianism in the reigns of William and Anne motivated others; but it seems as if there was also an innate propensity in the Ulster planters for movement and settlement. On nearly every American frontier, it has been said, the Scots-Irish were the defenders of the marches, advance agents and tamers of the wilderness (Tolles, 1960, 128). Moreover, the Ulster Scots 'kept the lamp of learning lighted on many an American frontier', remarks Tolles, who quotes Carl Wittke: 'the schoolhouse and the kirk went together wherever the Scotch-Irish frontier moved'. This, along with the fact that the Ulster society they came from was distinguished in Ireland by lively towns, chambers of commerce, libraries, clubs, private schools and newspapers (Foster, 1989), meant that the Scots-Irish were able to contribute to the intellectual growth of colonial America, including its natural history.

One of the early seats of scientific learning in colonial and post-colonial America was Philadelphia. This city was the destination port of choice for many Ulster emigrants; it has been calculated that 5665 Irish emigrants landed there during 1729, compared with a mere 43 Scots and 267 English and Welsh, and the flow continued until the end of the century (McGee, 1852). Belfast was a major embarkation point, and it was from there that in 1794 the Scotsman Alexander Wilson ('the father of American ornithology') took ship for Delaware; he came to live in Philadelphia, becoming yet another of that city's scientific luminaries (Brightwell, 1861).

Philadelphia was an intellectually active city decades before the Academy of Natural Sciences was founded in 1812. Benjamin Franklin had founded a club in 1727 called 'the Junto', and James Logan, a Quaker from Lurgan, Co. Armagh, was to advise on its library (Raistrick, 1968). Still intact, this has been called the best-chosen collection of books in colonial America (Tolles, 1960). Logan (1674-1751) emigrated to Philadelphia from Bristol in 1699 as William Penn's secretary. He rose to become the most influential statesman and most distinguished scholar in the Delaware Valley (Tolles, 1957). It was he who planted an Ulster Scots garrison on the Susquehanna as a buffer against restive Indians across the river. Logan was a botanist of repute, correspondent – in Latin – of Linnaeus (who named after him an order of herbs and shrubs, the *Loganiaceae*: Robert Brown also dedicated a genus, *Logania*), mentor to the young John Bartram, author of an unfinished treatise on ethics, translator of Cicero, commentator on Euclid and Ptolemy, and correspondent – again in Latin – with Fabricius, the greatest classicist of his age. In the words of an eminent nineteenth-century American scientist, 'To Logan belongs the honor of having carried on the first American investigations in physiological botany, the results of which were published in Leyden, in 1739' as *Experimenta et Meletemata de Plantarum Generatione* (Goode, 1901). Goode refers to a complete version in Latin of what had appeared in *Philosophical Transactions* in English abstract a few years before (Tolles, 1957) and was to appear in a dual Latin-English version in London in 1747 (Raistrick, 1968).

The Academy of Natural Sciences had by 1819 begun to rival the American Philosophical Society. Among the subscribers to the *Journal* of the Academy in Ireland were the Cork Institution, the Royal Dublin Society and the Royal Irish Academy (Stroud, 1995). The Academy had seven founders, one of these being Dr Camillus MacMahon Mann, about whom little is known. He was born in Ireland and took part in the 1798 rebellion. After a short exile in France he sought refuge in the United States. When he moved from Philadelphia to Baltimore to edit a paper (having been expelled from the Academy), he took the *Minutes* of the Academy with him and was denounced as a 'hot headed excentric Irish man ... some what crack brained' [sic] by the chemist Gerard Troost, a co-founder (Stroud, 1992).

A more reputable founder of the Academy of Natural Sciences, the naturalist Thomas Say, was like Logan a Quaker, a sect that has contributed disproportionately to science in Britain, Ireland and North America (perhaps in part because other avenues of professional advancement were either closed or unattractive to them). Quakerism was begun in Ireland by William Edmundson (1627-1712), an ex-Cromwellian soldier, who came in 1654 to live in Lurgan, Logan's birthplace two decades later (Myers, 1902). Among Ireland's early Quaker naturalists was John Rutty, author of the pioneering *Essay Towards a Natural History of the County of Dublin* (1772) and *History of the Rise and Progress of the Quakers in Ireland* (1751). Quakers participated in the westward emigration from Ireland, particularly to Pennsylvania between 1682 and 1750; back in Ireland they remained a force in natural history until well into the twentieth century.

Scientists of the Empire

Before the nineteenth century, fewer Irish southerners and Catholics than northerners and Protestants emigrated to North America, though there had been small Catholic emigrations to Maryland and Pennsylvania. There had been some exiles and fugitives after the failed rebellion of 1798. The trickle became a flood in the nineteenth century: between 1815 and 1845, before the Famine, at least a million Irish left the island; between 1845 and 1870 at least three million did so. They left chiefly for England or the White Dominions – Canada, Australia and New Zealand – and for the United States. The U.S. was the destination of 84 per cent of Irish emigrants between 1876 and 1921 (after which Canada tended to be the first choice of Protestants), but between 1946 and 1951 the U.K. was chosen by the same percentage of leavers (Foster, 1989); in such wise have the destinies of Britain and Ireland, as well as America and Ireland, been entwined.

By the nineteenth century the reasons for Irish presence overseas had multiplied: famine and economic disability at home, social and economic opportunity abroad. These reasons had also become confused with the British territorial expansion. This expansion accelerated the development of natural history (more territory, fresh flora and fauna; more exploration, fresh data), both in the colonies and in the home countries, including Ireland, whose scientists participated in the international traffic of specimens and information. For example, among the specimens sent to the Academy of Natural Sciences in Philadelphia in the early nineteenth century were one hundred shells from M.J. O'Kelly in Ireland (Stroud, 1995). It is no coincidence that the Victorian period registers the high water mark of both the British Empire and the pre-specialized study of nature. (Raby [1996] offers a readable guide to Victorian scientific travellers.) At this time the discipline was preoccupied with field collection, description and classification, and elementary biogeography.

In the beginning only the wealthy or those with patrons could take advantage of the overseas possessions. Sir Hans Sloane (1660-1753) is exemplary in this regard. Born in Killyleagh, Co. Down, he became a physician (like many early naturalists) and a pupil of Tournefort, a great naturalist of the day. He visited the West Indies in 1684 and was physician to the Governor of Jamaica, 1687-9. After his return to England he printed *Catalogus Plantarum quae in Insula Jamaica* (1696) and *Voyage to Madeira, Barbados ... and Jamaica* (1707-25). On his death, the plants he collected in the West Indies became the nucleus of the British Museum. Sloane was Secretary of the Royal Society from 1693 to 1712, and succeeded Isaac Newton as President in 1727.

Colonial administrators who were serious amateur naturalists were especially fortunate. Working for the Bengal Civil Service gave the Co. Longford-born botanist Michael Pakenham Edgeworth (half-brother of the novelist Maria Edgeworth) the opportunity to collect in India, Ceylon (Sri Lanka) and Aden.* The genus *Edgeworthia* is named after him. The botanist

---

* The balance of this essay is indebted to Robert Lloyd Praeger, *Some Irish Naturalists: A Biographical Note-Book* (1949) and Ray Desmond, *Dictionary of British and Irish Botanists and Horticulturists* (1994). The historical connections between natural history

John Zephaniah Holwell (b. Dublin 1711, d. 1798) worked for the Indian Medical Service, and the lepidopterist W.M. Crawford (1872-1941) for the Indian Civil Service. Crawford returned to Belfast in 1919 with a fine collection of Indian specimens, and was President of the Belfast Naturalists' Field Club in 1926-7. Another Quaker naturalist, W.H. Harvey (b. Limerick 1811, d. 1866), having secured the position of Colonial Treasurer in the British Cape Colony in 1836, seized the chance to botanize in South Africa, publishing *Genera of South African Plants* in 1838. After he left his colonial post in 1842 Harvey returned to Ireland where he became Professor of Botany, Royal Dublin Society. He embarked on a round-the-world trip in the mid-1850s, collecting in Sri Lanka, Australia, Tasmania, Fiji, Tonga and Florida. *Phycologica Britannica* appeared between 1846 and 1851, *Phycologica Australica* between 1853 and 1863. Praeger calls this student of marine algae 'the foremost phycologist of his day', and the genus *Harveya* bears his name; he was made a Fellow of the Royal Society in 1858. He rejected Darwin's theory of natural selection (Praeger, 1949; Nelson, 1992; Desmond, 1994).

John Ball's involvement in colonial affairs was more sedentary (he was Assistant Secretary of State for the Colonies), but this Dubliner (1818-89) was impressively mobile as a botanist. He collected with J.D. Hooker, the eminent English botanist, in Morocco and also collected in the Rocky Mountains, and travelled in South America. He published *Journal of Tour in Marocco* [sic] *and Great Atlas* (1878, with Hooker) and *Notes of a Naturalist in South America* (1887). He was especially interested in the topography and flora of the Alps and edited *Peaks, Passes, and Glaciers: A Series of Excursions by Members of the Alpine Club* (1859). The species *Erodium ballii* was named after him.

Other colonial appointees who pursued the pleasure of exotica and the possibility of pioneering collection and classification included Theodore Cooke (b. Tramore, Co. Waterford 1836, d. 1910), Director of the Botanical Survey of Western India; William Fawcett (b. Arklow 1851, d. 1926), Director of the Botanic Garden, Jamaica, author (with A.B. Rendle) of the *Flora of Jamaica* (1910-26), and namesake of the species *Columnea fawcettii*; and William Harris (b. Enniskillen 1860, d. 1920), Superintendent of Public Gardens and Plantations in Jamaica, then Government Botanist, who was commemorated in the genera *Harrisia* and *Harrisella*.

Geological surveys carried out in the colonies under official auspices and for military as well as scientific purposes (repeating the Irish experience) were invaluable opportunities, and at least three Irish geologists worked for

---

and the British Empire are explained in Miller and Reill (1996). It has been claimed that Cook's circumnavigation in the *Endeavour*, with Joseph Banks on board, inaugurated the British imperial-scientific alliance.

the Geological Survey of India: Thomas Oldham (b. Dublin 1816, d. 1878), who was appointed Superintendent in 1850; Valentine Ball (b. Dublin 1843, d. 1895, son of Sir Robert Ball); and Sir Henry Hayden (b. Londonderry 1869, d. 1923), who joined the Survey in 1895 and was Director 1910-20.

In the nineteenth century Britain had informal control of the Yangtze Valley and wished to extend her commerce throughout the Chinese Empire. The botanist William Hancock (b. Lurgan 1847, d. 1914) worked for the Chinese Imperial Customs, and collected plants in China, Formosa, Japan, Sumatra, Java, Jamaica, Guatemala and Mexico; the genus *Hancockia* commemorates him. Augustine Henry (1857-1930) also worked for the Chinese Imperial Customs; he became interested in botany and sent home large collections of specimens containing many new species. He wrote *Economic Botany of China* (1893) as well as *Trees of Great Britain and Ireland* (1906-13), published when he was Reader in Forestry at Cambridge. Although Praeger (1949) gives his birthplace as Cookstown, Co. Tyrone, Desmond (1994) offers Dundee; in any case, Henry received his M.A. from Belfast and was Professor of Forestry, College of Sciences, Dublin, 1913-26. Beyond the empire, William Bowles (b. near Cork 1705, d. 1780) became Superintendent of State Mines in Spain, travelled in that country and in France and published the much-translated *Introduccion a la Historia Natural, y a la Geographia Fisica de Espagna* (Madrid, 1775); the Peruvian genus *Bowlesia* was dedicated to him. (Reynolds [1997] has provided a summary of the life and achievements of this 'Eurogeologist'.)

Like clergymen at home, British soldiers overseas made an immense contribution to nineteenth-century natural history, and Ireland produced its share of them. Walter Synnot (b. Ballymoyer, Co. Armagh 1773, d. Tasmania 1851) was a Captain in the 66th Regiment of Foot who went to South Africa and sent 'more new and rare bulbs from the Cape of Good Hope at one time than was ever done by another individual' (R. Sweet, quoted in Desmond, 1994); Sweet named the genus *Synnotia* in his honour. An officer in the Bengal Artillery, Edward Madden (b. Ireland 1805, d. 1856) sent seeds from abroad to the Botanic Gardens, Glasnevin, and after his army career he collected plants in Aden, Suez, Cairo and Malta. He was President of the Botanical Society of Edinburgh and is remembered in the genus *Maddenia*. W.T. Alexander (b. Cork 1818, d. 1872) was a surgeon aboard the HMS *Plover* in the East Indies and China and he collected mosses and ferns on the Chinese coast and Ryuku Islands. S.M. Toppin (b. Clonmel, Co. Tipperary 1878, d. 1917) was a Major in the Royal Artillery and collected plants in Chitral and Burma. This soldier-naturalist, who met his death at Ypres, is honoured by the species *Impatiens toppinii*.

In this century, the most distinguished clergyman-naturalist to work out of Ireland and to sojourn in the empire was Rev. E.A. Armstrong, who was born in Belfast in 1900. He studied science, then philosophy, at Queen's University, and soon after was ordained in Cambridge as an Anglican priest. A curacy in Doncaster was followed by a three-year post as chaplain in Hong Kong, during which he studied Chinese. He spent eleven years in Leeds thereafter, as curate, then vicar (meanwhile earning his M.A. in Chinese Studies); he returned to Cambridge in 1943 to be vicar of St Mark's, Newnham, and retired in 1966, though continuing to write through debilitating illness.

The scientific study of bird behaviour, resulting in *Bird Display* (1942), *Bird Display and Behaviour* (1947) and *A Study of Bird Song* (1963), as well as a monograph, *The Wren* (1955), made Armstrong one of the most eminent ornithologists of the century. He combined intense study of the literature with independent fieldwork both at home and abroad. He travelled widely in search of knowledge and experience of birds, in Iceland, France, Holland, Italy, the West Indies, the United States, Central America, China and South America. His immense geographic experience found its intellectual counterpart in the polymathic breadth of his interests and publications. He was a folklorist (*The Folklore of Birds*, 1958), hagiographer (*Saint Francis: Nature Mystic*, 1973), biblical scholar (*The Gospel Parables*, 1967) and, as though these were not enough, literary critic, helping to pioneer the method of Shakespeare criticism called 'cluster analysis' (*Shakespeare's Imagination*, 1946, rev. 1963) and completing with Robert Patterson and H.C. Hart a trio of Irish naturalist-Shakespearians.

In *Birds of the Grey Wind* (1940), a neglected masterpiece, Armstrong captured memories of birdwatching in his native Northern Ireland in writing of eloquence and erudition. Acute observation acutely remembered, deepened by effortless reference to current ornithological knowledge and to the lives of Irish saints, led the celebrated American writer and zoologist William Beebe in 1944 to call *Birds of the Grey Wind* 'a volume which puts the author well in the forefront of natural historian *belles-lettres*'. Armstrong's work on avian psychology, Beebe went on to claim, 'assures him no uncertain position among the company of scientific ornithologists'.

Emigrant Naturalists

If much early emigration from Ireland occurred in waves stimulated by difficulties in the home country, later emigration tended to be orderly and personal, families and individuals simply seeking better lives for themselves, and scientists taking up professional and academic posts abroad. An early example was Charles Telfair (b. Belfast 1778, d. 1833), who emigrated to Mauritius where he became a surgeon and then Supervisor of the Botanic Garden. Like the other emigrant naturalists mentioned below, he did not return permanently to his native Ireland. Hooker named the genus *Telfairia* after him.

Rev. William Hincks (b. Cork 1794, d. 1871) was a member of the Hincks dynasty of Irish natural historians, which rivals the Balls and Pattersons in achievement. He emigrated to Canada (having been Professor of Natural History at Cork) to become Professor of Natural History, University of Toronto, 1854-71, and collected mainly in the area of his adopted city. Canada also welcomed John Adams (b. Ballymena, Co. Antrim 1872, d. 1950) who left his position as Professor of Botany, Royal Veterinary College, Dublin to take up the post of Dominion Botanist in Ottawa, the Canadian capital. He collected plants in Anticosti, the Gaspé peninsula, and Prince Edward Island, and was a student of photoperiodism and germination and an expert in algae, lichens and fungi in both Canada and Ireland. He was the author of general works in his science, including *Studies in Plant Life* (1907), *Elementary Botany* (1907) and *A Student's Illustrated Irish Flora* (1931) as well as the more specialized *Bibliography of Canadian Plant Geography* (1928-36).

Another Canadian immigrant is Bryan P. Beirne (b. Rosslare, Co. Wexford 1918). He was an accomplished field entomologist before entering Trinity College, Dublin, and graduating wih a doctorate in zoology. Before leaving Ireland in 1949, he wrote the definitive list of Irish microlepidoptera and ran a successful pest-control business in Dublin. In Belleville, Ontario, he became Director of the Department of Agriculture Research Institute, then Professor of Pestology at Simon Fraser University, British Columbia. He was the prime mover behind *A Bibliography of Irish Entomology* (1984) and in 1985 published *Irish Entomology: the First Hundred Years*, providing a valuable historical dimension to his own work and that of his contemporaries (O'Connor, 1988).

The most renowned emigrant naturalist working in Canada was John Macoun, who preceded Beirne in Belleville, Ontario, and who is profiled below. The Australian counterpart of Macoun (Canada's greatest all-round naturalist of the nineteenth century) was Sir Frederick M'Coy (b. Dublin 1817, d. 1899). Having carried out palaeontological investigation under Sir Richard Griffith for the geological map of Ireland and been Professor of Mineralogy and Geology, Queen's College, Belfast, M'Coy left in 1854 to occupy the Chair of Natural History in the new University of Melbourne. In that city he founded the National Museum of Natural History and Geology. He published zoological and palaeontological works, and, in Praeger's words, 'was recognized as the leading man of science in Australia'. Another emigrant naturalist, Philip MacMahon (b. Dublin 1857, d. 1911), flourished in Australia, where he was Curator of the Botanic Garden, Brisbane, then Director of Forests, Queensland. Before going to Australia, MacMahon collected in India.

New Zealand was also a favourite destination for British and Irish emigrants, and W.T.L. Travers (b. Castleview, Co. Limerick 1819, d. 1903) lived there from 1849 and died there. He practised law in New Zealand, having been trained as a lawyer in France, but was a founder member of the Botanic Garden, Wellington, studied alpine plants in the South Island, and was a keen ornithologist. The genus *Traversia* commemorates him.

Mention has already been made of distinguished naturalists who emigrated to the United States, before or after taking up their science. A later emigrant who left Ireland to take up an academic post in the U.S. was Thomas Antisell (b. Dublin 1817, d. 1893). Antisell was Lecturer in Botany, Peter Street School of Medicine, Dublin, but left for New York in 1848, the year of rebellion in Ireland where he was a prominent Young Irelander; Praeger speculates that his political allegiance might explain his emigration to the U.S. He was appointed Professor of Chemistry and Toxicology, Georgetown University, Washington, D.C. On the U.S. Department of Agriculture railroad survey in California and Arizona, Antisell was chief chemist for the geologist conducting the survey, and he took the opportunity to botanize in those western regions. He published many papers and Asa Gray named *Astragalus antiselli* in his honour. Robert Lloyd Praeger's brother William Emilius (b. Belfast 1863, d. 1936), also a naturalist, became Professor of Biology, Kalamazoo College, Michigan, in 1905, in which capacity he studied plant physiology and ecology.

Sojourners, Excursionists and Expeditionists

When closet naturalists (sedentary collectors and classifiers) gave way to field naturalists in the nineteenth century, travel became a component of nature study, and fieldwork became a pre-requisite for professional qualification in geology, botany and zoology. The expansion of transportation in many parts of the world made this logistically feasible. Some naturalists nowadays make excursions abroad to study and collect during institutional vacations and professional leaves of absence. Some remain outside Ireland for some time before returning, becoming resident aliens abroad. Some accompany expeditions, which are mounted to explore or survey unstudied regions or to solve particular and significant problems (or demonstrate important hypotheses). Irish naturalists have contributed their fair share of energy and expertise to overseas enterprises and come back to Ireland when the work was completed.

An early and controversial Irish sojourner abroad and explorer of the New World was John Brickell, who travelled to North Carolina in the 1720s and in 1730-1 was a member of an expedition that penetrated the western part of Carolina and possibly Tennessee in order to promote friendly relations with the Cherokee Indians (Urness, 1969). He was interested in animals and plants but especially birds, and in 1737 his book *The Natural History of North-Carolina* (a survey of the flora, fauna and aboriginals) was published in Dublin. The similarities between this lively book and John Lawson's pioneering *A New Voyage to Carolina* (1709, reprinted as *The History of Carolina*, 1714) have been debated. At the very least Brickell, a physician, added to Lawson's information, particularly fresh, and sometimes absurd, material on the medical properties of birds; he recommended distilled buzzard's feet for sciatica, crane's gall for palsy, passenger-pigeon dung for headache, and the dung of the 'goss hawk' ('drank while fasting in wine') for conception. Brickell appears to have returned to live in Ireland.

Another notable Irish explorer of the New World, likewise a physician, but whose reputation is beyond question, was Thomas Coulter (b. Dundalk 1793, d. 1843). This botanist, who collected in Mexico, California and Arizona from 1831 to 1833 but who sojourned in Mexico from 1824, is commemorated by both a genus, *Coulteria*, and a biography, *A Man Who Can Speak of Plants* (199?) by E.C. Nelson and A. Probert who print in full, from the hitherto unpublished original manuscripts, *Coulter's Notes of Upper California* (1835). Yet another physician-naturalist was Robert Templeton (1802-92), who painted shells and butterflies in Sri Lanka and who is profiled below. The number of physician-botanists, both inside and outside Ireland, who flourished in the eighteenth and nineteenth centuries testifies to the origins of botany in herbal medicine, and they are the counterpart in some ways of the British and Irish clergymen-ornithologists of the nineteenth and twentieth centuries (of which Armstrong and Fr P.G. Kennedy are examples), though the connection between ornithology and Christianity is not clear. In any event, all the established professions – the law, medicine, the church, the armed services – have contributed many naturalists seeking disciplined leisure or opportunities and finances for travel, and familiar with careful observation and the patient gathering of data.

A more extensive traveller than Coulter was Thomas Workman (b. Helen's Bay, Co. Down 1843, d. 1900), member of a distinguished Belfast shipbuilding family, whose travels included Egypt, India, China, the Philippines, and the Americas. He studied spiders and collected them in Ireland as well as abroad; and his valuable collection of specimens was presented after his death to the National Museum, Dublin, which in turn presented selected specimens to the British and Belfast Museums (Deane, 1924). Only one volume of his *Malaysian Spiders* (1896) – illustrated by his own hand – was published before he died in Minnesota. Two tropical spiders were named after him, *Damarchus workmanii* and *Theridium workmanii*. H. Lyster Jameson (b. Louth 1875, d. 1922), also a zoologist, contributed his first paper, on birds, to the first volume of *The Irish Naturalist* when he was seventeen. He later published papers on Irish bats. He studied in

London and Heidelberg before going to Sri Lanka to investigate the pearl-oyster fisheries and establishing the parasitic theory of pearl formation. He remained abroad, in the Transvaal, for health reasons, before returning to England where he died prematurely while Adviser on Inshore Fisheries to the Development Commission.

The story of Rev. William Spotswood Green (b. Youghal, Co. Cork 1847, d. 1919) has been entertainingly told by Clare Lloyd in her book *The Travelling Naturalists* (1985). Before becoming a Church of Ireland minister (rector of Carrigaline parish, Co. Cork), Green had been a mountain-climbing enthusiast, a member of expeditions to the Swiss Alps, Norway and the Lofoten Islands. A modest grant from the Royal Irish Academy enabled him to make the long voyage to New Zealand by way of Africa, Australia and Tasmania in the company of two alpine guides. His aim was to climb Mount Cook in the South Island, and after a series of well-recorded adventures he claimed to have done so. He was an energetic observer of wildlife and collector of alpine plants, among them a new Zealand species that Hooker at Kew Gardens pronounced to be new to science and named after its discoverer. Green's account of his expedition appeared in 1883 as *The High Alps of New Zealand*. His new reputation, enhanced by a paper on the Southern Alps read to the Royal Geographic Society, resulted in his being chosen as organizer of the Royal Irish Academy's deep-sea dredging operations. Green's involvement with the Irish fishing industry before and after his Canadian expedition in 1888 is explained in Moriarty's 'Fish and Fisheries' in this volume. Green and his cousin Rev. Henry Swanzy were commissioned by the Canadian government to survey the peaks and glaciers of the Selkirk range of the British Columbia Rockies. The survey, with its attendant adventures and natural-history observations, is recounted in Green's book *Among the Selkirk Glaciers* (1890). Lloyd quotes Praeger on Green after his death: 'He had satisfied the two chief desires of his life: he had explored the high mountain-snows of two continents, and also the depths of the ocean' (Lloyd, 1985).

E.W. McBride (b. Belfast 1866, d. 1940) was Professor of Zoology at McGill University, Canada, before returning to London where he was promoted to the professorship of Zoology at the Imperial College of Technology. He did distinguished work on the Echinodermata (starfishes, sea urchins, sea lilies and the like). Sir Nigel Ball (b. Dublin 1892, d. 1978) had a comparable career, holding the post of Professor of Botany, University College, Colombo, Sri Lanka, then returning to teach in King's College, London.

During the heroic age of seagoing exploration, between Cabot in the late fifteenth century, say, and Dampier in the early eighteenth century and even after, it was sea-captains and ships' surgeons who returned with collections and data (often confused and unclassified) from the ends of the earth. Natural history was then a by-product of nautical, military and 'hard science' exploration as late as those expeditions in which three of our pro-filed naturalists took part: the Arctic expeditions of 1818 and 1819-20, with Sir Edward Sabine as astronomer; the Euphrates explorations of 1835-7 led by Francis Chesney; and the search for Sir John Franklin's lost 1845 expe-dition, conducted by Francis Leopold McClintock. Later, the profile of nat-uralists on expeditions was raised. H.C. Hart (1847-1908) collected plants on the British Polar Expedition (Arctic) of 1875-6 and the Palestine Exploring Expedition of 1883-4, and is profiled below.

An Irish-led interior expedition worth remembering is the Palliser Expedition to western Canada, 1857-9. John Palliser (b. Comeragh House, Co. Waterford 1817, d. 1887) had his appetite for travel in North America whetted by a hunting tour to the Missouri area in 1847-8, recounted in *Solitary Rambles and Adventures of a Hunter in the Prairies* (1853). He sub-mitted a plan to the Royal Geographical Society to travel from Red River colony through the Rocky Mountains; to this agenda the Colonial Office added exploration of the old North-West Company canoe route west from Lake Superior. Under Palliser's command, there were an appointed geolo-gist and naturalist, a botanical collector, an astronomer and a magnetical observer. The explorers amassed astronomical, meteorological, geological and magnetic data, described the flora and fauna of the country, and assessed the region's capacity for settlement and transportation. The reports of the expe-dition were for some time the major source of information about the coun-try from Lake Superior to the Okanagan Valley in British Columbia and are still of value (Spry, 1963). Between them, then, Palliser and Macoun were responsible for generating through exploration a wealth of natural-history information about western Canada in the nineteenth century. Intermittent militia service between 1839 and 1863 involved Palliser at one point in a semi-confidential mission to the Caribbean and Confederate states (1862-3). Another daring exploration took him and his brother Frederick in 1869 to Novaya Zemlya and the Kara Sea in northern Russia in their specially rein-forced ship, the *Sampson*. Palliser's remaining years were devoted to running the heavily mortgaged estate in Co. Waterford and serving as a local Justice of the Peace (Spry, 1968).

It is worth recording the collecting abroad carried out by the botanist Daniel Macreight (b. Armagh 1799, d. 1857) who visited the Pyrenees and published *A Manual of British Botany*; the genus *Macreightia* remembers him. Isaac Carroll (b. Aghada, Co. Cork 1828, d. 1880), a lichenologist by special-ity, collected in Lapland and Iceland in the 1860s before his premature death ended a life devoted to the flora of his native country. Robert Lloyd Praeger (b. Holywood, Co. Down 1865, d. 1953), something of a presiding genius during much of the heroic age of Irish fieldwork (1863-1913), worked as a botanist outside as well as inside Ireland. In 1924 he went in search of sempervivums (houseleeks) to the Canary Islands and Madeira, and in 1926, in search of the same genus of plants, he botanized in the Balkans; he also spent time in the Austrian and Italian Tyrols (Collins, 1985). The innumerable references throughout this volume to one of the greatest all-round naturalists of these islands can be regarded as Praeger's composite profile.

It remains only to mention some of the naturalists who were not born in Ireland but who lived formative years of their scientific lives on the island and who staffed major expeditions. Sir Wyville Thomson (1830-82) was born in Scotland and lived in Ireland between 1853 and 1870, during which time he became, variously, Professor of Natural History, Queen's College, Cork; Professor of Natural History, Queen's College, Belfast; and Professor of Botany, Royal College of Science, Dublin. He took part in the famous deep-sea explorations known as the *Lightning, Porcupine* and *Challenger* expeditions. The latter vessel traversed over 68,000 miles of Atlantic and Pacific oceans in 1872 and the research accomplished radically augmented our knowledge of marine life. Thomson's book *The Depths of the Sea* (1873), an account of the *Porcupine* and *Lightning* voyages, bridged the gap between scientist and layman, a gap later to become a gulf as the study of Nature fragmented into highly specialized and technical branches of biology.

R.O. Cunningham (1841-1918), another Scot, succeeded Thomson as Professor of Natural History, Queen's College, Belfast (1871-1902). Like all college teachers of natural history in those pre-specializing days, he lectured on zoology, botany and geology. He was physician and naturalist on board the HMS *Nassau* expedition to southern South America (1867-9) and published *The Natural History of Magellan and Patagonia* in 1871. J.K. Charlesworth was born in Leeds and held the Chair of Geology at Queen's University, Belfast, from 1921. He was Geologist on the Scottish Spitzbergen expedition of 1919. He published distinguished papers on glaciation in Ireland and was awarded the Belfast Naturalists' Field Club Commemoration Medal in 1936. Like Thomson, Henry and Cunningham, Charlesworth contributed to the necessary and welcome infusion of outside energy and authority into the island; but that infusion has been balanced by the outward flow of enthusiasm and expertise that has always characterized the Irish study of nature.

References

Armstrong, E.A. 1942. *Bird Display: An Introduction to the Study of Bird Psychology*. Cambridge: Cambridge University Press.
Armstrong, E.A. [1947] 1965. *Bird Display and Behaviour*. New York: Dover.
Armstrong, E.A. 1955. *The Wren*. London: Collins.
Armstrong, E.A. [1963] 1973. *A Study of Bird Song*. New York: Dover.

Brightwell, C.L. 1861. *Difficulties Overcome: Scenes in the Life of Alexander Wilson*. London: Sampson, Low.

Burrage, H.S. (ed.). 1906. *Early English and French Voyages Chiefly from Hakluyt 1534-1608*. New York: Charles Scribner's Sons.

Chadwick, N. 1970. *The Celts*. Harmondsworth: Penguin.

Collins, T. 1985. *Floreat Hibernia: A Bio-Bibliography of Robert Lloyd Praeger 1865-1953*. Dublin: Royal Dublin Society.

Curtis, E. 1950. *A History of Ireland*. London: Methuen.

Deane, A. (ed.). 1924. *The Belfast Natural History and Philosophical Society: Centenary Volume 1821-1921*. Belfast: BNHPS.

Desmond, R. 1994. *Dictionary of British and Irish Botanists and Horticulturists*. London: Natural History Museum.

Doherty, C. 1991. 'Introduction' to 'Latin Writing in Ireland', in Seamus Deane (ed.), *The Field Day Anthology of Irish Writing*, vol. I. Derry: Field Day Publications.

Flower, R. 1947. *The Irish Tradition*. Oxford: Clarendon Press.

Foster, J.W. 1977. 'Certain Set Apart: The Western Island in the Irish Renaissance.' *Studies 66*: 261-74.

Foster, R.F. 1989. *Modern Ireland: 1600-1972*. London: Penguin.

Goode, G.B. 1901. 'The Beginnings of Natural History in America.' *Annual Report of the Smithsonian Institution 2 (1896/97)*: 357-406.

Hakluyt, R. 1907. *The Principal Navigations of the English Nation*, vol.6. London: Dent.

Innes-Smith, R.W. 1932. *English-Speaking Students of Medicine at the University of Leyden*. Edinburgh: Oliver and Boyd.

Joyce, P.W. (trans.). 1879. *Old Celtic Romances*. Dublin: Talbot Press.

Knott, E. and G. Murphy. 1966. *Early Irish Literature*. London: Routledge & Kegan Paul.

Lloyd, C. 1985. *The Travelling Naturalists*. London: Croom Helm.

McGee, T.D'A. 1852. *A History of the Irish Settlers in North America*. Boston: Patrick Donahoe.

McGee, T.D'A. 1857. *The Irish Writers of the Seventeenth Century*. Dublin: James Duffy.

Miller, D.P. and P.H. Reill (eds). 1996. *Visions of Empire: Voyages, Botany and Representations of Nature*. Cambridge: Cambridge University Press.

Myers, A.C. [1902] 1969. *Immigration of the Irish Quakers into Pennsylvania 1682-1750*. Baltimore: Genealogical Publishing Company.

Nelson, E.C. 1992. 'William Henry Harvey as Colonial Treasurer at the Cape of Good Hope: A Case of Depression and Bowdlerized History.' *Archives of Natural History 19*: 171-80.

Nelson, E.C. 1994. *Flowers of Mayo: Dr Patrick Browne's Fasciculus Plantarum Hiberniae 1788*. Blackrock: Edmund Burke.

Nelson, E.C. and A. Probert. 199?. *A Man Who Can Speak of Plants*.

O'Connor, J.P. 1988. 'Some Entomologists Associated with the Dublin Naturalists' Field Club.' *In the Field of the Naturalists: Proceedings of the DNFC Centenary Seminar*. Dublin: DNFC.

O'Loughlin, T. 1993. 'The Earliest World Maps Known in Ireland.' *History Ireland, Spring 1993*: 7-10.

Praeger, R.L. 1949. *Some Irish Naturalists: A Biographical Note-Book*. Dundalk: Dundalgan Press.

Raby, P. 1996. *Bright Paradise: Victorian Scientific Travellers*. London: Chatto and Windus.

Raistrick, A. 1968. *Quakers in Science and Industry*. Newton Abbot: David & Charles.

Ranelagh, J. O'B. 1983. *A Short History of Ireland*. Cambridge: Cambridge University Press.

Reynolds, G.A. 1997. 'William Bowles (1720-1780), Eurogeologist.' *European Geologist 5*: 67-70.

Seymour, St J.D. 1930. *Irish Visions of the Other-World*. London: SPCK.

Spry, I.M. 1963. *The Palliser Expedition*. Toronto: Macmillan.

Spry, I.M. 1968. *The Papers of the Palliser Expedition 1857-1860*. Toronto: Champlain Society.

Stroud, P.T. 1992. *Thomas Say: New World Naturalist*. Philadelphia: University of Pennsylvania Press.

Stroud, P.T. 1995. 'The Founding of the Academy of Natural Sciences of Philadelphia in 1812 and its Journal in 1817.' *Archives of Natural History* 22: 221-33.

Tolles, F.B. 1957. *James Logan and the Culture of Provincial America*. Boston: Little, Brown.

Tolles, F.B. 1960. *Quakers and the Atlantic Culture*. New York: Macmillan.

Urness, C. 1969. 'Introduction' to *The Natural History of North-Carolina* by John Brickell. New York: Johnson Reprint Corporation.

Zimmer, H. 1891. *The Irish Element in Mediaeval Culture*. New York: Putnam's.

Sir Francis Beaufort
1774-1857

SHEILA LANDY

Paradoxically, the British Navy's greatest hydrographer and map-maker was an indifferently educated Irishman. Best remembered as the originator of the Beaufort Scale, a measure of wind-force ranging from 0 to 12, and also of a system that indicates the weather's various states by letters of the alphabet, Francis Beaufort was born in Navan, Co. Meath, in 1774. His father, a descendant of Huguenots who settled in Dublin in 1738, was Church of Ireland rector of Navan, and also something of a polymath. The Rev. D.A. Beaufort included among his wide-ranging interests science, architecture, astronomy, topography and mapping, and was responsible for the best map of Ireland made prior to the appearance of the Ordnance Survey (Beaufort, 1792).

Francis, the third of six children, was educated in Dublin. He showed an interest in astronomy from a young age and was sent in his early teens for five month's study at Trinity College's Dunsink Observatory, which had been founded in 1785. Shortly after the family's move to London in 1788, the fourteen-year-old Francis began his seagoing career with a long trading and surveying voyage to the East Indies and China. During the passage the ship struck rocks and had to be abandoned by the crew who took to the boats and were rescued only after spending five days on the open sea. Undoubtedly this early experience of shipwreck, a consequence of the lack of reliable maps of routes taken by British merchant ships and men-of-war, was influential in shaping the young Beaufort's subsequent career.

During the next seven years he saw much active service in the Navy, survived a near drowning, and became a lieutenant at twenty-two. Beaufort at this time was spending most of his pay on expensive navigational instruments and, despite the difficult conditions on board ship, read voraciously, not just works of navigation and astronomy but also theology, philosophy and literature. His seagoing library in 1806 comprised more than two hundred books, with the result that, despite a mediocre schooling, Beaufort was able to transform himself into a learned man and scientist.

As a result of severe wounds sustained in battle with the Spanish in 1800, Beaufort, now a commander, spent the next four years ashore. Depressed by his inability to procure a ship to command, he wrote to his brother, '... thirty-two, and no employment, no wife, no shilling and no hope'. Lacking the patronage required for advancement in the Navy of those days, Beaufort found the preferment he deserved denied him. However, he was not long without employment on land. After a brief period in London he was reunited with his family in Ireland and soon became involved with a project devised by his brother-in-law, Richard Lovell Edgeworth. The 'ingenious Mr Edgeworth' was an inventor and radical educationalist, and father-to-be of Maria Edgeworth, one of the most famous novelists of the nineteenth century. Edgeworthstown, where the Edgeworth family had their home, was a cultural centre for local writers, publishers and intellectuals, and provided a new and stimulating environment for Beaufort after his years at sea. Edgeworth was obsessed with the idea of establishing a semaphore system that would transmit messages to Dublin from Galway, the purpose of which was to alert Dublin in the event of a French landing on the west coast. Unfortunately, despite the fact that the invention was probably the world's first telegraphic communication system, it proved to be clumsy, difficult to operate and vulnerable to adverse weather conditions, and was eventually abandoned.

In 1805 Beaufort was appointed to the command of the *Woolwich*, an armed store ship, and continued in service for the next five years. Interested in all aspects of modern science, and meteorology in particular, Beaufort, even as a midshipman, made weather reports every two hours rather than the required twelve to twenty-four hours. By 1806, and until his death, he was keeping a daily weather journal, noting wind direction and strength, temperatures and barometric readings. Unhappy with the weather recording systems then in use for ships' log-books, Beaufort was aware of the need for consistent and formal notation, rather than the subjective descriptions then in use. While waiting for a ship, Beaufort in 1806 devised a wind scale that classified the wind force at sea, ranging from 0 for dead calm to 13 for a full storm. The scale was originally based on the effect of the wind on a full-rigged man-of-war, and specified the amount of sail that a ship should carry in each situation. A little later he devised a system whereby the weather's various states, on sea and land, are indicated by letters of the alphabet, with dots beneath the letters to indicate intensity. The wind scale and weather notation tables were not adopted by the Admiralty until some thirty years later when they became mandatory for log entries in all ships of the Royal Navy. It is interesting to note that the first recorded use of the Beaufort scale was in the official log of HMS *Beagle*, which carried Darwin on his momentous voyage in 1831. The Beaufort wind scale achieved world-wide acceptance and is still used in shipping today.

On promotion to post-captain in 1810, Beaufort took command of the frigate *Fredricksteen,* and as a consequence of his reputation as one of the Navy's ablest surveyors, was selected from the whole Mediterranean fleet to survey an unknown part of the coast of Syria. The result was not only an excellent survey but also a detailed account of the geographical and archaeological aspects of the country. *Karamania, or a Brief Description of the South Coast of Asia Minor* (1817) was a learned and substantial work, of interest to both the scientist and the scholar, and became one of the major travel books of its day.

Beaufort's work in Asia Minor was brought to an abrupt end in 1812 by an attack on his ship by some Turkish fanatics. Seriously wounded, Beaufort returned to England when he had sufficiently recovered, and the *Fredricksteen* was paid off. Although he did not know it, this was the end of Beaufort's seagoing career. In the subsequent years he spent his time preparing for the Admiralty a very fine set of charts from the surveys he had made of the shores of Asia Minor, the Black Sea and Africa. These charts, engraved directly from his drawings, were sent to the Hydrographic Office. As late as 1972 Beaufort was quoted as a major authority for the surveys of the south coast of Turkey, and until 1976 was still given as the authority for its eastern part.

During the period 1812 to 1817 Beaufort began corresponding with the most prominent antiquarians, travellers and scholars of the day, and he continued this correspondence until the end of his life. In 1814 Beaufort was unanimously elected to the Royal Society, having been proposed by Richard Lovell Edgeworth. Six years later he became one of the founder members of the Royal Astronomical Society and in 1830 of the Royal Geographical Society. In 1826 he embarked on a project dear to his heart: the preparation of a series of maps to be sold by the Society for the Diffusion of Useful Knowledge. These maps, intended for purchase by the general public, were sold for sixpence each, a price made possible by Beaufort's producing them without any payment for himself.

The post of Hydrographer to the Admiralty was given to Beaufort in 1829, and he remained in that office for the next twenty-six years. During this time he set himself the mammoth task of planning detailed surveys of all unchartered coasts both at home and abroad. A total of almost fifteen hundred charts were produced during his term of office at an average rate of approximately sixty per year. These maps were unrivalled for accuracy and completeness, making the words 'admiralty chart' a synonym for excellence and reliability. His success as Hydrographer earned him a number of foreign honours from learned societies, including the American Philosophical

Society, the Académie Royale des Sciences de l'Institut de France, the Royal Irish Academy and the United States Naval Lyceum – a remarkable achievement for a man whose formal education ceased at the age of fourteen.

In addition to producing charts, the Hydrographic Office published non-cartographic nautical information. Beaufort was the originator of the *Nautical Magazine, Notices to Mariners and the Admiralty Time Tables*. As a result of his tremendous efforts the Hydrographic Office, previously no more than a map room, became a highly respected scientific department.

Beaufort's membership of the most important scientific institutions of the day brought him into contact with many eminent scientists. This enabled him to act as an influential link between geographers, astronomers, meteorologists, and the government department best able to support their research projects. It was Beaufort who secured funds for many of the great seaborne scientific expeditions of the latter part of the nineteenth century. For example, he succeeded in obtaining government support for the voyage in 1839 of James Clark Ross to the Antarctic, an expedition that resulted in the discovery of the Great Ross Ice Barrier and in the mapping of hundreds of miles of hitherto-unknown coasts of the Antarctic. An even more significant event in which Beaufort played an important role was his recommendation that Charles Darwin sail with Captain Robert Fitzroy on the momentous voyage in the *Beagle*. Beaufort was also a member of the Arctic Council and closely involved with the lengthy attempt, begun in 1847, to rescue Sir John Franklin, who had been lost in search of the North-west Passage.

In 1846 he elected to become Rear Admiral on the retired list rather than surrender his office; the mortification of his retirement was somewhat compensated for by his being made a Knight of the Bath two years later. He continued in the post of Hydrographer until 1855, only two years before his death at Hove, near Brighton, in December 1857 at the age of eighty-four.

Twice married – first to Alicia, the daughter of his first commander, Lestock Wilson, and then to Honora, a sister of Maria Edgeworth – Beaufort fathered four sons and two daughters. His youngest daughter, Emily, travelled extensively in the Middle East where she founded hospitals and organizations to provide medical aid to the poor. His second son, Francis Lestock Beaufort, became Attorney General of Calcutta.

The name Beaufort became synonymous in the Navy with hydrography and nautical science, and the Beaufort prize, awarded annually to the best student of navigation at the Royal Naval College, Dartmouth, is a fitting memorial to the British Navy's greatest scientist, and one who made the seas safer for all.

References

Anon. 1858. 'Biographical notice of the death of Rear-Admiral Sir Francis Beaufort.' *Monthly Notices of the Royal Astronomical Society 18*: 93-8.

Beaufort, D.A. 1792. Map of Ireland accompanying *Memoir of a Map of Ireland Illustrating the Topography of that Kingdom, and Containing a Short Account of its Present State, civil and ecclesiastical.* London.

Beaufort, F. 1817. *Karamania, or a Brief Description of the South Coast of Asia Minor.* London: R. Hunter.

Beaufort, F. 1820. *Memoir of a Survey of the Coast of Karamania made ... by Francis Beaufort in 1811 and 1812.* London: Hydrographic Department of the Admiralty.

Friendly, A. 1977. *Beaufort of the Admiralty.* London: Hutchinson.

Landy, S. 1985. 'Francis Beaufort: Hydrographer and Nautical Scientist,' in C. Mollan, W. Davis and B. Finucane (eds), *Some People and Places in Irish Science and Technology.* Dublin: Royal Irish Academy.

President of the Geological Society of London. 1858. 'Obituary of Rear-Admiral Sir Francis Beaufort.' *Quarterly Journal of the Geological Society of London 14*: xlvii-liv.

Sir Edward Sabine
1788-1883

PAUL HACKNEY

Edward Sabine was born in Dublin on 14 October 1788 of English parents. After education at Marlow he entered the Royal Military Academy at Woolwich in January 1803 and received a commission in the Royal Artillery in December of that year.

Following eventful military service in North America during 1813-16 he returned home and devoted his time to his interests in science, particularly astronomy and terrestrial magnetism. He was elected Fellow of the Royal Society in 1818 and in the same year was recommended by Sir Joseph Banks to be appointed as astronomer and naturalist to an expedition led by John Ross in search of the fabled North-west Passage between the Atlantic and Pacific Oceans.

Ross's instructions on his voyage of 1818 included that he

receive on board the *Isabella*, Captain Sabine of the Royal Artillery, who is represented to us as a Gentleman well skilled in Astronomy, Natural History and various branches of knowledge; to assist you in making such observations as may tend to the improvement of Geography and Navigation, and the advancement of science in general. You are to make use of every means in your power to collect and preserve such specimens of the animal, mineral and vegetable, kingdoms, as you can conveniently stow on board ... In this, as well as in every other part of your scientific duty, we trust that you will receive material assistance from Captain Sabine. (Ross, 1819)

Sabine disliked Ross, whom he referred to as a 'stupid fellow', and Ross in turn criticized Sabine's qualities as a naturalist in his account of the expedition (Ross, 1819; Berton, 1988). Ross, having referred to his instructions as quoted above, wrote to Sabine upon their return from the expedition to ask for a report of the natural-history results of the expedition. Sabine's reply suggests that he had little knowledge of natural history: 'I have no pretension to more than a very ordinary knowledge of any branch of it, excepting ornithology.' Sabine also said that he had communicated his specimens to Dr Leach of the Natural History Museum and implied that Ross should expect some sort of report from Leach direct, but in fact no report was forthcoming. The natural-history content of Ross's book is consequently sparse. What botanical information appears in the text was based on plants collected by Sabine and James Clark Ross (a midshipman and nephew of John Ross) from the shores of Baffin's Bay which were submitted to Robert Brown for identification.

Sabine was indeed knowledgeable about birds and had collected natural-history material on the voyage, including a specimen of a previously undescribed species of gull which his brother, Joseph, an eminent ornithologist, named *Larus sabini* in Edward's honour. Sabine had encountered the gull, which became known as Sabine's Gull, on islands off the west coast of Greenland. Sabine subsequently read a paper to the Linnean Society in April 1819 which recorded another twenty-three species of birds encountered by him on the expedition (Sabine, J., 1819).

Sabine's principal interests, however, were in the earth's magnetic field, and it is in this area that he was to make his name and greatest contributions to science. On his first voyage, with Ross's Arctic expedition of 1818, he made many observations on the declination and dip of the compass. Although it is now well known that the magnetic compass needle, upon which navigation had become so dependent, does not point to true north but actually deviates east or west of it, pointing towards the magnetic pole, this deviation, or declination, had not been discovered until the sixteenth century. At that time, in Britain, it had an 'easterly declination', meaning that the magnetic pole lay to the east of the true pole. It gradually decreased until about 1659 when the needle pointed exactly north and from then on the needle drifted westerly and the declination increased as the magnetic pole moved to the west of the true pole. The declination was also found to vary in different parts of the world, and since ship navigation relied so heavily on the magnetic compass it was vital to establish the size of compass error in the different parts of the globe. Sabine was also interested in the 'dip' or angle that a compass needle freely pivoting in a vertical plane would assume, and the strength of the magnetic field, both of which also vary from place to place. These also vary with time, and apart from long-term changes, Sabine identified cyclical changes associated with the sunspot cycle.

In 1819-20, at the age of thirty, Sabine made his second Arctic voyage, again as astronomer, on an expedition led by Edward Parry, who had been Ross's second-in-command in 1818. Their journey and scientific observations are described in Parry's own 1821 account, which shows that most of the observations were to test the accuracy of several types of chronometer and to compare their reliability for determination of longitude with longitudes obtained by lunar observation. The science of navigation was undergoing considerable scrutiny and refinement at the time, and Sabine was one of those closely involved.

His third Arctic voyage aboard the brig *Griper*, under the command of Captain Clavering, was to the northern parts of Norway, Spitzbergen and north-east Greenland. On 13 August 1823 he landed on an island off the east coast of Greenland that was subsequently named after him (Sabine Island c. 74°N). Another small island where he carried out pendulum observations, a little north of Sabine Island, was to be named Pendulum Island (Vahl et al., 1928-9).

Pendulum observations were seen as an important part of the scientific work of Arctic expeditions until the late nineteenth century (Greely, 1886). A pendulum takes longer to make a complete swing, or period, at the equator than at the poles. Sabine's experiments were an attempt to use the different periods of a pendulum to make an estimate of the differences in the force of gravity ('g') and thus calculate the degree of flattening of the earth; they were concerned with 'geodesy', measuring the form or shape of the earth. A pendulum clock was set up on land and allowed to run for several days, making due allowance for atmospheric pressure, altitude and temperature. (The Royal Society furnished the two clocks for use on the Parry voyage, the same instruments that had accompanied Captain Cook on his voyages.) In fact we now know that the variation in 'g' is too complex to be used to estimate polar flattening in this simple way, with the result that Sabine's estimate and those of his contemporaries underestimated the degree of flattening.

In 1827 Sabine obtained leave of absence to carry out scientific duties as long as he was not required by the Royal Artillery. However, Irish unrest in 1830 provoked an increased military presence; Sabine was recalled for duty and spent the next seven years serving with his regiment in Ireland. There he met and collaborated with Humphrey Lloyd, Professor of Natural and Experimental Philosophy at Trinity College, Dublin, who was also greatly interested in the study of magnetism.

Until this time scientists had difficulty obtaining accurate measurements of the parameters of the earth's magnetic field because of the inadequacies of the instruments and methods in use at the time. These difficulties were overcome successfully after 1834 by Lloyd's work, in particular his invention, with Sabine, of a single instrument designed to measure both dip and field intensity. In 1834 and 1835, together with James Clark Ross, Lloyd and Sabine carried out a magnetic survey of Ireland using, alongside older methods, their new instrument. The British Association for the Advancement of Science was largely responsible for research into terrestrial magnetism in the United Kingdom and their results were presented to the British Association at the Dublin meeting of 1835. Sabine and his collaborators went on to carry out similar surveys of Scotland, England and Wales.

Already the construction of permanent magnetic observatories had been urged by the leaders in the field of terrestrial magnetic studies, notably Karl Friedrich Gauss and Baron Friedrich von Humboldt who had set up the first, in the Russian Empire. Following a meeting with Sabine in Berlin, Humboldt contacted the Royal Society to urge the establishment of magnetic observatories throughout the British Empire. Subsequently, the first magnetic observatories in the British Isles were constructed at Greenwich and, more or less simultaneously, in the grounds of the Provost's House at Trinity College, Dublin. This was at Lloyd's instigation and was completed in 1838.

By the 1830s considerable advances had been made in the study of the earth's magnetic field, chiefly during the various Arctic voyages of Sabine and others. In 1831 James Clark Ross located the position of the north magnetic pole on the Boothian Peninsula in Arctic America, and the German physicist Karl Friedrich Gauss predicted that the south magnetic pole would be located around lat. 66°S long. 146°E (Kirwan, 1959; Ross 1982). Thus one of the principal objectives of a newly proposed British Antarctic expedition was to verify the exact location of the south magnetic pole, or even poles, since Sabine favoured the view of the Norwegian physicist Hansteen that there might be four magnetic poles. (This view, as we now know, was erroneous.)

The first public appeal to the British government to sponsor such a British Antarctic expedition was made at the 1835 Dublin meeting of the British Association, where Sabine was a dominant figure. In 1838, at the BA meeting in Newcastle-upon-Tyne, a formal resolution was carried again calling upon the British government to send out an expedition for making magnetic observations between Australia and Cape Horn. Eventually, through Sabine's exertions and those of Captain Washington RN (Secretary of the Royal Geographical Society), an expedition was organized and James Clark Ross was appointed to lead it. His ships were the *Erebus* and the *Terror* and his second-in-command was Captain Francis Crozier from Banbridge, Co. Down. Both James Clark Ross and Crozier had been members of Parry's second and third Arctic expeditions of 1821-3 and 1824-5 (Fluhmann, 1976).

The expedition departed from England in 1839. Magnetic observatories were set up, including one on Tasmania where Ross had the enthusiastic support of the Governor, Sir John Franklin. In 1841 Ross's expedition moved south to locate the magnetic pole and encountered the coast of Antarctica; a high mountain in what is now Victoria Land was named Mount Sabine by Ross. Although Ross was able to calculate the true position of the southern magnetic pole, it proved to be located in inaccessible mountainous terrain. In every respect Ross's expedition was notably successful and provided much information on the terrestrial magnetism of the southern latitudes.

Sabine was subsequently instrumental in ensuring the establishment of permanent magnetic observatories such as those at Hobart (Tasmania), the Cape of Good Hope and St Helena. The instruments and observational techniques used in these imperial observatories had been developed by Lloyd at his Dublin observatory. By the time of the International Geophysical Year in 1957/58 there were about 150 magnetic observatories widely distributed over the globe.

The importance of accurate and long-term observations of the earth's magnetic field remains to this day and Sabine was undoubtedly one of the great pioneers in the field, both with his own observations and in promoting the expeditions of others such as James Clark Ross. From 1840 onwards he contributed to *Philosophical Transactions of the Royal Society* a long series of papers under the title 'Contributions to Terrestrial Magnetism', which detailed the observations at the various British observatories. There were fifteen papers spread over thirty-six years, including magnetic maps, catalogues and tables. Sabine remained closely involved with the work of the BA and, for twenty years from 1839, he was its General Secretary and he occupied the presidential chair at the Belfast meeting in 1852 (at which an address was given by his old friend Francis Rawdon Chesney on his Euphrates Expedition). He also had close connections with the Royal Society, being its Foreign Secretary from 1845-50, then its Treasurer and became President from 1861-71.

Sabine still had a role in another British effort to find the Northwest Passage. In the 1840s the government decided to organize another expedition to the North American Arctic to make what was hoped would be a final successful attempt to locate a navigable passage between the two oceans. Sabine favoured his friend James Clark Ross as leader, but in the event, partly because of intense lobbying by his wife, Lady Jane Franklin, Sir John Franklin was given the command. Franklin was fifty-nine years old and Sabine and many others considered him too old for such a rigorous task. Despite his feelings about Franklin, Sabine gave scientific advice on the proposed expedition, which he regarded as a most important opportunity to complete the accumulated data on terrestrial magnetism (Cyriax, 1939), and consequently great importance was attached to the magnetic observations. Contributing to these observations would be a new instrument, called a deflection inclinometer, developed by Lloyd after 1842. This was a device for determining dip and absolute intensity of the magnetic field in high latitudes where existing instruments were inaccurate. The new instrument was carried on Franklin's Arctic Expedition of 1845 and that of Sir John Richardson and Sir James Ross in 1848. After some further modification it became the standard instrument for determining the strength of the magnetic field at sea (O'Hara, 1983).

Franklin, with Crozier as his second-in-command, left England in 1845 in the same ships as had served Ross and Crozier in their Antarctic voyage of 1839-43. By February 1847, with no news of the expedition, the government turned to Parry for advice. Parry conferred with Sabine and they assembled other experts, including Sir Francis Beaufort, to discuss the search for the Franklin Expedition. This was the beginning of the grand-sounding Arctic Council or Arctic Committee [*plate 13*], which in the event proved largely ineffective in its advice.

Sabine received several honours during his long life; as well as his Fellowship of the Royal Society, he received its Gold Medal and was elected an Honorary Fellow of several other learned societies and was a member of a number of foreign orders in Prussia, Italy and Brazil. His scientific activity corresponded almost entirely with his career as an officer in the army, from which he retired with the rank of General in 1870 having been knighted the previous year. His scientific output was prodigious; he contributed over a hundred papers to *Philosophical Transactions of the Royal Society* alone (Royal Society 1871, 1896). He reached the grand age of ninety-four and is buried in the family vault at Tewin in Hertfordshire, beside the remains of his wife, Elizabeth (formerly Laeves), who had worked closely with him and who also achieved prominence as a translator of scientific works, in particular those of Baron von Humboldt. They had no children.

References

Berton, P. 1988. *The Arctic Grail.* Toronto: McClelland and Stewart.

Cyriax, R.J. 1939. *Sir John Franklin's Last Arctic Expedition.* London: Methuen.

Fluhmann, M. 1976. *Second in Command: A Biography of Captain Francis Crozier R.N.* Canada: Govt. of the Northwest Territories.

Greely, A. 1886. *Three Years of Arctic Service: An Account of the Lady Franklin Bay Expedition of 1881-84.* 2 vols. London: R. Bentley.

Kirwan, L.P. 1959. *The White Road: A History of Polar Exploration.* London: Hollis and Carter.

O'Hara, J.G. 1983. 'Gauss and the Royal Society: the Reception of his Ideas on Magnetism in Britain (1832-42).' *Notes and Records of the Royal Society 38*: 17-78.

Parry, W.E. 1821. *Journal of a Voyage for the Discovery of a North-west Passage from the Atlantic to the Pacific performed in the Years 1819-20.* London: J. Murray.

Ross, J.K.S. 1819. *A Voyage of Discovery made under the Orders of the Admiralty in His Majesty's Ships* Isabella *and* Alexander *for the Purpose of Exploring Baffin's Bay and Inquiring into the Probability of a North-west Passage.* London: J. Murray.

Ross, M.J. 1982. *Ross in the Antarctic. The Voyages of James Clark Ross in Her Majesty's ships* Erebus *and* Terror *1839-1843.* Whitby: Caedmon of Whitby.

Royal Society. 1871. *Catalogue of Scientific Papers 1800-1863.* Cambridge: Cambridge University Press.

Royal Society. 1896. *Catalogue of Scientific Papers 1874-1883.* Cambridge: Cambridge University Press.

Sabine, E. 1819. 'A Memoir of the Birds of Greenland; with Descriptions and Notes on the Species observed in the late Voyage of Discovery in Davis's Strait and Baffin's Bay.' *Transactions of the Linnean Society 12*: 527-59.

Sabine, E. 1843 and 1851. *Observations on Days of Unusual Magnetic Disturbance made at the British Colonial Magnetic Observatories.* London: Longmans.

Sabine, E. 1851. *Observations made at the Cape of Good Hope Royal Observatory.* Volume 1. Magnetical observations 1841 to 1846. London: Longmans.

Sabine, E. 1845-57. *Observations made at the Toronto Magnetical and Meteorological Observatory.* 3 vols. London: Longmans.

Sabine, E. 1847, 1860. *Observations made at the St Helena Magnetical and Meteorological Observatory.* 2 vols. London: Longmans.

Sabine, E. 1850-3. *Observations Made at the Magnetical and Meteorological Observatory at Hobarton in Van Diemen Island and by the Antarctic Naval Expedition.* 3 vols. London: Longmans.

Sabine, J. 1819. 'An Account of a New Species of Gull lately discovered on the West Coast of Greenland.' *Transactions of the Linnean Society 12*: 520-3.

Vahl, M., C.C. Amdrup, L. Bobé, A.D.S. Jensen. 1928-29. *Greenland.* 3 vols. Copenhagen: Reitzel; London: Oxford University Press.

General Francis Rawdon Chesney
1789-1872

HELENA C.G. CHESNEY

Francis Rawdon Chesney has been called 'The Father of the Suez Canal' because his survey of the Suez region in 1830 was the first to establish the feasibility of a canal. He carried out further extensive surveys and mapping in the Middle East, including Turkey, Syria and Iraq, and commanded the 'Euphrates Expedition' (1835-7), sponsored by the British government, to survey another possible route to India and the Far East.

Chesney was born in 1789 near Annalong, Co. Down, the eldest of four sons of Captain Alexander Chesney, who had emigrated to America with his parents in 1772 but had returned to Ireland ten years later after being wounded in the American Revolution. Alexander Chesney placed a high value on discipline and learning, for he intended his sons to have military careers. Francis was named after his godfather Francis Rawdon, Earl of Moira, his father's commanding officer in South Carolina.

When Francis reached the age of fourteen, his godfather gave him a cadetship to the Military Academy at Woolwich. He was under the required height and thus initially failed admission but was later successful, aided by cork insoles in his boots. Like Edward Sabine, Chesney gained a commission at the age of sixteen with the Royal Artillery. He served in Portsmouth as a First Lieutenant and then in Guernsey as aide-de-camp to the governor until 1814. That year, when home on leave, Chesney first showed his courage and stamina by saving a local fisherman and the crew of a French vessel during savage gales that devastated the Annalong fishing fleet.

The Artillery, then part of the Ordnance Department, was involved with defences rather than with the active service Chesney would have preferred. Following the French defeat at Waterloo in 1815, an interest in military strategy led him to take leave to study Napoleon's battlefields. His three-thousand-mile walking tour started with the French campaign fields. Then he crossed the Alps to study Marengo and returned from Italy through Massena and descended the Rhine to Jena, Rossbach, Leipzig and finally Waterloo.

Another garrison posting, to Gibraltar, followed and in 1827 he was promoted to the rank of Captain. He later travelled to Turkey as a military observer to study Balkan battle strategies in the Russo-Turkish War. In 1830 his experience and aptitudes resulted in a posting to the Middle East, to investigate the alternative Egyptian and Syrian routes to India. The preservation of trade and military connections with India and the East were of immense economic and strategic importance to Britain. Chesney became interested in an idea, originally investigated by Napoleon's surveyors in 1798, of a canal connecting the Mediterranean and Red Seas. The French surveyors had concluded that a large difference in sea levels precluded the construction of a canal. Chesney surveyed Suez and Sinai, then travelled down the Red Sea and back through the Nile valley to Alexandria. His survey revealed that an insignificant difference in sea levels made construction of a canal feasible. However, the British government, taking advice from Lord Palmerston, the Foreign Secretary, failed to act on his results and some three decades later the French used Chesney's survey as the basis for the construction of the Suez Canal. At the opening of the canal on 17 November 1869, Ferdinand de Lesseps, their leading engineer, referred to Chesney as 'the Father of the Suez Canal'.

In December 1830 Chesney's good health and military training in surveying and astronomy encouraged him to apply for leave to pursue further exploration in the Middle East. Chesney was interested in the feasibility of securing a route to India through Syria and down the great Euphrates river valley, roughly along an ancient caravan road. The lower Euphrates had long been plied as far as Hilla, but the upper part, which flows from Beles for

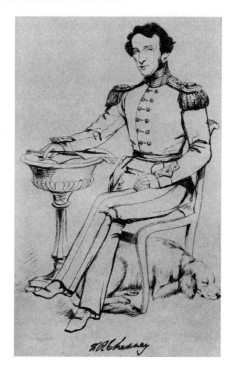

Drawing of Francis Rawdon Chesney by
C.Grey, RHA, 1838. (Royal Geographical
Society, London)

650 miles through the Syrian desert, was at that time a no man's land, inhabited by fierce Arab tribes who were a law unto themselves. Adopting Arab garb and accompanied by interpreters, Chesney travelled from Damascus through Syria to reach the Euphrates at Ana and descended the river on a kelek or raft. In this territory the hostility of Arab tribes frequently placed the party in danger, but Chesney sketched, made compass readings and secretly undertook soundings through a 'well' in the kelek. After successful completion of the survey, on the journey home he explored Persia, Eastern Anatolia and the Taurus Mountains on horseback, then travelled back to Constantinople and returned to London after a three-year exploration.

Armed with the results of his successful navigation Chesney started lobbying for an official survey of the Euphrates. Territorial gains meant that the Euphrates valley had by then become the frontier between the greatly expanded Egypt and Turkey, and Palmerston, the Foreign Secretary, was hesitant about igniting conflict in a region seething with local intrigue and hostility. Chesney persisted and in 1835, following an audience with William IV, Parliament voted £20,000 to fund a British expedition. This would investigate Chesney's contention that, if the Euphrates were navigable for most of the year, it could provide a viable commercial route and ensure a British presence in the region. Chesney was given command and a tight schedule that would not allow for many delays. Guest (1992) neatly describes the expedition as 'an attempt by the British government to achieve a geopolitical end by a technological means'.

Assigned the brevet rank of Colonel for the expedition, Chesney set about assembling an expeditionary force of fifty-three men. Several of the officers had Irish connections. The second in command was Lieutenant Henry Lynch from Co. Mayo, 'a clever diplomatist and expert in Oriental languages'. Lieutenant Hastings Murphy from Co. Kerry, originally of the Irish Ordnance Survey, was to direct the trigonometrical survey and Dr Charles Staunton, who studied medicine in Dublin, was appointed physician. The Duke of Wellington recommended Lieutenant Robert Cockburn to Chesney as an accomplished draughtsman and his old Woolwich friend Captain Edward Sabine recommended William Francis Ainsworth, a surgeon and geologist who had been engaged to deliver a course of public lectures by the Geological Society of Dublin in 1833. The two junior officers were experienced and able midshipmen, Edward Charlewood and James Fitzjames; the latter was to lose his life searching for the Franklin Expedition. Two specially commissioned iron-hulled paddle-steamers of 109 and 179 tons named the *Tigris* and the *Euphrates* were to be tested as a potential means of transport to service the route.

In April 1835 the expeditionary force landed at the mouth of the Orontes on the Syrian coast. Chesney widened the expedition's scope through his contact with Johann Helfer, a Prague doctor more interested in botany, entomology and homeopathic cures than in orthodox medicine, and his German-born wife Pauline, whom he invited to join the expedition at Aleppo. Surveys inland revealed that the river flowed in a series of rapids through several narrow gorges for ten miles before reaching the rolling plain that formed the watershed with the Euphrates. The *Tigris* was assembled but the engines proved to have insufficient power to traverse the raging gorges. After dismantling the *Tigris* the expeditionary force set out for Bir on the upper Euphrates, a distance of some 120 miles. The formidable difficulties encountered in transporting the expedition's ships and equipment may be judged by the fact that transport of a boiler weighing four and a half tons needed a team of 104 oxen with 52 local drivers, and required the construction of a hard-surfaced roadway. Delays at this stage produced serious difficulty with the expedition's overall schedule in a race against seasonal changes in water levels and local tribal difficulties, not to mention malaria which afflicted almost everyone, including Chesney.

The *Tigris* and *Euphrates* were assembled, trials were conducted to test their handling and they finally departed from Port William in March 1836. For two weeks both vessels steamed smoothly downstream as far as Is Geria, taking soundings and surveying as planned. There disaster struck when, after passing through a narrow gorge, an intense storm blew up. Tossed broadside the *Tigris* foundered and sank within minutes with the loss of twenty men, provisions, spare parts and cash. The *Euphrates* survived the ten-foot waves and the expeditionary team reassembled aboard her a few days later and proceeded downstream to Ana. On reaching Hit they inspected the tar springs that produced the dense clouds of smoke and steam which enveloped the town. Chesney discovered that a mixture of earth and bitumen provided good boiler fuel for the steamer! Downstream they stopped at Felluja, near the ancient Saklawiya Canal which joined the Euphrates with the Tigris, and undertook an adventurous journey overland to Baghdad to replenish the expedition and dispatch reports. A speedy departure followed threats from the local Shiite Arabs. They continued downstream for a hundred miles on the smooth river past dense groves of date palms and tamarisk trees, which harboured lions and wolves, to the treacherous fifty-mile stretch of the Lelum Marshes.

On 19 June 1836, ninety-one days after leaving Bir, the *Euphrates* reached the Shatt el-Arab waterway. Jubilant at having accomplished the main task of the expedition in mapping the area and proving that the Euphrates was navigable for steam vessels from Bir to Basra, they fired off a seventy-one gun salute to honour King William IV, who was seventy-one years old.

The planned ascent of the Euphrates was prevented by further mechanical breakdown which forced their return to Basra. With the expedition's main task completed and the termination date close Chesney disbanded the expedition. The men, who had achieved much while enduring considerable illness and discomfort during their explorations, returned home by various routes.

In the meantime Chesney travelled to Bombay to press the authorities to develop the new route as a viable alternative (without a canal at Suez) to the long journey round the Cape. Another expedition was planned, under the command of Lynch, to investigate the potential of running a steam flotilla on the river to safeguard this passage to India, but it was deferred due to the changing balance of power in the area. Chesney returned to London to start writing his account of the expedition.

The considerable entomological and botanical collections from this relatively unknown region were in large measure due to the enthusiasm of Johann and Pauline Helfer. Specimens from the expedition are now housed in collections in London, Edinburgh, Bologna, Berlin, Brussels, Florence, Munich and Vienna. Among the expedition's botanical collections, the species *Euphorbia chesneyii* (Klotszch and Garcke, 1860) and the genus *Chesneya* (Linley, 1840) were named after its commander. The Helfers eventually acquired a plantation in Burma where Johann Helfer discovered the Tenasserim coalfield, but he died shortly afterwards.

From 1843 to 1847 Chesney served as Commandant of Artillery in Hong Kong, then newly acquired from China as a result of the first Opium War (1839-42). He married for the third time in 1848 and returned to Ireland as Colonel Commandant of the Cork Division of the Artillery. He attained the rank of Major General in 1855 and General in 1868. Changing politics and commercial interests revived interest in the Euphrates route in the 1850s and 1860s, but the Foreign Office remained sceptical, and, rather ironically, British interest in the region was finally abandoned under pressure from the French following the opening of the Suez Canal in 1869.

Chesney published accounts of his explorations in *Expedition for the Survey of the Rivers Euphrates and Tigris* (3 vols) in 1850, which drew praise from such men as Retter and Humboldt; *The Russo-Turkish Campaigns of 1828 and 1829* (1854); and *Narrative of the Euphrates Expedition* (1868), besides a number of works of a military nature.

After his adventurous life he finally retired at the age of seventy-five to his family home, Packolet, near Annalong, and died there in 1872. He prized highly the various awards given in recognition of his achievements, including Fellowship of the Royal Society in 1834, the Gold Medal of the Royal Geographical Society in 1837 and an Honorary DCL from Oxford in 1850, but he declined any official honours.

References

Chesney, Lt. Col. F.R. 1850. *Expedition for the Survey of the Rivers Euphrates and Tigris.* 3 vols. London: Longman, Brown, Green and Longmans.

Chesney, Colonel F.R. 1854. *The Russo-Turkish Campaigns of 1828 and 1829: with a View of the Present State of Affairs in the East.* London: Longmans & Co.

Chesney, General F.R. 1868. *Narrative of the Euphrates Expedition.* London: Lane-Poole.

Guest, J. S. 1992. *The Euphrates Expedition.* London and New York: Kegan Paul.

Marshall-Cornwall, J. 1965. 'Three Soldier-Geographers.' *The Geographical Journal 131*: 357-65.

Sir Francis Leopold McClintock
1819-1907

PAUL HACKNEY

Francis Leopold McClintock, chiefly known for his involvement in the searches for the lost Franklin Expedition of 1845, was responsible for much of the new natural-history knowledge produced by those missions. The searches, initially financed by the Admiralty, were to continue throughout the late 1840s and 1850s; their story was detailed in contemporary issues of the *Illustrated London News* and has been told many times since (Lloyd, 1985). Briefly, Sir John Franklin and Francis Crozier (born in Banbridge, Co. Down), both accomplished explorers, sailed from England in 1845 with 127 officers and men in the *Erebus* and the *Terror* to seek a navigable passage from the North Atlantic to the Bering Straits – the elusive Northwest Passage. The expedition was last seen by whalers in the Davis Strait in late July 1845; they were never seen or heard of again by any Europeans. Search expeditions (initially regarded as 'relief expeditions' since it was hoped that the men were merely trapped somewhere in the Arctic) commenced in 1848 with an expedition commanded by Sir James Clark Ross, with F.L. McClintock on board HMS *Enterprise* as a second lieutenant.

McClintock was born in Dundalk, Co. Louth in 1819, the second son of Henry McClintock, an army officer who had become head of Dundalk Customs House, and Elizabeth, a daughter of the Archdeacon of Waterford. He had two younger brothers and four sisters; one brother became a distinguished physician who was elected President of the College of Surgeons of Ireland (Markham, 1909). His birthplace, in Seatown Place, Dundalk, still stands and is adorned with a plaque commemorating his birth. Nearby, writes Lloyd, 'the rolling farmland and woods of Co. Louth and Dundalk Bay with its vast flocks of wintering wildfowl must have given young Leopold McClintock a good introduction to wildlife'. All through his childhood he had wanted to go to sea and he entered the Royal Navy at the tender, but by no means exceptional, age of twelve in 1831. From 1848 to 1859 his naval duties were entirely associated with the Franklin searches. He is particularly well known in the annals of Arctic exploration for developing the skills of long-distance sledge journeys, using man-hauled sledges, during the unusually severe Arctic winters of that period (Dunbar, 1985; Alt *et al.*, 1985); one of his sledges used on the *Fox* expedition has survived intact in the family's care.

He is likewise famous for being the leader of the expedition that finally resolved the problem of Franklin's fate, when he and other members of the *Fox's* crew located various relics of the missing expedition on King William Island in 1859. These included the only document to survive from the lost expedition (McClintock, 1860). The document, which summarily described Franklin's death, the trapping of the ships in sea ice and their subsequent abandonment, had been hidden for safekeeping in a cairn. It was reproduced in facsimile in the supplement to the *Illustrated London News* of 1 October 1859 and also in McClintock's own account of the *Fox* Expedition (McClintock, 1860, 1861). The original is housed in the National Maritime Museum at Greenwich along with other Franklin relics found by McClintock and others.

Although the prime aim of the numerous search expeditions, by land as well as by sea, had been the determination of the fate of Franklin, there were important scientific and geographic results also. Much new territory was discovered, mapped and claimed for the British Crown; the territorial claim on the islands of the 'Arctic Archipelago' off the northern coast of America by modern Canada derives to a large degree from these search expeditions. McClintock himself discovered, explored and named Prince Patrick Island during a sledge expedition in 1851 and named more than seventy-five topographical features, such as capes, bays and small islands, during the later voyage of the *Fox* (Markham, 1909).

McClintock, a keen self-taught naturalist since childhood, took the opportunity on all four of his expeditions to collect large quantities of plant, animal and geological specimens. Working from the geological specimens brought back by McClintock from his first three Arctic voyages, Samuel Haughton, Professor of Geology in the University of Dublin, read a paper on the geology of the Arctic Archipelago to the Royal Dublin Society (Haughton, 1862). The published account (Haughton in McClintock, 1858) contains what must be the first geological map of the region, and describes and illustrates about twenty of the invertebrate fossils donated by McClintock to the Royal Dublin Society's Museum from his first three Arctic expeditions. McClintock had made the acquaintance of the Dublin men of science, such as Haughton, on visits to his mother's home. He became friendly also with William Henry Harvey, Professor of Botany at Trinity College, Dublin, who was a celebrated botanist with a particular interest in algae, and who had readily identified the Arctic plants in McClintock's collections. After McClintock's last voyage, that of the *Fox* in 1859, Haughton was able to revise his geological map, which was re-published incorporating the new information from specimens collected by McClintock and David Walker (appendix to McClintock, 1860).

The *Fox* expedition spent the first winter trapped in ice at Melville Bay. Apart from McClintock's usual duties his natural-history interests led him to consider how Arctic conditions affected wildlife in this harsh environment. In his journal for December 1857 he wrote:

Anything which illustrates the habits of these animals in such latitudes I think is most interesting, their instincts must be quickened in proportion as the difficulty of subsisting increases. Foxes, white and blue are very numerous; all the birds are merely summer visitors, therefore the hare is the only creature remaining upon which the fox can prey; but the hares are comparatively scarce: how then do the foxes live for 8 months of the year? Petersen [another expedition member] thinks they store up provisions during the summer in various holes and crevices and thus manage to eke out an existence during the dark winter season. (McClintock, 1860)

Palaeontology particularly engaged McClintock's attention and he became an avid collector of fossils. Many of these were of species new to science and some were later named in honour of McClintock himself, such as *Loxonema M'Clintockii* and *Ammonites M'Clintockii* (Haughton in McClintock, 1858). The specimens are now housed, along with other geological material collected by McClintock and David Walker, in the Natural History Division of the National Museum of Ireland, Dublin. In total there are about 360 fossil specimens from the four voyages (Haughton, 1862). In an interesting postscript to McClintock's collecting, a large cache of geological specimens left behind by him on Melville Island was discovered in 1960 by geologists from the Geological Survey of Canada, in whose collections they now repose (Colm O'Riordan, *pers. comm.*). There are also substantial amounts of bird, mammal and mollusc specimens from McClintock's voyages in the National Museum of Ireland. On a visit to Prince Patrick Island in 1853 he had the good fortune to obtain the first specimens of the eggs of the ivory gull, about whose nesting habits little was then known (Carte, 1856).

Search expeditions usually travelled by way of the Davis Strait between Greenland and Baffin Island and the North American mainland. Usually the ships called at the Danish settlements on the Greenland coast for coaling or shelter. McClintock became interested in the fossil flora of Greenland's west coast. In his journal for 31 July 1857 he described how, anchored at Godhaven on Disco Island, he met C.S.M. Olrik, the Danish government's Inspector of North Greenland. Olrik had an intimate knowledge of the country and had made a collection of fossil specimens. He gave McClintock several leaf fossils from the 'fossil forest' of Atanekerdluk. These, together with those he had collected, and those of David Walker and others, formed the basis of an account of the Miocene flora of Greenland by Professor Oswald Heer (1870). A new fossil genus of the Proteaceae, a flowering plant family now extinct in North America, was named *McClintockia* in his honour.

The voyage of the *Fox* was McClintock's final Arctic voyage. By now he was adjudged internationally as the undisputed expert on Arctic travel by sea and man-hauled sledge. Lady Jane Franklin, John Franklin's widow, had chosen him to command what was to be a privately funded expedition. He was accompanied by David Walker, a Belfast-born surgeon, who acted as naturalist and photographer and who collected large quantities of natural-history specimens. It is probably true to say that many, perhaps most, of the ships' surgeons on the various expeditions, as in the Royal Navy generally, were Irish or Scottish. Perhaps this can be attributed to the relatively poorer prospects of the average Irish or Scots medical man compared with his English counterpart.

From the *Fox*'s winter quarters (1858/9) at Port Kennedy in the Bellot Strait, McClintock devoted his available time to searches of the land within reach, while Walker undertook collecting and photography. On his return, Walker published a paper (1862) on the zoology of the expedition in which he listed the material brought back: forty-seven species of birds, four species of fish, one hundred species of crustaceans, eleven species of starfish or echinoderms, twenty-eight species of insects and spiders, and seven species of mammals including an adult polar bear, a young polar bear, specimens of ermine in winter and summer coats and a skull of a white (Beluga) whale. Apparently the insect and spider specimens were given to the Queen's College, now the Queen's University, Belfast, but these have all been lost. Among Walker's surviving photographs (Knight, 1977) is one of a dead polar bear on board the *Fox* – perhaps the same animal as that which survived, along with other expedition specimens, in the Zoological Museum of the Queen's University of Belfast until the 1940s, when the Department of Zoology moved to new premises and the museum was broken up. Another polar bear from the expedition and other specimens donated to the Royal Dublin Society were exhibited at the British Association meeting in Dublin in 1859 and are now incorporated in the collections of the National Museum of Ireland. Walker's botanical collections, also given to Queen's University, are now in the Ulster Museum, Belfast. He also sent plant specimens to J.D. Hooker of the Royal Botanic Gardens at Kew, who published an account of the collection (1861); these appear to have survived in the herbarium at Kew. Hooker was particularly interested in the specimens from Port Kennedy – a comparatively unknown area where Walker's collecting had provided fresh phytogeographical information. Walker also carried out physical observations and experiments such as trying to determine whether sea ice is salt or fresh (Walker, 1860). Subsequent to the Fox voyage, Walker emigrated to the United States and was living and practising medicine in Portland, Oregon, at the time of McClintock's death in 1907.

After his return from the *Fox* expedition, McClintock was knighted and lauded with honours including honorary degrees and the freedom of several cities (Royal Geographical Society, 1860). He wrote an account of the voyage which caught the public's imagination and became a best-seller (1860). His subsequent career included a spell as commander of HMS *Bulldog* in 1860, undertaking a survey of a possible north-Atlantic route for a submarine telegraph cable from Europe to North America. Although the cable was never laid by the company that had been formed for the purpose, the scientific information from the soundings was considerable (McClintock, 1861a). In 1865, in recognition of his scientific endeavours, he was elected to Fellowship of the Royal Society.

Until 1868 McClintock was Commodore at Jamaica, where he indulged his scientific interest again by collecting considerable quantities of marine animal life, again donated to the Royal Dublin Society's Museum (now in the National Museum of Ireland). He married Annette Dunlop of Monasterboice, Co. Louth in 1870 and became a Rear Admiral in 1871. In

1872 he was appointed Admiral Superintendent of Portsmouth Dockyard and in 1874-5 he was involved again with an Arctic expedition – that of Captain Nares (Nares, 1878), who is best known to naturalists as the commander of the *Challenger* expedition, which immediately preceded his Arctic expedition. For Nares, whose purpose was to try to reach the North Pole, McClintock selected and fitted out two ships, the *Alert* and the *Discovery*. The naturalist on board the *Discovery* was Henry Chichester Hart of Dublin (*see profile below*).

After his position at Portsmouth came to an end in 1879 and having by now reached the rank of Vice Admiral, McClintock spent three years as Commander of the Navy's North American and West Indian station, based on Bermuda. He retired in 1884, shortly after his return to England, with the rank of full Admiral, but retirement did not mean a cessation of work; he generously contributed from his knowledge and experience to many organizations. He became a member of the council of the Royal Geographical Society, a committee member of the National Lifeboat Institution, an active member of various Conservative Party bodies (he was a committed Unionist and had stood, unsuccessfully, for the Parliamentary constituency of Drogheda in 1868), an Elder Brother of Trinity House (the Lighthouse Service of Great Britain) and a member of numerous other organizations and societies. He was closely involved with the Royal Dublin Society for much of his career and his Arctic travels and scientific work were frequently reported in that Society's *Transactions*. After his return from the *Fox* Expedition he vividly recounted his exploits and scientific work to meetings of the Society.

McClintock died at his London home in November 1907 at the age of eighty-eight. He was held in such esteem that the mourners at his funeral included representatives of the King, the Prince of Wales and the Admiralty, together with the President of the Royal Geographical Society, the Deputy Master of Trinity House, the First Sea Lord and many brother officers and former shipmates. An alabaster slab was placed below the memorial to Sir John Franklin in Westminster Abbey with the inscription: 'Here also is commemorated Admiral Sir Leopold McClintock 1819-1907 – Discoverer of the Fate of Franklin in 1859.' His commemoration in England's national shrine might seem an attempt to 'hijack' the career of a distinguished Irishman and indeed such accusations were made by the editors of the *Natural History Review* in 1859:

It is a melancholy satisfaction to Lady Franklin to learn that her gallant husband died in comparative comfort and was spared the horrors of the fatal retreat from the *Erebus* and *Terror* but it must also be a bitter reflection that notwithstanding the noisy self-glorification of her countrymen she was left to solve the problem of her husband's fate without sympathy and without aid from those who are now most clamorous to appropriate to England the brave deeds of an Irishman.

The truth, however, is that McClintock always spoke in his journals and published writings with the overt pride of one who identified with the British tradition, especially that of the Royal Navy. He was, after all, from a class that scarcely distinguished itself from the English and proudly proclaimed the British connection. British patriotism is often today equated with jingoism, and there have been recent tendencies to emphasise the differences which separate the Irish and British traditions, but McClintock would, without doubt, have been proud of his Westminster Abbey memorial.

References

Alt, B.T., R.M. Koerner, D.A. Fisher and J.C. Bourgeois. 1985. 'Arctic Climate during the Franklin Era, as deduced from Ice Cores,' in P. Sutherland (ed.), *The Franklin Era in Canadian Arctic History*. Ottawa: National Museums of Canada, Mercury Series, Archaeological Survey of Canada Paper 131: 69-92.

Carte, A. 1856. 'Nidification of the Ivory Gull (*Larus eburneus*), Gmel.' *Journal of the Royal Dublin Society, 1*: 57-60, Pls. 1, 2.

Dunbar, M. 1985. 'The Effect of Sea Ice Conditions on Maritime Arctic Expeditions during the Franklin Era,' in P. Sutherland (ed.), *The Franklin Era in Canadian Arctic History*. Ottawa: National Museums of Canada, Mercury Series, Archaeological Survey of Canada Paper 131: 114-21.

Hart, H.C. 1898. *A Flora of County Donegal*. Dublin: Sealy, Bryers and Walker.

Haughton, S. 1862. 'On the Fossils brought home from the Arctic Regions in 1859, by Captain Sir F.L. McClintock.' *Journal of the Royal Dublin Society 3*: 52-8.

Heer, O. 1870. 'On the Miocene Flora of North Greenland.' *Journal of the Royal Dublin Society 5*: 70-85.

Hooker, J.D. 1861. 'An Account of the Plants collected by Dr Walker in Greenland and Arctic America during the Expedition of Sir Francis M'Clintock, R.N., in the Yacht *Fox*.' *Journal of the Linnean Society (Botany) 5*: 79-89.

Knight, R.J.B. (ed.). 1977. *Guide to the Manuscripts in the National Maritime Museum*. Vol. 1: The Personal Collections. London: Mansell.

Lloyd, C. 1985. *The Travelling Naturalists*. London: Croom Helm.

Markham, C. 1909. *The Life of Admiral Sir Leopold McClintock*. London: Murray.

McClintock, F.L. 1858. 'Reminiscences of Arctic Ice-travel in Search of Sir John Franklin and his Companions with Geological Notes and Illustrations by the Rev. Samuel Haughton.' *Journal of the Royal Dublin Society 1*: 183-250.

McClintock, F.L. (1860) 1908. *A Narrative of the Discovery of the Fate of Sir John Franklin and his Companions. The Voyage of the 'Fox' in Arctic Seas*. London: John Murray.

McClintock, F.L. 1861. 'Narrative of the Expedition in Search of Sir John Franklin and his Party.' *Journal of the Royal Geographical Society 31*: 1-13.

McClintock, F.L. 1861a. 'Surveys of HMS Bulldog.' *Proceedings of the Royal Geographical Society 5*: 61-70.

Nares, Sir G.S. 1878. *Narrative of a Voyage to the Polar Sea During 1875-6 in HM Ships 'Alert' & 'Discovery'*. 2 vols. London: Sampson, Low, Marston, Searle and Rivington.

Royal Geographical Society. 1860. 'Presentation of the Gold Medals to Lady Franklin and to Captain Sir F.L. M'Clintock.' *Journal of the Royal Geographical Society 30*: 94-9.

Walker, D. 1860. 'Ice Observations.' *Journal of the Royal Dublin Society 2*: 371-80.

Walker, D. 1862. 'Notes on the Zoology of the last Arctic Expedition under Captain Sir F.L. McClintock R.N.' *Journal of the Royal Dublin Society 3*: 61-77.

Robert Templeton
1802-92

HELENA C.G. CHESNEY AND ROBERT NASH

Robert Templeton, the only son of John and Katherine Templeton of Cranmore, Belfast, was born in December 1802, the second of five children. John Templeton (1766-1825), a prosperous Belfast wholesale merchant, was also an exceptional naturalist whose special interest was botany. He was elected an Associate of the Linnean Society of London in 1794 and knew and corresponded with eminent English botanists such as Joseph Banks, William Hooker, Dawson Turner and G.B. Sowerby. Throughout his life he was a 'strenuous and enlightened advocate of civil and religious liberty' and determined that his family should receive a sound schooling (Hincks, 1828, 1829). He was one of the prime movers behind the Belfast Academical Institution, which obtained its charter in 1807. The Institution opened its doors to pupils in 1814, and Robert, in the words of his sister Ellen, was 'one of the first boys marched into it'.*

Success at school led Robert in 1821 to the study of medicine in Edinburgh. From his school days, he had been especially interested in entomology; his 'cabinet' of insects is referred to in the entomological publications of George Crawford Hyndman, Robert Patterson and Alexander Haliday, all friends from childhood, and of English entomologists such as Joseph Obadiah Westwood. Indeed, because of the collections of Robert and his father John, the gardens and grounds of Cranmore and its environs are among the most cited Irish localities for many species of animals and plants. Robert's passionate interest in spiders and other arachnids led him to compile descriptions and figures of 'Irish Arachnida and Acari' (1833). The manuscript notes on spiders were eventually incorporated into one of the best-known and most exquisite spider books ever written, Blackwall's Ray Society monograph *A History of the Spiders of Great Britain and Ireland* (1861-4).

The bristle-tails and springtails, or Thysanurae, particularly interested him and, in 1836, he published 'Thysanurae Hibernicae', the first significant work in English on these primitive insects. He also undertook the compilation,

---

* A copy of Dubourdieu's *Statistical Survey of the County of Down* (1802) in the Ulster Museum Library was annotated, it would appear, by Ellen Templeton. A number of her comments provide interesting insight on some of the people, places and events mentioned in the text.

updating and publication (in the *Magazine of Natural History* between 1834 and 1837) of his father's copious manuscript notes on Irish marine and land worms, parasitic and intestinal worms, starfish, sea urchins, brittle-stars, jellyfish, sea anemones, hydroids, crustaceans, harvestmen, spiders and vertebrates. The groundwork had been laid for the meticulous observational and discriminatory skills that were to characterize his wide-ranging contributions to the zoology of the far-flung places where he served in the course of his duties.

In 1833 he was commissioned into the Royal Artillery as Assistant Surgeon in the Ordnance Medical Department and in the following spring took passage to Mauritius where, outside his medical duties, he found time to naturalize, before returning to England later in the year. Mauritius, or 'The Isle of France', furnished numbers of new insects, polychaete worms and crustaceans, of which he published illustrated descriptions. Early in 1835 he set out again, this time for Ceylon (Sri Lanka); on the voyage, via the Cape of Good Hope, he travelled first to Rio de Janeiro. During some months of service with the Royal Artillery in Colombo, he was elected a Corresponding Member of the Zoological Society of London.

In 1836 he journeyed to the Mediterranean, visiting Malta, then Corfu, other Ionian Islands and Albania. He took the opportunity to make collections of fish, beetles and other insects, some of which he sent back to Belfast Natural History Society Museum and to the Entomological Society of London.

By early 1839 Templeton was back in Ceylon and this time his stay was to be of twelve years' duration. Ceylon, sometimes then called 'Serendip' or 'The Land of the Hyacinth and the Ruby', had become a British colony in 1802. The island's luxuriant and varied natural history was still very poorly known, but naturalists, several of whom were army medical staff, were setting this to rights. Among these was Edgar Layard, who joined the Ceylon Civil Service in 1846. A passage from Tennent's *Ceylon* (1859) captures some of the beauty of the island:

At morning the dew hangs in diamond drops on the threads and gossamer which the spiders suspend across every pathway; and above the pool dragonflies of more than metallic lustre, flash in the early sunbeams .... Butterflies of large size and gorgeous colouring flutter over the endless expanse of flowers, and at times the extraordinary sight presents itself of flights of these delicate creatures, generally of a white or pale yellow hue, apparently miles in breadth, and of such prodigious extension as to occupy hours, and even days, uninterruptedly in their passage – whence coming no-one knows; whither going no-one can tell.*

---

* James Emerson Tennent (1804-69) of Belfast, born James Emerson, married Letitia Tennent, the only child of William Tennent, a prosperous Belfast banker. After William

Templeton's interest in the island's fauna enabled him to publish descriptions of two monkeys, a loris, a giant earthworm and several annelid worms, but he passed his accumulated details on a wide range of other invertebrates to other specialists to describe. Quite aside from his professional commitments, an assessment of Templeton's published work indicates scientific traits that partly explain this. His early writing on springtails, for example, is a most thorough piece of work in which previous literature on the subject is carefully discussed and great attention is paid to morphological detail. Not for Templeton, then, a rapid compilation, or the desire for personal glory that motivated many taxonomists.

Evidence of his generous personality comes from the pen of Layard in his autobiography: 'I was shortly after landing seized with a terrible illness and Dr Templeton of the Artillery ... came to see me. He quickly spied our butterfly nets and cross-examining my little wife, wormed out of her our history and pursuits and from that moment he was liken "one that sticketh closer than a brother" – not a fee would he ever take from me, he interested Sir J.E. Tennent – then Colonial Secretary, "a man of mickle might" in the colony, in my favour.' This resulted in Layard's appointment to Tennent's office. On another occasion Templeton visited when the Layards' finances were severely stretched, with three days of the month to go. Lamenting their problems he searched his pockets and found four sixpenny bits. 'There's one ... I have for cigars and must keep – my dinner I get at the mess, the three others you're welcome to.'

The amazing beauty and variety of Ceylonese Lepidoptera fascinated Layard and Templeton, and between them they collected 932 species of butterflies and moths, many new to science. They also turned their attention to the island's Mollusca, and the 630 species of shells in their collection comprised numerous new species, both marine and non-marine. Templeton published a privately printed list of 'Thysanura, Myriapoda, Scorpionidae, Cheliferidae and Phrynidae from Ceylon', but sent the bulk of his collections of beetles, Hymenoptera and Lepidoptera to the London entomologist Francis Walker for description.

Apart from his collecting activities Templeton also found time to pursue his interest in illustrating his finds. These were executed as aids to species identification, rather than for any artistic or decorative purposes;

Tennent died in the 1832 cholera epidemic, Emerson, who had served as an officer in the Artillery, joined Byron in the struggle for Greek independence, qualified for the Bar, and assumed his new name. A fine linguist and gifted public speaker, he became an MP and was appointed Civil Secretary to the Governor of Ceylon in 1845. During his five-year stay he wrote his compendious two-volume work on the island's history and natural history. He was knighted upon his retirement, and died two years later.

however, as with the finest scientific illustrations, they fulfil both these criteria. John Templeton had liberally illustrated his work and Robert, like his
four sisters, was trained in the art of illustration from an early age. The drawing master at the Academical Institution was Gaetano Fabrini, a native of
Florence, who worked in Belfast from 1804 and practised as a portrait- and
subject-painter for many years. From around the age of eighteen Robert
Templeton compiled a folio of ink drawings and watercolour paintings of
shells. These have proved to be accurate copies of illustrations from some of
the best-known shell books of the period, including *Historia Conchyliorum*
(1685-92) by Martin Lister, *Index Testarum Conchyliorum* (1742) by Niccolo
Gualtieri, *Encyclopédie Methodique* (1792) by Brugiére, *The Natural History of
British Shells* (1802) and *Naturalist's Repository* (1805) by Edward Donovan,
Introduction to the Study of Conchology (1815) by Samuel Brookes and *Genera
of Recent and Fossil Mollusca* (1821-34) by G.B. Sowerby. Comparison with
the originals demonstrates the development of his talent for illustration.

These skills were displayed in his folio of illustrations of Ceylonese
Lepidoptera, which rank among the best scientific illustrations of their time.
In these, the right dorsal surface of each insect is painted and a number is
allocated. The numbers link the figures to Templeton's butterfly collection,
Layard's paintings of the early stages and, presumably, to manuscript notes.
Templeton sent the sheets, along with the butterflies, to England to be studied by Frederic Moore and Francis Walker, both of whom, especially the
former, annotated them. Moore is celebrated for his prolific writings on oriental Lepidoptera and later published a compendious three-volume work,
The Lepidoptera of Ceylon (1880-7), illustrated by F.C. Moore, possibly a
son. The butterflies and paintings formed the basis for the addition of a considerable number of species to the known Ceylon fauna, augmenting knowledge based on the collections of the British Museum, the East India
Company and other collectors. For example, among the Papilionidae or
swallowtails, large and comparatively well-known butterflies, two new
species and a new sub-species were described by George Gray and Frederic
Moore. Since the illustrations aided the production of the final descriptions
they are called the *iconotypes* of these species.

Templeton's illustrations are scientifically important in another, less
obvious way: they reveal much about the state of zoological knowledge at the
time and about the expertise of Walker and Moore. Their annotations on
the sheets show that the complexity of the identity of some specimens was
being recognized, but not solved. This was the case, for example, with the
butterflies *Papilio polytes* and *Pachliopta aristolochiae*. There are three distinct forms of the female of *Papilio polytes*: namely *cyrus* Fabricius, which
looks like the male; *polytes* Linnaeus, which looks like *Pachliopta aristolochiae*; and *romulus* Cramer, which looks like *Pachliopta hector*. The butterflies

Pachliopta aristolochiae and *Pachliopta hector* are both poisonous and distasteful and are avoided by birds, which learn to associate their conspicuous colouring with an unpleasant experience. The *romulus* and *polytes* forms of *Papilio polytes*, which are not poisonous, 'mimic' the species *Pachliopta aristolochiae* and *Pachliopta hector* to avoid being eaten by birds.

The situation involving three female forms of one butterfly species, two of which look like other butterflies, was still defeating the experts in 1859. This sort of mimicry was not explained until 1870 after Bates, working on the butterflies of the Amazon, explained similar situations. The discursive notes on the illustrations reveal the discussions that Templeton's specimens and paintings provoked among those who examined them, and evidence of erasures shows that some were proving troublesome, even to the leading entomologists of the day. The annotations also proved the link between Templeton and Moore which led to the recent discovery of the type specimens in the Natural History Museum, London, since previously many of the butterflies named by Walker could not be associated with the butterfly species because it appeared that the original specimens were lost. The Walker annotations on paintings helped solve the problem of the 'missing' Templeton butterflies (Nash and Ross, 1980).

Templeton was recalled from Ceylon around 1852 due to the unrest that was to develop into the Crimean War in 1854. He served in the Crimea and was promoted to Surgeon-Major in 1855. Subsequently, he was stationed at the Hibernian Military School in Phoenix Park, Dublin and retired with the honorary rank of Deputy Inspector-General of Hospitals in 1860. He married Mary Slade of Brockley, near Bristol, in 1851, and two sons and a daughter were born of the marriage. On occasion he visited Belfast where his mother, sisters and other close relatives lived. (The family's links with Ceylon continued through his second son, Robert Stanster Templeton, who became Surveyor General of Ceylon.) He died in Edinburgh in 1892.

It was the closing of an age. A century of travel and exploration, duty and service – and, for natural history, a golden age of discovery – was nearly over. It was an age to which Templeton made a considerable contribution.

References

Blackwall, J. 1861-4. *A History of the Spiders of Great Britain and Ireland.* 2 vols. London: Ray Society.

Hincks, T.D. 1828/29. 'Memoir of the late John Templeton, Esq.' *Annals and Magazine of Natural History* 1: 403-6; 2: 305-10

Layard, E. n.d. Manuscript and biography (unpubl.). Blacker-Wood Library, McGill University, Montreal.

Nash, R. and H.C.G. Ross 1980. *Dr Robert Templeton Roy. Art. (1802-1892) Naturalist and Artist.* Belfast: Ulster Museum.

Templeton, R. 1836. 'Thysaurae Hibernicae.' *Transactions of the Entomological Society of London 1*: 89-98.

Tennent, Sir J.E. 1859. *Ceylon. An Account of the Island, Physical, Historical and Topographical.* London: Longman, Green, Longman & Roberts.

John Macoun *(1831-1920)*

MARY G. McGEOWN

John Macoun emigrated from Ireland to Canada at the age of nineteen in 1850. Although he had left school at thirteen, by 1869 he was Professor of Natural History at Albert College in Belleville, Ontario, and was widely known as a botanist and explorer. He explored vast tracts of north-west Canada and influenced the course of the Canadian Pacific Railway. This distinguished Ulsterman is still remembered in Canada: his exploits are recounted in recent histories of the Railway, his head appeared on a stamp in 1981, and his name is commemorated by no fewer than ten geographical features.* Forty-eight species of plants which he discovered bear his name.

John Macoun's ancestors settled in Maralin, or Magheralin, in the seventeenth century, probably coming from Linlithgowshire in Scotland. His son William Terrill Macoun traced the family to James Macoun, who was born in Linlithgow in 1639, married Elizabeth Montgomery of Lainshaw (Ayrshire) and emigrated to Ireland in 1672, and was killed at the Battle of the Boyne in 1690. However, the first Macoun may have come to Ireland before 1672. The name of Ensign James McEwne appears in the list of 'The Forty-nine Officers' – those who served in Cromwell's army in 1649 – along with several members of the McGill family from whom the Macouns later held leases of land in Maralin. Tombstones bearing the name Macoun still exist in the old graveyard near the ruins of the original church at Maralin, including one to James Macoun 'who departed this life the 15th March anno Dom 1706 aged 105 years and also his wife departed this life the 6th March 1706'. This James may have been the father of the James born in Linlithgow and killed at the Boyne.

John Macoun's father, also called James, became a soldier in the Seventh Dragoon Guards, fought in the Irish rebellion of 1798, and was wounded at the Battle of New Ross. After the death of his elder brother, James inherited the family home and small farm. He married Anne Jane

---

*The most significant of these is Mt Macoun (9998 ft) in Great Glacier Park, overlooking the Beaver River, a tributary of the Columbia River (Rayburn, 1981).

Nevin in 1824, but he died on 13 November 1836, leaving Anne Jane to bring up her young family of four during the terrible years of the failure of the potato crop in Ireland.

John Macoun's first schooling was given by an old woman who looked after five or six little ones. Later he attended the parochial school in Maralin which followed the Lancasterian method, with older pupils acting as monitors. After leaving school at thirteen, he helped his elder brother farm the family land and also worked on land belonging to a widowed aunt. The house had a large garden containing rare shrubs which his mother sold to eke out their income. She gave him and his brother flower-beds to look after and he would dig up plants in the fields to bring home to the garden. This love of plants may have been inherited from his mother and fostered by the proximity of the great gardens and park at nearby Moira, once considered amongst the finest gardens in Europe. In his autobiography, written when he was nearly ninety, Macoun tells of a chance meeting with the local squire, who gave him permission to play with his children in these gardens.

When Macoun's elder brother Frederick became twenty-one it was possible to sell the entailed property, for Mrs Macoun wanted to emigrate to Canada to join her brother, Alec Nevin, who had gone there some time before. The family party included the mother, the brothers Frederick, John and James, a sister Margaret and her husband, John Spence. After landing briefly at Quebec they disembarked at Montreal and boarded a smaller boat which took them to Kingston and then to Belleville where they lodged with a friend of their uncle Nevin, who lived at Seymour, about thirty-two miles away. Two days later, Frederick and John set out to walk there, arriving at their destination, a two-roomed shanty, late that evening. The following day a wagon was sent to fetch the rest of the family from Belleville.

During the voyage the family had planned that John was to become a farmer, but they found that almost all the land in the area was already taken up or was covered with trees. Macoun hired himself to a farmer named Ponton. Frederick bought a hundred acres, of which eleven were already cleared; this became the family home until it was replaced by the house Frederick built and made his home for the rest of his life. After working as a hired labourer for the summer Macoun helped his brother to clear his land over the winter, then took work as a clerk the following spring.

The following season he was able to buy 160 acres of land. He farmed for six years before deciding to become a teacher, partly because he wanted to study botany. Feeling that he was deficient in grammar, Macoun bought a grammar book; three days later he decided he was ready to see the county inspector and set out to walk the forty-three miles to where he lived. After discussing his ambitions the inspector (Rev. Joseph Hutton, originally minister of Eustace Street Unitarian Meeting House, Dublin) advised

Macoun to study for three weeks in the village school to learn how to govern a school, after which he could try for a post. After unsuccessful applications to schools in and around Seymour he found a post in Brighton, where he boarded with Simon Terrill, later to be his father-in-law.

He continued to read all he could obtain about plants, which he collected and described in his notebooks. During a summer session at Normal School in Toronto, he boarded with a lady whose son was a student at the University and prize man in botany. This man knew plants from books, Macoun knew them in the field, and they could teach each other. In his next post in Castleton, he became friends with the local doctor who was also a botanist. The turning point in his life came the next autumn when he obtained a teacher's post in Belleville. He learned to apply his knowledge and make his lessons in school interesting. His reputation as a teacher, and then as a botanist, began to grow.

In 1862 Macoun married Ellen Terrill. A son, James, was born in November of the same year, a daughter in 1866 and a second son, William Terrill, in 1869. James became a naturalist and botanist and while much of his life was spent understudying his father, he eventually became Chief of the Biological Division of the Geological Survey and became recognized as an international expert on seals. William became First Dominion Horticulturist and one of the world's greatest experts on pomology.*

As soon as he had established a home Macoun set about building a herbarium for his plant collection, as all his spare time was spent in collecting and studying plants. His reputation as a botanist increased and in 1868 he was offered the Chair of Natural History in Albert College, Belleville, newly created a university.

John Macoun began to spend his summers plant-hunting farther afield. At the beginning of the summer of 1872 he met Sandford Fleming, the engineer-in-chief of the Canadian-Pacific Railway Company, who was setting out by steamer across the Great Lakes to follow the route proposed for the new railway. Fleming asked him if he would care to come along and act as botanist to the party. The secretary was the Rev. George Monroe Grant, a Presbyterian minister who later became Principal of Queen's University, Kingston, Ontario, and famous for a book, *Ocean to Ocean*, based on this journey.

After crossing the lakes by steamer they travelled on wagons following the Dawson Route. Fleming aimed for at least forty miles a day, measuring the distance travelled by an 'odometer' attached to one of the carts, crossing lakes as they came to them by barge or canoe. Eventually they reached

---

*There is a Macoun apple named after William Terrill still retained in the U.K. National Apple Collection at Brogdale, Kent.

the immense prairie stretching about eight hundred miles from Portage Le Prairie to Fort Edmonton where the tall grass was bright with flowers, many of them new to Macoun. Some were later named after him.

Fleming decided that the party should split up at Fort Edmonton, with Macoun and Horetzky, the photographer of the party, following the Peace River to Fort St James, while Fleming and Grant went south to follow the route through the Yellowhead Pass. Macoun and Horetzky parted at Fort St James after a difficult journey. Macoun agreed to go south through the mountains to the Fraser River while Horetzky continued towards the coast. After a terrible journey through the mountains in the depth of winter, he eventually reached Victoria, British Columbia, on 12 December 1872, where he learned that his fifth child had been born. Following his return home to Belleville he prepared his account for Fleming's railway report (1874).

Over the next ten years Macoun made many long and strenuous journeys into the North-West Territories, the later ones on behalf of the Canadian government. His best-known book, *Manitoba and the Great North-West* (1882), was the result of these journeys. He says in his preface: 'In writing I have had the delight of revisiting in imagination many a cheery camp-fire, and many a scene of vast and lonely beauty on which memory loves to dwell.' One wonders what his wife thought of his love affair with the wilderness – she cannot have had much of his company throughout their long married life. When at home in Belleville he was often preoccupied with his attempts to obtain an official position with the Geological Survey of Canada, which was set up in 1842 to investigate and aid in the development of the mineral resources of the colony. The Survey did not provide for a naturalist or a botanist, and by 1871-2 its resources were already stretched by the need to map and report on the geology of the new territories of Rupert's Land and British Columbia.

While not originally in favour of extending the work of the Survey to include botany, its Director, Selwyn, after reading Macoun's report to Fleming, asked Macoun to accompany him to the Peace River area the following summer, 1875. This was a great opportunity for Macoun, and leaving Selwyn's party at Fort St John he journeyed down the Peace River. He noted that some areas bore good crops of all kinds, while just over the fence the ground was arid. He became convinced that when the ground was broken up by cultivation the rain could penetrate the hard crust and was adequate in amount and fell at the right time of year for most crops. Macoun's optimistic reports were at variance with those of earlier explorers, who had reported that South Saskatchewan was an extension of the Great American Desert and unsuitable for cultivation. However, his views were welcomed by the government and led to his being sent on further journeys to the west in 1879, 1880 and 1881. In 1882 he was appointed naturalist to the Survey, giving him the permanent post which had become his goal, and the family moved to Ottawa.

By this time the Prime Minister, John Macdonald, was committed to the building of the railway, partly as a political manoeuvre to bring British Columbia into Canada. When Macoun met with the railway executives they were planning to build the railway from Winnipeg to Fort Edmonton by a route long known as the Charlton Trail, and to cross the Rockies by the Yellowhead Pass. However, Macoun convinced them that South Saskatchewan was potentially very fertile, and they decided to abandon the route already surveyed at much cost in favour of a more southerly route crossing the Rockies by the Kicking Horse Pass. This decision was to change the map of Canada and influence the lives of millions as new towns grew up along the route of the railway across the prairies.

There is little doubt that Macoun was almost obsessed in his admiration of the southern plain of Saskatchewan, but nevertheless he was a careful, accurate and honest observer. Waiser's criticism (1989) that Macoun's evaluation of western Canada's potential was influenced by personal ambition seems unduly harsh. Indeed Waiser later grants: 'Extremely confident in his abilities, he genuinely believed that where other investigators had failed, his field work had scientifically demonstrated that the Peace River country and the southern plains were equal to the fertile belt. ... By concentrating on observation and generalising from it, Macoun, like the investigators before him, achieved a limited kind of truth.'

The truth appears to have been that the earlier explorers, Palliser and Hinds, had seen Saskatchewan under its 'normal' or dry conditions, whereas Macoun had visited several times during an unusually wet decade. The dry cycle returned in 1883 and many settlers who had eagerly bought land later abandoned their farms. The government once again sent Macoun to investigate but just as he arrived the rains began again and another prolonged wet period followed. The prairies were again filled with immigrant farmers and the area produced vast acres of wheat during the early years of the twentieth century. Great cattle ranches produced meat where wheat would not grow. Macoun's reputation remained undiminished until after his death, but in the 1930s the rains ceased, the hot dry winds returned and vast areas returned to desert once again.

In the meantime his son James, already an experienced botanist, had joined the summer expeditions in a voluntary capacity. On him was laid the burden of sorting, identifying and arranging to send off to experts outside Canada the large numbers of specimens (later including animal skins and bones as well as plants) they collected. Macoun did not have the knowledge, time or inclination to classify and identify all the numerous specimens himself and was content to send them to 'foreign experts' who were delighted to make use of his collections, often finding previously undescribed species. As early as 1862 he sent specimens to Sir Joseph Hooker at Kew, who responded by sending his book, *The British Jungermania*, as a present. All this contributed greatly to Macoun's international reputation.

Once in post as naturalist to the Survey, Macoun became responsible for listing the animal and bird life of Canada. His resources were minute in relation to his task, with only one part-time helper in the field and intermittent help from James. Little wonder that he needed and welcomed help from specialists outside Canada. Moreover, he was seeking a permanent home for his great herbarium, and growing collections of skins. He had already produced the first volume of his *Catalogue of Canadian Plants*, published in three parts between 1883 and 1886. A second volume in two parts appeared in 1890, and the third volume, part six, containing nearly a thousand species of mosses, including 237 previously unknown, appeared in 1892. This work was applauded on both sides of the Atlantic. His *Catalogue of Canadian Birds* was commenced in 1894.

All this explains why Macoun was invited as one of Canada's representatives to the Colonial Exhibition held in London in 1886, and was given facilities to study the collections at Kew. In his autobiography he describes the visit during which he was entertained at Sion House and Hatfield, and was a viceregal guest in Dublin. Subsequently he visited his relative, John Macoun of Kilmore House, near Lurgan – no doubt the beginning of a family friendship which led to his son William Terrill marrying the other John Macoun's daughter Lily.

While the published works nourished his reputation internationally, in Canada he became widely known as a lecturer, having the gift of communicating widely his enthusiasms and interests, this before the days of the mass media. He was ambitious and made use of the opportunities that his life afforded. A quick thinker and resourceful, he was a man who could sometimes be irascible and who did not suffer fools gladly, yet was innately kind and generous. He was a founder-member of the Royal Society of Canada and received many honours, perhaps the most unusual being a Resolution of Appreciation of his work passed by the Agricultural Committee of the Canadian House of Commons in 1903. The accolade he himself would have appreciated most came in 1927, after his death, when the government declared his museum in Ottawa to be the National Museum of Canada.

He suffered a stroke in 1912, but recovered and later that year moved to Victoria, British Columbia, not to retire but to continue as a botanist and writer. Remaining on the Survey's payroll, over the remaining years he collected plants on Vancouver Island and surrounding islets and presented a large collection of plants to the Herbarium in Victoria. He was writing his autobiography when he died at Sidney, Vancouver Island on 18 July 1920.

Sadly, his son James had died a few months before him and was buried in Patricia Bay Cemetery. His wife died some six months later and both were finally interred in the Macoun burial ground in Beechwood Cemetery, Ottawa, beside their son. The *Autobiography*, finished by their son William and his close friends, was published by the Ottawa Field Naturalists' Club in 1922. Macoun's portrait still hangs in their library.

References

Berton, P. 1970. *The Great Railway 1817-1881: The National Dream*. Toronto: McClelland and Stewart.
Berton, P. 1971. *The Great Railway, 1881-1885: The Last Spike*. Toronto: McClelland and Stewart.
McEwan, G. 1971. *Between the Red and the Rockies*. Toronto: University of Toronto Press.
McGeown, M.G. 1980. 'John Macoun – Botanist and Explorer from Maralin.' *Journal of Craigavon Historial Society 4*: 7-12.
McGeown, M.G. 1980. 'John Macoun.' *Alberta History 28*: 16-19.
Macoun, J. 1874. 'Report to Mr Fleming's Expedition,' in *Report of Progress on the Explorations and Surveys up to January 1874, Appendix C*, 56-98. Ottawa: MacLean, Roger and Co.
Macoun, J. 1882. *Manitoba and the Great North-West*. Guelph: The World Publishing Company.
Macoun, J. 1883-92. *Catalogue of Canadian Plants*. Montreal: Dawson Brothers, W.F. Brown.
Macoun, J. [1900-4] 1909. *Catalogue of Canadian Birds*. Ottawa: Government Printing Bureau.
Macoun, J. 1922. *Autobiography*. Ottawa: Ottawa Field Naturalists' Club.
Maralin Parish Vestry Records, 1703-1800.
Rayburn, A. 1981. 'Chief Geographer's Place-Name Survey, 1905-1909. 4: Manitoba.' *Canoma 7*: 1-25.
Waiser, W.A. 1983. 'Rambler: Professor John Macoun's Career with the Geological Survey of Canada, 1882-1912.' (Unpublished thesis, University of Saskatchewan.) Ottawa: National Library of Canada, Canadian Theses 60503, ISBN 0315-12619-1.
Waiser, W.A. 1989. *The Field Naturalist John Macoun, the Geological Survey and Natural Science*. Toronto: University of Toronto Press.

Henry Chichester Hart
1847-1908

IAIN HIGGINS

Henry Chichester Hart was born at Raheny, Co. Dublin, on 29 July 1847, and died 61 years later, on 7 August 1908, at Carrablagh, his home on Lough Swilly, Co. Donegal, having made an exceptionally diligent contribution to both the natural sciences and the humanistic scholarship of his day. He was educated at Trinity College, Dublin, where he studied for three years (1866-9), long enough to distinguish himself as the champion walker at the College Races, to come 'to love Shakespeare', and to earn an honours B.A. in Experimental and Natural Science. His degree earned, Hart did not go on to further study or to a regular occupation of any sort, and although in 1885-6 he served as lecturer in Natural Science at Queen's College, Galway, he avoided even an academic career such as that pursued by his father, Sir Andrew Searle Hart, a distinguished mathematician and Vice-Provost of Trinity College. The young man chose instead to become an amateur scholar, taking advantage of the privileges accruing to someone born into a landed Donegal family (he was High Sheriff of the county in 1895).

As an amateur scholar, Hart followed his own desires as well as the practice of his day, and devoted himself to natural history, above all to botany. He explored not only his native Ireland, but also parts of the Arctic and the Middle East. In or out of Ireland, alone or with others, he laboured long and hard in the field, where he was greatly aided by the superior physical strength and stamina that made him a champion walker and won the admiration of his contemporaries: a fellow Arctic naturalist called him 'physically ... the finest man I ever knew'. Much of Hart's botanical field work was pioneering, and in 1893 it earned him membership in the Royal Irish Academy; in 1895 he became a Fellow of the Royal Geographical Society. Towards the end of his life he left off his peripatetic botanizing to pursue sedentary but no less industrious work in the service of God and Shakespeare.

Hart began botanizing shortly before he entered Trinity College, and he published his first scientific writings in 1873. These were two 'short notes' in the *Journal of Botany British and Foreign*, a periodical open to amateur and professional botanists alike to which Hart contributed regularly until 1899. Two years after his first publication, he was made a Fellow of the Linnaean Society of London.

Hart was also honoured at this early date with an appointment as naturalist to HMS *Discovery* on the British Polar Expedition of 1875-6. Headed by Sir G.S. Nares, the expedition was the first wholly scientific British mission to the Arctic since the disastrous Franklin voyage of 1845. In the course of his duties, Hart visited some forty stations on Greenland between Egedesminde (lat. 68° 42') and Cape Joseph Henry (82° 50'), collecting specimens where conditions and the season allowed, but he did most of his work at Discovery Bay just north of the 80th parallel, where he was posted for almost a year. In addition to botanizing there, he experimented successfully with growing 'peas, beans, celery, wheat, mustard and cress', and dissected birds and land animals to determine their diet. Ill health prevented him from publishing his findings before 1880, when a synopsis appeared in the *Journal of Botany*; in the same year he published four brief notes on Arctic ornithology in the *Zoologist*. His collected specimens were deposited in the herbaria of Kew and the British Museum, as well as in the National Herbarium at Glasnevin.

Soon after his Arctic excursion, Hart found himself in an entirely different botanical and political world, engaged in a scientific undertaking that was part of the international scramble for power and influence in the Middle East. In 1883 he was asked by Edward Hull, Director of the Geological Survey of Ireland, to serve as a volunteer naturalist on the Palestine Exploration Society's geological expedition to the Sinai and Palestine. Aided by a grant from the Royal Irish Academy, Hart agreed to go, becoming one of the first botanists from the British Isles to work in the region. The specimens he collected there were deposited in the herbaria of Kew and the British Museum, while his detailed findings were published in 1885 in the *Quarterly Journal of the Palestine Exploration Committee* and the *Transactions of the Royal Irish Academy.* As on the Arctic expedition, Hart also did some zoological research, observing and collecting not only birds, but insects, molluscs, reptiles and mammals: 'As fast as I made gatherings, I was able to deposit them on the back of my admirable beast of burthen. For this purpose I had two sets of camel bags and drying boards, as well as multifarious swinging gear; guns, spy-glass, water-bottle, shoulder-bag, spirit-cylinder, portfolios, insect-box, *et hoc genus omne.*' His zoological findings were incorporated into a book revised from the Royal Irish Academy paper, *Some Account of the Fauna and Flora of Sinai, Petra and Wâdy 'Arabah* (Palestine Exploration Fund, 1891).

Like his Arctic paper, Hart's three reports on Palestine were organized according to the expedition's itinerary, but they differ from the former in that each is presented as a narrative based on extracts from his journal. The resulting document is more interesting to read than the standard scientific paper, and its interest is further enhanced by the occasional glimpse the journal extracts offer of both the botanist and the man. If such cameo self-portraits are to be believed, Hart would allow nothing to prevent him either from seeking out new specimens or from indulging his love of climbing:

On such excursions as these [up Mt. Sinai] the Bedouins grew much excited as I eluded their guardianship, and rushed into gullies or up cliffs after some coveted treasure of vegetation not seen before. With howls and gestures they besought of me to return to the track. They are, indeed, held to a certain extent responsible for the safety of the travellers in their charge. It was this reason which caused such screams of dismay amongst the Pyramid Arabs as I succeeded in dodging them, and ascending the second and dangerous pyramid without their troublesome escort, and, what was to them quite inexcusably unsafe, in my boots. In spite then of the Bedouins I followed the bent of my own botanical inclinations, and soon found out that they ceased to meddle when they saw they could not control.

Such overseas adventures notwithstanding, Hart's main interests and most important scientific contributions were in Irish botany. Year after year, he explored parts of his native country, especially his home county of

Donegal, recording and classifying plants wherever he went. In addition to his many notes and papers (some forty-five in all), he produced a pamphlet, *A List of the Plants found in the Islands of Aran* (Dublin, 1875), and two books, *The Flora of Howth* (Dublin, 1887) and *Flora of the County Donegal* (Dublin, 1898), the latter over four hundred pages long and the product of a lifetime's work. In favourable reviews in the *Journal of Botany*, the introduction to the former was held up as 'a model of what such essays should be'. But praise of Hart as a botanist was not confined to book reviews; the editors of the second (posthumous) edition of *Cybele Hibernica* (1898) singled him out as an exemplary field-worker, noting that he had 'done more to further our knowledge of Irish plant distribution than any other explorer of recent years' (More in Colgan and Scully, 1898).

Hart's botanical writings are not especially distinguished – he was no Irish Thoreau – but many of them can still be read with pleasure, for he preferred to offer his findings by way of a loosely narrative diary, whose manner was even more informal and informative than that of his Palestine reports. This style allowed him to intersperse his botanical observations with passing comments on matters of all sorts: the weather, local lore and habits, zoological and geological phenomena, natural beauty, good and bad lodgings, his own heavy labours, 'her Majesty's mail to Malin' ('From start to finish it is more or less a revel of chat and chaff'), and his publisher's mangling of a local map ('It makes Mulroy an inland lake! No doubt it commits other monstrosities.').

In addition to his botanical writings, Hart regularly published short zoological notes. Most appeared in the *Zoologist* in the years 1878-96, but a handful were published in the *Irish Naturalist* during the 1890s. His concerns here were mainly with the behaviour and the habitats of local birds, especially in Donegal, although he occasionally wrote notices of local land and water animals. In the 1880s he wrote a couple of zoological treatises for the common reader, *Voices from the Irish Woods* (Dublin, c. 1886) and *The Animals Mentioned in the Bible* (London, 1888).

The latter book took Hart outside Ireland once again, and represented the first of two scholarly undertakings on behalf of God; the second came a few years later when he assisted the Rev. W.C. Piercy in compiling *Murray's Bible Dictionary*. In the treatise on biblical animals, Hart made good use of his earlier experiences in the Holy Land. This curious study is the most readable of all of Hart's publications, and apart from its interest as a curiosity, it reveals a side of the man seen nowhere else in his writings. For him, science served faith; 'every fresh [scientific] observation lends a new force or adds an additional beauty to one or more [scriptural] passages; and at the same time that it explains a difficulty of the text, it increases in us a reverence and a faith for the inspired character of the Sacred Volume'.

Between nature and God Hart also found time for culture, turning his attention to Irish folklore, English philology, and Elizabethan literature. Apart from the material noticed in his botanical writings, Hart collected proverbs, songs, dialect words and other local lore from Ulster and elsewhere, but published virtually nothing; the collections were found amongst his papers after he died, and remain an untapped resource. Only the dialect studies have served further scholarship, being incorporated into *The English Dialect of Donegal: A Glossary* (Dublin, 1953) by Michael Traynor, who praised Hart for his 'amazing industry and acumen in collecting, collation, and annotation'. Hart's sole publication on Irish local culture was some 'Notes on Ulster Dialect, Chiefly Donegal' read to the London Philological Society in 1899 and concerned with words 'illustrative of English literature', philologically 'remarkable', or 'relating to natural objects, chiefly plants and animals'. Hart's rarely noticed sense of humour emerges here on several occasions: '"*She*" also represents "*he*," "*she*," or "*it*." I asked a Fanet man "How old is that bull?" "*She's* two years old, but *she's* not bullin' any yet, damn *her*." This is an Irish bull and no mistake.'

Hart continued his activities as a self-styled 'laborious word-hunter' into Elizabethan literature, a field in which he also worked as a literary historian and textual editor. Between 1902 and 1908, he published regularly in *Notes and Queries*, writing many short pieces on word usage, and two extended essays, both of which were republished as pamphlets by the Athenaeum Press in London. The second of these essays was on Robert Greene's prose works, the first on some literary quarrels associated with Ben Jonson, whose *Works* Hart edited in 1906. His labours here remained unfinished, and manuscripts relating to Jonson were found among his posthumous papers.

These papers also included Hart's editions of Shakespeare's *Henry VI, Pts. 1-3*, the last of seven plays that he had edited for the much-praised Arden *Shakespeare*, a series intended for student and scholar alike and still in use today, although now in revised editions. Hart's other Arden editions were of *Othello* (1903), which he thought 'the most perfect play that Shakespeare ever wrote', *The Merry Wives of Windsor* (1904), *Measure for Measure* (1905), and *Love's Labour's Lost* (1906). As an editor, Hart had to establish a proper text, write a general introduction (on matters of textual and reception history, sources and analogues, and literary appreciation), and provide a running commentary on the play, a triple task to which he brought the leisure of a gentleman, the patience of a botanist, and his own exceptionally wide reading in Elizabethan literature. As late as 1951 one of the Arden revisers thought Hart's notes on the parallels between Shakespeare and other Elizabethan writings to be 'still of the highest value'.

As a reader of Shakespeare, Hart was too much the botanist, and he rarely strayed from classifying into criticism, yet when he did he was at once decided and conventional in his views. Thus *Measure for Measure* had a 'painfully repugnant plot', but showed Shakespeare working 'with a high moral purpose and a stern sense of duty' and so producing 'some of the most beautiful passages of dignified poetry to be met with anywhere' in his writings. Beyond its poetic qualities, Hart found Shakespeare's language interesting in and of itself; indeed, his notes and introductions, especially to *Henry VI, Pt. 1*, show him to be deeply interested in philology and even claiming to have anticipated the *New English Dictionary* in recording elements of Elizabethan English.

In his editions of Shakespeare, then, Hart revealed glimpses of his personality, and the glimpses largely accord with the portraits sketched by the naturalists R.M. Barrington and R.L. Praeger. The latter, who knew him mainly through their correspondence, thought Hart a passionate and exceptionally energetic naturalist, but 'somewhat dictatorial, impatient, [and] difficult to handle'; when Praeger accidentally overlooked an invitation to visit Carrablagh to see the rhododendrons in flower, Hart wrote once to notice the slight and then broke off their correspondence altogether. As a close friend, Barrington sketched a slightly gentler portrait of Hart, but he too relates several anecdotes that show the same difficult man, someone who competed at virtually everything, especially the physical activities that he pursued throughout his life, walking and mountain-climbing. Hart was in fact a sufficiently distinguished climber to be asked in 1895 to contribute the Irish section of Haskett Smith's *Climbing in the British Isles*, and a competitive enough man to enjoy walks and climbs involving a wager. But he was also a dedicated enough botanist 'to remove [his] lower garments and wade the mouth of the Clonmany River' so as not to miss a single plant.

References

H.C. Hart's papers (1876-1908) are held by the library of Trinity College, Dublin (MSS 10901-22)

Barrington, R.M. 1908. 'Henry Chichester Hart.' *Irish Naturalist 17*: 248-54.
Colgan, N. and R.W. Scully. 1898. *Contributions Towards a Cybele Hibernica*. (2nd ed.). Dublin: Ponsonby.
Hart, H.C. 1887. *Flora of Howth*. Dublin: Hodges, Figgis.
Hart, H.C. 1888. *The Animals Mentioned in the Bible*. London: The Religious Tract Society.
Hart, H.C. 1898. *Flora of the County Donegal*. Dublin: Sealy, Bryers & Walker.
Praeger, R.L. 1886. 'Irish Topographical Botany.' *Proceedings of the Royal Irish Academy* (2nd ser.).
Praeger, R.L. 1950. *Some Irish Naturalists: A Biographical Notebook*. Dundalk, Dundalgan Press.
Scannell, M.J.P. 1990. 'Henry Chichester Hart,' in E.C. Mollan, W. Davis and B. Finucane (eds), *More People and Places in Irish Science and Technology*. Dublin: Royal Irish Academy.

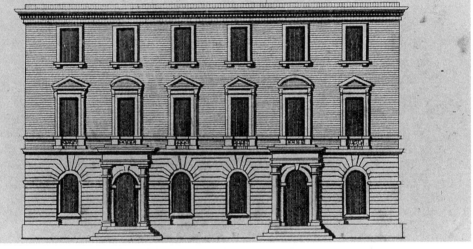

New Buildings at Dublin, for the use of the Dublin Society, & the Grand Canal Company.

Enlightenment and Education

HELENA C.G. CHESNEY

The European Enlightenment in Ireland

The eighteenth-century interest in natural history emanated from the tremendous progress in creative thought that had sparked the Scientific Revolution in the sixteenth and seventeenth centuries and impelled European civilization out of the Middle Ages. The seventeenth century was the golden age of the polymath; scholars took up religion, philosophy, natural sciences, history and many other subjects without specialized training and exhibited an enormous breadth of interest. Largely unaffected by the Renaissance, Ireland's scientific life sparked into being in the middle of the seventeenth century but remained some steps behind developments in Britain and continental Europe.

In England following the Reformation – which soon aroused a new intellectual interest in man's place in the world – science had grown into a fashionable pursuit. During the Commonwealth (1649-60) there was increased interest in the natural sciences. In 1660 impetus and focus were given to the practice and study of science with the establishment of the Royal Society of London. Its philosophy was based on Francis Bacon's vision that mankind's progress and fulfilment related to the practical application of scientific improvements. Prominent among its mainly Puritan fellows was Samuel Hartlib, 'who so consistently sought to introduce the new realistic, utilitarian, and empirical education into England' (Merton, 1970). In the field of natural philosophy, his influence was considerable in Ireland, as well as England, among those dedicated to replacing the mystic approach to science with academic study. The so-called 'Hartlib Circle' embraced the influential educational ideals of the Bohemian reformer Comenius, and linked these to the Baconian philosophy of – to quote Thomas Sprat in 1667 – 'the uses of all creatures to enrich mankind with all the benefits of fruitfulness and plenty' (Sprat, 1959).

Despite the large number of Puritans involved, the Royal Society's constitution, according to Sprat, opened it to 'Men of different Religions, Countries and Professions of Life … they openly profess, not to lay the Foundation of an English, Scottish, Irish, Popish or Protestant Philosophy; but a Philosophy of Mankind'. Clearly, neither a Christian nor a specifically Protestant outlook was considered necessary for the study of science. The Royal Society attracted an impressive selection of leading English intellectuals as members, along with a significant number of Anglo-Irish thinkers. As a result, current trends in scientific discourses and discoveries were quickly transmitted to Ireland, particularly to Dublin.

In Ireland, beyond the formal sphere of institutions, societies, lectures and publications, only tantalizing traces of this early activity now remain to aid the tracking of its development. Trinity College, set up as the first college of the University of Dublin in 1592, was funded with the primary aim of providing 'a civilising influence on a rebellious nation' (Robinson-Hammerstein, 1992). Undoubtedly England as the colonizer was alert to all possibilities for the exploitation of the country's resources. By 1650, many developments in natural history and the practical sciences had their origins in the acquisition of information for military, political and economic ends, which gave impetus to the accumulation of data and particularly promoted surveying and mapping.

Archbishop James Ussher of Armagh, intellectual and philosopher, funded publication of several works which, though not written by Irishmen, added to the growing fund of knowledge of Ireland's geology, landscape, flora and fauna (Clarke, 1973). Among these were John Arnold's *Philosophia Naturalis* (1641) and Gerard Boate's *Irelands Naturall History* (1652), the first modern scientific book on Ireland's nature prior to the Restoration. The army physician Sir William Petty, a graduate of Leiden, who became Surveyor General of Ireland, was also aided by Ussher with the Down Survey (1655-6) (Larcom, 1851), 'one of the most remarkable scientific works carried out in Ireland and considered to be one of the first modern surveys of the country' (Andrews, 1980).

In Ireland, although the study of natural sciences or the New Learning had started about the mid-seventeenth century, the first attempts at formalizing these arose only in 1683. Among the influential Anglo-Irish members of the Royal Society of London were Petty, mathematician, inventor and surveyor; William Molyneux, natural philosopher and astronomer; his brother Thomas, natural philosopher and physician; St George Ashe, mathematician; and Narcissus Marsh, founder of Marsh's Library in Dublin. Inspired by the principles of the Royal Society, they proposed that Dublin have a society with similar interests and aims: a society for 'the Improving Natural Knowledge, Mathematicks, and Mechanicks' that became best known as the Dublin Philosophical Society (Kelly, 1992). Most of the founders were part of the informal Hartlib circle and Petty, a former President of the Royal Society, became its President. One of the Society's founder members, the distinguished doctor and anatomist Allen Mullen, designed and set up a laboratory in 1684, 'the first of its kind recorded in Ireland' (Clarke, 1973). Mullen was also a Fellow of the Royal Society and had worked in London with Robert Boyle, the seventh son of Richard Boyle, Earl of Cork, and the best-known chemist of his generation.

By the early eighteenth century it was necessary for the 'philosophical' to become the 'practical' in order to keep pace with developments elsewhere. Trinity College, Dublin, the 'home' of the Society, had started the formal teaching of medicine in the 1650s and acquired its first chemical laboratory in 1710. Throughout the eighteenth century, especially in the second half, interest in natural history increased. Initially the study of both botany, which related to health, medicine and agriculture, and geology, with its important economic and strategic applications, received greater attention than zoology. However, no formal natural-history teaching existed in Dublin until 1711 when Trinity College appointed its first 'Professor in Botanie', who was also responsible for the Physic Garden on the campus (Nelson, 1993). This was Henry Nicholson, who had graduated from Leiden in 1709 and who published 'the first botanical treatise printed in Ireland, entitled *Methodus Plantarum in Horto Medico, Collegii Dublinensis* ...' (1712). The Quaker physician John Rutty, another Leiden medical graduate, published *The Natural History of County Dublin* in 1722. However, beyond medical needs, little natural history was taught in the university and it was to be a century before the first lectures devoted specifically to the subject were delivered by Whitley Stokes, later to be appointed Professor of Natural History. However John K'Eogh's *Zoologica Medicinalis Hibernica* (1739), a treatise on animals used in medicinal cures, supplemented his 1735 text on medical botany, bringing zoology into the realms of medicine.

Outside formal science, the appreciation of nature was a part of the fashionable intellectual activity associated with the Enlightenment. From 1734, the sociable Margaret Bentinck, Duchess of Portland, developed her passion for fine art and natural history and established a botanic garden and even a menagerie at Bulstrode in Buckinghamshire. Her close friend Mary Delaney, the wife of Patrick Delaney, Dean of St Patrick's Cathedral, Dublin, revealed in her famous diaries that the Anglo-Irish gentry indulged in similar activities (Day, 1991). Natural-history collecting and romantically landscaped gardens, shell grottoes and rustic summer-houses all became fashionable in Ireland, and contributed to the popularization of landscape and botanical study.

Eighteenth-century Dublin looked the part of a cultural capital and the second city of the Kingdom, after London. The Duke of Ormonde had extensively remodelled the city in a confident and ambitious attempt to emulate the grand avenues and quays of Paris. Dublin merchants had grown wealthy from their control of the export trade, and an increasing appetite for learning and discourse grew from the Enlightenment, with whose aims and philosophy the Irish intellectuals were fully conversant. The great work of the French philosopher and rationalist Pierre Bayle, *Dictionnaire Critique et Historique*, which had started publication in 1695, had considerable influence. Mc Cormack (1993) finds that Bayle's ideas were widely read in Ireland, for 'we can note the battered sets of his dictionary – usually in English translation – which still turn up in the dispersed libraries of Irish eighteenth-century houses'. Indeed Mc Cormack argues that 'without Bayle, the foundation of the Royal Irish Academy in 1785 would have been unthinkable'.

Between 1725 and 1760 science had waned in England when, without the inspiration of Newton who died in 1727, the Royal Society of London went into decline. In Ireland, however, 1731 saw the founding of the Dublin Society for Improving Husbandry, Manufactures and Other Useful Arts, whose aims were mainly practical rather than purely scientific, for landowners figured large in its membership and science was envisaged as the means of turning nature to their advantage. In pursuit of these aims, from 1734 to 1740 it leased a small botanic garden at Summerhill to run an experimental nursery of useful plants. One of the first links between the arts and sciences in Ireland was forged through the Dublin Society's interest in funding a wide range of artistic, craft and agricultural developments through financial grants or 'premiums'.

In 1785 the Earl of Charlemont and fellow enthusiasts founded another society, the Royal Irish Academy, to cultivate the fashionable subjects of science, polite literature and antiquities through holding meetings, publishing papers and helping to finance research. In the next one hundred years, 'the golden age of Irish science' according to Herries Davies (1985), these two Dublin societies championed the sciences. The Dublin Society evolved some innovative approaches to the promotion of science and in 1800 set up a committee to examine and compare its achievements with those of the Royal Institution in London. This committee reported that 'the Dublin Society had taken the lead of it and all other like institutions in Europe in everything except philosophical lectures'. In response a Chair of Natural and Experimental Philosophy was immediately established (Herries Davies, 1985). The Chair of Mineralogy and Chemistry, provided with a chemical laboratory or 'Repository' for research, was 'probably the first of its kind in the United Kingdom'. In another exemplary move, the Society funded lecture courses by notable English scientists to increase 'the spirit of philosophical enquiry' (Berry, 1915).

It seemed then that the Scientific Revolution had indeed produced developments that advanced man's place in the world through the harnessing of nature, aptly conforming to the original Baconian ideals of those who had first set the course of science in Ireland. These developments brought an increasing appetite for nature, one that 'parallels and interacts with currents in many similar fields, in gardening, in painting, in poetry' and led to 'shifts in attitude and taste, which enabled natural history to establish itself as a nourishment of the soul' (Porter, 1990). The practical and the sublime aspects perceived in the enlightened view of nature became linked through the philosophy of Edmund Burke, whose influential contributions *A Philosophical Inquiry into the Origin of Our Ideas of the Sublime and Beautiful* (1756) and *Reflections on the Revolution in France* (1790) illustrate the contradictory strands apparent in contemporary philosophy – the aesthetic and the political – in the second half of the eighteenth century. Also captivated by the aesthetic spirit of the age was James Usher, another Trinity graduate whose ideas on beauty and the sublime were expounded in *Clio, or a Discourse on Taste* (1769). In this, according to Kearney (1985), Usher insisted that 'our ideas of beauty, truth and the *summum bonum* are not reducible to empirical sensation or association'.

The Influence of European Education

Irish links with the Continent had long been strong on both the Catholic and Protestant sides. For two centuries, the Penal Laws denied Catholics and Nonconformist Protestants or Dissenters access to education at Trinity College and the English universities. Catholics were forced to travel to Irish colleges in Rome, Paris, Salamanca, Krakow and other continental cities. In part to make good this lack in Catholic education in Ireland, Maynooth College was founded in 1795 by an Act of Parliament exclusively for Roman Catholic education. This failed, however, to bring about many significant scientific contributions following in the European tradition. Gabbey (*pers. comm.*) considers that although science was in the curriculum, the Irish Jesuit tradition tended to concentrate on the sciences with a strong mathematical base, as evidenced by the specialization in electrical studies at Maynooth by the physicist Nicholas Callan, Professor of Natural History, and others. Unfortunately, the College sacrificed the teaching of natural philosophy because 'the demand for Roman Catholic Clergymen in Ireland is so urgent' (Anon., 1825).

Similarly, until 1845 the main educational links for Dissenters were also outside Ireland, mainly with Scotland and the Continent, although Trinity College had eventually been opened up to Presbyterians in 1783. With universities in Ireland and England closed to them, their tradition was to travel to universities in Edinburgh, Glasgow, Utrecht and Leiden to complete their education. However, many followers of the Established Church also preferred to educate their sons abroad, rather than send them to the University of Dublin. As a result a large proportion of those involved in Irish natural history were well informed on the latest continental thinking, discoveries and inventions in the natural sciences.

Probably the most notable example of the benefits of such an education is Sir Hans Sloane (1660-1753), who was born and received his early education in Killyleagh, Co. Down. An early member of the Royal Society who had studied medicine in Paris and Orange, he became Physician to Queen Anne and an influential proponent of science. The Temple Coffee House Botanic Club, considered to be the first natural-history society in Britain, if not the world (Allen, 1976), started in or around 1689 with Sloane and his scientifically minded friends as members. His personal collection containing many natural-history specimens was to form the basis of the British Museum.

His fellow-countryman and friend Sir Arthur Rawdon (1662-95) had been brought up and educated in France. Through Sloane, Rawdon was in contact with the leading English botanists of the time. In the midst of the enormous political upheavals resulting from the Williamite campaigns in which he fought, Rawdon confidently landscaped his grounds at Moira, Co. Down, with 'extensive walks, vistoes, a labyrinth, canals, ponds and groves laid out in the fashion of the time' (Smith and Harris, 1744). In 1689 his gardener, James Harlow, was dispatched to Jamaica to collect exotic plants for the gardens and returned some two years later with a superb collection of over a thousand living plants. By 1690, the year of the Battle of the Boyne, Rawdon had built a 'large stove' or greenhouse, among the first in the country. He is considered to have been one of the most important horticultural innovators in these islands. His wonderful gardens ranked high among the great plant collections of the period in the British Isles and Europe; sadly, scarcely any trace remains of them today at Moira (Nelson, 1981).

Close links arose between Leiden and Dublin Physic Gardens in the early eighteenth century with the appointment of William Hamilton (Nelson, 1982) and his successor in 1722, William Stephens, who also studied at Leiden. However, Thomas Molyneux who headed the School of Physic at Trinity College, and has been called 'the Father of Irish Medicine' (Lyons, 1990), had also been a medical student at Leiden from 1684 and there acquired an early *Hortus siccus* of dried plants. This had been examined and annotated for him by William Sherrard in 1693, during his stay at Moira with Rawdon. As Nelson (1982) notes, Sherrard had graduated in law from Cambridge and then had 'studied botany under such men as Tournefort in Paris and Hermann in Leiden'.

Richard Kirwan (c. 1733-1812), the Irish chemist, geologist and mineralogist, brought up in the Catholic faith and intended for the Jesuit priesthood, also had the benefit of education at Leiden. He renounced his Catholic beliefs in 1764, a prerequisite of being called to the Irish Bar, from which however he soon resigned to resume his scientific pursuits. Kirwan was President of the Royal Irish Academy and Inspector of Mines in Ireland, and became the most widely read Neptunist geologist and 'the Father of British Mineralogy' (Herries Davies, 1983). As a chemist, he was cited more frequently in European scientific journals than any other chemist of the age. Madame Lavoisier translated Kirwan's *Essay on Phlogiston and the Constitution of Acids* (1787) to make it available for French criticism. Incidentally, Kirwan also had a great taste for old Irish music, which he collected. The Catholic Robert Barnewall, later Lord Trimleston, also completed his education abroad, employing his time 'to advantage in studying botany and physic', before settling in his ancestral home in Co. Meath in 1746, which he furnished with 'rich cabinets and splendid gardens' (Maxwell, 1949).

These long-standing contacts with the Continent, and Leiden in particular, were to continue until well into the nineteenth century. Sir Frederick Moore, the Director of Glasnevin Botanic Gardens for over forty years, recalled in his autobiography the influence of his schooling in Hanover, Ghent and 'the School of Botany and the Botanic Gardens in Leiden' (Moore, 1940).

In the late eighteenth century the Irish naturalists, spurred on by the continental developments in taxonomy and systematics, or classification, greatly needed material on which to work, but there was a singular dearth of it in their country. This was to change dramatically in 1792 when Kirwan, through his extensive continental contacts, successfully acquired the Leskean natural history cabinet in Leipzig for the Dublin Society. N.G. Leske, formerly Professor of Natural History in Marburg, had been a pupil of Werner, one of the founders of geology, and his mineral collection was arranged on Wernerian principles; Karsten, who compiled the sale catalogue, was another eminent German mineralogist. Through this perceptive acquisition the Society's mineral collection grew to nearly 7500 specimens and became one of the largest and finest in the world. The Leskean acquisition also provided a large collection of shells and insects, a herbarium and several anatomical preparations (White, 1911). The value of such wide-ranging collections became evident and greatly encouraged naturalists to explore further contacts at home and abroad to assuage their need for specimens.

France was another source of inspiration and educational ideas for the Irish. William Paley's influential *Principles of Moral and Political Philosophy*, first published in 1785, was soon reprinted in Dublin. This work drew upon arguments related to events during the American War of Independence, and 'helped speed the change in attitude that resulted in the Acts for Catholic relief from the Penal Laws' (Mc Cormack, 1993). The Napoleonic Wars forced unstable alliances throughout Europe and engaged England in a desperate war with France, because Napoleon's insatiable quest for power constantly threatened from across the Channel. It is difficult to appreciate the great celebrations and enormous relief that followed Wellington's victory at Waterloo in 1815, resulting in a high level of anti-French feeling that was to last in England for nearly two decades. On the other hand, close connections with France and an empathy with revolutionary ideals existed in Ireland, particularly in the southern counties of Cork and Kerry. John Kane, the father of the educationalist and chemist Sir Robert Kane, was a Catholic and a United Irishman who had sought refuge in Paris, where he studied chemistry. On his return to Dublin he set up the profitable chemical works that funded his son's education. Among other notable Irish medical men and naturalists who received their education in France was John Hart, Professor of Anatomy at the Royal College of Surgeons in the 1840s. He had studied under the great zoologist Cuvier in Paris and later undertook the first description of the anatomy of the giant Irish deer (Bronte Gatenby, 1961). In 1835, a number of admirers of Cuvier founded The Cuvierian Society of Cork.

New developments and the changing spirit of the age were registered in a review of Irish science in 1825, which noticed that 'a great revolution' had taken place in the University of Dublin 'in which the "new science" is now cultivated with ardour and with every prospect of success' (Anon., 1825). The author went on to assert that Humphrey Lloyd had 'updated science teaching in Trinity College by broadening the syllabus and furnishing the best continental texts then available, with good results'. The review highlighted Maynooth College and Belfast [Academical] Institution as the other seminaries in Ireland that were successfully promoting science, and concluded: 'Let the men of science not relax in their exertions; and may no unseen obstacle oppose itself, to check the progress of the human mind, in this country, in one of its noblest spheres of action!' Adding further substance to these ideals were men such as Dionysius Lardner, a brilliant student in his days at Trinity College, Dublin, and a great popularizer of science. Taking inspiration from Denis Diderot's influential *L'Encyclopedie*, he conceived the *Cabinet Cyclopedia* (1830-49) to disseminate facts and opinions about science to an increasingly interested public. An influential educational reformer, he was to become the first Professor of Natural Philosophy and Astronomy at the newly formed University of London, which opened its doors to Dissenters, Roman Catholics and Jews alike (Davis, 1990).

Fortunately, or ironically, it would appear that the Penal Laws, which denied Catholics and Dissenters access to education at Trinity College or the

English universities and forced them to travel to universities in Scotland or Europe, furnished educational qualifications in medicine and the sciences at least the equal of those available to followers of the Established Church. More tellingly, it would appear also that through the broadening of their horizons, contacts and philosophy, their enlightened ideals and outlook combined to produce new approaches to the study of the natural sciences that rendered them more accessible to a wider audience than might have otherwise been possible at the time.

Education and Science in Belfast

The ability to contribute to science requires curiosity, imagination, education and the opportunity to exchange ideas, but in Ireland education was in short supply and very few schools existed before the nineteenth century. The hedge schools and travelling masters, as much a result of poverty as of the Penal Laws, were the only means of education for many, and even in the mid-eighteenth century 'many a ditchful of scholars' was to be found in the countryside. However, it appears that despite the large numbers of absentee landlords and 'rackrenters' who sorely exploited their holdings, some estate owners set up schools to improve the education of their tenants. At Killyleagh, Co. Down, the Hamilton family endowed a school of philosophy in the late seventeenth century, which under the Rev. John McAlpin flourished for many years 'to the great chagrin of the clergy of the Established Church because of its Presbyterian tendencies' (De Beer, 1953). In the 1770s Sir James Caldwell of Castlecaldwell, Co. Fermanagh, a Fellow of the Royal Society and a Count of the Holy Roman Empire, provided educational facilities for his tenantry and premiums for agricultural improvements (Maxwell, 1949). The inventor Richard Lovell Edgeworth of Edgeworthstown, Co. Longford, a member of the famed Lunar Society of Birmingham who had acquired liberal ideas during his travels on the Continent, was another of the landed gentry who attempted to improve the lives of their tenants through education (Edgeworth, 1820). According to Allen (1976), in many private Irish schools natural history was forming part of school syllabuses by 1790, especially where the schoolmasters were themselves naturalists. Some individuals contributed considerably, such as Adam Clarke (1760-1832), a scholar in Hebrew and the classics, who 'established several schools in Ulster and a small museum, and collected a valuable library' (Clarke, 1833). The considerable influence of Quaker philosophy and educational ideals in encouraging the study of natural history also emerges clearly. For example, the famous Ball family of naturalists and the botanist William Harvey received their schooling from the esteemed Quaker schoolmaster James White of Ballitore, Co. Kildare.

In 1783 the merchants in Belfast had seized the opportunity to export textiles directly to Britain and its empire and set themselves on course for a century of unparalleled industrial development, economic expansion and prosperity. The prosperity brought cultural development to what had been, until the early 1800s, a small provincial town whose population grew from 13,000 in 1782 to 50,000 in 1831. Living and working conditions were difficult for many of the workforce but the fast-growing town was fortunate in the number of citizens who pursued an ardent interest in natural history and in making education available to all sections of the community. Froggatt and Bridges (1985) observe that 'imparting and seeking knowledge were fundamental characteristics of society generally', and that 'enquiry into anything and everything from national culture and heritage to the wonders of the new factory machines ... blended with a puritan austerity to produce a disciplined intellectual vigour which ensured that many leading men were also prominent in the scientific and cultural life of Belfast'.

Several learned societies were established. The first with scientific aims was the Belfast Reading Society, founded in 1786. A decade later, having considerably extended its natural history collection through the purchase of scientific instruments, including a rain gauge, hygrometer and pyrometer, it became the Belfast Library and Society for Promoting Knowledge (Anderson, 1888). Science 'as a special object of cultivation' also concerned the Belfast Literary Society, founded in 1801 (Malcolm, 1851).

In the north great impetus to science arose in the educational field with the foundation of the Belfast Academy in 1786 and the Belfast Academical Institution in 1807. The Academy was closely modelled on Scottish educational ideals. Its first headmaster, Rev. Dr James Crombie, a St Andrews graduate, was one of the 'erudite and intellectually more inquisitive' New Light Presbyterian ministers (Stewart, 1985). Dr Reuben Bryce, who had graduated from Trinity College, Dublin, in 1776 before studying theology at Glasgow and Warrington Dissenting Academy, was the Principal from 1826 to 1880. He and his brother James, a geologist and mathematics master, took an exceptional interest in natural history: in 1828 they founded a natural history society, thought to be the first such school society in these islands, supplemented by a School Museum a year later (Drummond, 1831). Mineralogy became a popular subject of study; within two years the Museum, apart from shells and stuffed birds, had an impressive mineral collection, later described as the third or fourth finest in Ireland and detailed in a catalogue – *Tables of Simple Minerals, Rocks and Shells with Local Catalogues of Species for the use of Students of Natural History in the Belfast Academy* (Bryce, 1831).

Although the Principal, William Bruce, was not among them, from 1791 many of the Academy's patrons and their associates became closely involved in the Society of United Irishmen, whose *cri de coeur* was 'equality for all men regardless of creed' in a new attempt to harness and to utilize fully Ireland's human and natural resources. At this time many Scottish Presbyterian immigrants still spoke Gaelic and at the Academy Irish formed part of the syllabus. In 1795 the master Patrick Lynch prepared an Irish grammar to support its teaching (Stewart, 1985). Dr James McDonnell of the ancient Antrim clan, the first President of the Belfast Literary Society, was the moving force behind many literary, medical and scientific developments in the town. The founder of medical education in the town, he also played a leading role in organizing the first Belfast Harp Festival in 1792, and in 1830 McDonnell and James Bryce of the Academy became founder members of the Ulster Gaelic Society. Clearly the enlightened views of the founders of these Belfast institutions and the growing scientific community intended to encompass culture in all its forms.

As the population of Belfast expanded due to rapid industrialization, the lack of a university in the north of Ireland became a problem. Students had to travel to Dublin, Glasgow, Edinburgh, or farther afield to complete their studies. The Academy had failed to fill this gap and the Belfast Academical Institution was conceived in 1806 as a School with a Collegiate Department, whose philosophy and syllabus also approached those of the Dissenting Academies across the water. It opened in 1814 and, endowed with an annual government grant of £1500, it was to be furnished with a library and a museum for fossils and other specimens. The intention was to make a good education more accessible to pupils from the growing middle classes.

The Collegiate Department of the Institution planned to establish seven chairs, including a Chair of Natural Philosophy. Among the first Professors appointed were Thomas Andrews, James Marshall, Thomas Dix Hincks and James Lawson Drummond. Drummond taught 'a very wide field of natural history and a good deal of natural theology: there is scarcely a fact in Paley's Natural Theology that is not explained and illustrated' (Froggatt, 1976). Appointment of the Rev. Dr Thomas Dix Hincks to a chair at the Academical Institution brought an expert in Hebrew and Arabic and a keen naturalist to Belfast. He had been educated at Hackney Dissenting Academy in London (eventually forced to close in 1796, despite its considerable reputation, because of its sympathy for the French Revolution). Hincks then moved to Cork and was ordained in the Presbyterian ministry in 1792. There he started an Academy and helped found Cork Institution in 1806. In 1814 he moved to the Academy in Fermoy but shortly left for the new Academical Institution in Belfast (Bigger, 1924). His commitment to education was considerable and he served on the committees of various other Belfast educational establishments such as the Lancasterian School, established in 1814, and

Brown Street Daily School, established in 1821 (Anon., 1830). These 'Inst' professors, along with gifted amateurs such as John Templeton, George Hyndman, Robert Patterson and William Thompson, were enthusiastic proponents of another development that was to have far-reaching effects on science in the north.

This was the Belfast Natural History Society, founded in 1821, the first society in the north devoted entirely to the pursuit of natural history. 'Let us collect facts in order to have ideas' – the northern ledger-book naturalists fully endorsed Buffon and the Society attracted mainly middle-class businessmen, schoolmasters and the younger generation (Ross and Nash, 1986). Its first President, Drummond of the Institution, was a deeply religious man like so many of his contemporary naturalist friends and considered that 'conceptions of the power of Deity will be infinitely enlarged by the study of nature'. In 1820 he had published *Thoughts on the Study of Natural History and on the Importance of Attaching Museums of the Productions of Nature to National Seminaries of Education*, and the Society pursued its plans to widen access to natural history. These included lectures for both members and the public, and as a result of a rewarding public appeal the Society's Museum opened its fine building in 1831. The forward-looking Drummond, in his 'Presidental Address to Belfast Natural History Society at the Opening of its Museum' (1831a), commented:

With respect to museums I may now remark that they are considered, on the Continent, of such importance, that scarcely any town of considerable size is without one. The apathy on this head, which so long existed in the British islands, is every day wearing off, and I trust this museum when it comes into effective operation will be cherished and valued by a discerning public. I hope it will give a new and powerful impulse to the study of nature and physical science, that it will create and foster a taste for knowledge among all classes of our community, and that it will materially serve to raise the character of our town still higher, as a place favourable to the culture of literature and scientific pursuits.

The Natural History Society energetically set about acquiring material from many sources and published a detailed leaflet on 'Collecting Natural History Specimens' to encourage naturalists, relatives and acquaintances at home and overseas to send specimens. By 1831, when its Museum opened, it had 'about 2000 specimens of minerals; a nearly complete collection of native and a considerable number of foreign shells; 200 native and foreign birds; about 3000 insects; an extensive *Hortus siccus* of indigenous, American and other exotic plants; about 200 snakes and lizards ...' (Drummond, 1831a). From the first regular public access dating from May 1837, it attracted large numbers of citizens and within a decade was specifically targeting 'Mechanics and Operatives' in its advertising.

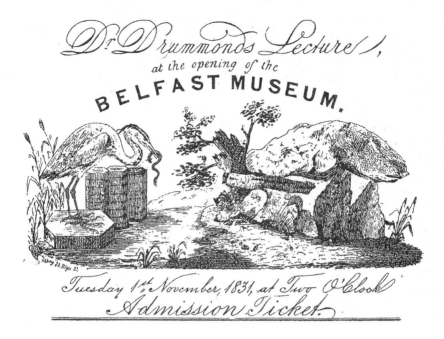

Dr Drummond's Lectures, at the opening of the **BELFAST MUSEUM.** *Tuesday 1st November, 1831, at Two O'Clock* **Admission Ticket.**

Ideas and ideals in support of the best museum practice obtained widely. In a copy of 'Directions for Preserving Subjects in Natural History' published by Belfast Museum about 1835, we find a handwritten addition that details the Smithsonian Institution's recommendations for collecting insects. By the 1850s, 'the accessible and lucid natural history exhibits that the eminent Belfast naturalists and antiquaries had produced in the Belfast Museum' were highlighted by Professor Edward Forbes in a lecture in London on 'The Educational Uses of Museums'.

Access to scientific texts was also seen as important. The *Catalogue of the Library at Belfast Museum* shows that in 1847 the library contained some 450 volumes and about the same number of pamphlets and reprints (Anon., 1847). Almost half the books were scientific works, with nearly a quarter of continental and American origin; of the pamphlets and papers, two thirds were of American origin, the majority of these being on natural science and education. The extent of these American publications reflects the close links with educational and scientific developments in the eastern-seaboard cities, Philadelphia, Boston and New York. Closely associated with the library's development was Ireland's foremost entomologist, Alexander Henry Haliday, a superb linguist, fluent in the classics, who maintained close contact with numerous European naturalists. His father, Dr Alexander Haliday, the town's best-known physician, was one of the founders of Belfast Academy. His grandfather, Rev. Samuel Haliday, had studied under the leading Leiden theologians, but joined the Non-subscribing New Light ministers in the

Antrim Presbytery, whose attitudes were more tolerant and liberal than those of the Old Light Presbyterians. A life-long friend of Samuel Haliday was the philosopher Francis Hutcheson (1694-1746) of Carryduff, who became Professor of Moral Philosophy at Glasgow in 1729 and was a notable contributor to the Scottish Enlightenment. Following its initial success, from 1842 the Natural History Society, in the fashion of the day, became Belfast Natural History and Philosophical Society and as such it continues to this day.

The dawn of a new era came in 1845 when the first Queen's Colleges of the University of Ireland opened their doors in Belfast, Galway and Cork to many of those not previously entitled to attend a university in Ireland. However, these colleges underwent a stormy history as church and state wrestled with the problem of satisfying educational, religious and political hopes and fears. By the 1850s no university degrees in science were being offered in Britain and the country faced the danger of losing its leadership in industry. It became obvious that the future basis of national wealth would depend on the application of science and technology. In response, the Department of Science and Art was set up in 1853 to organize and control a system of industrial education throughout the United Kingdom of Great Britain and Ireland – and as a result Irish science was to be much more closely controlled and financed than before.

Women and Natural History

In Ireland, as elsewhere, it was usually considered inappropriate and unnecessary to furnish women with a university education, and the universities were not open to them. The nobility and wealthy families often provided their daughters with private tutors in fields such as literature, moral philosophy, *belles-lettres* and the court languages of French and Italian. Natural philosophy was not usually added to their syllabus. In the north the influence of Francis Hutcheson's ideas, which had linked politics to morality and religion and gave prominence to the rights of women, took considerable hold (Scott, 1900). For the middle classes, education became a focus of their increasing affluence and natural philosophy acquired intellectual acceptability for both sexes. John Templeton and his friend the auctioneer George Hyndman were two of the growing number of liberally minded men closely involved with educational developments in Belfast who considered women's participation in natural history pursuits to be entirely appropriate, and from this time women became more involved in field collecting to augment their own collections and those of others. In 1810 Templeton listed his wife and daughters among nine women shell-collectors living within the environs of Belfast. Hannah Hincks, a daughter of Thomas Dix Hincks, became a keen

MUSEUM.

In order to afford the Working classes every facility for seeing such a rare specimen as the

LIVING CHAMELEON,

and for inspecting the otherwise extensive and interesting collection contained in this Institution, the Curator will be in attendance on

EASTER MONDAY,

From 9 in the morning till 6 in the afternoon.

Ordinary Admission Fee,   - - -   6d.
Mechanics & Operatives, (on this occasion only,) 2d.
Children (if accompanied by their Parents,) Half Price.

Robert F. Ward, Printer, 25, Waring-*Street*, Belfast.

Easter Monday attractions at Belfast Museum, 1832. (Ulster Museum, Belfast)

botanist and donated her fine herbarium to Belfast Natural History and Philosophical Society (Hackney, 1980).

In the first decades of the nineteenth century the two main Belfast schools, the Academy and the Academical Institution, paved the way for the further opening up of natural history to women. Reuben Bryce, a family friend of the Edgeworths, was greatly impressed with Maria Edgeworth's ideas of female education, which he 'carried out in the Belfast Academy with successful results' (Young, 1902). By 1836 'a good many girls attended classes' at the school and 'many adults, both ladies and gentlemen, attended the Academy Natural History Society meetings' (Stewart, 1985). Although the Academical Institution had been founded as a collegiate school for boys, it 'made public scientific lectures equally accessible and intelligible to both sexes' (Anon., 1818). By 1820 Drummond was recommending certain texts as 'admirably suited for somewhat advanced scholars, whether boys or girls', and lectures arranged for ladies at the Institution in 1831-2 included Moral Philosophy and Zoology. Belfast Natural History Society followed suit in 1833 and admitted its first two lady members: Mrs Bruce, the wife of Dr Bruce, Headmaster of the Academy, and Mrs Clewlow, one of John Templeton's shell-collectors. By the 1860s the vogue for field clubs opened up natural-history pursuits to ever greater numbers of women, 'as much for the novelty of the freedom they permitted, as for the acceptability of their involvement and contributions' (Allen, 1976). Geology, botany and conchology were to prove the most attractive studies for a new generation of women naturalists.

There had not always been such opportunities for women in natural history. In earlier times women were usually introduced to formal collecting and the study of natural history by male relatives or friends who were themselves naturalists. Rather brief glimpses of their early activity exist, such as evidence that in the 1690s Thomas Molyneux's wife Catherine joined him in collecting plants and in making extensive notes on natural history (Nelson, 1979). More glimpses appear in Trinity College where the Bursar's vouchers indicate that 'Mrs Rawdon', a sister of Sir Arthur Rawdon, presented her collection of insects and preserved animals, including reptiles, to the College in 1732 (Nelson, 1981). The publication of books such as *The Young Ladies' Introduction to Natural History* (1766) illustrates the trend of fashionable studies for women. By the end of the eighteenth century, seaweeds and shells, fishes and ferns were the new pursuits that filled leisure time for many.

Soon the naturalists of the boudoir were bent on becoming naturalists of the field and shore as many women discovered the freedom and satisfaction of open-air naturalizing. Ellen Hutchins of Bantry, Co. Cork, whose short life was troubled by illness, took up the study of seaweeds as a healthy open-air pastime. Around 1802 she met David Mackay, Curator of the Botanic Gardens at Glasnevin, who introduced her to the foremost English botanists, Hooker, Turner and Dillwyn, to whose publications she furnished information and accomplished illustrations (Ross, 1986). Mary and Anne Elizabeth, two sisters of the naturalist Robert Ball, also became expert naturalists. Both developed wide contacts abroad and each made considerable contributions to zoology and botany, which were usually published under their brother's name (Ross and Nash, 1986). Other female naturalists published anonymously, such as the writer of *Dialogues on Botany for the Use of Young Persons* ... (1819), who obviously knew personally John Templeton and his wonderful gardens at Cranmore.

Further changing perceptions of women are indicated in the responses of scientific organizations and natural history societies to the growing band of female enthusiasts. While not open to women members, the Royal Dublin Society occasionally relaxed its rules, and records show that in 1820 it 'allowed Lady Rossmore to choose a seat at lectures' (Berry, 1915). The Royal Irish Academy elected the notable astronomer Mary Somerville as an honorary fellow in 1834, giving her the distinction of being its first woman member. The meetings of the Royal Zoological Society of Dublin were open to women from its inception in 1830. By contrast, many leading British scientific societies were less liberal; for example, the Linnaean Society of London (founded in 1798) first admitted women in 1904, after it had been 'battered into submission by Mrs Ogilvie Farquharson' (Allen, 1976).

Postscript

It would appear that the early practitioners of science and natural history in Ireland drew many of their inspirations and ideas from the Continent, encouraged by the philosophy of the Enlightenment and ideas of revolutionary change. These they moulded and enlarged in pioneering directions that effectively opened up the study of natural history. Undoubtedly, the relatively small number of Irish naturalists enabled close contact, which facilitated the spread of new information and new ideas. The involvement of women, the young and amateurs in natural history was encouraged through widening access to education, and through the new societies, which added to their success and multiplied their numbers such that by 1845 some sixteen societies with scientific interests were flourishing throughout Ireland.

However, the times were changing and by the middle of the century the post-Enlightenment momentum in the Irish study of nature was to suffer a number of setbacks. Of the two worth remarking on here, one was natural in its origin, the other man-made, and both were political in their implications. A population of some four million in 1781 had doubled by 1841, but in 1845 potato blight struck with devastating, though entirely predictable effects: within five years half the population was lost through death or emigration. In north-east Ulster the thriving linen industry cushioned the worst effects of the disaster, but the social effects of the famine were enormous and many in the medico-scientific community were involved in helping to ameliorate its awful effects. Some of the blossoming scientific societies suffered fatal reductions in membership as a result. For instance, the Dublin Microscopical Society was incorporated into the Dublin Natural History Society in 1856. At the time the Treasurer reported that the Natural History Society had by the exertions of its members 'been kept alive in the time of the famine, and it was now beginning to return to its state of prosperity' (Anon., 1856).

For many of the societies and organizations that did survive the aftermath of the famine, a greater threat was looming on the horizon. Prior to 1850, as Jarrell (1983) observes, 'virtually every institution in Ireland touched by the Department of Science and Art had been founded by the Irish, with little or no sustenance from across the Irish Sea'. Shortly afterwards the major remoulding of Irish science directed from London was to bring about radical change in many scientific organizations, especially those based in Dublin.

By mid-century the Dublin Society had been astonishingly successful, having created six professorial chairs and its own museum, botanic garden, drawing school, library and courses of public lectures. The Society had even obtained government finance towards some of these developments and others that were even more innovative. The Society was linked to what Herries Davies (1983) describes as 'the unofficial geological survey' conducted by Sir Richard Griffith. Under the guise of his official post of Government Valuator, he and his staff undertook the survey work that eventually resulted in his wonderful geological map of Ireland published in 1839. Torrens (1982) considers that 'with the publication of this map the Royal Dublin Society was able to enter the field earlier and with more success than its equivalents in England'. It is difficult to imagine that it could have been carried out with such verve and subterfuge in any setting other than that of contemporary Ireland. However, such schemes did not please the government, as by 1852 more than a quarter of the funding for science and art in these islands was coming to Ireland (Jarrell, 1983). The beginning of the end came when they started reining in what they saw as a headstrong horse at full gallop and almost out of control in an exercise that was to be a 'careful, systematic and almost wholly bureaucratic takeover of key Irish scientific institutions by the Department of Science and Art in South Kensington' (Jarrell, 1983).

However, there were excitements to come, and all arguably derived originally from the Enlightenment, and all had their location in, or influence in, education. They include 'the evolution debate', discussed elsewhere in this volume and waged in part from within the schools, and the growth of the field clubs, whose activities stimulated nature study in schools and augmented the curriculum. The intricate story of the exploration of Irish natural history through the last two hundred years is composed of many threads. Examination of the various inspirations behind the trends and developments furnishes ample evidence of the blending of many cultural influences in the history and development of our relationship today with Ireland's nature.

References

Allen, D.E. 1976. *The Naturalist in Britain*. London: Allen Lane.

Anderson, J. 1888. *History of Belfast Library and Society for Promoting Knowledge, Commonly Known as the Linenhall Library*. Belfast: Linenhall Library.

Andrews, J.H. 1980. 'Science and Cartography in the Ireland of William and Samuel Molyneux.' *Proceedings of the Royal Irish Academy 80 C*: 231-50.

Anon. 1818. *The Uses of Natural History Study – Observations*. Belfast: 'Bookseller'.

Anon. 1825. 'State of Science in Ireland.' [in review of *A System of Algebraic Geometry*, 2 vols, by Rev. Dionysius Lardner] *The Dublin Philosophical Journal and Scientific Review 3*: 459-69.

Anon. 1847. *Catalogue of the Library at Belfast Museum.* Belfast: Belfast Natural History and Philosophical Society.

Anon. 1856. 'Report of Dublin Natural History Society A.G.M. 23 Nov. 1856.' *Natural History Review 4*: 37-9.

Berry, H.F. 1915. *A History of the Royal Dublin Society.* London: Longmans Green & Co.

Bigger, F.J. 1924. 'Thomas Dix Hincks' in A. Deane (ed.), *The Belfast Natural History and Philosophical Society. Centenary Volume, 1821-1921.* Belfast: Belfast Natural History and Philosophical Society.

Boate, G. 1652. *Irelands Naturall History.* London: Hartlib.

Bronte Gatenby, J. 1961. 'The History of Zoology and Comparative Anatomy in Trinity College, Dublin.' *Irish Journal of Medical Science*, September: 395-407.

Bryce, J. 1831 *Tables of Simple Minerals, Rocks and Shells with Local Catalogues of Species for the Use of Students of Natural History in the Belfast Academy.* Belfast: Simms & Mc Intyre.

Clarke, M. 1833. *Biography of Adam Clark.* London: Everett and Etheridge.

Clarke, D. 1973. 'An Outline of the History of Science in Ireland.' *Studies 62*: 287-302.

Davis, W.J. 1990. 'Dionysius Lardner; Physicist and Encyclopaedist.' In C. Mollan, W.J. Davis and B. Finucane (eds), *More People and Places in Irish Science and Technology.* Dublin: Royal Irish Academy.

Day, A. (ed.). 1991. *Letters from Georgian Ireland: The Correspondence of Mary Delaney, 1731-68.* Belfast: Friar's Bush Press.

DeBeer, G. 1953. *Sir Hans Sloane and the British Museum.* London: Oxford University Press.

Drummond, J.L. 1820. *Thoughts on the Study of Natural History and on the Importance of Attaching Museums of the Productions of Nature to National Seminaries of Education.* Belfast: Simms & Co.

Drummond, J.L. 1831. *Letters to a Young Naturalist on the Study of Nature and Natural Theology.* London: Longman, Rees, Orme, Brown & Green.

Drummond, J.L. 1831a. *Address of the President of the Belfast Natural History Society on the Opening of Belfast Museum, 1st November 1831.* Belfast: Hodgson.

Edgeworth, R.L. 1820. *Memoirs, begun by Himself and Concluded by his Daughter, Maria Edgeworth.* 2 vols. London: R. Hunter.

Froggatt, P. 1976. 'The Foundation of the "Inst" Medical Department and its Association with Belfast Fever Hospital.' *The Ulster Medical Journal 45*: 1-39.

Froggatt, P. and Bridges, B. 1985. *The Belfast Medical School 1835-1985.* Belfast: Queens University.

Hackney, P. 1980. 'Some Early Nineteenth Century Herbaria in Belfast.' *Irish Naturalist's Journal 20*: 114-18.

Herries Davies, G. 1983. *Sheets of Many Colours: the Mapping of Ireland's Rocks 1750-1890.* Dublin: Royal Dublin Society Historical Series in Irish Science and Technology.

Herries Davies, G. 1985. 'Irish Thought in Science,' in R. Kearney (ed.), *The Irish Mind.* Dublin: Wolfhound.

Jarrell, R.A. 1983. 'The Department of Science and Art and the Control of Irish Science in the Nineteenth Century.' *Irish Historical Studies 23 (92)*: 330-47.

Kearney, R. 1985. 'Introduction' to R. Kearney (ed.), *The Irish Mind.* Dublin: Wolfhound.

Kelly, P. 1992. 'From Molyneux to Berkeley: the Dublin Philosophical Society and its Legacy,' in D. Scott (ed.), *Treasures of the Mind.* London: Sotheby's.

K'Eogh, J. 1739. *Zoologia Medicinalis Hibernica: or a Medical Treatise of Birds, Beasts, Fishes, Reptiles or Insects, which are Commonly known and Propagated in this Kingdom ... .* Dublin: S. Powell.

Larcom, T. 1851. *The History of Ireland Commonly called The Down Survey by Doctor William Petty AD 1655-56.* Dublin: Irish Archaeological Society.

Lyons, J.B. 1990. 'Thomas Molyneux: Physician and Natural Philosopher,' in C. Mollan, W. Davis and B. Finucane (eds), *More People and Places in Irish Science and Technology.* Dublin: Royal Irish Academy.

Malcolm, A.G. 1851. *The History of the General Hospital, Belfast and other Medical Institutions of the Town.* Belfast: Agnew.

Maxwell, C. 1949. *Country and Town in Ireland under the Georges.* Dundalk: Dundalgan Press.

Mc Cormack, W.J. 1992. 'Edmund Burke: his Image in Painting and Literature,' in D. Scott (ed.), *Treasures of the Mind.* London: Sotheby's

Mc Cormack, W.J. 1993. *The Dublin Paper War of 1786-1788.* Dublin: Irish Academic Press.

Merton, R.K. [1938] 1970. *Science, Technology and Society in Seventeenth-Century England.* New York: Fertig.

Moore, F.W. 1940. 'Some Reminiscences.' *New Flora and Sylva 12*: 180-7.

Nelson, E.C. 1979. '"In Contemplation of Vegetables" – Caleb Threlkeld (1676-1728), his Life, background and Contribution to Irish Botany.' *Journal for the Society of the Bibliography of Natural History 9 (3)*: 257-73.

Nelson, E.C. 1981. 'Sir Arthur Rawdon (1662-1695) of Moira: His Life and Letters, Family and Friends, and his Jamaican Plants.' *Belfast Natural History and Philosophical Society Proceedings and Reports 10*: 30-52.

Nelson, E.C. 1982. The Influence of Leiden on Botany in Dublin in the early Eighteenth Century.' *Huntia 4:* 133-46.

Nelson, E.C. 1993. 'Botany and Medicine; Dublin and Leiden.' *Journal of the Irish Colleges of Physicians and Surgeons 22*: 133-6.

Paley, W. 1785. *The Principles of Moral and Political Philosophy.* Dublin: Exshaw White.

Porter, R. 1990. 'The New Taste for Nature in the Eighteenth Century.' *The Linnean 4 (1)*: 14-30.

Robinson-Hammerstein, H. 1992. 'Royal Policy and Civic Pride: Founding a University in Dublin,' in D. Scott (ed.), *Treasures of the Mind.* London: Sotheby's.

Ross, H.C.G. 1986. 'Ellen Hutchins, Botanist,' in C. Mollan, W. Davis and B. Finucane (eds), *Some People and Places in Irish Science and Technology.* Dublin: Royal Irish Academy.

Ross, H.C.G. and Nash, R. 1986. 'The Development of Natural History in early Nineteenth Century Ireland,' in *From Linnaeus to Darwin: Commentaries on the History of Biology and Geology.* London: Society for the History of Natural History.

Scott, W.R. 1900. *Francis Hutcheson: His Life, Teaching and Position in the History of Philosophy.* Cambridge: Cambridge University Press.

Smith, C. and W. Harris. 1744. *The Ancient and Present State of the County of Down.* Dublin: Reilly for Exshaw.

Sprat, T. [1667] 1959. *History of the Royal Society* (facsimile, appendix A). London: Cope and Jones.

Stewart, A.T.Q. 1985. *Belfast Royal Academy: The First Century 1785-1885.* Antrim: Greystone Press.

Thompson, W. 1849-56. *The Natural History of Ireland.* 4 vols. London: Reeve, Benham & Reeve.

Torrens, H. 1982. *In Review of Richard Griffith – 1784-1878.* G. L. Herries Davies and C. Mollan (eds). Dublin: Royal Dublin Society.

White, H.B. 1911. 'History of Science and Art Institutions, Dublin.' *Museum Bulletin of the National Museum of Science and Art 1 (4)*: 7-34.

Young, R.M. 1902. *In Belfast Literary Society 1801-1901. Historical Sketch with Memoirs of some Distinguished Members.* Belfast: The Linenhall Press.

Darwin in Belfast:
The Evolution Debate

DAVID N. LIVINGSTONE

Divine Visitation, Darwinian Vision

It is 22 September 1859 – the Thursday precisely eight weeks before the launch of Charles Darwin's *Origin of Species*. The annual meeting of the Evangelical Alliance has convened in Belfast. As one of its two secretaries approaches the rostrum, he is greeted by a derisive chorus of hissing and booing. Rev. William M'Ilwaine's reputation has preceded him. An evangelical Anglican who had been present at the inaugural meeting of the Alliance in 1846, a regular contributor to its annual proceedings, a member of the executive council since 1857,* and a local anti-Catholic controversialist of some notoriety (Hempton and Hill, 1992), M'Ilwaine had blotted his copybook in the eyes of the evangelicals gathered in Belfast, over an issue of momentous current concern. Since the early part of the year, and with even greater intensity since April, the north of Ireland had found itself swept by a tide of religious revival – a spiritual awakening accompanied in part by 'convulsions, swoons, visions, and other extraordinary effects that seemed to spread through the province of Ulster like an epidemic' (Donat, 1986). 'Monster meetings' in Belfast and Armagh presented the public face of a movement that transformed personal life, spawned prayer groups, and fostered family devotions.

William M'Ilwaine, the rector of St George's Church in Belfast, had welcomed these latter spiritual exercises. But he expressed his opposition to their physiological 'excesses' so vehemently that thereafter some evangelicals cast him as an enemy of God. In both popular print and medical treatise M'Ilwaine conducted his campaign against 'fanaticism of the wildest type' – a fanaticism, he charged, that had gripped 'the ignorant, uneducated, hard-

---

* I am grateful to Donald Patton for providing these details from his reading of early issues of the Evangelical Alliance's serial, *Evangelical Christendom*.

worked, and easily impressed class, and, in the proportion of nineteen out of every twenty, young and excitable females' (M'Ilwaine, 1859a). No doubt it was because this assessment had appeared some weeks earlier in September as a follow-up to sermons that M'Ilwaine had delivered on the subject in July (and which he subsequently pursued in the *Journal of Mental Science*), that he was the object of the Alliance's vilification (M'Ilwaine, 1859). But more: M'Ilwaine's Episcopalian convictions disposed him to query the laity-led character of this spiritual movement, which removed it from the sphere of clerical management. Appeals for financial support by earnest female converts only confirmed his judgments; M'Ilwaine condemned those who duly made monetary contributions as rendering 'a whole class of persons [unfit] for their lawful worldly occupations' (M'Ilwaine, 1859a).

There were, however, other voices to be heard. Whether because of his greater rhetorical finesse, or the sympathetic tone of his apologia, or his more democratic ecclesiology, James McCosh – the Scottish Presbyterian Professor of Metaphysics at Queen's College – found himself acclaimed as the Evangelical Alliance's intellectual champion of revival. The fact is, he too had considerable reservations over what he termed the Ulster revival's 'physiological accidents'. But his strategy on that same September Thursday, in his paper to the Alliance, was to relieve the revival movement of the burden of prejudice that its accompanying bodily manifestations had fostered in the minds of unsympathetic critics. Indeed to him these physical displays were mere 'accidents', explicable as purely natural reactions to extreme emotional experience and largely attributable to Irish ethnic temperament. But – and this is crucial – McCosh cast his diagnosis in the language of defence by insisting that the 'deep mental feeling' that induced somatic convulsions was itself 'a work of God' (McCosh, 1859). His address was well received; by late October one Belfast bookshop had sold some eight thousand copies of the pamphlet (Patton, 1993). So, despite their shared reservations, M'Ilwaine found himself cast as the villain of the piece, while McCosh emerged as the Revival's apologist.

This was not to be the last occasion on which M'Ilwaine and McCosh occupied different sides of a public controversy. In the following decades McCosh, who left Queen's in 1868 to assume the presidency of the College of New Jersey (later Princeton University), acquired a reputation as the foremost reconciler of evolution and Protestant theology.* Indeed, at the 1873 New York meeting of the Evangelical Alliance McCosh argued that instead

---

* McCosh's move to Princeton was merely one of a series of long-standing connections between Princetown Seminary and the Presbyterian College in Belfast. For generations, a considerable contingent of Ulster ministerial students crossed the Atlantic to study at Princeton, the publications of the Princeton theologians were staple diet for the Belfast

of denouncing the theory of evolution, 'Religious philosophers might be more profitably employed in showing ... the religious aspects of the doctrine of development; and some would be grateful to any who would help them to keep their new faith in science' (McCosh, 1874, 1871, 1888; Moore, 1979; Livingstone, 1987). Moreover, reminiscing on his twenty years as Princeton president, McCosh later confessed that he had devoted much of his time to 'defending Evolution, but, in so doing, [I] have given the proper account of it as the method of God's procedure, and find that when so understood it is in no way inconsistent with Scripture' (Sloane, 1896; Hoeveler, 1981).

The legacy of M'Ilwaine's encounter with Darwinism is altogether different. In the interim, and no doubt on account of his frosty reception at the 1859 Evangelical Alliance meeting, M'Ilwaine turned away from evangelicalism towards the very Catholic liturgy he had earlier denounced, and eventually succeeded in transforming St George's worship tradition into a more high-church style ('Death of Rev. Canon MacIlwaine'). But his controversialist instincts continued unabated, and were nowhere more clearly displayed than during the Belfast meeting of the British Association for the Advancement of Science in 1874. In the wake of the Association's Presidential Address by John Tyndall (*plate 15*), in which – as we shall presently see – Tyndall advocated his own version of materialism, M'Ilwaine entered the fray in the name of Church and creed.

His first foray occurred on Friday 4 September 1874, just over two weeks after Tyndall's goading speech. That day the *Northern Whig* of Belfast carried a letter from M'Ilwaine decrying the manner in which 'the holy name whereby we are called' had been deliberately assailed in that address, and asking for a document to be prepared and signed by British Association members and presented to its Council affirming traditional Christian beliefs. M'Ilwaine made it clear, moreover, that it was not 'the opinions of Darwin' or 'the doctrine of evolution' – contested and speculative though they were – that had caused him to lift his pen; rather it was the 'defiant challenge made' in the president's speech 'to religion on the part of science'. Within the week he had further stirred up matters by delivering an evening lecture at St George's with the pugilistic title, 'The Present Aspect of Infidelity, With Special Notice of Certain Recent Proceedings at the Meeting of the

---

students, and ties between key faculty in the two institutions were substantial (Allen, 1954). Peter Wallace and Mark Noll (1994) note that the 'Irish connection' was the 'most significant' element in Princeton's international student clientele. 'Over 340 Irish-born students attended Princeton Seminary prior to 1929. Of these, 87 returned to Northern Ireland as their principal place of service, of whom at least four became moderators of the General Assembly of the Presbyterian Church in Ireland.' The significance of this connection in the Belfast response to Darwin is examined in Livingstone (1994).

British Association', and a couple of months later chose to pursue the topic in his own presidential address to the Belfast Naturalists' Field Club. Here, pleading innocence to the charge of the *odium theologicum*, he dilated on the 'impropriety of debating a religious question in a scientific arena', and accused Tyndall – 'one of the high priesthood of science' – of propagating materialism and atheism under the guise of science, and of delivering an oration at once 'derogatory to Christianity' and 'most unphilosophical'. In so doing Tyndall had betrayed his own scientific heritage, for had not science's greatest heroes – Bacon, Newton, Boyle, Faraday – shown that 'real Christianity has ever proved, not the handmaid merely, but the elder sister and friend of true science?' (M'Ilwaine, 1874-5).

McCosh, of course, was every bit as unnerved by the naturalism of Tyndall's vision as M'Ilwaine, and thus devoted considerable intellectual energy to the task of producing an evolutionary teleology. But by lapsing into a Lamarckian evolutionism that conceived of organic progress along predetermined paths, he was able to couch his responses in terms of a sympathetic re-reading of the evolutionary story and thereby to do what he could to avert what one of his students, Rev. George Macloskie, called a potentially 'disastrous war between science and faith' (Sloane, 1896). So, whether speaking of divine visitation or Darwinian vision, rhetorical nuance counted for much, cognitive content for little. For it was style of communication rather than substance of argument that secured history's judgment on McCosh as the defender of religious revival *and* evolutionary theory, and on M'Ilwaine as arch-critic of both.

The Lull before the Storm

But what of the years between 1859 and 1874? Why was the initial response in Belfast to Darwin's ideas so muted?* Perhaps it was on account of the revival and its pastoral legacy; perhaps it was to do with the storm waves generated by the publication of *Essays and Reviews*, a collection of tracts by liberal churchmen which marked a growing tide of opposition to traditional orthodoxy (Rogerson, 1985); perhaps it was because no threat of epic proportions was perceived in the early reading of *The Origin* itself. Certainly some isolated comments had been made, though these were by no means of a universally hostile nature. George Macloskie, for example, had made some

---

* The absence of detailed studies on the response to Darwin in other British cities means that a regional geography of the British reaction to evolution theory is a real desideratum. Too often surveys of the reception of Darwinism operate at the national level ignoring provincial variation and leaving unexplored the reaction of urban intellectuals outside London.

tangential observations on the Darwinian theory in his consideration of 'The Natural History of Man' in 1862 – just a year after his ordination. Here, while expressing some hesitancy about the universal claims of the Darwinian system, Macloskie paused to confirm that the principle of natural selection could account for human racial differentation and provide good grounds for rejecting polygenism in favour of monogenism. Indeed, he insisted that he himself had 'already employed this principle, to explain the diversity that exists in the different tribes of mankind, whilst the specific unity is still pre-served' (Macloskie, 1862). To be sure, the deductive character of the Darwinian theory was, at this stage, bothersome to Macloskie, though in years to come – after he followed his teacher McCosh to Princeton University in 1875 – he would himself defend the necessity of scientific speculation and emerge as a major evangelical exponent of evolution among Old School Presbyterians in the United States (Livingstone, 1987).* For the meantime, Macloskie's piece was conspicuously bereft of the invective that would characterize debates in the aftermath of Tyndall's Belfast address.

On 3 November 1863 Rev. William Todd Martin provided his assessment of 'Our Church in its Relation to Progressive Thought' when he spoke to the Newry Presbyterian Young Men's Society. He had recently been installed as the minister of that congregation and later, after service in Newtownards, would succeed Henry Wallace as Professor of Ethics at Assembly's College (a.k.a. Presbyterian College) in 1887. The main thrust of his homily was to express concern at the inroads being made by *Essays and Reviews* and the pentateuchal criticism of Bishop Colenso and Principal Tulloch of the Established Church of Scotland – whose concessions to modern science and textual criticism, Martin believed, subverted the traditional authority of Scripture. Their strategies would, he forecast, 'make shipwreck of their faith'. To be sure, he did pause to lament that the 'Darwinian theory of development, and Sir Charles Lyell's theory of the Antiquity of Man, are conclusive proof that the tendency of philosophic thought is flowing away from evangelical truth, and towards scepticism' (Martin, 1863). But it was only later, in the aftermath of the Tyndall shock, and in the wake of Herbert Spencer's cosmic philosophizing, that he focused more specifically on the evolution question. For the time being, the implications of the Darwinian intervention were scarcely perceived, thereby bearing out the suspicion that, on the religious front at least, *The Origin* was 'upstaged' – to use Moore's word (1982) – by *Essays and Reviews*.

---

* While still in Belfast he wrote popular natural-science pieces for the Presbyterian Magazine *Plain Words* and published 'The Silicified Wood of Lough Neagh, with Notes on the Structure of Coniferous Wood', *Proceedings of the Belfast Natural History and Philosophical Society* (14 Feb. 1872), 51-74.

Doubtless other early Belfast evaluations of Darwin's theory lie buried in the archives of the city's intellectual past. Robert Watts (*plate 15*), for example, during his inaugural lecture at Assembly's College in 1866, hinted at Darwinism's irreconcilability with classical Paleyan natural theology and queried the naturalistic restrictions it seemed to impose on causality.* At this stage Watts's treatment of the subject was muted and cursory. By far the most considered and expansive appraisal of the new biology was made by Joseph John Murphy, a businessman who was secretary to the Church of Ireland's Diocesan Synod and Council, and a leading light in a variety of Belfast scientific and literary circles, twice occupying the presidency of the Belfast Literary Society and the Belfast Natural History and Philosophical Society (D'Arcy, 1934; Seaver, 1902). Murphy devoted much of his energy to elucidating the connections between science and Christianity. In 1865 he elaborated an evidentialist apologia for a consciously Protestant Christianity, defending the claims of the geologists for a long earth history and vigorously protesting the 'supposition that they are opposed to the teaching of the Christian religion'. Curiously perhaps, but certainly significantly, in this address to the Young Men's Society of the United Church of England and Ireland, Darwin's theory was entirely ignored.

In his 1866 presidential address to the Belfast Natural History and Philosophical Society, however, Murphy subjected Darwin's theory to considerable scrutiny, expressing substantial agreement with Darwin, but demurring on the all-sufficiency of natural selection to account for organic variation. In particular he queried its capacity to explain the development of the eye:

... it is probably no exaggeration to suppose that in order to improve such an organ as the eye at all, it must be improved in ten different ways at once. And the improbability of any complex organ being produced and brought to perfection in any such way is an improbability of the same kind and degree as that of producing a poem or a mathematical demonstration by throwing letters at random on a table.

This passage was to achieve considerable prominence. Darwin himself cited it in *The Variation of Animals and Plants under Domestication*, noted that a similar point had been made by Rev. C. Pritchard in his sermon at the Nottingham meeting of the British Association that same year, and presented his own resolution of the problem (Darwin, 1905, vol. 2). Sir Arthur Keith similarly excerpted what he called this 'just criticism' both in his Huxley lecture for 1923 and in his presidential address at the Leeds meeting of the BA in 1927, as did Archbishop D'Arcy of Armagh in his autobiographical reflections and in his Alexander Robertson Lectures at the University of Glasgow in 1932.

---

* Watts's lecture is reported in *The Banner of Ulster*, Thursday, 15 November 1866. I am grateful to Donald Patton for bringing this lecture to my attention.

Querying natural selection's ubiquity, however, did not mean denying its activity. And so Murphy deployed the Darwinian model in his account of 'The Origin of Organs of Flight' in a paper presented to the Field Club in 1869. Indeed that same year he had brought out the first edition of his two-volume *Habit and Intelligence*. Its title revealed the fundamental orientation of the work – illustrating the role of habit and intelligence in organic modification. Throughout, Murphy displayed a Lamarckian-sounding enthusiasm for the role of what he called 'self-adaptation', in conjunction with natural selection, in the history of life. But these twin mechanisms were insufficient of themselves to explain organic complexity without the role of an 'Organizing Intelligence'. That the law of natural selection had been 'proved' Murphy had no doubt; that 'all organic species have been descended from one or a few germs' he likewise had no cause to query; his only reservations were that the Darwinians were prone to claim near-omnipotence for the natural-selection mechanism and that recent geophysical research on the age of the earth required a more rapid evolutionary tempo than Darwin was ready to admit (Murphy, 1869, 1). Reservations notwithstanding, Murphy later insisted that in *Habit and Intelligence* he had gone 'about three-quarters of the way' with Darwin. Within less than half a decade the three-quarters, he admitted, had been reduced to half (Murphy, 1873-4).

Already by late 1872 Murphy's disquiet was mounting. In October of that year he put the finishing touches to *The Scientific Bases of Faith* (1873), a volume systematically reading Christian theology through scientific lenses. Dispensing with such cardinal evangelical doctrines as biblical inerrancy, plenary inspiration of scripture, the Fall, and the doctrine of a personal Devil, he made it clear that his brand of non-evangelical Anglicanism was fully compatible with evolution. Indeed, he called for a revamping of natural theology 'to suit the theory of evolution' and toyed with applying natural selection to history. But beyond that, discussion of Darwinism *strictu sensu* was conspicuous only by its absence. Before the book appeared in print, however, inattention had turned to opposition. His audience at the November meeting of the Belfast Natural History and Philosophical Society heard from their president that Kelvin's figures for the age of the earth presented 'a great difficulty in the way of Darwin's theory of the origin of species' and that 'eternity would not be long enough' for the Darwinian mechanism to derive all living beings 'from the simplest animalcules' (Murphy, 1872-3). By the time his next presidential address came around in 1873 he was vigorously contending for an anti-Darwinian account of evolution. Murphy could now concur with Darwin only on the *fact* of evolution. Other than that, he could not 'now agree with the distinctive parts of Darwin's theory at all'. To the contrary, he found it 'utterly paradoxical', and 'insufficient and unsatisfactory in every point'. What Murphy now enthusiastically endorsed was a *non*-Darwinian version of evolution 'guided by Intelligence' (Murphy, 1873-4).

Precisely why Murphy's attitudes began to change is unknown. But during the second half of 1872, as we will see, there had been considerable debate – involving Tyndall and Galton – on the issue of scientifically testing the efficacy of prayer. Their stance called forth a rebuttal from McCosh in the October issue of the London *Contemporary Review*. Both here and in Tyndall's querying of miracles, the naturalistic tendency of the new science manifested itself with increasing force. And yet for all that, there is little evidence to suggest that prior to 1874 evolutionary theory *per se* was causing any profound anxiety in Calvinist Belfast. To be sure, reservations – particularly over natural selection – were from time to time expressed. But these lacked both vitriol and vituperation. Things dramatically changed during the winter months of 1874/5, however, as an assault was orchestrated against the new biology. A massive departure from the seeming complacency of the previous decade and a half was hastily effected. What precipitated this turn of events?

The British Ass

The *Northern Whig* enthusiastically announced the coming of the 'Parliament of Science' – affectionately known as the British Ass – on Wednesday, 19 August 1874. It was 'no ordinary honour and privilege', the editorial told its readers, 'that Belfast should enjoy this year a renewal of the visit paid ... two-and-twenty years ago by the philosophers of the British Association'. Ironically, the meeting was being welcomed to the city as a temporary respite from 'spinning and weaving, and Orange riots, and ecclesiastical squabbles'. Nevertheless, 'some hot discussions' were predicted 'in the biological section' between advocates of human evolution and those 'intellectual people – not to speak of religious people at all – who believe there is a gulf between man and gorilla'. Nevertheless the editor was convinced that the 'Irish people ... will give a patient hearing to the philosophers notwithstanding'. The newspaper's enthusiasm for the coming event knew no bounds; the Association was welcomed to the city 'with all heartiness' and afterwards the resolution of a local workers' strike was credited to its presence.

The Belfast meeting was to be what Desmond and Moore call 'an X Club jamboree' with its priestly coterie of Huxley, Hooker, Lubbock, and of course Tyndall himself, all speechifying (Desmond and Moore, 1991). This 'Club' was a confraternity of like-minded scientists which had been meeting together for dinner for nearly a decade, and which included key members of the rising scientific establishment. All were committed to the emancipation of science from established civil and theological authorities, and they used their own collective political clout on every opportunity to advance naturalistic thinking. If an assault was to be mounted by the new scientific priesthood on the old clerical guardians of revelation and respectability, scripture and social status, then what better venue could there be for a call to arms than the BA's meeting in Calvinist Belfast?

Tyndall, himself a native of Co. Carlow and an Orangeman, was only too happy to favour a militant strategy. Indeed, his pugnacious reputation did not escape the notice of his native audience. A few hours before his evening speech, readers of the *Northern Whig* were introduced to the president-elect as 'a perfect Irishman in his controversies, flinging himself readily into the arena, and carrying on his wars with a thoroughly Celtic vehemence and good humour'. Tyndall's performance did not fall short of expectations. In an Ulster Hall garnished with accompanying orchestra, Tyndall delivered – with nothing short of evangelical fervour – a missionary call to 'wrest from theology the entire domain of cosmological theory'. He began by presenting his own history of the atomic theory since the time of Democritus, Epicurus, and Lucretius, suitably eliding those chapters in the story that did not serve his immediate purposes – which was to show how science had progressively routed the forces of metaphysical dogma. The implications were plain. All 'religious theories, schemes and systems which embrace notions of cosmogony ... must ... submit to the control of science, and relinquish all thought of controlling it' (Tyndall, 1874; Barton, 1987). The gauntlet had been thrown down.

Events moved quickly. On Sunday, 23 August, Tyndall's address was the subject of a truculent attack by Rev. Professor Robert Watts at Fisherwick Place Church in Belfast. Watts, the Assembly's College Professor of Systematic Theology – and an erstwhile student of Princeton Seminary – had good reason for spitting blood. He had already submitted to the organizers of the Biology Section of the Belfast British Association meeting a paper congenially entitled 'An Irenicum: Or, a Plea for Peace and Co-operation between Science and Theology' (Watts, 1888; Livingstone, 1992). They flatly rejected it.* It must have seemed to Watts that the scientific fraternity wasn't interested in peace, and that hostilities had been initiated by 'enlightened' scientists, not 'entrenched' clergymen, for the spurned lecture that Watts – not prepared to waste good words already committed to paper – delivered at noon the following Monday in Elmwood Presbyterian Church revealed just how enthusiastic he could be about science.* But the BA's rebuff had stung, and chagrin over his expulsion from the programme put him in a bad mood. Yet this was nothing to the anger that Tyndall's address aroused in him. So when on the Sunday following the infamous address he turned his big guns on Tyndall in a sermon preached to an overflowing

---

* *The Witness*, 9 October 1874.

evening congregation at Fisherwick Place Church, the irenic tone of the rejected paper was gone. Tyndall's mention of Epicurus was especially galling; that name had 'become a synonym for sensualist', and Watts baulked at the moral implications of adopting Epicurean values. To him it was a system that had 'wrought the ruin of the communities and individuals who have acted out its principles in the past; and if the people of Belfast substitute it for the holy religion of the Son of God, and practise its degrading dogmas, the moral destiny of the metropolis of Ulster may easily be forecast' (Watts, 1888a; also 'Truth versus Error', 1874).

Details of Watts's offensive were fully reported in the following week's edition of the Presbyterian newspaper, *The Witness* (28 August, 1874), and they proved so popular that the homily soon appeared as a pamphlet. Within a month *The Witness* (18 September 1874) reported that five thousand copies had been sold and a second edition called for. Its insistence that the tract constituted 'the most notable contribution to the controversial literature that has sprung out of the proceedings of the Belfast meeting of the British Association' enlarged at once Watts's reputation and the pamphlet's circulation. The refusal of both Tyndall and Huxley, moreover, to engage Watts in a local public debate – a challenge to which was issued in the *Northern Whig* on Tuesday, 27 August – only added to *his* standing and to *their* notoriety in Calvinist Belfast. 'Perhaps at no time since the Arian Controversy', Rev. R. Jeffery reflected in October, had 'the religious mind of Ulster been so deeply and indignantly stirred' (also Ross, 1874). Of course, not all Presbyterians were so indignant. 'An Orthodox Presbyterian' wrote to express his 'deep indignation at the ridiculous and undignified position in which [the Presbyterian] Church has been placed by the action of her self-constituted champion, Dr. Watts. ... Could the force of absurdity go further? Is it possible that the monstrous egotism which inspired such a proposal can escape the perception even of the simplest-minded among the orthodox admirers of Dr. Watts?'

Watts, however, was not a lone voice imprecating Tyndall-style science. On the very Sunday that he was arraigning atomism before the congregation of Fisherwick Place, the same message was buzzing through the ears of other congregations. Rev. John MacNaughtan at Rosemary Street Presbyterian Church, Rev. George Shaw at Fitzroy, and Rev. T.Y. Killen at Duncairn, all took up the cudgels. That evening W. Robertson Smith, Professor of Hebrew in Aberdeen (and a figure who would himself later be embroiled in a bitter public furore over his views on the pentateuchal documents, religious ritual and the anthropology of sacrifice [Leach, 1985]), found himself preaching from Killen's north Belfast pulpit. And while he did not speak

---

* *Northern Whig*, 25 August 1874, 8. Also *The Witness*, 9 October 1874.

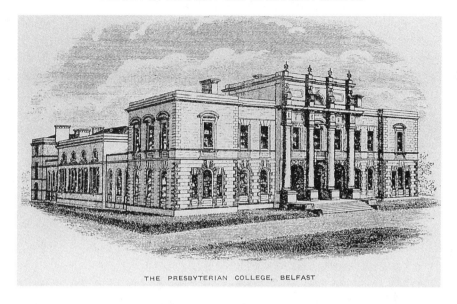

THE PRESBYTERIAN COLLEGE, BELFAST

out there and then on Tyndall's speech, he had certainly caught the prevailing mood, for he was moved within the week to write to the press challenging Tyndall's assertions about early religious history, castigating his
'pragmatic sketch of the history of atomism' and complaining that he was 'at
least a century behind the present state of scholarship' concerning the
Christian Middle Ages (Smith, 1874). Small wonder that Tyndall reflected:
'Every pulpit in Belfast thundered of me' (cited in Barton, 1987).

MacNaughtan, the Scottish minister of Rosemary Street, also tried to
put his flock right on 'Christianity and Science'; he too castigated the egre-
gious address and inveighed 'against [Tyndall's] erroneous teaching'. Again
the sermon was printed, this time at the request of his Kirk Session. The
entry in the Committee Minute Book of the Rosemary Street Presbyterian
Church for 3 September 1874 notes: 'the Committee cannot depart without
expressing their thanks to the Rev. John MacNaughtan and ... recording
their high appreciation of the promptness and ability with which he replied
to the materialistic doctrines and erroneous conclusions which were gratu-
itously advanced and covertly advocated by Professor Tyndall'.
MacNaughtan's strategy to avert hostilities was to declare that 'science and
Christianity have different spheres' and that therefore 'there is no reason
why they should ever come into collision'. The speculative materialism that
Tyndall had displayed *in excelsis* at the BA was not merely bad science,
MacNaughtan argued; it was contemptible moral philosophy. What hope,
the preacher mused, could cold materialism give a human sufferer in the
final throes of some fatal disease? (MacNaughtan, 1874). All this, of course,
was for popular consumption, as was recognized at the time; according to

397

one observer, the tract lacked 'that thoroughness and closeness of treatment such an address as that of Professor Tyndall's requires for its final and complete refutation' (Carswell, 1874).

For all the consternation stirred up by Tyndall's charge past the frontiers of science into the marchlands of religion, there was a sense that this act of aggression was ultimately to be welcomed, for it displayed to the world the machinations of the materialist school. It was precisely because Tyndall had spoken so plainly that the editor of *The Witness* could observe that 'We now know exactly the state of matters, and what is to be expected from Professor Tyndall and his school, and we shall be able to take our measures accordingly.'*

The Winter of Discontent

And measures the Presbyterian Church did take. When the Belfast Presbytery met for its monthly meeting on Wednesday, 2 September 1874, Rev. William Johnston, a recent Moderator of the Church's General Assembly, rose to address the gathering. The principles of Christianity, he began, had been subjected to an 'open and determined onslaught'. Two weeks ago that very day Professor John Tyndall had in the name of science assailed 'Christianity in its vital parts'. It pained him, Johnston went on, to hear the Professor thanked for his disquisition, and to discover, as had some of the newspapers, that 'in Belfast such materialism and atheism [could be] propagated without any protest on the part of the audience who heard it'.** But what bothered Johnston even more was the fact that while the British Association had pronounced its blessing on Tyndall's speculations, that same body 'had excluded a paper proposing to show how the inquiries of science could be conducted in thorough accordance with the principles of Christianity'. 'Thereby', he went on, 'the Association made themselves a party to a one-sided attack on Christianity.' Cries of 'hear hear' from the assembled company indicated that he had touched a raw nerve among the Presbyterian ministers present. The paper to which Johnston referred, of course, was by Watts, and before concluding Johnston 'proceeded to eulogise' Watts's riposte ('Belfast Presbytery').

---

* 'The British Association, *The Witness*, 28 August 1874.Rev George Macloskie, in a letter to the Northern Whig, for example, insisted that there was no desire in Belfast 'to stifle free scientific inquiry'. (27 August 1874, 8)
** This was also noted by the Dean of Manchester who was 'sorry to say' that Tyndall's Belfast address had been given 'without any protest on the part of the audience'. (*The Witness*, 4 September 1874.) Some general reflections on the intellectual scene in Belfast at the time are to be found in Brooke (1983).

Johnston had no intention of leaving the matter as a mere record of proceedings in the Presbytery's minute book. Some two weeks later he and a number of fellow clergymen met together to lay plans for a course of evening lectures to be given at Rosemary Street Church during the winter months on the relationship between science and Christianity ('Winter Lectures'). Arrangements were hastily finalized and in due course *The Witness* advertised their commencement in its columns on 27 November 1874. In time these addresses would be drawn together into a book, distributed on both sides of the Atlantic, under the title *Science and Revelation: A Series of Lectures in Reply to the Theories of Tyndall, Huxley, Darwin, Spencer, etc.*, with a preface by Johnston himself (1875).

During that 1874-5 winter of discontent, eight Presbyterian theologians and one scientist joined together to stem, from Rosemary Street pulpit, any materialist tide that Tyndall's rhetoric might trigger. Watts and MacNaughtan were, of course, among the coterie of apologists. But the first lecture, on 'Science and Revelation: Their Distinctive Provinces', was delivered by J.L. Porter, Professor of Biblical Criticism at the Presbyterian College. Having himself just presented a scientific paper to the recent British Association meeting on his 'Recent Journey East of the Jordan', he was happy to allow that 'no theological dogma can annul a fact of science'. But in an atmosphere still redolent with Tyndall's presence, he was moved to castigate 'crude theories and wild speculations', of which Darwinism was a prime case. As a piece of natural history, he conceded, *The Origin of Species* was 'one of the most important contributions to modern science'; in logic, it was 'an utter failure'. Because its author persistently confused fact and theory, the book had to be judged 'not scientific' (Porter, 1874).

Darwinism, moreover, spooked Porter on yet another front – education. Pedagogy, after all, formed the external fabric of his entire biography, for when he resigned his position at Assembly's College in 1878 it was to take up the position of Assistant Commissioner of Intermediate Education, and, later, to become President of Queen's College (Moody and Beckett, 1959). So it was not surprising that in his opening address to the Presbyterian students for the session 1874/5 he should refer to 'the evil tendencies of Recent Scientific Theories'. The spread of the Huxley-Tyndall cosmogony – though it was not real science – would 'quench every virtuous thought'. The need for theological colleges was thus more urgent than ever so that 'heavenly light is preserved and cherished' (Porter, 1875).

The concern for wider social and moral matters was also foremost in William Todd Martin's winter address a few days before Christmas. Earlier, in 1863, we recall, he had expressed grave concerns over the inroads being made by *Essays and Reviews* and pentateuchal criticism. What troubled him now was the impact the idea of an 'Impersonal Force' (a creative energy without personality) would have on morality and religion – and thus on the very foundations of the established social order. The new philosophy, he insisted, proposed 'the founding anew of society' and the reconstruction of 'the whole fabric of personal and social life'. This was the ultimate political goal of scientific naturalism, and it would be achieved by eradicating the very idea of sin from human consciousness. As a consequence, morality would be reduced to a mere survival strategy. Vice was eliminated; the pleasure principle reigned supreme. And that was not all. A Darwinian society was not merely one in which moral conscience had been anaesthetized; it was one in which all sorts of alarming practices could be legitimated in the name of science. Already detecting the sorts of policy that later eugenicists would advocate, he urged in 1875 that 'A State free from the "theological bias", and in the hands of philosophic legislators, would offer a tempting field for experiment in the direction of a higher development of organism and intelligence, by careful scientific oversight of the question of population. Utilitarian ethics could facilitate this great enterprise by abolishing the Christian sentiment which protects the purity of the family' (Martin, 1875).

If Tyndall's most recent excursion into public controversy was the main stimulus for the Presbyterians' winter lectures, his reduction of prayer to the language of energy was the subject of concern to Henry Wallace (1875). Back in June of 1872, Tyndall had received an anonymous letter from a member of the Athenaeum Club challenging Christians to subject prayer to experimental analysis (Turner, 1974). The Prayer Gauge Debate, as it came to be known, attracted numerous commentators, among them Francis Galton, who achieved notoriety for his attempt, as Theodore Porter (1986) describes it, 'to crush mystical piety under a heap of miscellaneous statistical facts'. Belfast Presbyterians were hardly prepared to stand idly by and witness prayer strangled by statistical methods and actuarial tables. And so Wallace, speaking in the Rosemary Street series on 18 January 1875, felt the need to search for some means of preventing the relentless laws of nature from choking the age-old Christian practice to death. Prayer needed some manoeuverability in a law-governed universe and Wallace worked hard to give it the scientific and theological space it needed.

Rehearsing the details of the other contributions to the winter lecture series need not further detain us; the shape of the project is by now plain. Throughout the exercise, the intellectual elite of the Belfast Presbyterian community was determined to gain control of the debate by setting the terms in which the conversation about evolution had to be conducted. In the post-Tyndall era, evolution came to be seen as irretrievably wedded to materialism; as such it required censure on every front. So it was necessary to re-survey the major theological landmarks in Presbyterian territory and to reaffirm those boundaries. Just as the villagers of medieval Europe and colonial

New England annually beat the bounds – marked out the village boundaries – so the Presbyterian hierarchy needed to re-establish its theological borders. Indeed, it is precisely for this reason, I would contend, that the winter lecture series at Rosemary Street Church included ministerial addresses – by A.C. Murphy on proofs of the Bible as divine revelation, by John McNaughtan on the reality of sin, by John Moran on the life of Christ, and by William Magill on the divine origin of scripture – that made no specific reference to Tyndall, Darwin, Spencer, or any version of evolutionary theory. That they were included in the series attests to the perceived need to reaffirm systematically the cardinal doctrines of the faith so as to ensure that Presbyterian theological territory remained intact.

Bishops' Move

If Belfast Protestants found the BA's recent meeting repugnant, Catholics had no less cause to squirm. Within days of the Belfast meeting Huxley would be describing the anonymous attack (by St George Mivart, the Catholic evolutionist) on *The Descent of Man* as replete with the 'misrepresentation and falsification [that] are the favourite weapons of Jesuitical Rome' and thus all too typical of 'the secret poisonings of the Papal Borgias'. With Darwin's complicity he secured Mivart's 'excommunication from the church scientific' (Desmond and Moore, 1991).

Just over a year earlier a Catholic serial, *The Irish Ecclesiastical Record*, had presented an evaluation of 'Darwinism' in which its correspondent castigated the 'Moloch of natural selection' for its 'ruthless extermination of ... unsuccessful competitors', for its lack of evidence for transitional forms, for its failure to account for gaps in the fossil record, and for its distasteful moral implications (J.G.C., 1873). As for the latest clash in Belfast, the Catholic archbishops and bishops of Ireland issued a pastoral letter in November 1874 in which they repudiated the 'blasphemy upon this Catholic nation' that had recently been uttered by the 'professors of Materialism ... under the name of Science'. This certainly was no new warfare, they reflected; but the Catholic hierarchy perceived that this most recent incarnation of materialism unveiled more clearly than ever before 'the moral and social doctrines that lurked in the gloomy recesses of [science's] speculative theories'. Quite simply it meant that moral responsibility had been erased, that virtue and vice had become but 'expressions of the same mechanical force', and that sin and holiness likewise vanished chimera-like into oblivion. Everything in human life from 'sensual love' to religious sentiment were 'all equally results of the play between organism and environment through countless ages of the past'. Such was the brutalizing materialism that now confronted the Irish people ('Pastoral Address', 1874).

The congruence between these evaluations and those of the Presbyterian commentators we have scrutinized is certainly marked. So why then should Watts, in a subsequent reprint of his pamphlet entitled 'Atomism: Dr. Tyndall's Atomic Theory of the Universe Examined and Refuted', incorporate in an appendix 'strictures on the recent Manifesto of the Roman Catholic Hierarchy of Ireland in reference to the sphere of Science'? That he wished to distance himself from their proposals is clear: it was 'painful', he noted, 'to observe the position taken by the Roman Catholic hierarchy of Ireland in their answer to Professors Tyndall and Huxley'. So, just what was the problem? Simply this – Watts felt that the Catholic willingness to compartmentalize science and religion would lead to 'the secularisation of the physical sciences'. Because Cardinal Cullen and his co-religionists seemed only too willing to follow Newman in restricting the physicist to the bare empirical, Watts insisted that since 'the Word of God enjoins it upon men as a duty to infer the invisible things of the Creator from the things that are made', the Roman Catholic hierarchy of Ireland had, by their declaration, 'taken up an attitude of antagonism to that Word, prohibiting scientists, as such, from rising above the law to the infinitely wise, Almighty Lawgiver' (Watts, 1875).

But then two of Watts's close Presbyterian allies in the anti-Tyndall campaign had themselves taken the very same line! J.L. Porter, in the very first lecture of the winter series, had appealed for a clear-cut boundary – in terms of both content and methodology – between the provinces of science and theology: for him it was a case of good fences makes good neighbours. And again, in an attempt to avert hostilities, Rev. John MacNaughtan, in his post-BA sermon, insisted that 'science and Christianity have different spheres' and that therefore 'there is no reason why they should ever come into collision'. To him the appropriate allocation of items to the respective regional geographies of science and religion would greatly assist in keeping the peace (MacNaughtan, 1874).

The sectarian traditions in Irish society doubtless had a key role to play in these machinations. The furore surrounding the Tyndall event merely became yet another occasion for Ulster Nonconformity to uncover its sense of siege. Watts had no desire to share his doctrinal space with Catholic bishops who were part of a tradition that had all too recently poured scorn on the New York meeting of the Evangelical Alliance and attacked his own hero, the Princeton theologian Charles Hodge. Moreover, though he may have privately agreed with their dismissal of the Alliance 'debate on the Darwinian theory' – in which McCosh had participated – as 'empty – nay, … almost childish', it was clearly important to Watts not to be seen in the company of such critics ('Evangelical Alliance', 1874). In his confrontation with evolutionary theory Watts wanted to cultivate and tend to his own tradition's theological space, and not engage in extramural affiliations. And by seeking to cast secularization and Catholicism as conspirators against the inductive truths of science and the revealed truths of scripture, he found it possible to conflate as a single object of opprobrium the old enemy, popery, and the new enemy, evolution.

The Catholic hierarchy did not miss the opportunity of firing its own broadsides at Protestantism. For the bishops and archbishops felt it would 'not be amiss, in connection with the Irish National system of education, to call attention to the fact that the Materialists of to-day are able to boast that the doctrines which have brought most odium upon their school have been openly taught by a high Protestant dignitary'. It only confirmed them in their uncompromising stance on the Catholic educational system. Had it not been for their own vigilance, an unbelieving tide would have swept through the entire curriculum. Such circumstances justified 'to the full the determination of Catholic Ireland not to allow her young men to frequent Universities and Colleges where Science is made the vehicle of Materialism'. Accordingly, the bishops and archbishops rebuked 'the indifference of those who may be tempted to grow slack in the struggle for a Catholic system of education' ('Pastoral Address'). Tyndall's speech, it seems, succeeded not only in fostering the opposition of both Protestants and Catholics to his own science, but in furthering their antagonism to each other.

No Surrender

In the aftermath of Tyndall's offensive, the Belfast religious community found it virtually impossible for at least a generation to find any rapprochement with Darwinian biology. One moment, a decade after the notorious BA meeting, will serve to illustrate how persistently antagonistic were the sentiments that lingered on in the city. The pan-Presbyterian General Council met in Belfast during the last week of June 1884. Several speakers called for the incorporation of evolution theory into the very fabric of Reformed Theology. The Scottish clergyman, hymnologist and author George Matheson, for example, told his fellow Presbyterians that he could detect the hidden hand of God behind Herbert Spencer's 'Unknowable' – the creative impulse behind the universe that Spencer believed to be beyond comprehension – a viewpoint he further elaborated the following year in his volume *Can the Old Faith Live with the New? Or, The Problem of Evolution and Revelation*. Spencer's Force, as Matheson encountered it, was none other than the Spirit of God, and the doctrine of Evolution nothing less than a revelation of the workings of Providence. Indeed he was prepared to suggest that 'in the production of the human race there may have co-operated the factors called Natural Selection, Heredity, Concomitant Variation, and

Environment' (Matheson, 1884). Professor Jean Monod, who followed Matheson on the programme, concurred in his judgments about the 'possibility of harmonizing with the leading doctrines of Christianity, the system of Evolution rightly understood'; and the Scottish Presbyterian moral philosopher Henry Calderwood (supported presently by Professor Salmond from Aberdeen) threw his weight behind Matheson's proposals, insisting that 'Evolution theory is a theory teaching Creation'.

Local delegates, however, were not so sanguine in their judgments. The redoubtable Watts told them outright that evolution was a 'mere hypothesis' with 'not one single particle of evidence' to support it. The need for embarking on any doctrinal reconstruction did not exactly commend itself to him. Indeed, he had long been campaigning, in both Belfast and Scotland, against Spencer's system because to him it was explicitly designed 'to overthrow the Scripture doctrine of special creations', as he claimed in *An Examination of Herbert Spencer's Biological Hypothesis* (1875a). In a letter to his wife on 26 September 1877, Watts observed: 'My lecture in Perth on Herbert Spencer's Biological Hypothesis came off very well.'* To hear latter-day Scottish Calvinists divinizing the 'Inscrutable Ultimate' – attributing divinity to what Spencerians considered to be beyond knowing – must have sounded like the grossest act of doctrinal betrayal. Others concurred. In the wake of Matheson's flirtation with a Spencerian theology, Todd Martin (1887) issued a book-length criticism of Spencer's Cosmic System, expressing typically inductivist suspicions of the entire project. Cosmic evolutionists, he judged, were forever going on about their far-flung empire and the comprehensiveness of their claims, and thereby persistently committed the cardinal error of elevating the particular into the universal. Their claims simply had to be relegated to the class of spurious, untestable hypotheses. If ever there were a group who persistently read their own metaphysics into the data it was the cosmic evolutionists. To reconstruct theology along Matheson's lines would be flagrantly irresponsible.

In the aftermath of the gathering, the ever-watchful Robert Watts continued to keep an eye on things. Henry Drummond's *Natural Law in the Spiritual World* (1883) had already fallen under his gaze, and as soon as *The Ascent of Man* (1894) appeared on the horizon Watts had it in his sights. Drummond's extravagant evangelical efforts to evolutionize theology and to import Spencer's evolutionary laws into the supernatural realm created a sensation at the time; yet, taken overall, published reactions were remarkably mild (see Moore, 1985; Smith, 1902; Lennox, 1901; Simpson, n.d.). But there were critics. 'Deadly poison', snorted Horatius Bonar. Watts concurred:

---

* From unpublished 'Family Letters of Revd Robert Watts, D.D., LL.D' compiled by his wife. I am grateful to Dr R.E.L. Rodgers for making this typescript available to me.

the Drummond project was a mess – theologically and scientifically. To be sure, his aim of removing 'the alleged antagonism' between science and religion was a worthy objective. But the Drummond strategy ultimately was 'not an Irenicum between science and religion or between the laws of the empires of matter and of spirit' at all. Rather it only displayed the expansionist character of natural law. Watts found the whole project so bizarre that, as he worked up to his conclusion, he felt 'inclined to apologise for attempting a formal refutation of a theory which, if it means anything intelligible, involves the denial of all that the Scriptures teach, and all that Christian experience reveals' (Watts, 1888b, 1894). And it was not just testy Calvinists who prickled under Drummond's touch. J.J. Murphy – who in the mid-1880s continued to adhere to his non-Darwinian version of evolution, employing it in accounts of human language and moral freedom, and who believed that it provided a firm foundation for Christian theism – issued his own impeachment of Drummond in a review for the *British Quarterly Review* in 1884 (reprinted in Murphy, 1893).

Tyndall's BA speech cast a long shadow over intellectual life in Victorian Belfast. The flavour of his 'materialist manifesto' lingered on, and made it far more difficult for local churchmen to negotiate the sort of conceptual accommodations to evolutionary theory that were able to be effected in other places. In such an atmosphere they could only see the folly of acceding to the accommodationist strategies of a Drummond or a Matheson. These newer compromises only seemed to confirm them in the rightness of the belligerent path on which they had embarked a decade and more earlier.

References

Allen, R. 1954. *The Presbyterian College Belfast, 1853-1953.* Belfast: William Mullan.

Anon. 1875. *Science and Revelation: A Series of Lectures in Reply to The Theories of Tyndall, Huxley, Darwin, Spencer, etc.* Belfast: William Mullan.

Barton, R. 1987. 'John Tyndall, Pantheist: A Rereading of the Belfast Address.' *Osiris 2nd series, 3*: 111-34.

'The Belfast Presbytery and the British Association.' *The Witness*, 4 September 1874.

Brooke, P. 1983. 'Religion and Secular Thought, 1800-75,' in J.C. Beckett et al., *Belfast: The Making of a City 1800-1914.* Belfast: Appletree Press.

Carswell, R. 1874. Review of *Christianity and Science* by John MacNaughtan. *The Witness*, 18 September.

D'Arcy, C.F. 1932. *Providence and the World-Order.* The Alexander Robertson Lectures delivered before the University of Glasgow, 1932. London: Hodder & Stoughton.

D'Arcy, C.F. 1934. *The Adventures of a Bishop, A Phase of Irish Life: A Personal and Historical Narrative.* London: Hodder & Stoughton.

Darwin, C. 1905. *The Variation of Animals and Plants under Domestication.* 2 vols. London: John Murray.

'Death of Rev. Canon MacIlwaine, DD.' *Irish Ecclesiastical Gazette*, 15 August 1885: 690-1.

Desmond, A. and J. Moore. 1991. *Darwin.* London: Michael Joseph.

Donat, J.G. 1986. 'British Medicine and the Ulster Revival of 1859.' Ph.D. thesis, University of London.

Drummond, H. 1883. *Natural Law in the Spiritual World*. London: Hodder and Stoughton.

Drummond, H. 1894. *The Lowell Lectures on the Ascent of Man*. London: Hodder and Stoughton.

'The Evangelical Alliance.' 1874. *Irish Ecclesiastical Record 11* (January).

Hempton, D. and M. Hill. 1992. *Evangelical Protestantism in Ulster Society: 1740-1890*. London and New York: Routledge.

Hoeveler, J.D. 1981. *James McCosh and the Scottish Intellectual Tradition*. Princeton: Princeton University Press.

J.G.C. 1873. 'Darwinism.' *Irish Ecclesiastical Record 9*: 337-61.

Jeffrey, R. 1874. 'Scientific Giants v. Theological Pigmies.' *The Christian Banner 2 (5)* (October): 43-5.

Keith, Sir A. 1923. 'The Adaptational Machinery Concerned in the Evolution of Man's Body.' [12th Huxley Memorial Lecture.] *Nature*, Supplement, No. 2807 (18 August): 257-68.

Keith, Sir A. 1927. *Concerning Man's Origin. Being the Presidential Address Given at the Meeting of the British Association Held in Leeds on August 31, 1927, and Recent Essays on Darwinian Subjects*. London: Watts & Co.

Leach, E. 1985. 'Anthropology of Religion: British and French Schools,' in N. Smart, J. Clayton, P. Sherry, and S.T. Katz (eds), *Nineteenth Century Religious Thought in the West, Vol. III*. Cambridge: Cambridge University Press, 215-62.

Lennox, C. 1901. *Henry Drummond. A Biographical Sketch (With Bibliography)*. London: Andrew Melrose.

Livingstone, D.N. 1987. *Darwin's Forgotten Defenders: The Encounter between Evangelical Theology and Evolutionary Thought*. Edinburgh: Scottish Academic Press.

Livingstone, D.N. 1992. 'Darwinism and Calvinism: The Belfast-Princeton Connection.' *Isis 83*: 408-28.

Livingstone, D.N. 1994. 'Science and Religion: Foreword to the Historical Geography of an Encounter.' *Journal of Historical Geography 20*: 367-83.

Macloskie, Rev. G. 1862. 'The Natural History of Man.' *The Ulster Magazine 3*: 217-37.

McCosh, J. 1859. *The Ulster Revival and Its Physiological Accidents. A Paper Read Before the Evangelical Alliance, September 22, 1859*. Belfast: C. Aitchison.

McCosh, J. 1871. *Christianity and Positivism: A Series of Lectures to the Times on Natural Theology aned Christian Apologetics*. London: Macmillan.

McCosh, J. 1872. 'On Prayer.' *Contemporary Review 22*: 777-8.

McCosh, J. 1874. 'Religious Aspects of the Doctrine of Development,' in S. Irenaeus Prime (ed.), *History, Orations, and Other Documents of the Sixth General Conference of the Evangelical Alliance*. New York: Harper, 264-71.

McCosh, J. 1888. *The Religious Aspect of Evolution*. New York: Scribner's.

M'Ilwaine, Rev. W. 1859. *The 'Revival Movement' Examined*. Belfast: Wheatcroft & Henry.

M'Ilwaine, Rev. W. 1859a. *Revivalism Reviewed*. Belfast: T. M'Ilroy.

M'Ilwaine, Rev. W. 1874-5. 'Presidential Address.' *Proceedings of the Belfast Naturalists' Field Club* (Winter): 81-99.

MacNaughtan, J. 1874. *The Address of Professor Tyndall, at the Opening of the British Association for the Advancement of Science, Examined in A Sermon on Christianity and Science*. Belfast: Aitchison, Reed, & Henderson.

Martin, W.T. 1863. *Our Church in its Relation to Progressive Thought*. Newry: James Burns.

Martin, W.T. 1875. *The Doctrine of An Impersonal God in its Effects on Morality and Religion*. Belfast: William Mullan.

Martin, W.T. 1887. *The Evolution Hypothesis: A Criticism of the New Cosmic Philosophy*. Edinburgh: James Gemmell.

Matheson, G. 1884. 'The Religious Bearings of the Doctrine of Evolution,' in G.D. Mathews (ed.), *Alliance of The Reformed Churches Holding the Presbyterian System. Minutes and Proceedings of the*

Third General Council, Belfast, 1884. Belfast: Assembly's Offices.

Matheson, G. 1885. *Can the Old Faith Live with the New? or, The Problem of Evolution and Revelation.* Edinburgh: William Blackwood & Sons.

Moody, T.W. and J.C. Beckett. 1959. *Queen's, Belfast 1845-1949: The History of a University.* London: Faber & Faber.

Moore, J.R. 1979. *The Post-Darwinian Controversies: A Study of the Protestant Struggle to Come to Terms with Darwin in Great Britain and America, 1870-1900.* Cambridge: Cambridge University Press.

Moore, J.R. 1982. '1859 and All That: Remaking the Story of Evolution-and-Religion,' in R.G. Chapman and C.T. Duval (eds), *Charles Darwin, 1809-1882: A Centennial Commemorative.* Wellington, N.Z.: Nova Pacifica, 167-94.

Moore, J.R. 1985. 'Evangelicals and Evolution: Henry Drummond, Herbert Spencer, and the Naturalization of the Spiritual World.' *Scottish Journal of Theology 38*: 383-417.

Murphy, J.J. 1865. *The Grounds of Belief. A Lecture Read Before the United Church of Scotland and Ireland Young Men's Society.* Belfast: Phillips & Sons.

Murphy, J.J. 1866. 'Presidential Address to the Belfast Natural History and Philosophical Society.' *Northern Whig*, 19 November.

Murphy, J.J. 1869. *Habit and Intelligence in their Connexion with the Laws of Matter and Force: A Series of Scientific Essays.* 2 vols. London: Macmillan.

Murphy, J.J. 1869-70. 'The Origin of Organs of Flight.' *Proceedings of the Belfast Naturalists' Field Club,* 7th Report.

Murphy, J.J. 1872-3. 'Presidential Address on Some Questions in Cosmological Science.' *Proceedings of the Belfast Natural History and Philosophical Society*: 1-19.

Murphy, J.J. 1873. *The Scientific Bases of Faith.* London: Macmillan.

Murphy, J.J. 1873-4. 'Presidential Address on the Present State of the Darwinian Controversy.' *Proceedings of the Belfast Natural History and Philosophical Society*: 1-24.

Murphy, J.J. 1893. *Natural Selection and Spiritual Freedom.* London: Macmillan.

Orthodox Presbyterian. 1874. 'Letter.' *Northern Whig*, 28 August.

'Pastoral Address of the Archbishops and Bishops of Ireland.' 1874. *Irish Ecclesiastical Record 11.*

Patton, W.D. 1993. 'James McCosh, The Making of a Reputation: A Study of the Life and Work of the Rev. Dr. James McCosh in Ireland, from His Appointment as Professor of Logic and Metaphysics in Queen's College Belfast 1851 to His Appointment as President of Princeton College, New Jersey and Professor of Philosophy, in 1868.' Ph.D. thesis, Queen's University, Belfast.

Porter, J.L. 1874. *Science and Revelation: Their Distinctive Provinces. With a Review of the Theories of Tyndall, Huxley, Darwin, and Herbert Spencer.* Belfast: William Mullan.

Porter, J.L. 1875. *Theological Colleges: Their Place and Influence in the Church and in the World; with Special Reference to the Evil Tendencies of Recent Scientific Theories. Being the Opening Lecture of Assembly's College, Belfast, Session 1874-75.* Belfast: William Mullan.

Porter, T.M. 1986. *The Rise of Statistical Thinking 1820-1900.* Princeton: Princeton University Press.

'Professor John Tyndall, D.C.L., LL.D.' 1874. *Northern Whig*, 19 August, 5-6.

Rogerson, J.W. 1985. *Old Testament Criticism in the Nineteenth Century: England and Germany.* Philadelphia: Fortress Press.

Ross, R. 1874. 'Professor Tyndall's Theory of Life and Organization.' *The Christian Banner 2 (5)*: 41-3.

Seaver, R.W. 1902. 'Joseph John Murphy,' in A. Deane (ed.), *Belfast Literary Society, 1801-1901. Historical Sketch, With Memoirs of Some Distinguished Members.* Belfast: McCaw, Stevenson & Orr.

Simpson, J.Y. n.d. (c. 1901). *Henry Drummond.* Edinburgh: Oliphant Anderson & Ferrier.

Sloane, W.M. 1896. *The Life of James McCosh: A Record Chiefly Autobiographical.* Edinburgh: T. & T. Clark.

Smith, G.A. 1902. *The Life of Henry Drummond.* London: Hodder and Stoughton.

Smith, R. 1874. 'Letter.' *Northern Whig,* 27 August.

'Truth versus Error.' 1874. *Ulster Echo,* 27 August.

Turner, F.M. 1974. 'Rainfall, Plagues and the Prince of Wales: A Chapter in the Conflict of Religion and Science.' *Journal of British Studies 13*: 46-65.

Tyndall, J. 1874. *Address Delivered Before the British Association Assembled at Belfast, with Addition.* London: Longmans, Green, and Co.

Wallace, H. 1874. 'Teachings of the British Association.' *Plain Words,* October 1874: 253-7.

Wallace, [H.]. 1875. *Prayer in Relation to Natural Law.* Belfast: William Mullan.

Wallace, P. and M. Noll. 1994. 'The Students of Princeton Seminary, 1812-1929: A Research Note.' *American Presbyterians 72*: 203-15.

Watts, R. 1875. *Atomism: Dr. Tyndall's atomic theory of the universe examined and refuted. To which are added, Humanitarianism accepts, provisionally, Tyndall's impersonal atomic deity; and a letter to the presbytery of Belfast; containing a note from the Rev. Dr. Hodge, and a critique on Tyndall's recent Manchester recantation, together with strictures on the late manifesto of the Roman Catholic hierarchy of Ireland in reference to the sphere of science.* Belfast: Mullan.

Watts, R. 1875a. *An Examination of Herbert Spencer's Biological Hypothesis.* Belfast: William Mullan.

Watts, R. 1888. 'An Irenicum: Or, a Plea for Peace and Co-operation between Science and Theology,' in *The Reign of Causality: A Vindication of the Scientific Principle of Telic Causal Efficiency.* Edinburgh: T. & T. Clark.

Watts, R. 1888a. 'Atomism – An Examination of Professor Tyndall's Opening Address before the British Association, 1874,' in *The Reign of Causality: A Vindication of the Scientific Principle of Telic Causal Efficiency.* Edinburgh: T. & T. Clark.

Watts, R. 1888b. 'Natural Law in the Spiritual World,' in *The Reign of Causality: A Vindication of the Scientific Principle of Telic Causal Efficiency.* Edinburgh: T. & T. Clark.

Watts, R. 1894. *Professor Drummond's 'Ascent of Man,' and Principal Fairbairn's 'Place of Christ in Modern Theology', Examined in the Light of Science and Revelation.* Edinburgh: R.W. Hunter.

'Winter Lectures in Belfast.' *The Witness,* 25 September 1874.

Nature and Nation in the Nineteenth Century

JOHN WILSON FOSTER

Romantic Nationalism

What Karl Alfred Von Zittel (1901) saw as the 'Heroic Age of Geology', the period from 1790 to 1820, coincided with that cultural movement we know as European Romanticism. The notion of the sublime – together with the enthusiastic travel to the peripheries that it tempted – energized both the science and the cultural movement. The aesthetics of nature, developed in the eighteenth century, were expanded and intensified to permit a profound interaction between the observer and nature. If the earth contained remote, immense and wild places, these were matched by the emotional intensities and vicissitudes in mood of the traveller; the human being was less observer of, than participant in, the natural world. As Samuel Taylor Coleridge put it in 'Dejection: An Ode' (1802):

> O Sara! we receive but what we give,
> And in our life alone does Nature live.

Much Romantic literature is a lament for those occasions when the reciprocity between nature and humanity breaks down.

The Romantic period saw a shift in the tectonic plates of European intellect and the perception of nature. The pre-eminence of reason, measurement and objectivity was questioned. A toned-down version of the Romantics' belief in what Coleridge called the 'Shaping Spirit of Imagination' was taken on board by the most cultivated scientists of the nineteenth century, including the Irish-born physicist, alpinist and evolutionist John Tyndall, as his 1870 essay 'Scientific Use of the Imagination' demonstrates (1907, II).

A key Romantic text, Mary Shelley's *Frankenstein* (1818), was stimulated by the author's contemplation of both the geological features and formidable prospects of the Alps and the contemporary experiments of chemists and physicists.* The name of the benevolent Irish magistrate in *Frankenstein*, Mr Kirwin, might well have been suggested by the name of Richard Kirwan, the famous Irish chemist and mineralogist who appears as a rather Romantic figure in the portrait (1802-8) by H.D. Hamilton (and finished by his daughter Harriet after his death); although it is unlikely Shelley ever saw it, she and her husband, the poet Percy Bysshe Shelley, were intensely interested in contemporary experiments in chemistry and physics and would have doubtless been familiar with Kirwan's name.

Until recently, the Romantics were generally supposed to have been antagonistic to science, and Romanticism to have been a radical widening of the gulf between the Two Cultures. Nature, it seemed, was imaginatively liberated by writers from the natural historians. But this was only partially true, as the cases of the Shelleys and Coleridge, with his great interest in Humphry Davy, demonstrate. As for Wordsworth, Wyatt has demonstrated the poet's later enthusiasm for geology, his friendship with geologists who like him were great walkers, and the presence of geological allusions in his poetry. Science, after all, could evocatively explore the awful mysteries of physical life and of the wondrous Earth that mirrored the mysteries of the human heart and imagination.

Moreover, many of the Romantics, especially Percy Shelley and the young Wordsworth and Coleridge, were passionate admirers of the French Revolution before the Terror. These poets were all lovers of nature, in part because nature bespoke liberty. For them, nature's creatures, including human beings, were properly conceived of as sovereign and 'republican', owing allegiance only to nature itself and to the kind of society that developed itself on natural principles of freedom and justice. Whereas life in the aggregate, life classified (in poetic diction and perceptions of society alike), remained important chiefly in the rhetoric of political revolution, it was individualism that helped to signal the break with the uncompromising rationalism of the Enlightenment. In the depiction of nature, individualism took the extreme forms of nature's limitless grandeur and of nature's particularities (Dr Johnson's famous streaks on the tulip petals) both being recorded with intensity of feeling. Even in natural history, the taxonomy of the century of Carl Linnaeus, Mathurin Brisson, Jacob Klein and other systematists, became less of a central preoccupation in the following century.

---

*The interest of Mary and Percy Shelley in electromagnetism paralleled the interest of F.W.J. Schelling (1775-1854) – the German theorist of *Naturphilosophie* – in Faraday's work on the same subject. The vitality and unity of nature and being were key concepts for both sets of writers and thinkers. For *Naturphilosophie* see Bynum et al. (1985). For aspects of relations between Romanticism and natural history, see Wilshire (1968), Gaull (1988), Butler (1993) and Sacks (1993).

The atheist and radical poet Shelley spoke on Dublin platforms and published *An Address to the Irish People* (1812) – the title suggesting revolutionary aggregation in action – and must have taken prisoner some sympathetic ears, for there were those from the native population and even from the Protestant Ascendancy who wanted to see in Ireland after the Act of Union (1800) not renovation or reform but revolution and an end to the modes of thought that issued in the science of the Anglo-Irish tradition. These radicals had already been crushed in the rebellion of 1798 and the failed rising of 1803, but these failures seeded future physical-force Irish nationalism; both uprisings had been inspired by the French Revolution and the rebels had entertained hopes of decisive French support.*

There was an Irish Romantic literature but it had little of the coherence of England's two waves of Romantics (Blake, Wordsworth and Coleridge followed by Shelley, Byron and Keats). Irish Romanticism exhibited an instability of programme as well as of mode (the picturesque, the sublime, the sentimental, the gothic, the macabre) that was probably due to the colonial situation in which Irish writers found themselves. Irish Romantic literature has been described as 'intensely and undisguisedly political' (Dunne, 1988), preoccupied with nation-building through claims of cultural distinctiveness and ancientness that would weaken the case for the maintenance of the Act of Union, but this is true later rather than earlier in the nineteenth century. Some of the Romantic writers are political only by implication, their costume-drama celebration of the Irish past and their aesthetic celebration of the Irish landscape amounting to a kind of cultural nationalism: oblique tributaries feeding into a larger current. The more cogent anti-Union claims were advanced chiefly by liberal Protestants, and were followed (logically – given the militant rhetoric of some – but hopelessly) by a revolution of sorts in 1848 led by the Young Ireland group, a literary and political set, to whose chief thinker, Thomas Davis, I will return.

In either kind of Irish Romantic literature, there was, under the circumstances, little celebration of Irish nature for its own sake, none of the self-rewarding sensuousness of Keats or the personal enrichment or pantheistic spirit Wordsworth found in the Lake District. There are no Irish poets of the time to whom we might refer as 'nature poets' in the way we might

---

*Wordsworth outlived his youthful revolutionary fervour, though it is likely that as regards Ireland he never experienced it. He early absorbed the views of the Elizabethans on Ireland, especially Spenser and Campion. He visited Ireland in the autumn of 1829 and that year wrote a letter to the Bishop of London, in which (echoing Spenser and others) he alleged that Ireland's misery was caused by the papacy and by wrongful tenure and management of landed property that were the legacy of 'imperfect conquest'. Wordsworth opposed reform legislation at the time Daniel O'Connell was campaiging for Catholic Emancipation (see Marjarum, 1940).

refer to Wordsworth and Clare as nature poets. (The words 'nature', 'landscape' and 'scenery', in fact, have among the bulk of the Irish people to this day a somewhat effete connotation and evoke an Anglo-Irish world view.) Nor was there that interest in cutting-edge experimental science we find in Shelley or Coleridge.

Nevertheless, nineteenth-century romantic Irish nationalism (and its eighteenth-century roots) had elements that are of interest to the historian of natural history. There was the Celtic primitivism taking Irish form with Sylvester O'Halloran's *Antiquities of Ireland* (1772) and his god-daughter Charlotte Brooke's *Reliques of Irish Poetry* (1789). Irish landscape was perceived as vestigial, ancient and ruined – not cultivated or tasteful in configuration or prospect like the Anglo-Irish demesne, but nonetheless picturesque in its ruination. What was important was that the ruined landscape bore witness to a dignified pre-conquest culture. So too did the expressive remains of the elder Gaelic society, its songs and sagas. The 'hardware' and 'software' of an ancient civilization – i.e. the material and immaterial remnants – fired the imagination both of Romantic writers (drawn to the Gothic version of the picturesque) and of antiquarians of a cultivated bent. Only some of these truly wished to see the elder culture reanimated, since in its vestigial form it had the attractiveness of the lamentable. Picturesque and pre-conquest Irelands could fuse in the imagination of the writer, as they do in Lady Morgan's Romantic novel *The Wild Irish Girl* (1806), which draws on the author's familiarity with Sligo.* Wolff remarks that 'Romantic melancholy amidst romantic scenery cluttered with romantic ruins provided for the audiences of the time the perfect background for the political and social message' (Morgan, 1979). Morgan uses her visiting narrator to redeem Ireland from its demeaning portraiture by Elizabethan sojourners, and does so in part through the island's picturesque qualities: Dublin Bay is 'one of the most splendid spectacles in the scene of picturesque creation'. The narrator's journey from Dublin to the west shows a poverty of agriculture but ample compensation:

To him who derives gratification from the embellished labours of art, rather than the simple but sublime operations of nature, Irish scenery will afford little interest; but the bold features of its varying landscape, the stupendous attitude of its 'cloud-capt'

---

*An adequate account of the depiction of nature in Irish literature would require a book in its own right. For the primary material of the nineteenth century, readers could consult the relevant sections of *The Field Day Anthology of Irish Writing* (Deane, 1991, II) and the Garland facsimile series of seventy-seven novels and collections of shorter stories by twenty-two Irish and Anglo-Irish novelists issued under the title *Ireland from the Act of Union 1800 to the Death of Parnell 1891* and selected by R.L. Wolff. For secondary sources, consult McKenna (1978).

mountains, the impervious gloom of its deep embosomed glens, the savage desola-
tion of its uncultivated heaths, and boundless bogs, with whose rich veins of a picturesque champagne, thrown at intervals into gay expansion by the hand of nature,
awaken in the mind of the poetic or pictorial traveller, all the pleasures of tasteful
enjoyment, all the sublime emotions of a rapt imagination. And if the glowing fancy
of Claude Loraine would have dwelt enraptured on the paradisial charms of English
landscape, the superior genius of Salvator Rosa would have reposed its eagle wing
amidst those scenes of mysterious sublimity, with which the wildly magnificent landscape of Ireland abounds. (Morgan, 1979)

This echoes earlier English Gothic fiction and both English and Irish
topographical writing (see 'Encountering Traditions' in this volume), and
anticipates passages of *Frankenstein*, but Morgan does not have Shelley's
republican convictions. Her work exhibits at most what Wolff calls 'her
Whiggish political principles'; in English literature the picturesque landscape
(as an idealized landscape) is more often than not a flamboyant disguise for
a fundamentally conservative outlook, which in the Irish context is a unionist outlook.

The perception of the Irish landscape as strewn with incomplete signs
of the pre-conquest past, to be read like manuscripts as well as to be appreciated like paintings, was sharpened by antiquarianism, on which Lady
Morgan drew in her novel. A great advance was made when John
O'Donovan (a founding member of the Ossianic Society) and the scholars
Eugene O'Curry and George Petrie mapped the antiquities of Ireland in the
1830s for the Historical Department of the Ordnance Survey under the
direction of an English army officer, T.A. Larcom (Andrews, 1975).

The English mapping of Ireland required the translation of Irish placenames or the coining of placenames in English and was a colonial enterprise.
However, it is an irony that the cultural work of the mappers, discreetly conducted at the same time as their scientific cartography, resurrected impressive and stimulating evidence of Ireland's pre-conquest culture. For a while,
this was consonant with unionism: Sir Samuel Ferguson, for example, tried
to accommodate ancient Irish poetry into the British literary canon, as he
sought to accommodate ancient Irish culture into British culture, the under-
pinning of his unionism (Deane, 1991). Later in the century, however, antiquarianism was to quicken into serious cultural nationalism that helped support the twentieth-century independence campaign (O'Connor, 1967;
Thompson, 1967). Liam and Máire de Paor interpret the Ordnance Survey
of Ireland as the fruitful union of Anglo-Irish antiquarianism and the Gaelic
learning and tradition of the past.

Petrie gave a position on the Survey to James Clarence Mangan, and
discovered this 'shadowy figure' (O'Connor, 1967) as a poet. Mangan is as
close as anyone to an Irish Romantic poet on the early nineteenth-century

English model. His best-known poem was and is 'Dark Rosaleen', a para-phrase of an old Gaelic song. Mangan's dark rose is Ireland. In Ireland a potent symbolism was generated from the rose (ironic given this flower's association with England); Zimmermann has illuminating paragraphs on its recurrence in the popular Irish imagination and in the imagination of lesser Irish writers, and of course its importance to Yeats's complex symbolism is well known to literary critics.* A curious feature of nineteenth-century Irish nationalist culture is the way the rose and certain other natural elements are invested with political symbolism. The black bird turns up again (see 'Encountering Traditions' in this volume), this time in an anonymous broad-side, 'The Royal Black Bird', an allusion to the Old Pretender, the son of James II. The speaker fears a fowler has taken his blackbird, which once flourished in England. The broadside appeared around 1715 but was popu-lar in the following century (Zimmermann, 1967; Coleborne, 1991). New words to this air in 1881 made Charles Stewart Parnell 'the Blackbird of Avondale', likewise the quarry of a base fowler (Zimmermann, 1967). Zimmerman reminds us that Patrick Dineen in his famous Irish-English dic-tionary translates *londubh* as 'a blackbird; a Jacobite, a rapparee, a hero'. It was in this tradition that the Irish poet Francis Ledwidge, who was killed in the First World War, imagined the executed leaders of the Easter 1916 rebellion as Ireland's blackbirds.

The use of nature symbolism was not just a poetic fancy; it was also a precaution in dangerous political weather, when secret meanings could be conveyed by its means. Participating in a European folksong tradition, the speaker of the Irish ballad frequently begins by taking to the field:

> By a pleasant grove as for pleasure I strayed,
> One calm dewy evening in spring ...
>   (Zimmermann, 1967)

This is not just an 'establishment shot', as the film-makers would say; one goes abroad, not as a field naturalist (as Protestants were wont to do from the mid-nineteenth century onwards), but 'to view the state of the country', as one song has it (ironically echoing the title of Spenser's famous book on Ireland). 'How's poor ould Ireland/And how does she stand?' asks

---

*James Joyce, Yeats's opposite number in terms of literary style and vision, seemed to mock Irish patriotic biomorphism when he had his hero, Stephen Dedalus, famously define Ireland as a sow that eats its own farrow. Flann O'Brien, like Joyce an anti-Romantic modernist, likewise engaged in mockery: in his dark 1941 novel *An Béal Bocht* (trans. as *The Poor Mouth*), the novelist introduces a threatening monster that turns out to bear a similarity to the map of 'the pleasant little land which is our own' turned side-ways (O'Brien, 1975).

the United Irishman Napper Tandy when he meets the speaker of the street-ballad, 'The Wearing of the Green'. The nature, or condition, of the country – the nation, not countryside, though the countryside is the most authentic habitat of the nation – is the object of the sortie. One goes abroad to take the political temperature (is it hot enough yet for insurrection?) or measure the political climate of Ireland. In the cumulation of such ballads, there is the suggestion of a real Irish landscape, mostly invisible to the ruling formations, unstudied and unstudiable, a second and secret nature beyond the jurisdiction of natural history, waiting in abeyance.

There is also implied a relationship between nationalism and unspoilt nature, the freedom that might be, an idea found among the English Romantics. This relationship took its rise in Germany around the end of the eighteenth century. With the success of a Romantic liberationist nationalism (such as Ireland's), nature would resurge to overwhelm the superficial cultivation of the established order. In the poem 'The Spirit of Irish Song' (a tribute by its author, Thomas Furlong, to Hardiman's epoch-making *Irish Minstrelsy* [1831], for which he was a chief translator), Irish ballads and songs are regarded as artless and the products of 'Nature', very different from the 'forms of art' which are to be flung aside. The equation was made explicitly nationalist in the famous song of the 1798 rebellion, 'The Croppy Boy', in which wild creatures are in coded compact with the rebels: 'It was early, early in the spring,/The birds did whistle and sweetly sing,/Changing their notes from tree to tree/And the song they sang was "Old Ireland Free".'* Nature as freedom is neatly symbolized in the Tree of Liberty. The image in the street-ballad 'Ireland's Liberty Tree' of freedom as a tree that needs watering with tears of the (presumably defeated) brave (Zimmermann, 1967) becomes in Patrick Pearse in the early twentieth century a freedom that requires watering with one's own – and others' – blood. Yeats remembered this when he combined the rose and the liberty-tree in his ballad-like poem 'The Rose Tree' and had Pearse say to James Connolly (another Easter 1916 martyr):

> There's nothing but our own red blood
> Can make a right Rose Tree.

The Orange enemies of Irish nationalism had their own Tree of Liberty ('planted' in Ireland by William III), and Zimmermann tells us that loyalist writers often parodied nationalist zoomorphism. In a re-writing of 'The Royal Black Bird', William is an eagle, King James a vulture, and Daniel O'Connell a mockingbird. On the other hand, the conceptions of freedom

---

*Croppies got their name from their cropped hairstyle, borrowed from the French revolutionists' fashion.

that were so powerful in the early nineteenth century had strong roots in religious Dissent, including Presbyterianism; it was later in the century that they were appropriated by Catholic nationalists, for whom Irish nature became symbolic while for Dissenters it became objective (in the attraction of many of them to science), and untroublingly so until evolutionism aroused Dissenter consternation (see Livingstone in this volume).

The plant referred to in Ireland as shamrock (*seamróg*) is, as Praeger tells us, either the lesser trefoil (*Trifolium minus*) or white clover (*Trifolium repens*). Paraphrasing Colgan, Praeger tells us that the shamrock was a common Irish food until the late seventeenth century, when it was overtaken by the potato; English colonists and travellers recorded the name 'shamrock' as early as 1571. In the fate of the shamrock as a political emblem we witness the descent from folk protest through symbolism to the Irish-American sentimentality of today. A fairly recent legend (first recorded in 1727) has it that St Patrick demonstrated the trinity with a trefoil; whatever the truth of this, the plant had become a religious emblem and badge of nationality by 1700. In 1778 the Cork Volunteers sang 'The Shamrock Cockade'. John Keegan Casey, Fenian poet, published *A Wreath of Shamrocks: Ballads, Songs and Legends* in 1866; it contained the now-famous rebel song 'The Rising of the Moon'. *The Shamrock* was a nineteenth-century magazine that published nationalist poetry. (See Ardagh [1933] for a shamrock bibliography.)

By the end of the eighteenth century, the colour green itself had acquired a political meaning (Zimmermann, 1967), culminating in the street-ballad already referred to, 'The Wearing of the Green', which Yeats wove into his famous poem 'Easter 1916'. Ireland is nowadays everywhere associated with the colour green; against this association the colour orange – being not nearly as 'natural' a colour (like a partitioned Ireland, some would no doubt say) – makes little headway in the affections of those who are not Ulster unionists. The orange lily is the loyalists' shamrock, but its cultural association is little known outside Ulster and enclaves of loyalist sympathy abroad.

Despite the symbolic use of nature, and the patriot's love for the countryside (often abstractly conceived), natural history in the scientific sense had little appeal for Irish nationalism. To the exclusively political nationalist, science is of little use. As Clarke puts it (echoing popular belief), the scientist, 'unlike the writer, artist or patriot, is rarely a mere nationalist but always has been and always will be an internationalist'. Although thoughtful nationalists in Ireland might easily derive some patriotic pride from Irish achievements in science, such nationalists have frequently been inclined to literature and the arts but not (ill-advisedly) to science. Nationalism – though it fitted an international pattern established in various European movements: the French revolution, English and German Romanticisms – necessarily emphasized what is distinctively Irish in the island's culture in order to justify political separatism: mentality, language, folklore, spirituality, literature, and the survivals of a material culture from before the 'Conquests'.

Pride in Irish nature, if not in Irish natural history, is of course compatible with nationalism. In an essay for *The Nation* entitled 'Irish Scenery', the Young Irelander Thomas Davis challenges Irish travellers to postpone trips to the Continent in favour of travels through their own land: we might say that the Grand Tour of the Continent (a unionist itinerary very different from the nefarious journey of rebels to the Continent for military aid) is to become the National Tour. (Molly Ivors, fervent Irish nationalist, was later to challenge Gabriel Conroy to do the same thing in James Joyce's great story 'The Dead', written in 1907.) In 'Irish Scenery', Davis might be seen as a patron saint of the future Bord Fáilte (Davis, 1889). But it is not just the picturesque and antiquarian riches he promotes; he remarks that 'The Entomology, Botany, and Geology of Ireland are not half explored', not to speak of its ethnography, folk music, and social history. Although he reads here as a patron saint too of the naturalists' field clubs (the first of which started up less than two decades after he published his essay), Davis describes the landscape as scenery, a kind of cloak for the soul of Ireland. To travel amidst the scenery will instil love in the traveller, and love of country will advance the nationalist cause. The scientific study of Ireland per se does not seem greatly to appeal to Davis.

It has been pointed out (Jones, 1997) that in some countries science has been embraced by nationalists as a way of resisting colonialism, but this would not have been easy in nineteenth-century Ireland, even if it had been contemplated. The Anglo-Irish presence in science was dominant, and in the second half of the century the natural-history enthusiasm of northern Protestants (mostly of Dissenter tradition) might have further discouraged Catholics. In Ulster there may also have been a kind of displacement of energy at work: Brooke (1983) suggests that a sizeable volume of Catholic energy may have gone into the attempts by Gavan Duffy and others from the 1830s onwards (when the organized study of nature emerged in Ulster) to develop a distinct political voice in Belfast and elsewhere.

Nature and the Famine

Within a year of Davis's death in 1845, the potato crop in Ireland failed. The Great Famine had effects that far exceeded the death and starvation of those unlucky enough to fall prey to it. Suddenly, musings on Irish scenery would have seemed desperately beside the point. Through mortality and emigration, the population of the island – which had doubled between 1780 and 1845 (Connell, 1950/1) – shrank back to 1780s figures; the nearly six million inhabitants in 1811 had become eight and a quarter millions by 1845, but after the Famine the population rapidly diminished and was still diminishing steadily in 1908, as Murray noted in his report on 'The Depopulation of Ireland'. Swift had bemoaned the rural waste caused by the widespread conversion of arable land to pasturage in the early eighteenth century; Murray recorded a widespread change from pasturage back to tillage after Forster's Corn Law in 1784 and yet another reversal after the abolition of the corn laws (which Murray thought affected Ireland after 1846 more than the potato famine). All of these large-scale agricultural changes would have had enormous ecological effects, not to speak of the cultural effects.*

More immediately, the landscape altered in appearance when agriculture was neglected as the Famine took its grip, holdings lying idle, fields and hedgerows stripped of edible greenery and berries. William Steuart Trench, in *Realities of Irish Life* (1868), remembered that when the potato blight became endemic, luxuriant growths of potato plants were belied by the almost unbearable stench that rose from the fields. The land reverted to an unfruitful wildness, as Sir John Davies had warned in 1612 it would if husbandry and good seed failed. The Irish roaming for food resembled 'famishing wolves' (Woodham-Smith, 1962) – a disturbing echo of the lupine natives portrayed by the Elizabethans. William Carleton in his novel *The Black Prophet* (1847) re-created the landscape he had seen during the famines of 1817 and 1822 in order to represent the Famine of 1847: he offered a picture of 'the country, with its waste, unreaped crops, lying in a state of plashy and fermenting ruin, and its desolate and wintry aspect ...'. The Famine could permit among the writers a kind of anti-picturesque and anti-pastoral mode that was its own swerve from realism.

The effects of the changes in human population and landscape on Irish wildlife populations and distributions and on wildlife utilization, during and after the Famine, must have been considerable. One comes across scattered data. For example, Ussher tells us that the quail (*Coturnix coturnix*) was abundant before 1845, 'possibly owing to the growth of wheat' (after the 1784 corn law).

The extensive growth of wheat, leaving stubbles full of weeds, in the early part of the century, and the multiplication of potato-gardens up to the time of the famine ... were facts in favour of this bird at that period, and bevies of Quails used to be met with commonly through the winter months in every cultivated district .... After the famine, much of the tilled lands were turned into pasture or reverted into moor; and about 1850-53 I heard an old sportsman remark that Quails were then much less fre-

---

*The Famine was a disaster for the Irish language – survivors abandoning it because of the bad luck associated with it – and in the short run for cultural nationalism. It has been claimed by Emmet Larkin that it was only after the Famine that 'the mass of the Irish people became practising Catholics' (Evans, 1992).

quently met with in co. Waterford than they had been, while the Rev. C. Irvine dated their decrease in co. Tyrone from 1848' (Ussher and Warren, 1900).

Michael Viney (1986) has claimed to detect one far-reaching cultural effect of the Famine that is of moment to the historian of natural history. He is of the opinion that the Famine caused the native Irish (who suffered more than their northern Dissenter fellow-islanders) to distrust nature: 'In the biological treachery of the Famine, nature was disgraced.' It would be intriguing to seek documentary evidence for this in memoirs, tour-guides, travel accounts, novels, diaries and letters. Certainly a sense of the inadequacies of the Irish countryside would have been a motive for post-Famine emigration. Yet when that countryside was remembered by the emigrant (or the returned emigrant) in a song or poem, homesickness would usually dictate an ambivalence: the countryside is beautiful even when beggaring; see, for example, John Francis O'Donnell's 'The Return'. Ambivalence was often abandoned for an unabashed and stylized idealism: if Lady Dufferin's 'The Irish Emigrant' was not written by an impoverished emigrant, its popularity made it by proxy the sentimental expression of such emigrants.

Nature and the Irish Countryman

Before and after the Famine, the inhabitants of the Big House and its demesne exercised a surplus biblical dominion over nature (stretching beyond utility and necessity into aesthetics, leisure and connoisseurship) with their agriculture, horticulture, natural history, and field sports (see Viney and Reeves-Smyth in this volume). But the native population had more pragmatic anxieties; in J.M. Synge's famous play *The Playboy of the Western World* (1907), an inappropriate appreciation of nature (particularly of birds: 'felts and finches') is what marks Christy Mahon as a half-wit, according to his father. ('Felts' was a colloquial Irish word for thrushes.) Land-hunger and land-greed are what motivate the relationship of Synge's peasants to nature.

Patrick Kavanagh's *The Green Fool* (1938) and *Tarry Flynn* (1948), set in counties Cavan and Monaghan, corroborate the Syngean picture and likewise present title characters whose love of nature is seen by their fellows as proof of near-idiocy. This was the survival of an earlier attitude outside Ireland. The first professional biologist to visit the New World, Peter Kalm, found on his travels of 1748 to 1751, that among the inhabitants there was 'little account made of Natural History ... science being here (as in other parts of the world) looked upon as a mere trifle, and the pastime of fools'.*

---

*It is to be remembered that up until recently bird-watchers were regarded by many Britons and Irish people as rather eccentric persons of obscure motive. It was the

Paradoxically, the real Irish depicted by Synge and Kavanagh were closer to nature than the cultivators of demesnes, but they seemingly could not distance, objectify or appreciate it. Even though their experience of nature was also cultural, mediated through husbandry and their own informal field sports, the distinction between nature and culture does not appear to have pressed urgently or philosophically upon them.

This, and the attendant ambiguities when the distinction is attempted, is what make the diary of Amhlaoibh Ó Súilleabháin (Humphrey O'Sullivan, 1780-1837) so interesting. O'Sullivan was the son of a schoolteacher who taught in a sheepshed, then a sod-wall schoolhouse. He lived in Callan, Co. Kilkenny, and taught school himself after his father's death in 1808 and also became a drapery shopkeeper. He kept his diary in Irish between 1 April 1827 (with retrospective entries from January) and July 1835. The diary has been called by its editor 'a document not only modern but, in Irish literature, unique of its kind' (O'Sullivan, 1936); it is said to rank 'as one of the most significant of the non-imaginative Irish prose writings in the nineteenth century' (Williams and Ford, 1992).

Of interest to the natural historian are the entries that cover botany, birds, agriculture, floods, moving bogs, and the weather. O'Sullivan can inhabit the world of folklore: 'This, the twelfth day of April [1827], is the first of the three days of the old brindled cow, namely three days which the weather of Old March took from the beginning of Old April.' (There follows the story.) But there is plenty of serious natural history, far more so than in Tomás Ó Crohan's much later *The Islandman* (1929 in Irish, 1934 in English). This entry for 30 April 1828 is an example:

The fourth day, Sunday. Morning showery; afternoon, clouds and bright intervals: a hard west wind. I see the cowslip. Its calyx and leaf are just like those of the primrose; but [the flowers of the] cowslip are in clusters, while those of the primrose are all apart. There is a great difference between the crowfoot and the buttercup. One of them, the crowfoot, is hirsute, and the other, the buttercup, smooth. There are five lobes in the calyx of the crowfoot, and only three in that of the buttercup; and, in the crowfoot, the male organs are more numerous than they are in the buttercup; moreover, in the crowfoot the leaf is long like grass; in the buttercup, it is like a heart; though both of them have a yellow corona, there is a great difference in the parts [of the corona], for they are oval in the crowfoot and elongated, like the blade of a knife in the buttercup .... What I have been calling the crowfoot is really the buttercup. I do not know the name of that which I call the buttercup.

Americans who reversed this unflattering perception, doing so by changing the name of the activity (from the passive bird-watching to the active birding, cf. hunting or fishing) and by making obligatory an impressive and even armour-like apparatus for the activity (scopes, binoculars, special rain gear, plastic-covered field-guides, fashionable hiking-boots, etc.), commanding the respect of at least American passers-by.

It would be interesting to know where O'Sullivan got his sexual classification, his interest in detailed distinctions between plants, and his sense of
nature as an ecosystem (though this concept would have been at best blurred
for him, and the term beyond him in the distant future). It is hard to know
how unusual O'Sullivan was in his attention to the particularities of nature.
It may be that the dismissive, utterly pragmatic attitude dramatized in Synge
was most in evidence in the west of Ireland with its peculiarly disobliging
landscape.

Nature and Colonization: The Waste Places

The most disobliging landscape of all, the 'waste' landscape of Famine
Ireland, was not an entirely new phenomenon. Spenser referred in the 1590s
to the 'Irish deserts' and the 'waste wild places' to which rebels and outlaws
repaired, and Swift too, a century and a quarter later, bemoaned the uncultivated expanses. In his article 'The Colonization of Waste Land in Ireland,
1780-1845', K.H. Connell gives us the remarkable fact that two hundred and
fifty years after Spenser, despite the hugely expanded population and land-
hunger, 'there remained idle at the time of the Famine nearly four million
acres which agriculturists and engineers were convinced were capable of economic development': more than a fifth of the cultivable area of the island
(Connell, 1950/1).

This would have been good news for many species of plant and animal, though it is a pity we have no population censuses by which to chart
the changes in species diversity and numbers between 1780 – when some
serious land reclamation began – and 1845, and between 1845 and the present. To take an almost random example for amusement: riding between the
villages of Somerford and Ocksey in Wiltshire during thistle season in 1826,
Richard Cobbett on horseback flushed parties of goldfinches until at last
there was a flock of what he estimated as ten thousand birds in front of him
(Cobbett, 1912, II). One wonders if such an experience of this (or some
other) species of bird was available at that time to the traveller in the unreclaimed regions of Ireland.

There is of course semi-anecdotal, semi-scientific evidence of numbers
in Ireland of obvious species between 1780 and 1845, for example the gold-
en and white-tailed sea eagles, though in the case of these birds, human persecution rather than human habitation or habitat changes appears to have
been the decisive factor in this decline (Thompson, 1849-56, I). Reclamation
probably resulted in fewer species of plant and animal being extinguished
and more species expanding their range, because cultivation meant greater
habitat diversity.

In discussing how birds reacted to 'the operations of man', Thompson gives the example of a mid-nineteenth-century marsh near Belfast, five hundred feet above the neighbouring sea. It was drained and the only avian inhabitant, the snipe, vanished. But 'as cultivation advanced, the numerous species of small birds attendant on it, became visitors, and plantations soon made them inhabitants of the place'. Corncrakes haunted the meadows, quail and partridge the grain-fields; an artificial pond attracted mallard and teal and a pair of sandpipers; planted willows by the water's edge brought the kingfisher, heron, moorhen, and pied and grey wagtails. The snipe returned; swallows and martins hunted flies above the pond; the sedge-warbler and willow-warbler became seasonal visitors; planted alders brought redpolls in winter, the larches various tits and the goldcrest. And so on (Thompson, 1849-56, I). By contrast, quail in the nineteenth century were found on the edges of bogs, and not in the bogs themselves: 'consequently their haunts were circumscribed in those western counties which are chiefly unreclaimed' (Ussher and Warren, 1900).

The colonization of waste ground went on apace in the years Connell analyses. Between 1841 and 1851, 1,330,281 acres had been added to the cultivated area of Ireland, but the Famine had devastated the population and slowed down the colonizing process. Nevertheless, the habitat alteration and the corresponding alterations in animal and plant populations must have been striking. Reclamation was furthered by, and simultaneously resulted in, the building and improvement of roads, and it is interesting that road-books first became popular when the colonization of waste ground was in full swing. These roads must have been useful to the growing numbers of amateur naturalists who took to the field in the later nineteenth century.

Yet in 1845 a fifth of the country remained mountain or bog, some of it simply not worth reclaiming. Acreage was further wasted during the continuing depopulation of the west after the Famine. It is noteworthy that the west was the symbolic site of Ireland's real (and belated) Romantic movement – the Irish Literary Revival between the 1880s and the founding of the Irish Free State (Foster, 1987). Yeats and Synge in particular 'cultivated' in their writing – 'reclaimed' for Anglo-Irish literature, we might say – the 'desolate places' (Yeats's phrase), amid a general celebration of Irish nature, which they suffused with mysticism, charm and poetry. The transformation of poverty and neglect into stark beauty (for example, Synge's Aran Islands) and western lushness into pastoral (for example, Yeats's Innisfree) was a species of cultural colonization that paralleled the colonization of waste ground by various agencies.

Indeed, the effort of waste-land reclamation in Ireland could be regarded as an element of colonization in the political and economic senses, and much of the reclamation was conducted on the demesnes and properties of Anglo-Irish landlords. Of course, in another sense Irish nature had already been profoundly colonized; for example, the majority of Irish lake and river fish species were introduced by the Anglo-Irish down the centuries, and several species of mammals and birds.

It should be noted, however, that the reclamation of waste ground was not merely an Irish project; it was a British project as well. Chambers's *Information for the People*, a nineteenth-century encyclopedia that included natural history, devotes numerous pages to the subject of 'Culture of Waste Lands – Spade Husbandry'. The writer estimates that there were thirty million acres of waste land in the British Isles at the time of writing. The reclamation of waste ground in England, Scotland and Wales would surely have had some knock-on effects in the neighbouring island in terms of animal populations and even distributions, though sufficient data may not exist for us to assess the scale of these. Yet Ussher and Warren in their important 1900 survey, *The Birds of Ireland*, pointedly offered their readers a map of Ireland with the sizeable areas of unreclaimed land indicated in brown, most of them on the western seaboard. They regarded the unreclaimed land as 'a division which is important in determining the character of the avifauna, especially as such lands are chiefly tracts of peat' (Ussher and Warren, 1900).

Natural History and Colonization: Places of Knowledge

It has been claimed that the energetic setting up of museums, including natural history museums, in the nineteenth century in the British colonies and dependencies was a form of cultural colonialism and a way of 'civilizing by nature's example' (Sheets-Pyenson, 1981). The claim would be reinforced by the belief of Richard Owen, the famous Victorian naturalist, that museums furthered British imperialism; when he was Superintendent at the British Museum (Natural History), South Kensington, naturalists in the colonies had to send their specimens back to the imperial capital for cataloguing. The museum in South Kensington opened its doors in 1881; there were two thousand scientific museums in existence by 1910, serving to enlighten and entertain a burgeoning middle class with increased mobility and wealth (Sheets-Pyenson, 1981). By the late nineteenth century colonial legislators were supporting public museums: these in turn gave work to British and Irish naturalists (see 'Naturalists Abroad' in this volume) and presumably stimulated the profession of 'naturalist' in the twentieth century. Much of the data and many of the specimens collected abroad were returned to the mother country and the metropolitan museums, but the colonial museums also adapted themselves to local circumstances and sometimes protected local material from transfer to European institutions (Sheets-Pyenson, 1981, 1988).

Certain scholars have interpreted the rise of natural-history institutions in nineteenth-century Ireland (societies, museums, government departments) by means of this colonial model (Jarrell, 1981; Yearley, 1989), and have done so using the concept of dependency central to the understanding of colonial culture as well as colonial politics. Jarrell has recounted what he regards as the careful, systematic, bureaucratic takeover of key Irish scientific institutions in the nineteenth century by the Department of Science and Art in London, and interprets this as a colonialist strategy. The extent to which Ireland then was rather different in its relationship to Britain from Australia, Canada and New Zealand, certainly from India and South Africa, complicates matters: unlike these other countries, Ireland was at once a colony and a partner country in the United Kingdom. Jones (1997) has suggested the limitations of the colonial model of interpretation of nineteenth-century natural history in Ireland, but the usefulness of the model is undeniable.

Dependency, as far as it exists, can cause the resentfully dependent (as distinct from 'the gratefully oppressed', to quote James Joyce's stinging phrase) to turn actively in another direction from the colonizers, and to seek a different independence: perhaps, in the Irish case, a cultural independence that excluded science. If nationalism inclines to neglect science for being insufficiently rooted in place, it can also neglect science when the latter is perceived as rooted in the wrong place and by the wrong people. Of the nineteenth century, Jarrell remarks: 'There were two Irelands, and almost all the scientists were Anglo-Irish. Trinity College, the Royal Dublin Society, and the Royal Irish Academy were near exclusive preserves of the minority .... In centres outside Dublin, especially in Cork and Belfast, the scientific leaders were equally Anglo-Irish. Were there scientists in the "other" Ireland? There were, of course, but few in number.' (The distinction between the Anglo-Irish and the Ulster Scots that Jarrell neglects somewhat complicates his picture.)

Certainly there were at work in Ireland perceptions of ethnicity that were more significant than their counterparts in England and Scotland. Science was itself in danger in Ireland of being ethnicized as foreign and an imposition (not truly Irish), as well as being categorized as anti-religious (not acceptably Catholic) and socially remote.

One way for the self-perceived nationalist (not to be regarded as synonymous with the Catholic) to pursue science under the rankling circumstances of political dependency, was to cultivate 'ethnic' natural history. A rare attempt to marry science to Celtic nationalism was Michael Moloney's curious book, *Irish Ethno-Botany and the Evolution of Medicine in Ireland* (1919). It essays a history of a national (or indigenous) medicine, claims that the study of 'Celtic nature creeds' should enter the economy and the educational curriculum, that the centre of Irish medicine should be ethno-botany, and that 'a study of ... native flora in his own tongue [i.e. the Irish language] will enable the student to inherit some of the scientific, literary, aesthetic, and religious possessions of the race'. Long before the French cultural theorist

Michel Foucault (see Outram in this volume), Moloney believed that science is 'situated' and socially and even politically mediated. Despite Matthew Arnold and before C.P. Snow (see 'The Culture of Nature', this volume), Moloney saw no essential or necessary division between science and literature, and it was the nationalist project that enabled him to do so.

Moloney's contribution to nationalism seems to have petered out: *Irish Ethno-Botany* does not appear to have been emulated in other fields of natural history. Corrigan, however, has re-opened for discussion that branch of ethnobotany ('the study of the relationship between man and his ambient vegetation') he calls ethnopharmacology, and suggests that, with scientific caution, the inter-disciplinary subject could be pursued. A history of the subject would include the contribution of Aodh Mac Dómhnaill (Hugh McDonnell, 1802-67), whose *Fealsunacht* (Philosophy) is said to rank along-side Amhlaoibh Ó Súilleabháin's diary as the best non-imaginative Irish prose work of the nineteenth century (Williams and Ford, 1992). Born in Co. Meath, McDonnell became involved in helping Protestant societies use the Irish language for proselytizing purposes. He worked in the field in the Glens of Antrim and became an associate of the versatile Shipboy McAdam, Belfast folklorist, Irish-language enthusiast, inventor and foundry-owner. McDonnell's *Fealsunacht* was written in Belfast (Beckett, 1987); it includes extensive lists of Irish plants (many of them of medicinal repute), of fishes, and of birds, both in Irish and 'with their names in western Europe' (Beckett, 1967). McDonnell's natural history appears to have been largely overlooked by historians of the subject. It is, of course, for cultural reasons an itinerant record-keeping, very different from the institutional natural history of eighteenth- and nineteenth-century Anglo-Ireland.

The situation Jarrell depicts was a function of political and class power inside Ireland as well as between Ireland and England, and the Anglo-Irish had their 'places of knowledge': estates, gentlemen's houses, observatories, botanical gardens, rooms of curiosities. And so what Yaron Ezrahi says would seem vividly to apply to the Irish case: 'the place of knowledge is implicated in the network of relations between knowledge and power, in the distribution of knowledge in society, in perceptions of its validity and legitimacy' (Ophir and Shapin, 1991).

But there were those among the Anglo-Irish whose activities and opinions complicated the situation. Thomas Davis, a Protestant, stood in the historical sequence of Anglo-Irish leaders of Irish nationalists. He believed that in order to attain nationality, it was necessary 'to increase and economise the exertions of the literary class in Ireland'. In his essay 'Institutions of Dublin', he claimed that this could be helped by a thorough institutional reorganization. He suggested reducing the city's numerous institutions – the Royal Dublin Society, the Royal Irish Academy, the Irish Archaeological Society, the Royal Zoological Society, the Geological Society, the Dublin Natural History Society, the Dublin Philosophical Society, the Royal Agricultural Society, etc. – to just three. They would be the Royal Irish Academy, the Royal Dublin Society, and a new Natural History Society or Academy with a 'specially Irish museum'. (In the cases of the first two, he wished to abandon the adjective of patronage, 'Royal'; interestingly, it was dropped in neither case even when the Irish Free State became the Republic of Ireland in 1949.)

He particularly wished the Royal Irish Academy to 'divorce' itself from its scientific department, retaining its interest only in antiquities and literature (both of which can further the project of nationality). Science (i.e. the 'hard' sciences) would revert to Trinity College, which would be 'required' to form a voluntary organization for the purpose. Housed in a new Academy, natural history was clearly in Davis's mind reclaimable for cultural nationalism, whereas the exact sciences were to be returned to their original enclave where Irish nationality was of small matter.

What actually happened in the nineteenth century is as complicated as any institutional history. Apart from the normal exchanges that took place between scientific institutions, including those between Irish and English institutions, there was correspondence (in the scientific fashion) between Irish scientists and the major British associations (to which I will return), and an impressive set of Irish serial publications to which British as well as Irish scientists contributed. The journals offer evidence both of the level of Irish activity and of the participation of Irish scientists in the international exchange of data, methods, and results, since bodies abroad subscribed to the major Irish serials. The National Academy of Sciences, Philadelphia, for example, holds the following: Royal Irish Academy, *Transactions* (1787-1906) and *Proceedings* (1836-); Royal Dublin Society, *Journal* (1856-), *Scientific Proceedings* (1877-1957, 1960-) and *Scientific Transactions* (1877-1909); Belfast Natural History and Philosophical Society, *Proceedings and Reports* (1852-1956); Dublin University Zoological and Botanical Association, *Proceedings* (1857-60); Dublin Natural History Society, *Proceedings* (1860-4); Belfast Naturalists' Field Club, *Annual Report and Proceedings* (1865-); Dublin Biological Association, *Proceedings* (1875-); *Irish Naturalist* (1892-1924).

Amidst all this activity, by 1900 a clear pattern of devolution in the institutional control of science had established itself, with the newly created Department of Agriculture and Technical Instruction for Ireland assuming responsibility for the Inspectorate of Irish Fisheries, for example, then taking over from South Kensington 'all the scientific intitutions which the [British] government had acquired in the previous century: the National Museum, the Botanic Gardens, the Royal College of Science and from 1905 the Geological Survey as well' (Whyte, 1997). Indeed, devolution was such as to pose a dilemma of loyalty for English scientists working in Ireland, one

which some resolved by pressing the claims of Irish science. Whyte has identified an upsurge in Irish scientific activity (including zoology and botany)
in the period 1900-14, a period disrupted by the outbreak of the Great War.

On the other hand, the ambiguous identity of the relevant metropolis
(was it to be Dublin or London?) created discomfiture among Ireland's
administrative scientists, and lapses in loyalty to Ireland among English scientists assumed a political tinge in the years approaching 1922, the year
Home Rule was achieved for part of the island. It was impossible to keep
the conduct of science innocent of the serious political developments that led
to the creation of the Free State and Northern Ireland. Whyte recounts
Timothy Corcoran's attempt to set up a National Academy of Ireland in
response to the Royal Irish Academy's refusal to re-admit Eoin MacNeill as
a member after his expulsion following the Easter Rising. (MacNeill was a
leader of the Irish Volunteers, though he countermanded the order to rise.)
The proposed National Academy sank without trace in 1922; the RIA rein-
stated MacNeill and has continued since then to receive Irish government
financial support (Whyte, 1997).

Natural History and Catholicism

It was just such a casting off of science as Thomas Davis seemed to advocate that John Cardinal Newman apparently counselled against. He did so
not as a nationalist or an Anglo-Irishman, but as a Roman Catholic. Newman
was invited in 1851 to become the first Rector of the Catholic University in
Dublin, established because of Catholic dissatisfaction with the constitution
of the three existing Queen's Colleges. This institution was the forebear of
today's National University of Ireland. Newman set out his views on the
ideal curriculum of a Catholic university – and the place of science in it –
in a series of lectures and addresses to the university in Dublin before and
after it opened its doors in 1854; these eventually comprised *The Idea of a
University* (1873).

Newman is at pains to dispel the popular idea that the physical sciences
are essentially or even contingently at odds with Revelation (theology, i.e.
Catholicism). The two are employed upon the two different kinds of knowledge – the natural and the supernatural; and their methods are unlike, one
inductive, the other deductive. By 'nature', Newman means 'that vast system of things, taken as a whole, of which we are cognizant by means of our
natural powers'. Revelation, on the other hand, is the 'direct interference
from above, for the introduction of truths otherwise unknown'. Therefore
'Theology and Science ... in their own actual fields ... are ... incapable of
collision and [need] never to be reconciled.'

This admission of complementarity of disciplines, this intellectual rendering unto Caesar, as it were, that which is Caesar's, is a strand of Newman's famous educational liberalism. There is, however, an impression of reluctance when Newman comes to science, as my biblical allusion suggests. This stems from the domination of modern science by Protestants up until Newman's day. Protestant scientists are acceptable teachers qua scientists but not qua Protestants: that is, should they exceed the strict bounds of their science. It would, of course, be preferable if scientific textbooks written by Catholics were available, but the existing situation is workable as long as the intellectual partition between theology and science is rigidly maintained. The rigidity of this maintenance is the other side of Newman's liberalism, for he regarded himself as engaged in a crusade against the 'liberalism' of secular thought in Britain and Ireland.

'Catholic Theology has nothing to fear from the progress of Physical Science', Newman asserts; still, he does not positively encourage the practice of science by Catholic students. Indeed, it is even implied in his lectures that if the work of the sciences has to be conducted, better it be conducted by Protestants lest the partition ever prove porous. This 'default mechanism' remained operative in Catholic Ireland long after Newman and well into the twentieth century. Certain appointments of Catholics to scientific posts to the contrary (Jones, 1997), science appears to have been culturally 'ceded' to the Anglo-Irish and the Ulster Scots by the powers that were; there was no official proscription but no official encouragement either. Newman set the agenda in the 1850s.

Newman muses on the intellectual intercourse between science and revelation historically practised by some Protestants. This is a reference to natural (or physical) theology, and he derives it from William Paley. He confesses to viewing it 'with the greatest suspicion', and finds its theological deficiencies decisive. 'What does Physical Theology tell us of duty and conscience? of a particular providence? and, coming at length to Christianity, what does it teach us even of the four last things, death, judgment, heaven, and hell, the mere elements of Christianity? It cannot tell us anything of Christianity at all.' It is 'a naturalistic, pantheistic' religion and to be rejected outright. This kind of stricture would have made anxious one of Newman's young admirers. The 'nature poet' Gerard Manley Hopkins, a convert like Newman to Roman Catholicism, was worried by his own passionate attraction to the shapes, sights and sounds of nature. It was not just the difficulty of leaving Anglicanism that perplexed Hopkins, but the difficulty of being attracted to literature with its inevitable elements of paganism (especially that of Ancient Greece, but also Wordsworth's), humanism (especially Arnold's) and aestheticism (especially Walter Pater's). After becoming a Jesuit in 1868 (and burning his poems) and preaching or ministering in

England and Scotland, Hopkins was appointed in 1884 to the Chair of Classics at University College Dublin, then a Jesuit college, descendant of Newman's Catholic University.

Though tortured and exalted by nature and poetry, Hopkins painstakingly fashioned his own intense brand of natural theology both in verse – which he resumed in some guilt – and in the prose of his notebooks and letters. He was a strikingly original observer of nature, interpreting the form and coherence of plants and animals in terms of organic force in a way that combined Romantic subjectivity with the naturalist's objectivity, aesthetic appreciation with a fieldworker's intense scrutiny. Consult any selection of his poems, letters and notebooks for copious examples; his description of an oak tree is as good an example as any (Gardner, 1953). Hopkins might even be regarded as a patron saint of biodiversity (see his poem 'Glory be to God for dappled things'), of conservation (see his poem 'Binsey Poplars') and of environmentalism (as long as it is underpinned by a respect for the otherness and lowlinesses of nature):

> What would the world be, once bereft
> Of wet and of wildness? Let them be left,
> O let them be left, wildness and wet;
> Long live the weeds and the wilderness yet.
>
> ('Inversnaid')

Newman held that 'Reason cannot but illustrate and defend Revelation', and this paradoxically anti-Enlightenment stance can be taken as characteristic of the Catholic Church in Ireland after the mid-nineteenth century. His fond recall of medieval Catholic universities was, *mutatis mutandis*, shared by the native Irish churchmen, and the medieval element in modern Irish culture remained significant until the time of Joyce and even after. In his Prefaces to a reprint of his *Address Delivered before The British Association Assembled at Belfast* (1874), John Tyndall, the physicist and champion of Darwinism (b. Co. Carlow, 1820), responding to the outrage that greeted his speech, remarked that it was in the Middle Ages that scientists had essentially won their battle against obscurantism.

But it was of course the issue of organic evolution that had aroused the wrath of the clergy, led in Ireland by Cardinal Cullen who, when Archbishop of Armagh, had invited Newman to Dublin. Newman's unease about the possibility that science, dominated by Protestants, would transgress its boundaries and infect the piety of his students, seems to have hardened in his successors into a determination that such an event could not take place. Tyndall is happy to agree with Cardinal Cullen that – in Tyndall's words – 'the Catholic youth around [Cullen] are not proof to the seductions of science', and happy to disagree with Cullen's belief that science can be held at bay. Tyndall cites 'a Memorial addressed by Seventy of the Students and Ex-students of the Catholic University in Ireland to the Episcopal Board of the University'. According to Tyndall 'it expresses the profoundest dissatisfaction with the curriculum marked out for the students': the faculty, the memorialists pointed out, 'did not contain the name of a single Professor of the Physical or Natural Sciences'. They claimed that 'Irish Catholics are writhing under the sense of their inferiority in science' and will seek training in it at the other Irish colleges should it continue to be withheld from them at the Catholic University. (It was precisely to prevent this that Newman contemplated science as a university subject in the first place.) Tyndall is hopeful that after centuries of obedience, 'the Irish intellect is beginning to show signs of independence'; 'The youth of Ireland will imbibe science, however gradually.'

Tyndall's speech raised Protestant hackles too, and he refers acidly to the resolution passed by the Presbytery of Belfast accusing Huxley and him, in their explication and defence of Darwinism, of 'ignoring the existence of God, and advocating pure and simple materialism'. (It is an historical irony that the year that saw the publication of Darwin's *Origin of Species* – 1859 – also saw a great Protestant revival in Ulster – 'the Year of Grace' – that spread to other parts of the United Kingdom [Gibson, 1860].) But in one of his Prefaces Tyndall re-phrases what he said in his speech, which was this: 'In the course of scientific investigation, then, as I have tried to impress upon you, we make continual incursions from a physical world where we observe facts, into a super- or sub-physical world, where the facts elude all observation, and we are thrown back upon the picturing power of the mind' (Tyndall, 1874).

If this is yet compatible with materialist explanations of the universe (science simply overcoming its inadequacies without relapsing into supernatural explanations; the human imagination itself an evolved capacity), it is a materialism compatible with the achievements of art and literature: one of Tyndall's epigraphs is a set of lines from Wordsworth's 'Tintern Abbey' (1798) that refers famously to the motion and spirit that rolls through all of nature, including 'the mind of man'. And Tyndall was, after all, the author of an 1870 essay, 'Scientific Use of the Imagination', to which I have already referred.

But the ranks of Protestantism were disordered against Tyndall and Darwinism (see Livingstone in this volume), because many devout Protestants were also practising scientists, keen naturalists and sophisticated theologians. This was not the case with the spokesmen of Irish Catholicism. The Church that saw off the threat of modernism around the turn of the twentieth century (Foster, 1987) was unlikely to advance the cause of Enlightenment science, much less Darwinism. Clarke reminds us that

Maynooth College, Catholic Ireland's venerable chief seminary, 'has had a strong scientific tradition in what used to be called applied science': this claim seems beyond dispute. But what is one to make of Jarrell's claim (1981) that he has been 'unable to detect any significant antiscience bias on the part of the clergy in … Ireland during the nineteenth century'? The situation changed, of course, in the later decades of the twentieth century. Outram (1988) has briefly discussed some doctrinal difficulties for Catholicism presented by science in general and natural history in particular. But any remaining opposition to the methodology and practice of the natural sciences and natural history on the part of the Irish Catholic Church has become primarily historical or has dwindled to mere reservations – reflecting the shrinking role of the Church in Irish society – and Catholic (or lapsed Catholic) naturalists now play their full part in these disciplines, thus fulfilling Newman's cautious educational hopes for the future.

Aspects of Evolution

Natural theology was not proof against the threat posed by the theory of evolution to the alliance Protestantism had forged with natural history. There had been Christians opposed to natural theology before evolution appeared on the horizon, Thomas Burnet and Joseph Butler among them, for whom Nature and Revelation were essentially mysterious (Willey, 1957). And it was before publication of *Origin of Species* in 1859 that peace between religion and science was actively sought. There were those who saw a serious disparity between revealed religion and the alleged evidence of nature. At the time of Charles Lyell's challenging geological syntheses, the celebrated geologist Hugh Miller saw his task in *The Testimony of the Rocks* (1857) as the uncovering of 'that scheme of reconciliation between the Geologic and Mosaic Records which accepts the six days of creation as vastly extended periods'. The celebrated naturalist Philip Henry Gosse attempted a reconciliation the same year: *Omphalos: An Attempt to Untie the Geological Knot*.

The existence of fossils connected the geological issues of the age of the Earth and the profound changes in the Earth unaccounted for in the Bible with the zoological issues of the age of life and its profound changes likewise unaccounted for in the Bible. It was the organic evolution of Wallace and Darwin that had the most immediate impact on religion, society and even politics. However much the theory was denied by naturalists as respected as Philip Henry Gosse and Richard Owen, it was the scientists associated with evolution – Lyell, Darwin, Wallace, Tyndall, Haeckel, Huxley – who brought the submerged rivalry between science and religion to the surface where it had to be faced. Henceforward, culture in Britain and Protestant

Ireland was a divided empire. Indeed, it was divided three ways – among science, religion and literature – and there is no more graphic portrait of the triangular contest in the mind of one individual than the masterly memoir by Gosse's son Edmund in *Father and Son* (1907).

That memoir includes a poignant account of the dismay and mockery that greeted *Omphalos*, particularly its theory of prochronism, the idea that God had created and placed the fossils amidst the geological record as though the Earth had existed, and species had lived and died, before the Creation. A later essay in reconciliation was Samuel Kinns's *Moses and Geology; or, The Harmony of The Bible with Science* (1882, rev. 1884). This large book accepts the evolutionists' notions of cultivation (or improvement) by artificial selection; natural selection (survival of the fittest); development by use; and variation; yet still constructs ingenious arguments that form a baffle between these and the master idea of organic evolution. As for fossils, they are evidence of revelation, not evolution – 'this must have been one of the many providential arrangements to reveal to us the "story of His hand-iwork"', a divinely deposited narrative of the past. Besides, the discontinu-ity of the fossil record, like the persistence of organs and characters (the eye of the bee resembling fundamentally that of the trilobite, say, in the arrange-ment of nerves), argue against Darwin's notion of unbroken evolution.

I mention Kinns partly because of the manifesto signed by 617 scien-tists at the British Association 1865 meeting, which he reproduces along with the list of signatories. 'We, the undersigned students of the Natural Sciences,' the manifesto read, 'desire to express our sincere regret that researches into scientific truth are perverted by some in our own times into occasions for casting doubt upon the truth and authenticity of the Holy Scriptures. We conceive that it is impossible for the Word of God as writ-ten in the book of Nature, and God's Word written in Holy Scripture, to contradict one another; however much they may appear to differ.' Eventually, it affirmed, the manner in which the two records can be recon-ciled will be revealed to us by God. The pressure to sign such a manifesto much have been enormous, apart from the intrinsic merit it would have struck some signatories as having. Among the signatories (Gosse of course is there) can be found the Acting Palaeontologist of the Geological Survey of Ireland (W.H. Baily); the late Demonstrator of Anatomy in the University of Dublin (C.H. Bowdler Bell); and Gen. F.R. Chesney, subject of a profile in this volume ('Naturalists Abroad'). Undoubtedly there are other names on the list associated with Ireland.

This was a dispute largely between believing and lapsed Protestants. As was not the case in Ireland, the parties to the dispute in England sprang from a common culture. The dissimilar situation in Ireland perhaps explains why the evolution debate did not occupy centre stage in Catholic Ireland:

the strength of the pre-scientific culture in Catholic Ireland and of the Catholic Church did not permit this to happen.

Tyndall was a major player in the evolution debate; he was, says Irvine, 'Huxley rarefied and intensified', capable both of pugnacious argument – as in his Belfast address: 'more important than the Huxley/Wilberforce clash in 1860', according to Cosslett (1984) – and of popular writing of a Wordsworthian flavour and flair. He was the son of an Orangeman and was himself an opponent of Home Rule for Ireland. Indeed, Di Gregorio reminds us that 'like many of the "progressive" scientists of his time, such as Tyndall, Lubbock, and Stokes, Huxley was a convinced Unionist'. Gladstone, who supported Home Rule, was an opponent of Huxley's on political as well as theological grounds. The political coloration of the scientists, particularly of Tyndall – who because he was born a Protestant in Ireland was, he professed, 'taught to hold my own against the Church of Rome' (Tyndall, 1874) – must surely (however fractionally) have stiffened the resistance of the Irish Catholic hierarchy to science in general and biology in particular. To Newman's concerns over the anti-theological inclinations of science could be added Irish concerns over the anti-nationalist and anti-Catholic inclinations of British scientists.

While it would be rash to suggest that the internationalism and co-operativism of science might incline the individual to Irish unionism rather than Irish nationalism, it would be less rash to suggest that the involvement of (mostly Protestant) Irish scientists in the British science scene might cause the notion of political and institutional separatism to provoke anxieties on the parts both of the British and Irish workers. Each *Report of the British Association for the Advancement of Science* indicates the depth of that involvement. As expected, the involvement is deepest in the Reports of those years in which the BA met in Ireland: 1835 (Dublin), 1843 (Cork), 1852, 1874 (Belfast), 1908 (Dublin). Among the authors of major or section reports across those years we find names familiar to historians of Irish natural history – Thompson, Tyndall, Bryce, Forbes, Griffith, Jukes, McAdam, Dickie, McCosh, Hyndman, Stewart, Cole, Patten, Welch, Green. The British scientific community was a warp and weft of connections: shared data, correspondence, mutual guided visits, overlapping society and club memberships.

The immediate career of evolutionism in British culture would not have allayed Catholic, especially Irish Catholic, anxieties. Evolutionary theory inserted *Homo sapiens* into the order of nature, and made of him the object of natural history, ethnology and anthropology. Humanity, in first making an impact on nature and then dominating it, was acting as a species in nature; one of Huxley's books was entitled *Evidence as to Man's Place in Nature* (1863). Yet in the direction of culture, it became difficult to keep the ethnological interest of Huxley and others separate from contemporary politics.

Home Rulers frequently spoke of Scotland and Ireland as separate ethnic nationalities, but Huxley and his associates were convinced that there was an admixture of Celtic and Germanic blood throughout the British Isles and that ethnicity did not support dissolution of the Union (Di Gregorio, 1984).

Huxley regarded most of the Irish (wrongly, in his opinion, called Celts) as of the 'Melanchroic' type of humanity; that is, a hybrid of the major 'Xanthochroic' (European) and 'Australoid' types. The Irish could be no more Celtic than the Cornish, and if certain virtues were claimed for the latter (intelligence, perseverance, thrift, industry, sobriety, lawfulness), they must logically be claimed for the former. Huxley's unpleasant assumption is that clearly no one would claim most of those virtues for the Irish. Despite Huxley's apparent anti-Irishness, his conviction of admixture (Celtic blood flows in English veins) translated itself politically into liberal unionism, but unionism nevertheless.

Others in England were unionists of an illiberal and anti-Irish stripe, for whom the Union had to do with English hegemony rather than Protestant rights in Ireland. These often portrayed the Irish in terms derived from evolutionism. The Irish had before been harshly depicted by their political enemies and racial detractors in terms deriving from natural history. Political readers of Mary Shelley's *Frankenstein* (1818) appropriated the rampaging monster as the embodiment of republicanism, be it Godwinism in England or Jacobinism in France, and their interpretation was reinforced by Burke's frequent representation of revolution as monstrous (Sterrenburg, 1979). Behind such political demonization was the pre-evolutionary perception of nature as consisting of fixed species, a divinely ordained order occasionally violated by monsters, hybrids originating from the devil. (Victor Frankenstein reads Pliny and Buffon, and the former's natural history is full of the monstrous.) Late eighteenth-century naturalists were enthralled specifically by reports of monstrous 'men of the woods'.

Because of the 1798 rebellion and the uprising in 1803, it was easy to equate the monster of Irish insurrectionary republicanism with the monster of Jacobinism. This monster took the form of Frankenstein's creation after the Phoenix Park murders of 1882 and the Irish agrarian outrages: the 'created' or 'slave' Irish are depicted as turning upon their masters (Sterrenburg, 1979).* It also took the form of the missing link, the ape-like ancestor that Bishop Wilberforce repudiated (as a blasphemy and a caricature) and that Darwin's theory required. The simian Irish, studied in Victorian caricature by Curtis (1971), succeeded the lupine Irish and man-of-the-woods Irish ('*Satyrus sylvestrus*') in English political caricature, and did so in the context

---

*The first slaves transported to the West Indies by the British were Irish.

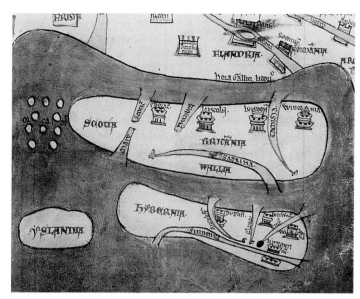

Detail from Giraldus Cambrensis's map of Europe circa 1200 in *Topographia Hiberniae*.

Stephen Pearce, *The Arctic Council*. Francis Beaufort is seated; Edward Sabine is fourth from right, wearing the full-dress uniform of a colonel of the Royal Artillery.

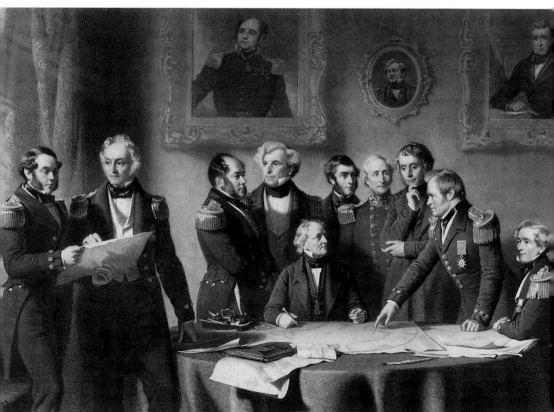

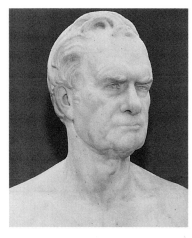

Left: Sir Richard Griffith, who produced a splendid geological map of Ireland (1838-55) based largely on the observations of his surveyors for the General Valuation of Rateable Property.

Below: A portrait (1802–8) of Richard Kirwan, begun by H.D. Hamilton and finished by his daughter Harriet after his death.

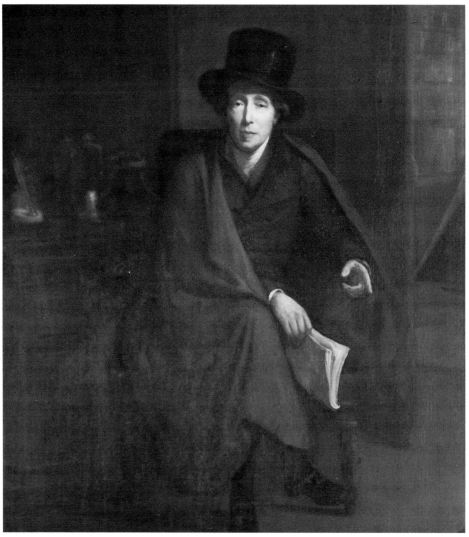

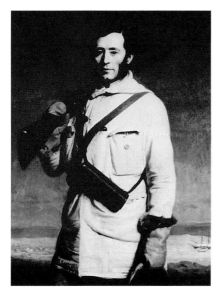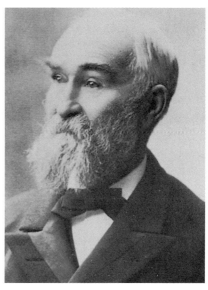

Sir Francis Leopold McClintock by Stephen Pearce, 1859 (*left*), and John Macoun in 1902 (*right*).

Opponents in the evolution debate: Rev. Robert Watts (*left*), and John Tyndall, from *Punch* (*right*).

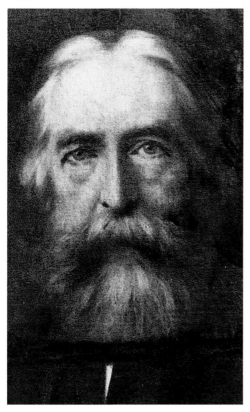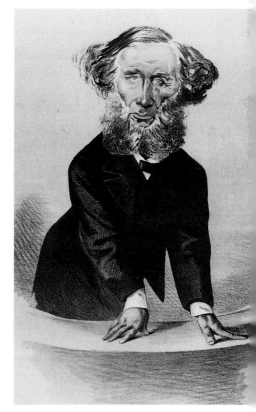

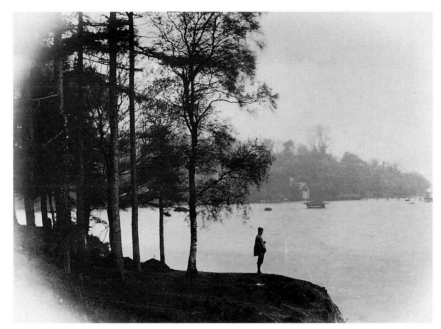

Robert Lloyd Praeger as a young man at Kenmare, Co. Kerry, July 1898, photographed by R.J. Welch.

Beaters at Mount Juliet, Thomastown, Co. Kilkenny.

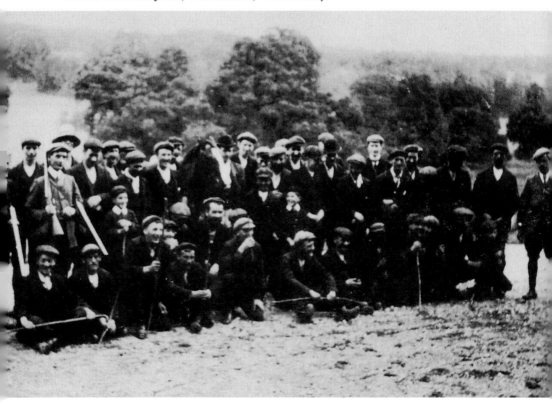

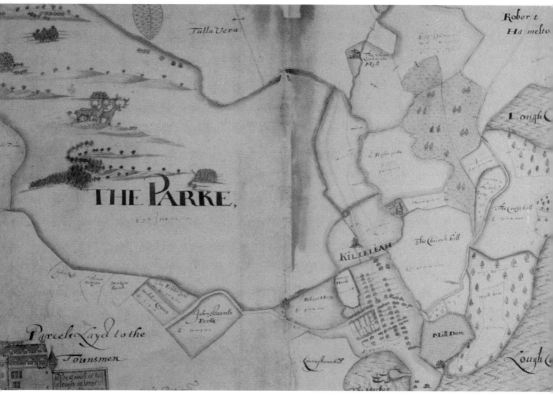

Raven's 1625 map of the Killyleagh demesne, Co. Down, showing the deer park, with deer pictorially depicted. The castle is in lower left corner.

A sad sight encountered too often in Ireland today: an eighteenth-century landscape park that has been completely devastated. The demesne park at Headford, Co. Galway, was noted by travellers in the west of Ireland for its 'well-planted and well-kept' parkland setting. Little now remains, save the ruins of some buildings.

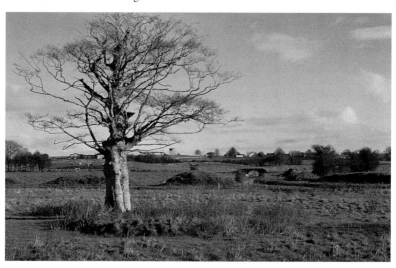

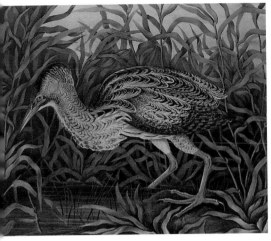
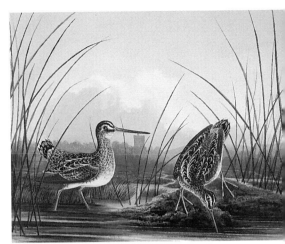

Above: Two paintings by Richard Dunscombe Parker (1805-81): *The Bittern (Botaurus stellaris)*, and *Snipe, Male and Female, with Blarney Castle*.

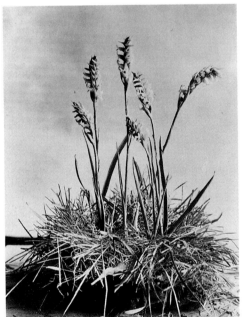

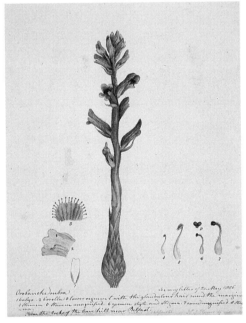

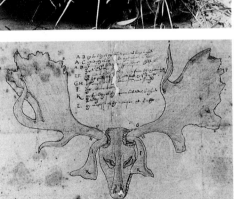

Above, left: R.J. Welch's photograph of *Spiranthes stricta*, Irish lady's tresses, from Robert Lloyd Praeger's *The Way That I Went* (1937).

Above, right: John Templeton, *Red Broomrape (Orobanche alba* var. *rubra)*.

Left: Unknown artist, *Skull of the Great Irish Deer*. The drawing was made for Adam Loftus between 1588 and 1597.

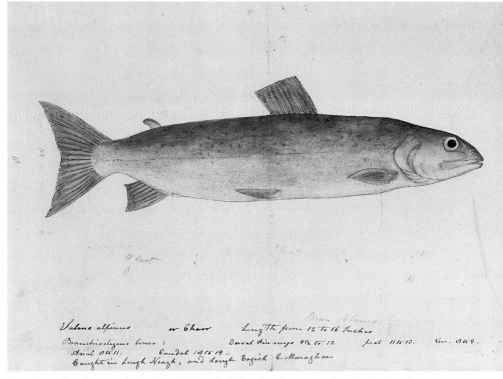

Drawing of a char caught in Lough Neagh. The char is now extinct in the lough.

Andrew Nicholl (1804-86), *A Bank of Flowers, with a View of Bray and the Valley of the Dargle, Co. Wicklow.*

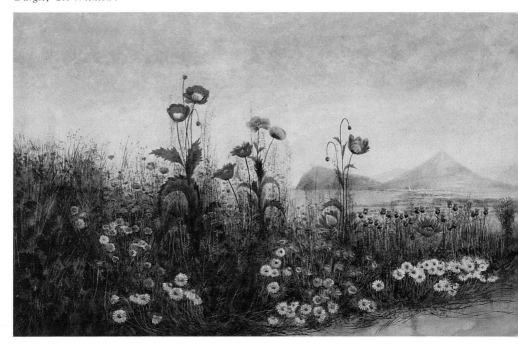

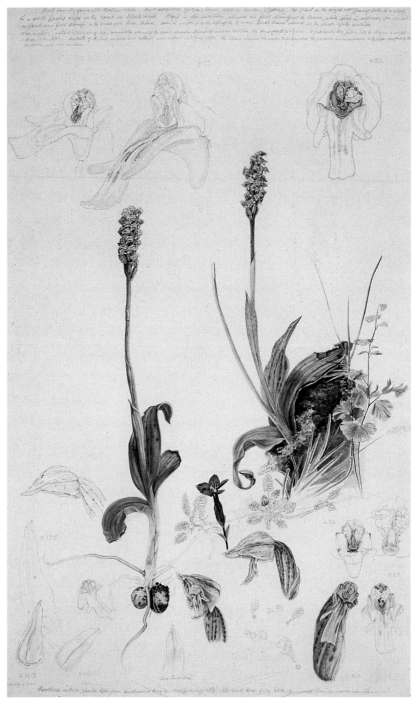

Raymond Piper (b. 1923), *Neotinea maculata* var. *maculata*
(Dense-flowered orchid), pencil and watercolour on white paper.
This orchid, formerly *Neotinea intacta*, occurs in the west of Ireland.

of evolution and Victorian interest in physical anthropology (including the popular pursuit of phrenology).*

The likening of the Irish to apes did not occur only in political caricature of the *Punch* variety. In 1860 the naturalist and writer Charles Kingsley was staying at Markree Castle, Co. Sligo, and was excited by the fishing (he killed his first salmon on this visit). In a letter home, having recorded that 'This place is full of glory – very lovely, and well kept up', he wrote:

But I am haunted by the human chimpanzees I saw along that hundred miles of horrible country. I don't believe they are our fault. I believe here are not only many more of them than of old, but that they are happier, better, more comfortably fed and lodged under our rule than they ever were. But to see white chimpanzees is dreadful; if they were black, one would not feel it so much, but their skins, except where tanned by exposure, are as white as ours. Tell Rose I will get her plants. (Kingsley, 1877, II)

As other letters from Ireland attest, Kingsley's attitude to the Irish is a not wholly cruel colonial paternalism.** The unpleasant racialism it consorts with is directed, almost unconsciously, against black people. But the chimpanzee resemblance was surely prompted by Darwinism as well as African exploration and unfortunately accorded with outright anti-Irish racialism in Britain.

From Giraldus to the late nineteenth century, the English attitude to the Irish was on one level of political and racial distaste a popular species of cryptozoology. At one end of the spectrum would be Charlotte Yonge's flippant reference to house sparrows as 'the Irishmen of birds, with their noise and their squabbles, their boldness and ubiquity' (Thomas, 1984). At the other end is something approaching a popular teratology, the science of the monstrous; joining the wild man and the man-wolf are the tailed Irish who, according to a captain in General Ireton's regiment, were among the slaughtered of an Irish garrison in Cashel in 1647 (Thomas, 1984). (Could such an idea have suggested, ironically or not, Swift's Yahoos?)

Teratology was a science, incidentally, by which Oscar Wilde was fascinated. Wilde was an Irishman who knew his science, particularly his biology,

---

*Yet even Huxley in *Man's Place in Nature* drew on reports of monstrous man-apes, not to discuss the role of mutations in evolution, but to ambush readers, familiarizing them with a monstrous idea, one might say, so that they would be less shocked by the claim that the ancestors of humanity were anthropoid.

**Kingsley is gratified to see farms growing up in post-Famine, wasted Mayo and farmers cultivating roots and grasses 'instead of the horrid potato in black bog'. Nine years later, writing from Kenmare, Kingsley counsels justice for Ireland and 'personal love and care' for the Irish – more colonial paternalism – and indicts British policy in the island, which he sees as aimed fundamentally at preventing the growth of population.

very well indeed, and he was a life-long Darwinian (Foster, 1993/4). His dazzling but brief career offers not just this irony but other ironies in the light of what I have just been discussing. From his home city of Dublin, Wilde crossed to London to colonize culturally the capital and metropolis. There he produced his own shimmeringly witty anti-English satires, in which bourgeois English society is depicted as a lowly life-form and the cultivated Celt a higher life-form, akin to the Greek of old. It was a revenge so rarefied that Wilde himself was famously accused by the German critic Max Nordau of being so cultivated that he had like the other aesthetes collapsed backwards into degeneration.* Certain English made Wilde pay a cruder and severer penalty.

On his death-bed Wilde embraced the Catholicism he had been flirting with for many years, and we assume he would have squared it with his Darwinism on grounds of the superior (because more highly evolved) aesthetic appeal of Catholicism over the constitutional religion of England. His death in 1900 brings our story to a formally pleasing conclusion, before which his abbreviated life brilliantly assorted the essential cultural elements in a century which he said had been made by two men, the Catholic Celticist and biographer of Christ, Ernst Renan, and Charles Darwin.

---

*The concept of evolution paradoxically stirred a widespread interest in its opposite, degeneration (Chamberlin and Gilman, 1985). H.G. Wells dramatized the idea in his scientific romance, *The Time Machine* (1895), and seemed to satirize the Wildean aesthetes, having already written an essay on zoological retrogression (Philmus and Hughes, 1975)

References

Andrews, J.H. 1975. *A Paper Landscape: The Ordnance Survey in Nineteenth-Century Ireland*. Oxford: Oxford University Press.

Ardagh, J. 1933. 'The Shamrock: A Bibliography.' *Irish Book Lover* 21: 37-40.

Beckett, C. 1967. *Fealsunacht Aodha Mhic Dhomhnaill*. Dublin: An Clochomhar Tta.

Beckett, C. 1987. *Aodh Mac Domhnaill*. Dundalk: Dundalgan.

Brooke, C. 1789. *Reliques of Irish Poetry: Consisting of Heroic Poems, Odes, Elegies, and Songs*. Dublin: Bonham.

Brooke, P. 1983. 'Religion and Secular Thought 1850-75,' in J.C. Beckett *et al.*, *Belfast: The Making of the City 1800-1914*. Belfast: Appletree Press.

Butler, M. 1993. Introduction to M. Shelley, *Frankenstein, or The Modern Prometheus (1818, 1831)*. London: Pickering and Chatto.

Bynum, W.F., E.J. Browne and R. Porter (eds). *Dictionary of the History of Science*. Princeton: Princeton University Press.

Carleton, W. 1847. *The Black Prophet, A Tale of Irish Famine*. London and Belfast: Simms & McIntyre.

Chamberlin, T. and S. Gilman (eds). 1985. *Degeneration: The Dark Side of Progress*. New York: Columbia University Press.

Chambers, W., and R. Chambers. 1848. *Chambers's Information for the People*. Multivolume. Edinburgh: W. and R. Chambers; London: W.S. Orr.

Clarke, D. 1973. 'An Outline of the History of Science in Ireland.' *Studies 62*: 287-302.

Cobbett, W. [1830] 1912. *Rural Rides*. 2 vols. London: Dent.

Coleborne, B. 1991. 'Anglo-Irish Verse 1675-1825,' in S. Deane (ed.), *The Field Day Anthology of Irish Writing*, vol. 1. Derry: Field Day Publications.

Colgan, N. 1896. 'The Shamrock in Literature: A Critical Chronology.' *Royal Society of Antiquaries of Ireland Journal 26*: 211-26, 349-61.

Connell, K.H. 1950/1. 'The Colonization of Waste Land in Ireland, 1780-1845.' *Economic History Review. Ser.2. 3*: 44-71.

Corrigan, D. 1984. 'The Scientific Basis of Folk Medicine: The Irish Dimension,' in R. Vickery (ed.), *Plant-Lore Studies*. London: The Folklore Society.

Cosslett, T. (ed.). 1984. *Science and Religion in the Nineteenth Century*. Cambridge: Cambridge University Press.

Curtis Jr., P. 1971. *Apes and Angels: The Irishman in Victorian Caricature*. Washington, D.C.: Smithsonian Institution Press.

Davis, T. 1889. *Prose Writings: Essays on Ireland*. London: Walter Scott.

de Paor, M. and L. 1978. *Early Christian Ireland*. London: Thames and Hudson.

Deane, S. 1991. 'Poetry and Song 1800-1890' and 'The Famine and Young Ireland,' in S. Deane (ed.), *The Field Day Anthology of Irish Writing*. Vol. 2. Derry: Field Day Publications.

Di Gregorio, M.A. 1984. *T.H. Huxley's Place in Natural Science*. New Haven and London: Yale University Press.

Dufferin, Lady. [1894] 1991. 'The Irish Emigrant,' in Seamus Deane (ed.), *The Field Day Anthology of Irish Writing*, vcl. II. Derry: Field Day Publications.

Dunne, T. 1988. 'Haunted by History: Irish Romantic Writing 1800-50,' in R. Porter and M. Teich (eds), *Romanticism in National Context*. Cambridge: Cambridge University Press.

Evans, E.E. (1971) 1992. *The Personality of Ireland: Habitat, Heritage and History*. Dublin: Lilliput Press.

Foster, J.W. 1987. *Fictions of the Irish Literary Revival: A Changeling Art*. Syracuse: Syracuse University Press; Dublin: Gill and Macmillan.

Foster, J.W. 1993/4. 'Against Nature? Science and Oscar Wilde.' *University of Toronto Quarterly 63*: 328-46.

Gardner, H. (ed.). 1953. *Gerard Manley Hopkins: A Selection of his Poems and Prose*. Harmondsworth: Penguin.

Gaull, M. 1988. *English Romanticism: The Human Context*. New York: Norton.

Gibson, W. 1860. *The Year of Grace: A History of the Ulster Revival of 1859*. Edinburgh: Elliott.

Gosse, E. [1907] 1986. *Father and Son: A Study of Two Temperaments*. Harmondsworth: Penguin.

Gosse, P.H. [1857] 1984. *Omphalos: An Attempt to Untie the Geological Knot*. London: Van Voorst.

Irvine, W. 1963. *Apes, Angels, & Victorians: The Story of Darwin, Huxley, and Evolution*. New York: Time Inc.

Jarrell, R.A. 1981. 'Differential National Development and Science in the Nineteenth Century; The problems of Quebec and Ireland,' in Nathan Reingold and Marc Rothenburg (eds), *Scientific Colonialism: A Cross-Cultural Comparison*. Washington, D.C.: Smithsonian Institution Press.

Jones, G. 1997. 'Science, Catholicism and Nationalism.' *The Irish Review*, no. 20: 47-61.

Joyce, J. 1914. 'The Dead,' in *Dubliners*. London: Grant Richards.

Kalm, P. [1770] 1987. *Travels in North America*. Trans. J.R. Forster, rev. A. Benson. New York: Dover.

Kavanagh, P. 1938. *The Green Fool*. London: Michael Joseph.

Kavanagh, P. 1948. *Tarry Flynn*. London: Pilot Press.

Kingsley, C. 1877. *Charles Kingsley: His Letters and Memories of his Life*. Ed. Mrs Kingsley. 2 vols. London: Henry S. King.

Kinns, S. 1884. *Moses and Geology, or The Harmony of the Bible with Science*. London: Cassell.

McKenna, B. 1978. *Irish Literature, 1800-1875: A Guide to Information Sources*. Detroit: Gale.

Marjarum, E.W. 1940. 'Wordworth's View of the State of Ireland.' *PMLA 55*: 608-11.

Miller, H. 1857. *The Testimony of the Rocks: Or, Geology in its Bearings on the two Theologies, Natural and Revealed*. New York: Hurst.

Moloney, M. 1919. *Irish Ethno-Botany and the Evolution of Medicine in Ireland*. Dublin: M.H. Gill.

Morgan, Lady. [1806] 1979. *The Wild Irish Girl*. Introduction R.L. Wolff. New York: Garland.

Murray, R.H. 1908. 'The Depopulation of Ireland.' *Report of the British Association for the Advancement of Science*. London: BAAS.

Newman, J. (Cardinal). [1873] 1982. *The Idea of a University, Defined and Illustrated*. Notre Dame, Indiana: University of Notre Dame Press.

O'Brien, F. (1941) 1975. *The Poor Mouth*. Trans. from *An Béal Bocht* by Patrick C. Power. London: Picador.

O'Connor, F. 1967. *A Short History of Irish Literature: A Backward Look*. New York: G.P. Putnam's Sons.

O'Donnell, J.F. 1991 (1891). 'The Return,' in Seamus Deane (ed.), *The Field Day Anthology of Irish Writing*, vol. II. Derry: Field Day Publications.

O'Halloran, S. 1772. *An Introduction to the History and Antiquities of Ireland*. Dublin: Ewing.

Ophir, A. and S. Shapin. 1991. 'The Place of Knowledge: A Methodological Survey,' *Science in Context 4*: 3-21.

O'Sullivan, H. [A. Ó SÚilleabháin] 1936. *Cinnlae Amlaoib Ui Suileahain: The Diary of Humphrey O'Sullivan*. Ed., trans. M. McGrath S.J. London: Simpkin, Marshall for The Irish Texts Society.

Outram, D. 1988. 'Heavenly Bodies and Logical Minds,' *Graph* (Spring): 9-11.

Philmus, R. and D.Y. Hughes. 1975. *H.G. Wells: Early Writings in Science and Science Fiction*. Berkeley: University of California Press.

Praeger, R. L. [1937] 1969. *The Way that I Went*. Dublin: Allen Figgis.

Rupke, N.A. 1994. *Richard Owen: Victorian Naturalist*. New Haven: Yale University Press.

Sacks, O. 1993. 'The Poet of Chemistry [Humphry Davy.]' *New York Review of Books*. 4 Nov.: 50-6.

Sheets-Pyenson, S. 1981. 'Civilizing by Nature's Example: The Development of Colonial Museums of Natural History,' in N. Reingold and M. Rothenburg (eds), *Scientific Colonialism: A Cross-Cultural Comparison*. Washington, D.C.: Smithsonian Institution Press.

Sheets-Pyenson, S. 1988. *Cathedrals of Science: The Development of Natural History Museums during the Late Nineteenth Century*. Kingston, Ont.: McGill-Queens University Press.

Spenser, E. [1596] 1970. *A View of the Present State of Ireland*. Ed. W.L. Renwick. Oxford: Clarendon.

Sterrenburg, L. 1979. 'Mary Shelley's Monster: Politics and Psyche,' in G. Levine and U.C. Knoepflmacher (eds), *The Endurance of Frankenstein*. Berkeley: University of California Press.

Thomas, K. 1984. *Man and the Natural World: Changing Attitudes in England 1500-1800*. Harmondsworth: Penguin.

Thompson, W. 1849-56. *The Natural History of Ireland*. 4 vols. London: Reeve, Benham and Reeve; (vol. 4) Henry G. Bohn.

Thompson, W.I. 1967. *The Imagination of an Insurrection: Dublin 1916*. Oxford: Oxford University Press.

Trench, W.S. [1868] 1991. *Realities of Irish Life*, extracted in Seamus Deane (ed.), *The Field Day Anthology of Irish Writing*, vol. II. Derry: Field Day Publications.

Tyndall, J. 1874. *Address Delivered before The British Association Assembled at Belfast, With Additions*. London: Longmans, Green & Co.

Tyndall, J. [1870] 1907. 'Scientific Use of the Imagination,' in *Fragments of Science*. 2 vols. London: Longmans Green.

Ussher, R.J.and R. Warren. 1900. *The Birds of Ireland*. London: Gurney and Jackson.

Viney, M. 1986. 'Woodcock for a Farthing: The Irish Experience of Nature.' *The Irish Review*, no.1: 58-64.

Von Zittel, K.A. 1901. *History of Geology and Palaeontology*. Trans. M.M. Ogilvie-Gordon. London: Scott.

Whyte, N. 1997. 'Science and Nationality in Edwardian Ireland,' in P.J. Bowler and N. Whyte (eds), *Science and Society in Ireland: The Social Context of Science and Technology in Ireland 1900-1950*. Belfast: Institute of Irish Studies, Queen's University of Belfast.

Willey, Basil. [1940] 1957. *The Eighteenth Century Background*. London: Chatto and Windus.

Williams, J.E.C. and P.K. Ford. 1992. *The Irish Literary Tradition*. Cardiff: University of Wales Press.

Wilshire, B. (ed.). 1968. *Romanticism and Evolution: The Nineteenth Century*. New York: Capricorn.

Woodham-Smith, C. 1962. *The Great Hunger: Ireland 1845-9*. London: New English Library.

Wyatt, J. 1996. *Wordsworth and the Geologists*. Cambridge: Cambridge University Press.

Yearley, S. 1989. 'Colonial Science and Dependent Development: The Case of the Irish Experience,' *Sociological Review 37*: 303-31.

Zimmermann, G.-D. 1967. *Songs of Irish Rebellion: Political Street Ballads and Rebel Songs 1780-1900*. Hatboro, Pa.: Folklore Associates.

Contrasting Natures: The Issue of Names

SEÁN LYSAGHT

Language, Nationalism, Nature

At first sight, the flora and the fauna of Ireland would in themselves appear to be immune to the kinds of political and cultural disputes that mark Irish history. Biological boundaries are not the same as political ones; the birds and the animals are innocent of our concerns and our guilt. Yet immediately we are forced to concede that in writing a scientific and cultural history of nature in Ireland, we are dealing with our conceptions and our interpretation of nature. This is true even of something as apparently neutral as the name for a seagull or a species of fern.

The reason for this is that before we can consider anything in nature we have got to have a name for it, whether that name is *Larus ridibundus*, black-headed gull or *Faoileán ceanndubh*. Indeed, in the biblical account of the creation, Adam's first act in this world was to give names to the wild animals; it was his way of controlling nature and subordinating it to his understanding (Genesis 2: 19-20). The act of naming, whether in a peasant vernacular or in modern scientific nomenclature, is a vital record of our relationship with nature: names register the level of our awareness of the variety and abundance around us, and the benefits and threats we perceive nature to represent.

Part of the task of a history of natural history is to renew our awareness of the variety and abundance in nature and give ourselves enhanced access to it. In Ireland, however, there is a particular obstacle to our relationship with nature which has to do with the fact that the old Gaelic vernacular has been lost to most of the country – and with it a range of names for plants and animals, the key to the old Gaelic community's relationship with the natural world. The decline of that primitive relationship with land and sea, and the extinction of its vocabulary, have given rise to a powerful nostalgia. It is as if the loss of the language carried with it the loss of the objects themselves. In a brief poem, 'The Death of Irish' (1983), Aidan Mathews articulates a recurrent feeling:

> The tide gone out for good,
> Thirty-one words for seaweed
> Whiten on the foreshore.

In his *Literary History of Ireland* (1899), Douglas Hyde estimated that following the influence of the British national schools system the vocabulary of the Irish child was reduced from a sophisticated three thousand to a paltry 'six hundred English words, badly pronounced and barbarously employed'. He considered that 'the unique stock-in-trade of an Irish-speaker's mind' was 'gone forever, *and replaced by nothing*'. Part of that stock-in-trade would of course have been the terms for the plants and animals that were known to the Gaelic community.

The national schools system to which Hyde refers was designed to improve literacy and numeracy, to the detriment of other subjects. The system dated from 1831, but reached its most mechanical, unimaginative form in the 'payment-by-results era' of 1872 to 1899. In 1900, however, a Revised Programme for National Schools became operational under the newly formed Department of Agriculture and Technical Instruction. This programme gave a new emphasis to local and environmental studies: teachers were encouraged to visit sites of local historical interest with their pupils, and to promote the study of natural history in the classroom. The gains of the new reforms were to be short-lived, of course, because of the troubled era Ireland entered from 1914 onwards. With the foundation of the Irish Free State, educational policy was radically overhauled to provide for the teaching of the Irish language and to foster an intensely nationalist sense of culture and identity. The crucial report of the Irish National Teachers' Organisation conference of 1922 on national education policy recommended the elimination of drawing, elementary science, hygiene, nature study, and needlework as obligatory subjects. In the early decades of the Free State, 'Mastery of the Irish language was the primary goal of education policy' (Coolahan, 1981).

The Irish heritage promoted by the Gaelic League and the Free State national schools was composed of history, antiquities, folklore, games, music and dancing. Natural history does not seem to have figured, presumably because flora and fauna were not specifically 'Irish'; and in any case natural history, in the form of field clubs and scientific associations, had traditionally been the preserve of the Protestant gentry and professional middle class. An enthusiasm for Ireland's natural history had been a component of the cultural revival of the 1890s, but its associations with the Ascendancy meant that it did not survive through to the new Gaelic cultural agenda of the Free State. The institutions, the personnel and the terminology of natural history were all thoroughly implicated in the phase of 'constructive unionism' that lasted from about 1890 to the First World War; the scientific tradition they represented was characterized by discretion after independence.

At the other extreme to the scientific elite, we have the primitive communities in the Gaeltachts in the west of Ireland that were to serve as the cradles of the new culture. The terminology for nature, if it were to survive at all, would have to be active here. A great deal of sentimental capital was invested in the future of the Gaeltachts, with the mixed results that have by now become familiar. In a keynote article on 'The Last Years of the Gaeltacht' published in 1981, Desmond Fennell summarizes the situation as follows:

The Gaelic which is spoken today in the Gaeltacht, and which is gradually being abandoned, is a very thin language compared with the spoken Gaelic of three hundred, a hundred, or fifty years ago. While the Gaeltacht has been shrinking, territorially, its language has been shrinking in vocabulary. Among the first sets of words to go, I suppose, were those connected with Brehon law, the aristocracy and the Gaelic political structure. These were replaced to some extent, but not in the same abundance, by new terms referring to the corresponding English realities. Much nearer to our own time, a huge loss of vocabulary occurred when the craft industries largely disappeared from the countryside in face of competition from factory-products ... today you see people working in the fields, fishing, gathering seaweed, building houses and making boats. Eighty years ago there were coopers, nail-makers, sail-makers, weavers, tailors, cobblers and so on .... The technical vocabularies connected with all of these and other crafts are completely gone, and nothing equivalent has replaced them. Most of the new technical terms are the raw English words, not even phonetically Gaelicized. Similarly, with the disappearance of herbal medicine and its practitioners, a huge wealth of medical and botanical terms has gone.

Analysing the same situation more specifically from the point of view of biological terminology, Michael Viney agrees with Fennell's assessment, and observes:

The vocabulary of the Gaeltacht is dwindling. In my own corner of Connacht, where Irish is no longer spoken as a language, Irish names for natural things linger on – the only names, very often, by which some birds and plants are known, and that uncertainly: *scraith-chloch*, the lichen the 'old people' used for a yellow dye; *meacan* or the comfrey they used as a herbal poultice. Name and utility survive together, but in a past tense. I doubt very much if many of these names are being passed on to the children: they hold Irish in such contempt ... the intimacy with nature that the 'old people' knew has, indeed, been overtaken by 'a sort of silence' (1986).

In the same essay, Viney argues that this has contributed to low environmental awareness in contemporary Ireland. The Famine, the long memory of deprivation on the land, and the loss of names for nature, all combine to stifle that more romanticized view of the natural world that we get in England. We can express the problem as a series of stereotypes: English culture has given prominence to a sentimental, pastoral view of nature and countryside based on continuity, belonging, and fruition; Irish experience has been marked by the opposites: discontinuity, exile, and sterility.

Seamus Heaney, particularly in *Wintering Out* (1972), takes as his poetic territory the interface between these stereotypes. In poems like 'Fodder', 'Bog Oak', and 'Land', the results display a startling alertness to different nuances of Irish rural experience. Among the poems of this collection are two elegies for the lost relationship with nature resulting from the extensive spoliation of native Irish woodland ('Midnight') and the loss of the Gaelic vernacular ('The Backward Look'). The second poem includes, in italics, transliterations of Gaelic names for the snipe (*Gallinago gallinago*):

> A stagger in air
> as if a language
> failed, a sleight
> of wing.
>
> A snipe's bleat is fleeing
> its nesting ground
> into dialect,
> into variants,
>
> transliterations whirr
> on the nature reserves –
> *little goat of the air,*
> *of the evening,*
> *little goat of the frost.*

Heaney is here combining two phenomena in one: the marginalization of the snipe by drainage and modern agriculture into 'nature reserves'; and the marginalization of the national language into the cultural reserves of the Gaeltachts, denoted here by 'dialect' and 'variants'. In 'Midnight', the poet's tongue is restrained by the forces that exterminated the wolf and cut down the Irish woodlands, leaving a natural environment characterized by absences:

> Rain on the roof to-night
> Sogs turf-banks and heather,
> Sets glinting outcrops
> Of basalt and granite,
> Drips to the moss of bare boughs.
> The old dens are soaking.

The pads are lost or
Retrieved by small vermin

That glisten and scut.
Nothing is panting, lolling,
Vapouring. The tongue's
Leashed in my throat.

There is a restraint upon the language and the voice of these poems
because they express, in English, the fact of the loss of Gaelic, among other
things. In these, and in several other poems in the same collection, Heaney
grounds his literary vocabulary in the Irish landscape. The luxuriant vocabulary of the pastoral genre, implying a fruitful, accommodating environment,
is quite out of place in Heaney's sparse, rather comfortless landscape; at the
same time, his fidelity to the peculiar texture of that landscape marked by
history constitutes one of the cardinal strengths of his poetry.

Heaney is usually alert to the ambiguities of a situation where the special circumstances of Irish experience, including its depleted landscape and
wildlife, provide an English-speaking literary tradition with distinct subject-
matter. There are moments, however, when he yields to the stereotype, as
when he claims that Robert Lloyd Praeger's eye for landscape 'is regulated
by laws of aesthetics, by the disciplines of physical geography, and not, to
borrow a phrase from Wordsworth, by the primary laws of our nature, the
laws of feeling' (Heaney, 1980). In this 1977 lecture on 'The Sense of Place',
Heaney objects to the scientific attitude of mind as one that is cut off from
primal patterns of feeling. In its stead, Heaney wants to restore the relationship with place through an understanding of placenames and the history
they register.

This broadly nationalist, atavistic attitude also manifests itself as the
claim that languages are untranslatable, and that the special relationship with
nature in Gaelic Ireland can never be retrieved. It is implied that there was
a quality to the peasant's speech as he named the seabirds in Gaelic – *crosán,
colúr toinne, puifín* – which translation can only imperfectly recapture.
Heaney expands on the idea of tone in a review of Kinsella and O'Tuama's
An Duanaire, An Irish Anthology 1600-1900: Poems of the Dispossessed (1981),
a collection of Gaelic poems in translation: 'As a translator, Kinsella is most
interested in tone, to try to carry the tone of Irish across the linguistic
divide. Tone is the inner life of a language, a secret spirit at play behind or
at odds with what is being said and how it is being structured in syntax and
figures of speech. It has subtly to do with the deepest value system that the
group speaking the language is possessed by' (Heaney, 1988). The point is
a fine one – and Heaney is not denying the wisdom or efficacy of translation – but it is obvious that a passage such as this courts oversimplification:

because the language is lost, the community is lost; so is its folklore, its view of nature, its whole distinguishing 'tone'. Heaney situates himself here well outside the reach of active understanding with an obscurantist terminology: 'the inner life'; 'a secret spirit'; 'subtly'; 'deepest'. At its worst, this emphasis on tone leads to the cult of placenames, where a totemic, sectarian value is placed on the history as recorded in the name of a place. The squabbles about (London)derry are a case in point.

But if we return to the innocent landscape again, we find surprisingly that Heaney himself has been there ahead of us, for example in a poem from *Door into the Dark* (1969), 'The Peninsula'. Tired of historical disputes, the poet drives off to the peninsula and rediscovers the attractions of the seashore and its wildlife. For once they do not carry the burden of history but are imagined in a pure state by the poet. This time physical geography will be the key to a new relationship:

> And drive back home, still with nothing to say
> Except that now you will uncode all landscapes
> By this: things founded clean on their own shapes,
> Water and ground in their extremity.

There is a similar return to the natural landscape at the end of the 1977 lecture where Heaney quotes J.C. Beckett, who says that in Ireland it is to 'the stable element, the land itself, that we must look for continuity'.

Heaney has therefore courted two different attitudes to naming and identification. The first of these is tribal and territorial, implying that the place and its name have a peculiar flavour that can only be savoured and safeguarded by the natives; this carries with it the implication that names are ultimately untranslatable. The second view is more universal, taking its cue from geology and natural history, and transcending the confines of sectarian or cultural disputes. In his 1983 Field Day pamphlet, *An Open Letter*, Heaney objected to the inclusion of a selection of his work in an anthology of British poetry and illustrated his objection with a story inherited from Miroslav Holub, where a man in a thronged cinema makes loud disruptive objection to a beaver being called a muskrat on the screen: 'Names were not for negotiation./Right names were the first foundation/For telling truth.' Holub himself, who combines poetry with a scientific vocation as an immunologist, has said that

Nobody can tolerate crookneck squash being called turnips, or Sirius Aldebaran. The right name is the first step toward the truth which makes things things and us us. Which conjures away any perils of the nameless things, and helps us live. And such hairsplitting in natural history is on the one hand a phenomenon of essential human features, and an element of science on the other (quoted in Heaney, 1988).

The 'right name' is a concept that can, of course, have a variety of uses, conservative or progressive. For a Gaelic sentimentalist, the 'right name' of *Anthus pratensis* might be *giolla cuaiche* (the cuckoo's servant), and not the less expressive English meadow pipit, or even the standard Irish *riabhóg*. Scientists, on the other hand, will tend to favour the Latin Linnaean form because it avoids the inaccuracies that occur in the application of vernacular names. In no instance will science deny the possibility of translation because scientific nomenclature is grounded in objective differences and distinctions that remain unchanged from culture to culture. The dignity of Heaney's objection to the adjective 'British' in *An Open Letter* is that it is not validated by an appeal to vagueness; instead it is vindicated by a natural distinction.

Culture versus Science?

Heaney's adaptation of Holub notwithstanding, there would appear to be a conflict of sentiment here between the modern scientific namers of nature and those who cherish the older relationship with nature represented by the Gaelic vernacular. The scientific register can appear cold or newfangled compared with the expressive traditional names; it is also more productive: science has explored, identified and named thousands of life forms that were unknown to any peasant dialect, and it has produced new names (for species, subspecies and races) where previously there was only one. Of the 5269 fauna species listed in the Clare Island Survey (Collins, 1985), only a fraction would have been known to the Gaelic vernacular, and these would have comprised mostly the higher categories: birds, mammals, some insects. But the Gaelic names for plants and animals express a primitive community living from the land and the sea, intimate with seasonal cycles and alert to the aspects of the natural world that were beneficial or detrimental to themselves, whereas the Latin scientific names for obscure or unappealing plant and animal groups seem to lead no further than the taxonomist's laboratory.

We find ourselves once again confronted with the figure of the scientist as someone who is alien to the native affections. Such a stereotype is not peculiarly Irish; it is indeed a commonplace in Romantic culture and has an even older lineage in the Faust tradition. The figure of the inhuman scientist, as much a literary phenomenon as anything else, comes into prominence as Mary Shelley's Frankenstein, and the mad scientists of Victorian Gothic, including Dr Jekyll. Arthur Koestler, in his history of modern astronomy, *The Sleepwalkers* (1959), considers that this marginalization of science away from the ethical centre of culture has its roots in the seventeenth-century row between Galileo and the Vatican, when ethical authority and empirical science parted company. Nowadays, with the work of Stephen Hawking,

John Banville* and Koestler himself, to name only three, this gulf between culture and science seems more apparent than real, and it remains to be seen to what extent that gap can be bridged in the history of Irish culture as well.

The Case of Robert Lloyd Praeger

In the Irish context, the career of Robert Lloyd Praeger (1865-1953) is exemplary. The bulk of Praeger's work was in botany, although he made a number of significant forays into other fields, such as quaternary studies, archaeology, and geology. One can search through his entire published output, which stands just short of eight hundred articles, books and reviews in the available bibliography (Collins, 1985), and find scarcely a reference to political events or cultural disputes. He would appear to be a scientist whose work places him outside the jurisdiction of 'Irish culture', if by culture we mean something local or exclusive.

There are certainly large areas of Praeger's work in systematic botany, geology and quaternary studies that were addressed to an international scientific community and where local issues appear to have little or no purchase. But elsewhere, especially with his work in topographical botany, Praeger was operating closer to home. His work is structurally similar to the regional and local loyalties of the poets and antiquarians, even though its conventions largely exclude the language of human feeling. Whereas the folklorists and antiquarians saw each locality as having its distinctive fund of human stories, Praeger collected and recorded the place's botanical lore. Instead of the traditional *dinnshenchas* of placenames, with each name revealing something of the past history and the identity of the place, in Praeger's work we get flower names in association with place, where the botanical names are felt to constitute the area's identity.

Praeger's early associations were with the Belfast Naturalists' Field Club, in which his appetite for fieldwork was stimulated by men like his maternal grandfather Robert Patterson (who edited the final volume of Thompson's *Natural History of Ireland* after Thompson's death), his uncle William Hugh Patterson, and the botanist Samuel Alexander Stewart. The members of the BNFC had been enthusiastically engaged in exploring the wildlife, plants, and antiquities of the north-east since the foundation of the club in 1863, and there were still many virgin fields for botanical exploration when the young Robin Praeger came on to the scene in the 1880s.

Praeger's first substantial publication was a twenty-six page paper on the ferns of Ulster, published jointly with William Phillips in the BNFC's

---

* Banville has described modern physics as 'one of the most beautiful, moving and poetic enterprises man has ever devised' (*The Irish Times*, 1 Feb. 1992).

Proceedings in 1887. During these early years the quaternary history of the north-east was also an interest of his, and he published analyses of molluscan and human remains in gravels and estuarine clays at Larne, Belfast, and elsewhere. But botany came to predominate thereafter, especially following his move to Dublin in 1893 to a post at the National Library offering, as he saw it, 'unbounded facilities for scientific work' and 'long holidays which I can spend among my favourite spots in the "black north"'.*

In 1893 the new journal *The Irish Naturalist* – of which Praeger was a founding editor – published his 'Flora of County Armagh', and two years later Praeger and Stewart published their major supplement to Stewart and Corry's *Flora of the North-east of Ireland* (1888) in the BNFC's *Proceedings*. The supplement was a summary of several years of botanical work by BNFC members, making the north-east by far the best-explored region in the country. Like most of the regional floras in this period, Praeger and Stewart's supplement was basically a systematic list of plants, giving an indication of the occurrence of each species in the area concerned. Although the supplement gave Praeger 'more trouble than anything else I ever wrote',** it paved the way for an even more grandiose scheme: a survey of the flora of the entire country. Praeger was exercised by the fact that in Hewett Cottrell Watson's *Topographical Botany* (1883), a regional survey of the plants of the British Isles, Ireland had been given only marginal treatment, and he was concerned to correct the balance in Ireland's favour. The resulting work, *Irish Topographical Botany* (1901), followed the model of his own supplement, and of Colgan and Scully's national survey of plant distribution, *Cybele Hibernica* (1898), by listing plant species with their relevant localities. In the course of the introduction, Praeger noted with satisfaction that he had managed, with a single exception, to reach his target of five hundred species for each of the forty divisions he had devised, whereas 'Watson published "Topographical Botany" when for nine vice-counties no information was available but scattered notes of rarer plants'.

It is clear that Praeger's involvement with his region and his country was impelled by a sense of locality every bit as keen as the parochialism we are familiar with in the Monaghan poet Patrick Kavanagh and the veneration of place in Heaney's poetry of the early 1970s. The genre of topographical botany tends, of course, to conceal the affective dimension, but we

---

* Robert Lloyd Praeger to Mary Isabella Leebody, 17 June 1893, National Botanic Gardens. Mrs Leebody, a keen amateur botanist, was married to Professor J.R. Leebody of Foyle College, Derry.
** Robert Lloyd Praeger to Mary Isabella Leebody, 15 Feb. 1896, National Botanic Gardens.

find that dimension there nonetheless (not to speak of the evidence of great labour and dedication that these researches represent). In the introduction to *Irish Topographical Botany*, having explained his fieldwork methods, Praeger paused to take stock of five years' experience in some of the less travelled parts of the country:

The long summer days spent in the Limestone Plain, where the gentle undulations of the ground only occasionally hid the distant rim of brown and blue hills; the marshy meadows, heavy with the scent of flowers; the great brown bogs, where the curlews alone relieved the loneliness; the bare limestone pavements and gaunt grey hills of Clare and Galway; the savage cliffs of the Mayo coast; the flower-filled sand-dunes which fringe the Irish Sea; the fertile undulations of southern Ulster; the swift brown current of the Barrow; the fretted limestone shores of the great western lakes; the towering cones of the Galtees: all have left memories that can never be effaced.

Each of these areas was distinguished in Praeger's memory for the abundance, variety, and specificity of its flora; here we have names in connection with places, particularly where Praeger found a plant in a new locality. In 1899, for instance, he discovered *Neotinea intacta* (now *N. maculata*, plate 20) near Lough Corrib, thus extending its known range: 'The headquarters of this rare orchid are on the Burren limestones, where it is frequent over an area extending from near Athenry to Castle Taylor, and thence westward to the Atlantic. Outside this continuous area, the only known station was near Cong, where Dr [David] Moore found it many years ago. My pleasure at discovering a connecting link between these widely separated localities may be imagined' (Praeger, 1900). It should be emphasized that this satisfaction was not incidental to the study he was undertaking, but constituted its very substance.

The connection between plant names and localities is at the centre of Praeger's work as a topographical botanist, both in *Irish Topographical Botany* and in the extensive summary of work that he published in 1934, *The Botanist in Ireland*. Throughout his work on topographical botany, Praeger's affection for place manifests itself in a series of plant names, as in the following passage celebrating the Ben Bulben area, from *The Way that I Went* (1937):

While this Ben Bulben region is beloved of all seekers of the picturesque, it is to the botanist a special place of pilgrimage, on account of the profusion of alpine plants which cling to the grey cliff-walls, and the presence among them of some of extreme rarity. The fringed Sandwort, rather widespread about Glendale and Gleniff, grows nowhere else in Ireland, nor is it found in Britain, while the Clustered Alpine Saxifrage and Chickweed-leaved Willow-herb have no other Irish station; the rocks are decked with Mountain Avens, Cushion Pink, Yellow Mountain Saxifrage, Green Spleenwort, Holly Fern, and many other plants of the hills. The Canadian Blue-eyed Grass occurs on the lower grounds; the Maidenhair Fern in limestone chinks both on the cliffs and down by the sea.

Linnaean System, Gaelic Vernacular: Attempts at Reconciliation

The vernacular and scientific plant names that provided the foundation for this work were of course based on the species of Linnaean convention. (Not that this in itself excluded the affections: Praeger wrote to Mary Isabella Leebody – a field botanist living in Derry – in July 1893 to confirm her finding of the Irish Lady's Tresses, *Spiranthes romanzoffiana*, saying that the plant 'is nothing less than my own dear *Spiranthes Romanzoviana*'.)* But we find, running parallel to the main thrust of work within the scientific convention, a current of interest in the Gaelic plant and animal names.

In the eighteenth century, Threlkeld (1727) and K'Eogh (1735) had recorded Irish names for plants in their floras, but it was John White who first confronted the problem of trying to reconcile Linnaean and native Gaelic names, in *An Essay on the Indigenous Grasses of Ireland* (1808). During his travels around Ireland under the sponsorship of the Royal Dublin Society in search of plants, White collected many of the Irish names. 'Upon looking over these names some time after, and seeing the confused, irregular manner in which they stood, when compared with the Linnaean method, I thought from the language there could be a regular system formed.' Some time after this, a reading of one of the works of General Charles Vallancey – probably his *Essay on the Antiquity of the Irish Language* (1772) – relaunched the project in his mind: 'I was roused by the accounts given of this language, its copious and expressive terms, to carry on my former design of compiling the generic and specific names after the manner mentioned, following the Linnaean method as closely as possible.' White accordingly published a Latin, an English, and an Irish name for each species in his essay. His vernacular names are remarkable in that they conform to the binomial system: *Agrostis pumila* / dwarf bent-grass / *taenfhér abhac*; *Agrostis minima* / least bent-grass / *taenfhér robheg*. The results are at times quaint – *Panicum sanguinale* becomes cocksfoot panic-grass or *Panicfhér coschoiligh* – but this was in keeping with contemporary practice: the coinage of vernacular names for plant species became widespread in Victorian times, with plants such as the distant-spiked sedge and the Tunbridge filmy fern entering the language.

Later in the century, the question of Gaelic names again attracted the interests of botanists as well as folklorists. In his *Flora of the County Donegal* (1898), Henry Chichester Hart provided an appendix listing popular plant names in Irish and in English, but considered that there were many local inaccuracies. Nathaniel Colgan, who published his *Flora of County Dublin* in

---

* Robert Lloyd Praeger to Mary Isabella Leebody, 21 July 1893, National Botanic Gardens.

1904, was more actively involved with the question of native Gaelic names, and advertised the rich plant lore in the Gaelic vernacular in the introduction to his book. He reported collecting thirty-five native plant names in a day in the Carlingford Hills in 1901, 'all in common use amongst the unlettered peasantry and all applied by them to definite species'. Colgan went on to speculate that in 'the extensive Gaelic areas of Western and Southern Ireland, this native plant vocabulary might be increased ten-fold for in spite of the exaggeration or misrepresentation of uncritical or uncandid writers on this subject, Irish plant lore is remarkably rich'.

In a similar vein, in a lecture to the Limerick Field Club in January that year, Helen Laird celebrated the rich awareness of nature reflected in Gaelic names. 'Any Irish botanist', she declared, 'who gets caught into the swirl of the Irish Revival which is flowing so rapidly around us, and finds himself face to face with the subject of Irish plant names, and plant lore, has a field of research before him truly fascinating to the Celtic mind, strewn as it is with infinite possibilities.' Her lecture dealt mainly with the combinations of fairy lore, accurate observation and simple utility that were found in the Gaelic names; but it contained an additional dimension of great significance: Laird was not only looking back nostalgically to an irretrievable past, she was also looking forward to the future.

Laird was interested in the contemporary scientific developments which included, for amateurs, the field clubs, for farmers, the Department of Agriculture and Technical Instruction, and for scientists, the construction, from 1904, of the new Royal College of Science at Merrion Street in the splendid building that now houses the Taoiseach's office. She voiced the hope that one of the Gaelic terms for Ireland, *Inis na bhfidhbhadh* (the island of woods), would again be applicable, and that the trees would 'wave aloft their green plumes again'. She continued: 'The pamphlets on flax growing [i.e. of the Department of Agriculture and Technical Instruction] may call up a vision of blue fields varying the green banks of the Shannon, and in our imagination we may taste the glowing fruit of many an Oola, abounding in apples.' (Laird's audience would have been familiar with Oola, the name of a village in Co. Limerick.)

This blend of patriotic fervour and scientific confidence is again reflected in a little-known book published in 1919, *Irish Ethno-Botany and the History of Medicine in Ireland*, by Michael Moloney, a medical doctor practising in Waterford. In this work Moloney sets out to demonstrate that early Irish herbal lore was extensive and effective, with 'wonderful results accomplished by ... hereditary healers, who were acquainted with and used the materia medica of their own country'. While he did not set out 'to decry orthodox medicine', the author also insisted that 'a study of the Ethno-Botany of the Celts allied with the Pharmacology of to-day may win back some of the fame of the Irish Physicians of long ago, and help at the same time the common cause of humanity'. Moloney also confronted the question of whether 'English and Cymric' plant lore were not adequate to account for the pharmacological properties of Irish plants; and here he makes a claim about the special features of the Irish flora that we find repeated many times throughout Praeger's writings: 'It is true that the flora of Ireland is on the whole a reduced British flora. Yet we have a number of species very rare or altogether unknown in Great Britain. Besides, just as we are a distinct national entity, so we possess a specific herb lore, and one which will bear comparison with that of any other country.' Apart from the unusual biological nationalism of its introduction, Moloney's book is noteworthy for its systematically organized list of plants, including marine forms, with scientific, English and Gaelic names, and traditional medicinal uses.

Laird wanted to restore the meaning of certain key names through technical innovation; on the level of biological nomenclature, the combination of patriotic sentiment and scientific sensibility resulted in the desire to correlate Gaelic names and Linnaean terms. We see this also in White's *Essay*, in Colgan's *Flora of County Dublin*, and in Moloney's *Irish Ethno-Botany*.

Colgan returned to the subject again in a series of articles on folklore and Gaelic nomenclature in *The Irish Naturalist* in 1914 and 1915. In the first of these, 'Field Notes on the Folk-lore of Irish Plants and Animals', Colgan supplied an anecdote that demonstrates the difficulties encountered by the gentleman naturalist trying to tie the countryman down to accuracy. Colgan was interested in the rural belief that each plant species occurred as male and female individuals; in this case the plant he wanted to know more about was the ragwort, or 'bulkishawn'. On a drive in north County Dublin in 1905, his informant was the car driver:

The She-Bulkishawn, he told me, was an ingredient in a famous horse medicine, which appeared to be quite as potent as Don Quixote's Balsam of Fierabras, and far more complex in its constitution. No less than twelve 'erribs' went to the brewing of this medicine. There was Garlic and Fetherfew, and Yarrow and Broom, and He-Bulkishawn and She-Bulkishawn, and six other 'erribs,' he disremembered the names, but the She-Bulkishawn was the best of them. He wouldn't say himself that all the twelve 'erribs' were indispensable, but I gathered from him that not even the most advanced thinkers would venture to omit any of them. 'What is the She-Bulkishawn like?' I inquired. 'Oh,' he answered, 'it's something like the He-Bulkishawn, the Ragweed that grows everywhere, but it hasn't any flowers and it's a sight harder to find.' He was instructed to keep a sharp look-out for her, and, finally, as we approached Ballyrothery, he stood up and, pointing eagerly with his whip to a tuft of the Common Tansy growing on a roadside bank near a field gate, cried out – 'There she is!'

Notwithstanding difficulties such as these, Colgan and R.F. Scharff continued to explore the issue, and it was Scharff in particular who pushed ahead during the Great War (and the build-up to Irish independence) with the work of publishing lists of bird and animal names in Irish in the *Irish Naturalist*.

Colgan was especially alert to the problem of localism in the application of vernacular names. A jellyfish that he landed on to a boat off Rush around 1910 was called by the fishermen 'sun jelly' or 'swalder'; swalder was also the name at Howth, but at Dun Laoghaire the name became 'squalls', while the bigger specimens were called 'parliament men'. The same problem beset the Gaelic names. *Crosán* (for starfish) at Skerries became *crosóg* at Dalkey; *faochan* (for periwinkle) on Clare Island became *faochóg* on the mainland four miles away. Colgan cautioned that 'the name changes, and often quite rapidly, with change of locality ... A mountain range, a river or an arm of the sea may serve as a linguistic no less than a biological barrier' (Colgan, 1915).

Colgan also considered that several names for a single species was the rule rather than the exception. This is fully borne out by the lists Scharff published (1915, 1915a, 1916), as well as by the list of Irish bird names that Sean Mac Giollarnaith later compiled as an appendix to Kennedy, Ruttledge and Scroope's *Birds of Ireland* (1954). In his list of bird names, Scharff gave seven different names for kingfisher; according to Mac Giollarnaith, the chough was called *Chathóg dheargchosach* on the Aran Islands, *coróg* in west Mayo, and *cosdhearg* in Kerry. The linguistic map of Gaelic nomenclature was clearly a fractured one, and even where the available names had been recorded there remained the problem of their application to the species known to science.

The solution to this problem was to standardize the Gaelic names themselves in line with scientific convention, as White had attempted in 1808 in his essay on Irish grasses. This has been largely achieved now with the publication, by the Department of Education, of a standard lexicon of Irish plant and animal names, *Ainmneacha Plandaí agus Ainmhithe* (1978); in botany, Maura Scannell and Donal Synnott produced a second edition of their *Census Catalogue of the Flora of Ireland* in 1987 with a standardized Gaelic nomenclature. The names in this definitive – and exemplary – work are a pragmatic blend of available vernacular names and new coinages. The basic framework for this, as for all definitive registers of biological names, is of course the standard Linnaean nomenclature: it is scientific taxonomy that decides on the boundaries between species and on the necessity for new names. The need for a stable vernacular is obvious in the case of the higher forms, the birds, animals, and plants; but the points that discriminate between, say, species of moss and lichen are so technical that the scientific name is all that is ever likely to be needed. This is reflected in Scannell and Synnott's *Catalogue* where, for instance, the plants of the Hieracium hawkweeds are bracketed under a single vernacular name – hawkweed, *lus na seabhac*; the finer discriminations of this critical genus are a matter for specialists only.

Shortcomings of Vernacular Nomenclature

Accurate naming is a practice central to the scientific tradition. It affirms a correspondence between the language we use and the world in which we live; it forms part of that empirical spirit which came to the fore in the seventeenth century and insisted that the objective world was the goal of knowledge and enquiry, and that no power group had a right to interpose its own interests between the understanding and its objects. The conflict between scholasticism and the scientific tradition on this score is captured beautifully by John Banville's historical novels *Doctor Copernicus* (1976) and *Kepler* (1981), in which the key issue is the accurate identification of things in themselves: Nicolas Copernicus and Johannes Kepler completely overturned a medieval order where models of the universe were designed only to 'save the phenomena' or superficially conform to the observed motions of the planets, and where the accurate description of the heavens was inhibited by the proscriptions of the Church.

The growth of the scientific sensibility inevitably carried with it the need to find new or standardized names for things; the names needed to be empirically accurate and to have a universal application. This entailed sorting out the confusion that existed in pre-scientific vernaculars over the application of names, as in the biological nomenclature that we are considering. The predicament of the early-modern scientist in this regard is captured by one of the pioneers of the new movement, Francis Bacon, in his account of empirical method in *Novum Organum* (1620):

... men believe that their reason governs words; but it is also true that words react on the understanding; and this it is that has rendered philosophy and the sciences sophistical and inactive. Now words, being commonly framed and applied according to the capacity of the vulgar, follow those lines of division which are most obvious to the vulgar understanding. And whenever an understanding of greater acuteness or a more diligent observation would alter those lines to suit the true divisions of nature, words stand in the way and resist the change.

In Bacon's England, the standardization of names for objects in nature saw the replacement of a motley fund of regional terms with a new and generally applicable set of names, so we should remember that the decline of a peasant vernacular with its superstitions and folk beliefs was not a specifically colonial issue. The case of English in England has been discussed by

Keith Thomas in *Man and the Natural World* (1983), where the establish-ment of a standard nomenclature involved the loss of a colourful but irreg-ular lexicon of plant and animal terminology.

Nostalgia for the pre-modern past has found strong reinforcement in Ireland, however, because of Gaelic nationalism and a concomitant tenden-cy to totemize the old, dialectal name as the 'right name'. On the question of names for nature, there is a persistent belief that the Gaelic vernacular could rival, in accuracy and completeness, Linnaean nomenclature, although the concepts of accuracy and completeness within the framework of system-atic classification are derivative of the Linnaean model itself. The native Gaelic names for plants as investigated by Colgan, Hart and others reflect-ed the material situation and superstitions of a pre-modern rural culture. The only systematic view of the natural world which might be inferred from the old terminology was reported by Colgan along with the idea of sexes in plants already quoted (Colgan, 1914). Colgan describes, somewhat whimsi-cally, the doctrine of 'transmogrification of species':

In accordance with the Transmogrification Doctrine, a species is held to have an innate capacity, within the life-time of a single individual, of producing another species belonging to a distinct genus or even to a distinct Order or Class. The new species is usually held, and not unjustly, to be the old species gone wild. For instance, at Feenone between Louisburgh and the Killary, in 1911, a man pointed me out the Royal Fern, and said, 'We call them Wild Rannyocks,' the Rannyock proper, the sane and steady Rannyock, being here, as everywhere in Gaelic Ireland, the Common Bracken. Again, in Clare Island, Sparganium or the Bur-Reed is held to be the Wild Shellistring or Flagger. A countryman near Kilbarrick, Co. Dublin, once assured me that the common *Centaurea nigra* or Blackhead grew out of the Plantain or Ribwort, and, to cap these instances, a farmer near Cocles Bridge at Garristown was quite positive that a flowering plant of Angelica which I pointed out to him in a ditch had originated in the Flaggers or Yellow Iris that grew alongside. 'Sometimes,' he said, 'them Flaggers blossom out that-a-way; more times they don't. Wild Flaggers they call them.'

Colgan knew that findings such as these had little more than anecdotal value; at most, they reflect a pre-scientific view of the natural world where the peasant's husbandry was pitted against chaotic forces in nature for which he had no explanatory model (Thomas, 1971). Such a world-view sees wild nature as the degeneration of civilized order: the idea is widely reflected in the literature of Renaissance England, in Shakespeare's *King Lear* and *The Tempest* and in Milton's *Comus*, for example.

D.A. Webb's critical examination of Irish names for his standard *Irish Flora* (1977) led him to exercise great caution in the linking of the Irish name with the scientific species; he gives the Irish name only where he feels that the attribution is precise, and applies the same criteria when dealing with English vernacular names, excluding the 'book-names' invented in the nineteenth century. His discussion of the validity of Irish names includes a remarkable sentence: 'The predominance of the spoken over the written language for some centuries, *coupled with the fact that the Irish are more interested in words and names than in material objects* [my italics], has made the application of popular plant names in Ireland extremely fluctuating and obscure' (Webb, 1977).

This is an extremely suggestive point which could take us into fields of linguistic theory and collective psychology far removed from the present topic. It is sufficient in this context to observe that the issue of nomenclature in natural history has wider ramifications, which relate to the value we give to the English vernacular we now practise and to the older Gaelic language. Conservationists and excursionists can all too easily imagine that the paucity of the rural community's present linguistic relationship with nature is the residue of a once-sophisticated knowledge of the natural world. On the other hand, the detailed knowledge of natural species which Linnaean names describe is unprecedented in any pre-modern vernacular; and it can hardly be claimed that this knowledge alienates us from the affections and the imagination, as Praeger's career demonstrates.

Furthermore, the process of description, classification and naming that Linnaeus systematized for the first time has since that time been subject to continual modification. The natural groupings are constantly being modified within changing conventions. Praeger himself had a part to play in this process of evolution with his two monographs on the stonecrops and houseleeks, 'An Account of the Genus Sedum as Found in Cultivation' (1921) and *An Account of the Sempervivum Group* (1932), which were responsible for securing him a European reputation as a botanist. Praeger applied extreme meticulousness to resolving the daunting complexities of both groups: the results are monuments to empirical science. They are also linguistic achievements, in the sense that language is operating here at the limit of its potential to register the complexities of the natural world, and as such they offer suggestive parallels to the work of poets and philosophers as they confront language with the texture of experience.

Nature and Science as Agents of Reconciliation

As we saw in Heaney's poem 'The Peninsula', nature offers relief from the confinement of human affairs. A drive in the country is a way of getting away from it all – from domestic, marital, or professional disputes. But the equation is not that simple, because nature itself has in turn been the subject of quarrels about nomenclature, conservation, land-ownership, and so on. The conflicts involve differences of interpretation of a common resource, but at present there are signs that we are willing to broaden the scope of that interpretation to go beyond nostalgia for a peasant culture that was destined to be transformed anyway by the process of modernization. The growth of interpretative centres and tourist offices around the country for the use of Irish and foreign visitors alike is an affirmation of the fact that most of us are now excursionists on the landscape rather than natives to it. By virtue of our life-style, we are likely to have more in common with the Victorian tourist than with the ageing Gaelic speaker, whose worth as the repository of a marginal culture has been diluted by obsolescence.

The history of natural history in Ireland must inevitably put into focus that remarkable era of exploration between the 1880s and the First World War when biological nomenclature was the mode, as well as the motive, of discovery. Localities revealed themselves as plant and animal names, and the record of scientific or vernacular English names marked the opening up of the Irish landscape as a virgin frontier by pioneers such as Praeger, Colgan and Hart. Their relationship with Ireland was that peculiar blend of unionism and regionalism which now seems so remote to those who have been brought up in the nationalist tradition (although it is still alive and well in the north-east).

Placing on record their achievement and their patriotism is part of the rehabilitation of science within Irish culture which Dorinda Outram called for in a memorable article in *The Irish Review* in 1986. 'Irish history has always focussed', she argued, 'on a narrowly conceived version of the transactions of power .... But for Irish history to deprive itself of the history of science is also to deprive itself of some valuable tools for critical reflections on the nature of power and authority, and the capacity of man to gain that power and authority through contact with sources which, like the natural world, stand outside the human group.' 'Irish history', in these terms, dwelt on conflicts between power groups while leaving out the history of Irish science, which deals with the history of the encounter between man and the natural world. We find parallel complaints elsewhere about the importance attached to the past in Ireland to the detriment of scientific enquiry.

In *The Way that I Went* (1937), Praeger voiced the hope that 'a person of ordinary intelligence would find as much to interest him in the ground he walks on, the air he breathes, the myriad lower creatures, large and small, which share the earth with him, as in the present activities of populous human hives, or in the memorials of bygone piety or warfare which are everywhere with us'. Two hundred and ten years earlier, in his first treatise of Irish botany, *Synopsis Stirpium Hibernicarum* (1727), the dissenting clergyman Caleb Threlkeld was urging similar things on the nation:

... although we are not the same Nation of Men, who dwelt here a thousand Years ago, yet the spontaneous Plants are the same as they were in the time of the Danes and Bryan Boro, and in my Opinion it had been more Benefit to Mankind to have made stricter enquiries into the Natural Growth of the Soil ... than to have trifled away Pains and Time, in amusing us with fabulous Stories concerning the Generations of Men preceding us ...

Helen Laird quoted these remarks to that meeting of the Limerick Field Club in 1904.

It is perhaps most helpful to read these arguments, from Threlkeld to Outram, as a call, not to abandon history, but to put Ireland's military and political history in due perspective. While it may not leave power transactions and contestations behind, 'natural' history does focus our mind on the endurance of the natural world as a locus of enquiry and analysis. Given Ireland's conflicts of language and tradition, the most telling instance of the encounter between man and the natural world is in the selection of names for things in nature. But ultimately, the context of the problem extends to the history of ideas on a European scale and it is unwarranted and unduly restrictive to give a special privilege to the Gaelic terms of a primitive rural community.

In the narrative of Irish natural history that this volume is seeking to reconstruct, botany is the most fertile single discipline because of the importance of plants in agriculture, herbal lore and medicine since ancient times. Since plants continue to have pharmacological, agricultural and aesthetic significance, there is a remarkable potential for narrative and cultural continuity in this area. Anyone who explores this tradition becomes aware that although the object of botanical study is ostensibly merely empirical, each new act of scientific compilation requires speculative and intellectual exertions that we normally associate with metaphysical and literary discourses. The lack of institutionalization of metaphysics in Ireland before the establishment of modern university departments of philosophy, as well as the discontinuity of the literary traditions, have given rise to assumptions of discontinuity or absence in Irish cultural experience. The study of nature, on the other hand, offers the prospect of transcending these assumptions.

References

Bacon, F. [1620] 1905. *Novum Organum. The Works of Francis Bacon.* Vol. 1. Trans. R. Ellis and J. Spedding. London: Routledge.

Colgan, N. 1904. *Flora of County Dublin.* Dublin: Hodges, Figgis.

Colgan, N. 1914. 'Field Notes on the Folk-Lore of Irish Plants and Animals.' *Irish Naturalist 23*: 53-64.

Colgan, N. 1915. 'On Irish Animal Names.' *Irish Naturalist 24*: 166-9.

Colgan, N. and R.W. Scully. 1898. *Contributions towards a Cybele Hibernica, being Outlines of the Geographical Distribution of Plants in Ireland.* Second edition Founded on the Papers of the late Alexander Goodman More. Dublin: Edward Ponsonby.

Collins, T. 1985. *Floreat Hibernia: A Bio-bibliography of Robert Lloyd Praeger 1865-1953.* Dublin: Royal Dublin Society.

Coolahan, John. 1981. *Irish Education: Its History and Structure*. Dublin: Institute of Public Administration.

Department of Education. 1978. *Ainmneacha Plandaí agus Ainmhithe: Flora and Fauna Nomenclature*. Dublin: Stationery Office.

Fennell, D. 1981. 'The Last Years of the Gaeltacht.' *The Crane Bag 5*: 8-11.

Hart, H.C. 1898. *Flora of the County Donegal*. Dublin: Sealy, Bryers and Walker.

Heaney, S. 1969. *Door into the Dark*. London: Faber and Faber.

Heaney, S. 1972. *Wintering Out*. London: Faber and Faber.

Heaney, S. 1980. *Preoccupations: Selected Prose 1968-1978*. London: Faber and Faber.

Heaney, S. 1983. *An Open Letter*. Field Day Pamphlets, no. 2. Derry: Field Day.

Heaney, S. 1988. *The Government of the Tongue*. London: Faber and Faber.

Hyde, D. 1899. *A Literary History of Ireland*. London: Fisher Unwin. New ed. with an Introduction by B. O'Cuív. London: Ernest Benn, 1967.

Kennedy, P.G., R.F. Ruttledge and C.F. Scroope. 1954. *The Birds of Ireland*. London and Edinburgh: Oliver and Boyd.

K'Eogh, John. 1735. *Botanalogia Universalis Hibernica, Or: A General Irish Herbal [...]*. Cork: G. Harrison.

Koestler, A. 1959. *The Sleepwalkers: A History of Man's Changing Vision of the Universe*. London: Hutchinson.

Laird, H. 1904. 'A Bohareen of Irish Botany: Gaelic Plant Names and Animal Lore.' *Journal of the Limerick Field Club 2*: 196-210.

Mathews, A. 1983. *Minding Ruth*. Oldcastle: Gallery.

Moloney, M.F. 1919. *Irish Ethno-Botany and the Evolution of Medicine in Ireland*. Dublin: Gill.

Morton, A.G. 1981. *History of Botanical Science*. London: Academic Press.

Nelson, E.C. and W. Walsh. 1991. *The Burren: A Companion to the Wildflowers of an Irish Limestone Wilderness*. Aberystwyth and Kilkenny: Boethius Press and the Conservancy of the Burren.

Outram, D. 1986. 'Negating the Natural: or why Historians Deny Irish Science.' *Irish Review 1*: 45-9.

Phillips, W.H. and R.L. Praeger. 1887. 'The Ferns of Ulster.' *Proceedings of the Belfast Naturalists' Field Club 2(2)* (Appendix 1): 1-26.

Praeger, R.L. 1900. 'Botanical Exploration in 1899.' *Irish Naturalist 8*: 135-49.

Praeger, R.L. 1901. *Irish Topographical Botany*. Dublin: Royal Irish Academy.

Praeger, R.L. 1921. 'An Account of the Genus Sedum as Found in Cultivation.' *Journal of the Royal Horticultural Society 46*.

Praeger, R.L. 1932. *An Account of the Sempervivum Group*. London: Royal Horticultural Society.

Praeger, R.L. 1934. *The Botanist in Ireland*. Dublin: Hodges Figgis.

Praeger, R.L. 1937. *The Way that I Went*. Dublin: Hodges Figgis.

Praeger, R.L. and S.A. Stewart. 1895. 'A Supplement to the 'Flora of the North-east of Ireland' of Stewart and Corry.' *Proceedings of the Belfast Naturalists' Field Club 4(2)* (Appendix 5): 133-236.

Scannell, M. and D. Synnott. 1987. *Census Catalogue of the Flora of Ireland*. Dublin: Stationery Office.

Scharff, R. 1915. 'On the Irish Names of Plants and Animals.' *Irish Naturalist 24*: 45-53.

Scharff, R. 1915a. 'On the Irish Names of Birds.' *Irish Naturalist 24*: 109-29.

Scharff, R. 1916. 'On the Irish Names of Reptiles, Amphibians and Fishes.' *Irish Naturalist 25*: 106-19.

Scharff, R. 1916a. 'On the Irish Names of Invertebrate Animals.' *Irish Naturalist 25*: 140-52.

Synnott, D. 1979. 'Folk-lore, Legend and Irish Plants.' *Irish Gardening and Horticulture 3*: 37-43.

Thomas, K. 1971. *Religion and the Decline of Magic: Studies in Popular Belief in Sixteenth- and Seventeenth-Century England*. London: Weidenfeld and Nicolson.

Thomas, K. 1983. *Man and the Natural World: Changing Attitudes in England 1500-1800*. London: Allen Lane.

Threlkeld, C. 1727. *Synopsis Stirpium Hibernicarum, being a Short Treatise of Native Plants, Especially such as Grow Spontaneously in the Vicinity of Dublin; with their Latin, English and Irish Names: and an Abridgement of their Virtues*. Dublin: Davys, Norris and Worrall. Facsimile reprint with an introduction by E.C. Nelson and a glossary of Irish plant names by D. Synnott. Aberystwyth and Kilkenny: Boethius Press, 1988.

Viney, M. 1986. 'Woodcock for a Farthing: The Irish Experience of Nature.' *Irish Review* *1*: 58-64.

Webb, D. [1943] 1977. *An Irish Flora*. Sixth rev. ed. 1977. Dundalk: Dundalgan Press.

White, J. 1808. *An Essay on the Indigenous Grasses of Ireland*. Dublin: The Dublin Society.

The History of Natural History: Grand Narrative or Local Lore?

DORINDA OUTRAM

Of what history is the history of natural history in Ireland a part? In 1966 the French philosopher Michel Foucault (1926-84) attempted to insert the history of natural history in the West into a 'grand narrative' of changes in the underlying structures of thought in Europe since the Renaissance. The purpose of this essay is to question the extent to which Foucault's conceptualization of the history of natural history in general is helpful in understanding the history of natural history in Ireland, and whether other available conceptualizations of natural history might perform differently or better than Foucault's in aiding our understanding of the Irish context.

Classical vs Modern Natural History: Foucault's Theory

Foucault's account of natural history is largely contained in his 1966 book *Mots et Choses*, translated in 1970 as *The Order of Things*. Here, Foucault put forward an influential account of the changes that proceeded in natural history between what he describes as the 'Classical Age' (roughly the seventeenth and eighteenth centuries) and the 'Modern Age' (roughly the period from the end of the eighteenth century to the present, the period dominated by evolutionary ideas). These changes, according to Foucault, were concurrent with similar developments in linguistics and economics. Natural history is thus firmly fastened to an account of deep-level change occurring in major structures of European thought as a whole. Foucault describes these changes as 'archaeological'.

To understand these changes is to employ an approach to the history of thought (an 'archaeology') that eliminates the fundamental role of the human subject as the agent of history. As an historical method that decentres the human subject, Foucault's analyses tend to deal with historical periods of such length that they cannot be understood as the result of individual action. This approach by Foucault has often seemed incoherent. How can there ever be a history of thought which is not essentially a history of thinkers? To try to answer such criticism, Foucault has produced a history that thinks about historical evidence as monuments indicating the basic 'archaeological' structures of thought behind cultures. Foucault calls these basic structures 'discursive formations'. In his analysis a scientific discipline such as natural history may, for example, be just one part of a discursive formation that also includes various sorts of non-scientific discourse (for example, legal, literary, philosophical or common-sense statements) which are governed by the same rules and concerns. This is why in *The Order of Things* Foucault searched the three sciences of grammar, natural history, and economics for similarities, noting that each of them underwent a sharp break between what he calls 'classical' and 'modern' ways of thinking.

In the case of natural history, Foucault asserts that whereas before the Classical Age living beings had been fastened in a web of largely verbal knowledge including legends and fables, mixing direct observation and hearsay, in the Classical Age natural history was concerned only with a limited range of easily observable characteristics, being 'a meticulous examination of things themselves for the first time, and then of transcribing what has been gathered in smooth, neutralized, and faithful words ... natural history is nothing more than the nomination of the visible'.

In this way, classical natural history freed itself from the veil of verbal description so as 'to bring ... the things observed as close as possible to words'. Natural history, according to Foucault, increasingly became concerned with focusing visual attention on the 'character' of the plant or animal, the feature that conveyed the essential nature of each organism. For Linnaeus, for example, that 'character' lay in reproduction, which was used as the basis of determining the degree to which the plant was more or less similar to others described on the same basis. This is what Foucault describes as the general project of natural history in this period of 'defining identities by means of the general grid of differences'.

Because of the postulates that lay behind this approach to classification, Foucault argues, natural history had to assume a continuity in nature that was entirely at variance with man's actual experience of nature as a 'confused wealth of representation'. Foucault asserts that naturalists of the Classical Age endeavoured to make sense of this wealth of representation by producing schematic views of the natural relationships often expressed in tables of taxonomic orders. As well, there are 'temporal' groupings of natural beings that result from interruptions in the order of nature by the events of climate and geological change. Foucault argues that attempts by such eighteenth-century thinkers as the Swiss naturalist Charles Bonnet, the French writer Denis Diderot and the French scientist Pierre-Louis Moreau de Maupertuis to discuss the transformations of living beings are to be understood merely as offshoots of the central project of the Classical Age, which is to construct a 'permanent tabulation' for the beings of nature. He thus denies that there can be any continuity between the natural history of the Classical Age and the natural history of the Modern Age, which is dominated by evolutionism: 'There is not and cannot even be the suspicion of an evolutionism or a transformism in Classical thought.' The reason for this is that for classical natural historians, time was not integral to the nature of the beings they described. This makes them very different from what, Foucault alleges, is the nature of living beings described by 'genuine' evolutionary theory of the modern era.

Another important difference is that although the natural history of the Classical Age dealt with living beings, it did not, according to Foucault, deal with a concept of 'life'. 'Life does not constitute an obvious threshold beyond which entirely new forms of knowledge are required.' In other words, only the Modern Age was able to transform natural history into biology, the science of life: this is why Foucault claims that before the nineteenth century 'biology did not exist ... life itself did not exist. All that existed were living beings.' Foucault describes this change as a rupture with past thinking of startling finality:

One day, towards the end of the eighteenth century, [Baron Georges] Cuvier was to topple the glass jars of the Museum, smash them open, and dissect all the forms of animal visibility that the Classical Age had preserved in them. This iconoclastic gesture ... does not reveal a new curiosity diverted towards a secret that no-one had the interest or courage to uncover, or the possibility of uncovering before. It is, rather ... a mutation in the natural dimension of western culture: the end of 'history' in the sense in which it was understood by Tournefort, Linnaeus, Buffon and Adanson ... and it was also to be the beginning of what, by substituting anatomy for classification, organism for structure, internal subordination for visible character, the series for the tabulation, was to make possible the precipitation into the old flat world of animals and plants, engraved in black and white, a whole profound mass of time to which men were to give the renewed name of 'history'.

According to Foucault, it was then that nature and living beings could be identified as living, dynamic and changing systems, as 'economies'. This is an idea that has been taken up by historians such as Bernard Balan (1975) and Karl Figlio (1966), who have pointed to the overlap of concepts and vocabulary between science and social analysis through such key words as 'economy'. Economy, meaning a complex system obeying its own ends, was also an important concept in detaching natural history from its theological interpretation, where nature was seen as organized by God for his ends and primarily as a habitat for man, his creation. Nature was no longer confined to a grid defined by the human observer; it escaped, entered its own history, and worked out its own teleologies. The renewal of 'natural history' as 'biology' in the nineteenth century was the result of this transformation (Gutting, 1989). Nature was seen as a collection of resources at man's disposal; creation had been ordered by a benevolent God so that all other creatures should serve man's purposes, and 'wilderness' was there to be 'developed' for human needs.

Problems with Foucault's Theory

In spite of the criticism to which much of Foucault's work has been subjected by historians such as A.P. O'Brien (1989), his account of 'natural history' has become virtually paradigmatic, and has found followers throughout Europe. Historians such as Wolf Lepenies (1976, 1979) and Giulio Barsanti (1979), to cite two, have reproduced Foucault's theory of a sharp break in the way in which nature itself was conceptualized between the Classical and the Modern periods, including the growth of historical, i.e. non-static, ideas of the development of nature. Foucault's account, in spite of its ambiguities, in spite of its focus on a limited range of material drawn from the work of scientists alone, has achieved this degree of acceptability perhaps because it appears to argue for a definitive 'modernity' for post-1800 life-sciences.

However, Foucault's analysis presents us also with many problems. It is, first of all, an analysis undertaken specifically in opposition to historians of individual 'disciplines' in science. Foucault sets out to provide a radically new approach, and attempts to link different disciplines (e.g., economics, linguistics, natural history) by showing similarities in basic levels of concepts (an archaeology). This is one major difficulty in applying his work to the history of a particular discipline, since Foucault's entire line of argument is devoted to undermining the concept of disciplines as autonomous intellectual entities.

Nor does Foucault's analysis link up very well with other ways of conceptualizing the history of natural history. Increasingly since the 1970s, the emergence of a form of history specifically devoted to the environment has seen the relationships between the life sciences and nature as a political one where the life sciences exist to describe and legitimate man's power and exploitation of nature (Worster, 1988; Cronon, 1992). This insight, consciously or not, parallels claims by the German philosophers Max Horkheimer and Theodor Adorno that the Enlightenment, which Foucault is content to characterize as the 'Classical Age' of natural history, was one in fact that saw the legitimation of human domination and exploitation of nature. It may be no accident that the era that sees the emergence of 'natural history' also sees the first large-scale extinctions of species in nature wherever white settlement took place (Lyon, 1991). Closer to home, entire forests were devastated in Ireland to build the British navy in the eighteenth century, thus neatly exemplifying how political relationships between human groups are rapidly translated into 'political' or exploitative relationships with nature. This power-relation between man and other living beings is not one that emerges from Foucault's account.

Thirdly, and just as seriously, Foucault's account, while explicitly aimed at undermining disciplinary boundaries, and re-situating the changes in natural history against deeper changes in structures of thought, uses a range of original sources based entirely on the writings of French naturalists, a range of sources entirely the same as would be used by a historian of ideas working on a narrowly conceived disciplinary basis. Foucault, while deeply critical of actual structures of ideas, is less so of the status of his primary sources. These are analyzed as accurate transcriptions of assumptions in natural history. They are never treated as strategic statements, produced more in response to specific circumstances than as representing absolute truths (Outram, 1986).

If we turn to a consideration of the local and national context of natural history in Ireland, Foucault's approach to the history of natural history poses many obvious problems. The nature of Foucault's sources makes obvious his assumption that the patterns of French natural history are repeated elsewhere, indeed that they are the paradigm. He has little to say about possible national divergences from this model. Another way of making this point is to say that there are problems with any model of intellectual development that makes implicit (or explicit) claims to universality. What does the model 'explain' or 'situate' if it does not apply in the particular case? From within the heart of Foucault's analysis, we may note the extent to which the Classical Age in natural history was conceived as one where words and things 'were brought as close together as possible'. But in the context of Ireland, where English and Irish persisted side by side at least into the early nineteenth century, and there were many truly bilingual individuals, just whose words do we mean? In spite of his overtly anti-disciplinary position, Foucault's analysis still reads as though his definition of what 'natural history' actually was has been taken from a twentieth-century disciplinary viewpoint. In particular, Foucault's idea of what he must understand as 'natural history' completely excludes the theological dimension so strong in the English, and hence Anglo-Irish tradition. Here again, we see the insensitivity of universalistic accounts to the differences between 'cultural domains'. For all these reasons, Foucault's emphasis on 'natural history' seems to have little purchase on the cultural context of 'natural history' in Ireland in the period of the Enlightenment and after. In thus providing a model that has no hold on the cultural insertion of 'natural history', Foucault avoids the question of the actual meaning that the practice of natural history had to either practitioners or audience within a specific context.

All this might be read as saying in a rather prolonged way what has been apparent for some time: that Foucault's insights have often sat uneasily with historical practice. But other models of how we might understand natural history also present their own problems. In *Purity and Danger* (1966), for example, the English anthropologist Mary Douglas puts forward the view that the way in which a society orders its view of nature depends on the 'boundary lines' that society draws between insiders and outsiders, good and bad, high and low. In other words, the very different ways in which 'natural histories' have been thought of in the past are analogous to social structures. For example, Douglas notes how the classification of the animal world into clean and unclean creatures in the Book of Leviticus allowed Judaism a set of meanings around which Temple worship, holiness, the structure of food consumption, and the distinction between Hebrew society as settled and Nomadic hunters who ate wild game, could be made.

There are obvious attractions to this view. It seems to allow for an easy marriage between historical insight and the structure of ideas, a fruitful interplay between related fields of anthropology, history and history of ideas. The problems begin when we consider the process by which analogies are made between social and natural categories. Who is to say what the 'deep structure' of society is? Who is to say what features of the society are salient enough to be translated into interpretations of the natural order? Why these and not others? What means are supplied for verifying that the analogy between society and nature is in fact visible to the members of that society? Can we generalize from the experiences of non-Western societies to that of our own where knowledge of nature has become an area of activity called 'science', separated out from the rest of life to a degree unknown in more 'traditional' societies? What criteria, to sum up, do we have for assessing the validity of the analogy between natural knowledge and social structure?

Objections in Practice to Foucault's Theory

There are thus serious problems in the use of many available theoretical positions about approaches to the history of natural history. How might we proceed to construct a questionnaire that would allow us to characterize the structures of natural history in Ireland and link them to changes happening elsewhere? It is clear that universalistic 'grand narratives', such as Foucault's, are of little assistance. They provide us with too little leverage at the level of specific national and regional situations; and they also often contain within themselves assumptions about what agendas are important. These assumptions are themselves often based only on one national experience, in Foucault's case that of the French.

But we might get somewhere by challenging one of the most basic assumptions in Foucault's account: that the transformation in 'natural history' occurred as a result of a changing relationship to time. Why time? Why not space? Given the rapid destruction of habitats and extinction of species occurring throughout the European-settled world in the eighteenth century, Foucault's assertion that 'natural history' changed into 'biology' through the invention of the notion of 'life' and its insertion into 'time', must surely be read today with a grim irony of which Foucault was unaware at the time of writing, but which certainly is to the fore in current thinking about the history of our relationship with natural history. Authors such as Keith Thomas (1984) and Donald Worster (1988), for example, have highlighted the exploitative character of attitudes towards nature in western Christianity.

Foucault's analysis also overlooks the extent to which natural history defined itself in relation to 'place'. 'Natural history' contains many different strands of thought and varieties of practice. Particularly strong in the Anglo-Irish case was a kind of natural history that treated the debates about taxonomy (with which Foucault is so concerned) as secondary to its interest in connecting the natural organisms of a particular place with the history, geology and antiquities of that place. In this respect, the county histories of Ireland produced by Charles Smith (1746, 1750) or Walter Harris (1744), which recounted the history, historical monuments, topographical features, antiquities, archaeology, geology, natural and industrial products and natural history, all within the same covers, differed little from the works of natural history being produced in the contemporary North American colonies by Mark Catesby (1731-43) or Thomas Jefferson in 1784. As Keith Thomas has pointed out, this sort of 'natural history', which aimed to give a unified account of human and natural activity within a particular region rather than describe taxonomic conflicts, was the Anglo-American norm.

This alone should cast doubt on Foucault's other main assumption: that changes in natural history can largely be defined through shifts in taxonomy. Certainly it was the case that conflict between important figures such as Buffon and Linnaeus over the nature and purposes of the classification of living (and non-living) beings, assumed a high profile for some strands of natural history in the eighteenth century (Lyon and Sloan, 1981). But while Foucault treats taxonomy as defining the Classical Age, it would be more accurate to say that in fact it divided it. Chaos and division in classification was such as to prevent any consensus emerging; even the division between the Classical and Modern Ages over this point is debatable (Outram, 1986).

All this means that there is no way in which a singular history of natural history defined as a taxonomy in relation to 'time' can be constructed, that there is no one lens that will allow us to see the whole of 'natural history' between the eighteenth and nineteenth centuries. Such universalistic models seem peculiarly inappropriate to apply to the Irish situation of divided language between English and Irish and cultural difference between town and country, modernity and tradition, frontier and settled areas, within and beyond the Pale, divided religion between Catholic and Protestant, and divided perceptions of the natural world between improving landlord, peasant farmer, gentleman naturalist, and academic scientist. We need to be able to construct an account of 'natural history' that will take account of the divided culture in which it was embedded, a culture that involved practitioners and audience alike in continuous negotiation between different traditions carrying different perceptions of the natural world. To do otherwise is to subsume natural history under universalistic accounts such as that of Foucault, or under the assumptions of Mary Douglas that there is a singular 'social structure' which represents the diversity of experience in each situation of cultural interchange. It is also to subsume natural history within the frameworks of nineteenth-century nationalism with its assumption of monolithic congruence between land, people, language and nature. We need, in other words, a different way of articulating the relations between 'culture' and 'nature' and place. Let us try to do this from the basis of the specific history of natural history within Ireland.

The Irish Situation

Irish natural history developed features of its own that fit badly with Foucault's account. Firstly, it faced problems common to Irish science in general, problems that prevented Ireland from developing the 'big science' characteristic of late-nineteenth-century and twentieth-century Germany, for example.

The reasons for this have often been rehearsed; institutional weakness in science due to the poverty of the state's finances, absence of expanding industry, and the low cultural acceptance of science due to its identification with a declining Protestant elite of industrialists, improving landlords, and administrators, were factors at work. As Seán Lysaght (1989) has noted, for the period from 1922 in Southern Ireland, 'The scientist is dramatised in Irish cultural lore as a homologue of the colonist.' Along with this went the hostile reaction of Catholicism itself to science, a reaction that was intensified in Ireland by the association of Catholicism with the struggle against the Protestant Ascendancy. The relationship between Irish Catholicism and science in Ireland still awaits serious exploration. The hostility between the two can be gauged by the 1874 decision by the Catholic hierarchy to exclude physical science from the programme of Maynooth College. Actions such as these indicate that the response of Irish Catholicism was very different from the response to science of the international Catholic Church, which began a slow accommodation with science, and Darwinism in particular, from the 1890s onwards (Glick, 1974), at precisely the time when the Irish Catholic church was becoming more strongly bound up with the nationalist anti-colonial and thus anti-scientific agenda.

However, the position of science in Southern Ireland was not due to purely Irish religious factors, such as the rise of conservative Catholicism in the nineteenth century. For example, in spite of the fact that Ulster Presbyterianism had its own problems with science in the nineteenth century, these problems did not result in the cultural exclusion of science itself. Rather, the specifically Southern Irish relationship between science and religion was due to the specific cultural consequences of nationalist mobilization in the South.

The construction of the Irish 'nation' as a monolithic alliance between nationalism and Catholicism left little space for the moral systems that had accompanied both science and the Enlightenment. Values such as objectivity, rationality, and individual autonomy, central to the ethos of science, were discarded (Outram, 1988, 1989). Since the heroic naturalists like the explorers Alexander von Humboldt and Pierre-Simon Pallas, at the end of the Enlightenment, the field study of nature had been much supported by the culturally acceptable creation of a vocational identity that marked the ideal naturalist in his lonely travels through nature: an identity of invincible rectitude, indifference to social contrivance and corruption, and absolute personal autonomy. This vocational identity for the ideal man of science itself mirrored the increasing concern of the late Enlightenment to provide an account of the order of nature as a self-sufficient system, outside social construction.

But a mythology of science outside social production is a luxury of lands with settled histories where the society that produces science is not itself in question. It did not answer the question: what sort of a land was Ireland? Was it a 'wilderness' or a 'frontier', or an area containing a population of organisms basically similar to that of the British Isles? (Yearley, 1992; Baker, 1990). The great difficulties in conceptualizing the nature of the land in which the order of nature lay embedded had negative consequences for attitudes towards that order, and for the very project of understanding it through natural history (Snyder, 1984), and may well have laid the roots of the comparative indifference towards ecological issues that many recent commentators have discerned in Ireland (Baker, 1990; Yearley, 1992).

None of this prevented the continuance of a strong fieldwork tradition in Ireland from the late nineteenth century into the twentieth (Deane, 1924; Campbell, 1938; Collins, 1992); what it did prevent was the full integration of Irish natural history fieldwork into the emerging laboratory-based disciplines increasingly dominant in other states such as France and Germany, where the scientific profession was larger, cultural acceptance of science stronger, and government financing more generous. In that sense, Irish natural history, especially in Southern Ireland after 1922, does operate in a cultural universe where full integration with the Darwinian paradigm, which fuelled so much fieldwork, was difficult.

It is clear that many interpretations both of the history of natural history and of the relationships between social 'structures' and images of the natural world, have only a limited purchase on the problem of constructing a cultural history of natural history in Ireland, or indeed in any society where different cultural traditions are brought into proximity in a relationship of conflict. How then are we to proceed in the future? Is there a potential for a remaking of the relationship between the natural order and its conceptualization in Ireland? Maybe such a remaking could come from a return to a framing concept of locality. This would allow us to take in the particularities of the overlap of cultural and geographic space, to attend to what has been called the 'historical geography' of cultural development, and provide ourselves with a more balanced account of the interaction of local responses and grand narrative outlines of conceptual change. This approach might also draw upon recent concerns in cultural geography and the sociology of science with the ways in which particular forms of scientific knowledge migrate. This interest is conceptually important because it allows science, once seen as the paradigmatically 'universal' endeavour, to recapture its local roots (Berndt, 1976; Livingstone, 1992; Ophir and Shapin, 1991; Thrift, 1985). In doing so, we also incorporate one of the central pre-suppositions of eighteenth-century field natural history itself, that of the embeddedness of the natural order in a particular land.

References

Baker, S. 1990. 'The Evolution of the Irish Ecology Movement,' in Rudig (ed.), *Green Politics One* 1990. Edinburgh: Edinburgh University Press.

Balan, B. 1975. 'Premières Recherches sur l'Origine et la Formation du Concept de l'Economie Animal.' *Revue de l'histoire des sciences et de leurs applications* 28: 289-326.

Barsanti, G. 1979. *Dalla storia naturale alla storia della natura: saggio su Lamarck.* Milan: Feltrinelli.

Berndt, R.M. 1976. 'Territoriality and the Problem of Demarcating Socio-Cultural Space,' in N. Peterson (ed.), *Tribes and Boundaries.* Canberra: A.N.U. Press.

Campbell, A.A. 1938. *Belfast Naturalists' Field Club: Origins and Progress.* Belfast: Hugh Greer.

Catesby, M. 1731-43. *The Natural History of Carolina, Florida and the Bahama Islands.* 2 vols. London: author.

Collins, T. 1992. 'Women Naturalists in Ireland.' *Bulletin of the UCG Women's Studies Centre 1*: 1-19.

Cronon, W. 1992. 'A Place for Stories: Nature, History and Narrative.' *Journal of American History* 78: 1347-76.

Deane, A. 1924. *The Belfast Natural History and Philosophical Society.* Belfast: BNHPS.

Douglas, M. [1966] 1989. *Purity and Danger: An Analysis of the Concepts of Pollution and Taboo.*

London: Routledge.

Figlio, K.M. 1966. 'The Metaphor of Organisation: An Historiographical Perspective on the Bio-medical sciences of the early nineteenth century.' *History of Science 14*: 17-53.

Foucault, M. 1966. *Mots et Choses*. Paris: Gallimard. Translated by Alan Sheridan as *The Order of Things*. 1970. London: Tavistock. [Citations are from this edition.]

Glick, T.F. 1974. *The Comparative Reception of Darwinism*. Austin, Texas: University of Texas Press.

Gutting, G. 1989. *Michel Foucault's Archaeology of Scientific Reason*. Cambridge, U.K.: Cambridge University Press.

Harris, W. and C. Smith. 1744. *The Antient and Present State of the County of Down ... with the Natural and Civil History of the Same*. Dublin: A. Reilly.

Jefferson, T. [1784] 1955, 1981. *Notes on the State of Virginia*. Chapel Hill: University of North Carolina Press; New York: Penguin.

Lepenies, W. 1976. *Das Ende der Naturgeschichte: Wandel Kultureller Selbstverständlichkeiten* in der *Wissenschaften des 18 und 19 Jahrhunderts*. Munich: Surkamp.

Lepenies, W. 1979. 'De l'Histoire Naturelle à l'Histoire de la Nature.' *Dix-huitième Siècle 11*: 175-84.

Livingstone, D.N. 1992. 'Darwinism and Calvinism: The Belfast-Princeton Connection.' *ISIS 83*: 408-28.

Lyon, J. and P. Sloan (eds). 1981. *From Natural History to the History of Nature: Readings in Buffon and his Critics*. Notre Dame, Indiana: University of Notre Dame Press.

Lyon, T. J. (ed.). 1991. *This Incomperable Lande: A Book of American Nature Writing*. New York: Viking Penguin.

Lysaght, S. 1989. 'Heaney vs. Praeger: Contrasting Natures.' *The Irish Review 7*.

O'Brien, A. P. 1989. 'Foucault's History of Culture,' in L. Hunt (ed.), *The New Cultural History*. Berkeley: University of California Press.

Ophir, A. and S. Shapin. 1991. 'The Place of Knowledge: A Methodological Survey.' *Science in Context 4*: 3-21.

Outram, D. 1986. 'Uncertain Legislator: Georges Cuvier's Laws of Nature.' *Journal of the History of Biology 19*: 323-68.

Outram, D. 1988. 'Heavenly Bodies and Logical Minds: Banville, Science and Religion.' *Graph: Irish Literary Review 1*: 9-11.

Outram, D. 1989. 'Holding the Future at Bay: The French Revolution and Modern Ireland.' *The Irish Review 2*: 1-7.

Smith, C. 1746. *The Antient and Present State of the County and City of Waterford: Being a Natural, Civil ... and Topographical Description thereof.* Dublin: A. Reilly.

Smith, C. 1750. *The Antient and Present State of the City and County of Cork*. 4 vols. Dublin: A. Reilly.

Snyder, G. 1984. *Good, Wild, Sacred.* Hereford, U.K.: Five Seasons Press.

Thrift, N. 1985. 'Flies and Germs: A Geography of Knowledge,' in D. Gregory and J. Urry (eds), *Social Relations and Social Structures*. London: Macmillan.

Thomas, K. 1984. *Man and the Natural World: A History of the Modern Sensibility*. London: Pantheon.

Worster, D. 1988. *Nature's Economy: A History of Ecological Ideas*. Cambridge: Cambridge University Press.

Yearley, S. 1992/93. 'The Social Shaping of the Environmental Movement in Ireland,' in L. O'Dowd et al. (eds), *Ireland: A New Sociological Profile*. Dublin: Institute of Public Administration.

Essential Texts in Irish Natural History

DAVID CABOT

The Invisible College

An act of the English parliament in 1642 allowed Dutchmen to subscribe to a fund for the 'reduction of the Irish'; in exchange, grants of land confiscated from the Irish were made to subscribers. One of the subscribers was a Dr Gerard Boate, born at Gorcum in 1604. Boate invested £180 in the expectation of 'a reward' of 847 acres (Bottigheimer, 1971). He studied medicine at the University of Leyden, then settled in London in 1630 where he was appointed physician to the King. He was an enthusiastic supporter of the fund and wrote a book to describe the advantages of Ireland's natural resources for 'adventurers' and other contributors to the fund planning to settle in Ireland. Thus was born the first regional natural history written in the English language: a small duodecimo volume, published in London in 1652, entitled *Irelands Naturall History*. Boate died three years before the publication of his book. His widow obtained in 1667 a grant of land in Tipperary in return for his payments to 'the funds for the reduction of the Irish'.

Gerard Boate – according to a letter from his brother Arnold to Samuel Hartlib, the book's publisher, printed in a note 'To the Reader' – 'begun to write that work at the beginning of the year of our Lord 1645 and made an end of it long before the end of the same year; wheras he went not to Ireland untill the latter end of the year 1649 and dyed at Dublin within a very short while after he was arrived there'. Before Gerard started writing, Arnold Boate went to London and spent six months with Gerard 'reasoning about Ireland ... chiefly about the Naturall History of the same'. Gerard set down in writing what he heard from Arnold and then 'he conferred afterwards about the same with several of those Gentlemen', principally Sir William Parsons and his son Richard Parsons, who had been driven out of Ireland and were living in London (Boate, 1652).

Gerard sent his draft to Arnold, now back in Dublin, for comment, corrections and emendations. Arnold had resided in Dublin for eight years and 'made very many journeys into the Countrie and by meanes therof saw a great part of it, especially of the Provinces of Leinster and Ulster'. Arnold recounts that Gerard had intended to add more 'Books' to *Irelands Naturall History* to have made it a 'compleat Naturall History'. One was to have been on 'all kinds of plants', another on 'all sorts of living Creatures' and the third on 'the Natives of Ireland and their old fashions, Lawes, and Customes'. Alas, these were never written. Indeed, Gerard's manuscript was thought to have been mislaid before he moved to Dublin. The manuscript and other papers came into the possession of Samuel Hartlib, a German living in London.

Hartlib and the Boates were part of the 'Invisible College', which was 'an assembly of learned and curious gentlemen, who, after the breaking out of the civil wars, in order to divert themselves from those melancholy scenes, applied themselves to experimental enquiries, and the study of nature, which was then called the new philosophy, and at length gave birth to the Royal Society' (Boyle, 1744, quoted in Webster, 1974). The Boates displayed characteristic attributes of the Invisible College – enthusiasm for Baconian natural history, and anti-authoritarianism in both natural philosophy and medicine (Webster, 1974). They followed Bacon's advice to take advantage of the accumulated experience of artisans to compile exhaustive histories of trade and nature. *Irelands Naturall History* was a major departure from the antiquarian and anecdotal chorographical tradition.

The approach adopted by Boate was one of scientific pragmatism, in keeping with his training at Leyden and the Baconian New Philosophy. He was one of the first authors to exclude descriptions of marvels, supernatural events and apocryphal accounts of weird and wonderful things.

The full title of the book in the first edition, underlined in red ink, is: *IRELANDS NATVRALL HISTORY. Being a true and ample Description of its Situation, Greatness, Shape, and Nature; Of its Hills, Woods, Heaths, Bogs; Of its Fruitfull Parts and profitable Grounds, with the severall ways of Manuring and Improving the same: With its Heads or Promontories, Harbours, Roades and Bayes; Of its Springs and Fountaines, Brookes, Rivers, Loghs; Of its Metalls, Mineralls, Freestone, Marble, Sea-coal, Turf, and other things that are taken out of the ground. And lastly, of the Nature and temperature of its Air and Season, and what diseases it is free from, or subject unto. Conducing to the Advancement of Navigation, Husbandry, and other profitable Arts and Professions. Written by Gerard Boate, late Doctor of Physick to the State in Ireland. And now Published By Samuell Hartlib, Esq; for the Common Good of Ireland, and more especially, for the benefit of the Adventurers and Planters therin. Imprinted at London for John Wright at the Kings Head in the Old Bayley. 1652.*

The 'Epistle Dedicatory' to Oliver Cromwell and Charles Fleetwood by Hartlib occupies eight pages, followed by five pages 'To the Reader' by Arnold Boate. There are twenty-four chapters on 186 pages followed by 'A table of the principal Heads contained in this Book'. Complete copies have an erratum leaf.

The success of the book was signalled by a French edition published by Robert De Ninville in Paris in 1666. It was again a small duodecimo, five pages of Preface and one with the Imprimatur of the King, followed by 334 pages of main text and ending with four pages of 'Table Des Chapitres'. A new Dublin edition in quarto was published by George Grierson, Dublin, in 1726, with the title page *A Natural History of Ireland, In Three Parts by Several Hands*. In this new edition there is much new and extraneous material contained in Part II, consisting of 'A Collection of such Papers as were communicated to the Royal Society, referring to some Curiosities in Ireland', and Part III, which is 'A Discourse concerning Danish Mounts, Forts and Towers in Ireland; never before published. By Thomas Molyneux, M.D. F.R.S. in England'. This edition was later re-issued by Geo. and Alex. Ewing in Dublin in 1755 but with a new title-page giving authorship credit to 'Dr. Gerard Boate, Thomas Molineux, M.D. F.R.S. and Others'. The preface entitled 'The Bookseller to the Reader' on pages iii and iv has been rewritten and the contents pages have been reset. *A Natural History of Ireland* was later included in the first volume of *A Collection of Tracts and Treatises Illustrative of the Natural History, Antiquities and Polictical and Social State of Ireland*, published in Dublin, 1860.

The first chapter describes the situation and shape of Ireland, followed by details of the provinces, the counties of the English Pale and the main towns of Ireland. About one third of the book is devoted to a remarkably accurate description of Ireland's coastline. Boate could be claimed with good justification as one of the first geomorphologists. Working inland Boate discusses springs, fountains, lakes, rivers and mountains. With an eye to the 'adventurers', considerable attention is given to agricultural potential. Bogs, regarded as of recent origin, were classified: 'places barren through superfluous moisture are bogs called by the Irish Moones' (from the Irish *móin*, meaning 'a bog'). Like all early commentators on bogs, Boate viewed them as waste lands, ready for draining and agricultural improvement. He was full of admiration for the ability of the Irish to traverse the deepest bogs: 'in which nimble trick, called commonly treading of the Bogs, most Irish are very expert, as having been trained up in it from their infancy'.

Boate describes the destruction of woods and forests, and attributes this principally to the use of wood as a source of charcoal used in iron smelting which had been started by the English. So great was the destruction that he wrote: 'in the space of many years, yea of some ages, that a great part of the woods, which the English found in Ireland at their first arrival there, are quite destroyed, so as nothing at all remaineth of them at this time'. Boate also dealt with the potential of minerals, and recorded information from a credible source about the collection of a small amount of gold from a 'certain rivulet in the county of nether-Tyrone, called Miola', and concluded that 'rich gold mines do lye hidden' in the mountains. Boate also had a particular interest in iron ore and other mineral deposits. He was one of the first observers to distinguish between surface deposits of rocks, minerals and soils and those of earlier origin under the ground. He repudiated the notion that it was the property of the waters in Lough Neagh to convert wood into stone and iron.

The 1726 edition of *A Natural History of Ireland* contains many additional papers, letters and notes from other scientists of the time, thrown together in a somewhat incoherent manner. The most significant is a paper by Sir Thomas Molyneux on the giant red deer, the first detailed publication on the remains of this magnificient beast, for a long time incorrectly called 'the Irish elk' when it was neither an elk nor an Irish subspecies.

With *A Natural History of Ireland*, scientific analysis or 'true experimental natural philosophy' was to supersede a previous admixture of observed facts, mythology and gullibility, as demonstrated in *Topographia Hiberniae* by the twelfth-century travel writer Giraldus Cambrensis. Boate had set the trend for careful surveys and inventories. In 1682 Moses Pitt, a London bookseller, was preparing his *English Atlas*. Sir Thomas Molyneux was approached to supply information from Ireland, which, *inter alia*, was to include data on 'plants, animals, fruits, mettals or other natural productions'. Molyneux apparently collected the information on questionnaires sent to colleagues, but the project fell through when Pitt was arrested for unpaid debts. Many of Molyneux's papers from this episode reside in the library of Trinity College, Dublin.

One of Molyneux's important informants was the historian and scholar Roderic O'Flaherty of Galway. O'Flaherty had written *A Chorographical Description of the Territory of West or H-Iar Connaught* in 1684. It was one of many similar learned treatises compiled at about the same time with the objective of illustrating the celebrated Down Survey of Ireland by William Petty. However, it was not until nearly two hundred years later, in 1846, that the Irish Archaeological Society published the O'Flaherty manuscript, based on a copy in the library of Trinity College, Dublin, and edited by James Hardiman. For his time O'Flaherty was an accurate recorder and provides an important natural-history commentary, albeit of a particular western area (County Galway, basically), to complement Boate's more national survey.

O'Flaherty describes H-Iar Connaught as follows:

The country is generally coarse, moorish, and mountanous, full of high rocky hills, large valleys, great bogs, some woods, whereof it had abundance before they were cut. It is replenished with rivers, brooks, lakes, and standing waters, even on the tops of the highest mountains. On the sea side there are many excellent large and safe harbours for ships to ride on anchor; the climate is wholesome, soe as divers attain to the age of ninety years, a hundred and upwards. The land produces wild beasts, as wolves, deere, foxes, badgers, hedgehogs, hares, rabbets, squirrells, martins, weesles and the amphibious otter, of which kind the white-faced otter is very rare. It is never killed, they say, but with loss of man or dog, and its skin is mighty precious. It admits no rats to live any where within it, except the Isles of Aran, and the district of the west liberties of Galway.

When discussing the sea he writes:

It now and then casts ashore great whales, gramps, porcupisses, thunies. Both sea and land have their severall kinds of birds. Here is a kind of black eagle, which kills the deere by grappling him with his claw, and forcing him to run headlong into precipices. Here the ganet soares high into the sky to espy his prey in the sea under him, at which he casts himself headlong into the sea, and swallows up whole herrings in a morsell. This bird flys through the ship's sailes, piercing them with his beak. Here is the bird engendered by the sea out of timber long lying in the sea. Some call them clakes and soland-geese, some puffins, others bernacles, because they resemble them. We call them *girrinn.*

Apart from swallowing the barnacle goose myth, O Flaherty's seventeenth-century text is a valuable contribution to the natural history of Ireland.

Some forty years before O'Flaherty wrote his work, a botanist was at work in the Irish landscape. Richard Heaton, usually considered the source of the earliest records of Irish flowering plants, was a Dublin clergyman, later Dean of Clonfert, who explored not only County Dublin but also the west coast from 1633 until his death, sometime about Christmas 1666. He is credited by Charles Nelson (1978) with the first systematic study of the Irish flora. From Caleb Threlkeld we know that Heaton was busy before 1641: 'As to the Irish Names I copied them from a Manuscript, which bears great Authority with me, and seems to be written sometime before the civil Wars in 1641 and probably by that Revd. Irish Divine Mr. Heaton, who is quoted by Dr. How in the *Phytologia Britannica*, for the *Ros Solis, Hyacinthus Stellaris* and *Pyrola*' (Preface to *Synopsis Stirpium Hibernicarum*). Eight species recorded by Heaton were reported in Dr William How's *Phytologia Britannica*, a duodecimo volume of some 130 pages, published in London in 1650.

The Eighteenth Century

By the turn of the eighteenth century, writers of Irish natural history were putting more emphasis on direct observation and less on hearsay.

Edward Lhwyd, Keeper of the Ashmolean Museum in Oxford and eminent Welsh natural historian, visited Ireland briefly in 1699 and 1700 in search of antiquities and natural features. He published his findings in the form of a letter dated 25 August 1700 to Dr Tancred Robinson, FRS, which was printed in the *Philosophical Transactions* of 1712. Lhwyd visited Sligo, the Burren, the Aran Islands, Antrim, and the mountains of Mayo, Galway and Kerry, recording several plant species new to the country. He also discovered some interesting manuscripts: 'I have in divers Parts of the Kingdom picked up about 20 or 30 Irish Manuscripts on Parchment: But the Ignorance of their Criticks is such, that tho' I consulted the chiefest of them, as O'Flaherty (Author of the *Ogygia*) and several others, they could scarce interpret one Page of all my Manuscripts; and this is occasioned by the want of a Dictionary, which it seems none of their Nation ever took the trouble to compose.'

The first original book on botany published in Ireland was *Methodus plantarum in horto medico Collegii Dublinensis jam jam disponendarum; In dua partes divisa; quarum prima de plantis, altera de fruticibus & arboribus agit*. It was printed and published in Dublin in 1712. The author was Dr Henry Nicholson, first Professor of Botany at Trinity College, Dublin, and the book is basically a catalogue of plants growing in the Physic Garden, i.e. the medicinal garden, located within the walls of that institution. Dr Nicholson's successor was William Stephens who, in 1727, published his lecture notes as *Botanical Elements*.

Two years after Nicholson's catalogue, a very noteworthy book was printed in Belfast by James Blow. It was *The Experienced Huntsman* by Arthur Stringer, a small, little-known text, of which a second edition was published in Dublin in 1780. The earliest treatise on hunting in Ireland, it is the first reliable work on the wild mammals of Britain and Ireland (Fairley, 1975). Stringer is curiously not mentioned in Praeger's *Some Irish Naturalists* (1949), and there is no reference to him in William Thompson's *The Natural History of Ireland* (1849-56) either. Even James Fairley overlooked the work when compiling his 1972 edition of his *Irish Wild Mammals: A Guide to the Literature*. Amends were made in 1977, when the 1780 Dublin edition was re-issued in Belfast by the Blackstaff Press with an introduction by Fairley.

Arthur Stringer was no armchair naturalist stitching plausible copy gleaned from other people's works. Employed as a huntsman by the Conway family, who had been granted an estate east of Lough Neagh by James I in 1610, he was a practical man who knew his mammals, their habits and behaviour. When the time came to write his book he drew upon a wealth of information accumulated as notes for more than thirty years – his style is remarkably fresh and bouncy, coming straight from the thicket as it were. He drew upon his own experience and notes covering more than thirty years.

The book bears the subtitle 'Upon the Nature and Chace of the Stagg, Buck, Hare, Fox, Martern [marten] and Otter With some particular Directions concerning the Breeding and Entring of Hounds'. Stringer has a short, unflattering account of the badger: 'a very melancholy fat Creature, Sleeps incessantly, and naturally (when in Season) very Lecherous'. Of the otter he writes:

When the Bitch or Female Otter is in Season for the Dog, her Box swelleth and is much larger than at other times, as that of a Hound Bitch; and if in a River or Lough where Otters are plenty, there will be sometimes two or three Brace of Dogs or Male Otters following her, yea, and they will fight and tear each other till they leave Blood on the River Banks; their Noise when they fight so is very loud and shrill, not much unlike the Noise of Cats when fighting, but you may hear the Otters much further; how long they carry their Young I cannot truely inform you, but in my Opinion the Otter does much resemble the Ferrit in that thing of Generation ...

One of the most significant publications during the eighteenth century was the earliest book on the flora of Ireland, compiled by an English Dissenting minister and physician, Caleb Threlkeld. The title of the first edition was: *Synopsis Stirpium Hibernicarum Alphabetice Dispositarum. Sive Commentatio de Plantis Indigenis praesertim Dublinensibus instituta. Being A Short Treatise of Native Plants, especially such as grow spontaneously in the Vicinity of Dublin; with their Latin, English and Irish Names: And an Abridgment of their Vertues. With several new Discoverys. With An Appendix of Observations made upon Plants. By Dr. Molyneux, Physician to the State in Ireland. The first Essay of this Kind in the Kingdom of Ireland. Dublin: Printed by S. Powell, for F. Davys in Ross-lane, Richard Norris in Essex-street, at the Corner of Crane-lane, and Josiah Worrall opposite to the Swan-tavern on the Blind-key, MDCCXXVI.*

The first edition of *Synopsis* was published in 1726 in Dublin (Nelson, 1978). Only two copies have been traced – one in the National Library of Ireland, the other in the Bodleian Library, Oxford. The second edition was published in 1727 with only a change of date on the title-page. The third edition was also released in 1727, when the title-page was reset with minor changes.

In his Preface Threlkeld says: 'During the Summer Months I used to perambulate in Company of ingenious Men, both of the Clergy and Laity, to have ocular Demonstration of the Plants themselves in their native Soil, where Nature regaled our Senses with her Gaiety and Garnishes, which makes some Resemblance of the paradisiacal State. From twelve Years Observation I collected Specimens for an Hortus Siccus, and set down the Places where they grew, besides I made Inquiries of ingenious Men, and now I have reduced our Plants into the Model you here see.'

Until Threlkeld's work appeared there had been little previous botanical work in Ireland (Mitchell, 1975). Threlkeld wrote in the Preface: 'The only Reasons I know why this Branch of Learning has been dormant in Ireland, and no publick Advances made towards its Illustration, are that the Wars and Commotions have laid an Imbargo upon the Pens of the Learned, or Discord among petty subaltern Princes has render'd Perambulation perillous, least they should be treated like Spyes, as I was once my self at Tinmouth-Castle near Newcastle upon Tine, the Year of the Union 1707, because I clambered up the Rocks, and kept not the High-road ....'

The core of the *Synopsis* is a list of over five hundred groups or species, listed alphabetically, of fungi, algae, mosses, ferns, and flowering and non-flowering plants. The English, Latin and Irish names (often with regional variations) are given. Details of distribution and medical 'virtues' are also stated.

The importance of the *Synopsis* as a landmark in the history of Irish botany and natural history writing has attracted scholarly attention from, amongst others, Michael Mitchell (1974) and Charles Nelson (1979). Mitchell concluded that Thelkeld's account of the Irish flora is derived from several sources: a manuscript catalogue of Irish plants believed to have been written in the first half of the seventeenth century and attributed by Threlkeld to Richard Heaton; his own personal observations in the Dublin area and those of his friends and associates from other parts of the country; records from, in particular, William Sherard, who was in Ireland from 1690 to 1694 as tutor to Sir Arthur Rawdon's son at Moira, Co. Down, which were printed in the second (1696) and third (1724) editions of John Ray's *Synopsis Methodica Stirpium Britannicarum*; records from Richard Heaton published in William How's *Phytologia Britannica*; and finally from several of John Ray's own writings. Mitchell concluded that most of Threlkeld's material was drawn from other people, much of it unacknowledged, and that a description of him by Nathaniel Colgan, author of *Flora of the County Dublin* (1904), as 'A candid Author and plain Dealer' was questionable.

On the other hand, Nelson claims that Threlkeld could not be accused of plagiarism, 'though he was careless in citing the sources of information'. According to Nelson, Threlkeld's own collections of plants contributed the bulk of the information in the book. This view is strengthened by a recent examination of twenty-two early eighteenth-century herbarium sheets in the Herbarium, Trinity College, Dublin, by Declan Doogue and John Parnell (1992), who suggested, on the balance of evidence available, that they belonged to Threlkeld, possibly from his *Hortus Siccus* mentioned in his Preface.

In 1720, six years before the publication of Threlkeld's *Synopsis*, Dr Patrick Browne was born at Woodstock, Co. Mayo. As a student at Leyden

University, he was friendly with Linnaeus and other eminent men, and became an active naturalist. In 1774 he published catalogues of the birds and fishes of Ireland in *The Gentleman's and London Magazine*. His manuscript 'Fasciculus Plantarum Hiberniae' has survived in the possession of the Linnean Society, London, and contains many important botanical records derived from specimens collected in Mayo and Galway in 1788.

Herbals, designed as textbooks for physicians or indeed anyone wanting to concoct cures, were different from floras, which aimed to catalogue plants in the interest of 'science'. Despite references to the medicinal virtues of certain plants, Threlkeld's *Synopsis* was definitely a flora underpinned by the author's desire, typical of eighteenth-century men, to take stock. So, to a lesser extent, was Browne's *Fasciculus*. A representative of the other trend was John K'Eogh, who published the first Irish herbal in 1735, the same year as Linnaeus brought out *Systema Naturae*. K'Eogh's effort was somewhat belated, as Linnaeus's binomial classification turned out to mark the beginning of modern botany and the demise of herbalists (Kritch, 1976). Viewed by the enlightened mind, herbalism must have already reeked of superstition and archaism. As a form of applied science, seeking primarily to relieve and fortify the body, it had to be removed to the realm of medicine proper, or the culinary art or even gardening. Botany, left to its own devices, could start organizing the world of flowers and plants along intellectual lines.

John K'Eogh was probably born in Co. Roscommon, where his father was a minister. He was educated at Trinity College, Dublin, and was appointed Chaplain to James King, fourth Lord Kingston, and later obtained the living of Mitchelstown, Co. Cork (Praeger, 1949; McCarthy and Sherwood-Smith, 1992). The title of K'Eogh's herbal is *Botanalogia Universalis Hibernica, Or, A General Irish Herbal Calculated for this Kingdom, Giving an Account of the Herbs, Shrubs, and Trees, Naturally Produced therein, in English, Irish, and Latin; with a true description Concerning the Chalybeat Waters, Shewing their Origin, Situation, Medicinal Virtues, & Another of the prophylactic, Or, Hygiastic Part of Medicine, Shewing how Health may be preserved, and Distempers which human Bodies are subject to, prevented.*

K'Eogh argues the case for an Irish Herbal in the preface: 'the necessity of Compiling a particular Herbal for this Kingdom, for such as have been Composed for England, France, Germany, &c. will not in all respects be sufficient for us here, for the virtues of Herbs Differ according to the Climate, or Soil in which they grow ...'. K'Eogh later states his qualifications: 'When I was writing on the Subject, I had the Advantage daily of Viewing the Gardens belonging to the Right Honourable James Lord Baron of Kingston; wherein were Contained near two hundred different Species of Herbs and Trees. I was not aquainted with any Garden, which could show so many, this was no small advantage, or Conveniency to forward this Undertaking.'

Botanalogia lists the species of plants alphabetically, each with its English, Latin and Irish names, together with its medicinal properties. The localities for some of the more unusual species are also given. In the preface K'Eogh writes: 'I hope the next Edition will make a Sufficient Compensation or Amends' as he 'had to put it in the Press sooner than I intended'. There was no other edition until 1986.

In 1739 John K'Eogh followed his *Botanalogia* with a similar treatise concerning the medicinal properties of animals. This was *Zoologia Medicinalis Hibernica: or, A Treatise of Birds, Beasts, Fishes, Reptiles or Insects, which are commonly known and propagated in this Kingdom [...].* In his four-page preface, following a five page Dedication to the Right Honourable William, Lord Baron of Howth, K'Eogh says:

There is not a bird, beast, fish or reptile, but has some medicinal virtue for the service of man, if found out; so it is incumbent upon all lovers of knowledge, all who have a regard for their country, and the preservation of their healths, to endeavour, by making experiments, to find out the medicinal arcana's of nature undiscovered, whether proceeding from vegetables, animals, or minerals ... My principal intention in publishing these treatises on vegetables and animals, was to contrive to cure all the diseases, which the natives of this kingdom are afflicted with, by simple, easy, and safe methods, such as by herbs, or parts extracted from animals, which are prepared either by pulverization, decoction, infusion, distillation, etc.

Unlike K'Eogh's herbal, where comments on plant habitats and distributions were given, there is no similar information in the *Zoologia*. The treatise of the birds, beasts, fishes, reptiles and insects ranges over 103 pages with an amusing rag-bag list of animals as diverse as silk-worm, hoglouse, whale, woodpecker, periwinkle and sturgeon. Followers of K'Eogh's advice would find under Sparrow: 'The flesh, and brains of sparrows being frequently eaten excite venery and clear the sight.' Under Otter: 'The Testicles made into Powder, and drank, help to cure the Epilepsy.' The fat of a heron mixed with oil of amber 'being dropt warm into the ears, cures deafness'. The prescriptions in *Zoologia* draw heavily upon early scholars, with acknowledgements to Pliny, Albertus Magnus, Avicenna, Horace, and others. It is curious that a pharmacopoeia published as late as 1739 should draw upon such early writers, especially as their approach was generally out of fashion.

In 1744 the Physico-Historical Society of Ireland was established in Dublin, thirteen years after the founding of the Dublin (later Royal Dublin) Society. One of the main objectives of the PHSI was the publication of a series of monographs on the 'ancient and present state' of each county in Ireland. Walter Harris came first with his survey of the *County of Down* (1744), followed by Charles Smith's *County and City of Waterford* (1746),

County and City of Cork (1750) and *County of Kerry* (1756). These volumes can be looked upon as the forerunners of the county and regional natural histories that were to flourish in the second half of the nineteenth century. The County Down survey contained two small lists of plants, the first attempt at a county flora in Ireland. The records were collected in May 1743, probably by Isaac Butler, employed as a surveyor by the Physico-Historical Society. Some of the records were erroneous, while others referred to unknown species (Stewart and Corry, 1888). The Kerry survey contains a list of 104 species in pre-Linnaean format. Reviewing this list in his *Flora of Kerry*, Scully (1916) considers that twenty of the flowering plants were 'set down in error'.

The volume on County Dublin was assigned by the Physico-Historical Society to Walter Harris and Dr Lionel Jenkins, who then engaged Isaac Butler, described by Colgan (1904) as 'Judicial Astrologer, Discoverer of Losses, and Calculator of Nativities', to carry out botanical surveys. For reasons unknown, Dr John Rutty, an English physician who had been living in Dublin since 1724, and an active member of the Society until its demise in 1747, took over the work.

Rutty's two-volume work, *An Essay Towards a Natural History of the County Dublin, Accommodated to the Noble Design of the Dublin Society*, was published in 1772. It was the first real county natural history in Ireland, and as such a landmark. The volumes covered flora, fauna, geology, meteorology, minerals, agriculture, air, water, mineral waters, soils of Dublin, and mortality of Dubliners. The book had a particular emphasis on the practical uses, medicinal or culinary, of the flora and fauna. There are five copperplate engravings of birds – the first serious attempt to provide natural-history illustrations in an Irish book. The first volume is mainly devoted to 'vegetables' or botany, including a 'Kalendarium Botanicum Hibernicum' dated May 1758, giving the flowering seasons of plants observed in county Dublin. Rutty added twenty-eight new species of plants to the county flora. Strangely, he did not use the Linnaean system of binomial classification although it had been used in England ten years previously. Under this new system, each species was given both a generic and a specific name instead of an often long and rambling description. For example, water mint is *Mentha aquatica* under the Linnaean system, but in Rutty it is still *Mentha rotundifolia palustris seu aquatica major.*

Rutty also added more than thirty species of birds and twenty species of fish to the lists published in the earlier county surveys. He cleared up many 'vulgar errors' concerning the poisonous nature of newts and viviparous lizards. Of the Magpye or Pianet Rutty writes: 'It is a foreigner, naturalised here since the latter end of K. James the IId's reign, and is said to have been driven hither by a strong wind.' Rutty, who thought that 'House

Swallows' were migrants – contrary to those who thought they hibernated in the mud of estuaries – found confirmation in number 483 of the *Philosophical Transactions* of 'their not being Sleepers as, some have supposed … so they leave us at the approach of winter, probably to go to warmer climates for food'.

Botany Comes of Age

Until the end of the eighteenth century it was clear that Ireland was lagging behind in the study and publication of natural history compared with the rapid progress being made in England. During these times, travel in Ireland was more difficult, indeed hazardous in a country that was often in turmoil. Also, there was less wealth in Ireland and consequently less leisure time, as well as a weaker institutional infrastructure to encourage, promote and publish scientific findings. However, at the end of the century and beginning of the nineteenth century, the pace of development of Irish natural history study began to quicken. Initially the development of science was centred on Dublin, which was the focus of wealth, political power and learning. Gradually it trickled out, first to the North, where the first provincial scientific society in Ireland – the Belfast Natural History Society – was formed in 1821.

Towards the end of the eighteenth century Dr Walter Wade, a medical doctor practising in Dublin and Professor of Botany at the Dublin Society, was the prime force in the establishment of the Society's Botanic Garden at Glasnevin in 1795. A year earlier Wade had published his *Catalogus Systematicus Plantarum Indigenarum in Comitatu Dublinensi Inventarum. Pars Prima*. It was a descriptive flora of the plants in County Dublin, written in Latin, and, for the first time in Ireland, arranged according to the Linnaean system. It is a small octavo, 286-page book that is seldom encountered outside libraries today. Wade made a point of seeing every species recorded, and was the first amongst Irish botanists to study grasses, adding thirty-two new species to the Dublin list. The intended *Pars Secunda*, which would have contained the sedges and non-flowering plants plus fungi, never appeared.

In 1802 Wade published in the *Philosophical Transactions* his 'Catalogus Plantarum Rariorum in Comitatu Gallovidiae, praecipue Cunnamara inventarum: or a systematic account of the more rare plants principally found in the County Galway; but more particularly in that part of it called Cunnamara'. In the preface he writes that he willingly seized the opportunity of undertaking a botanical tour 'for several weeks during August in Cunnamara'. He claims he was the first serious botanist to examine this area.

In 1804 Wade published his paper, *Plantae Rariores in Hibernia Inventae; or Habitats of Some of the Plants, Rather Scarce and Valuable,*

Found in Ireland; with Concise Remarks on the Properties and Uses of Many of Them. It is an important list of flowering plants, lichens, bryophytes and marine algae and contains many records from the west of Ireland where Wade spent some time exploring under the aegis of the Dublin Society. Fifty-five species new to the Dublin flora are listed. There is a hand-coloured plate of the moss *Buxbaumia aphylla*, which Wade claimed to have discovered.

Also in 1804, the first book entirely devoted to the mosses of Ireland, *Muscologiae Hibernicae Spicilegium*, was published in Yarmouth, England. Its author, Dawson Turner, was a wealthy Norfolk banker. A member of the Geological Society of London, founded in 1807, he published with Lewis Weston Dillwyn, in 1805, *The Botanist's Guide through England and Wales.* Later came a comprehensive monograph on British seaweeds. In the *Muscologiae* Turner describes 231 species that he had seen himself in Ireland or had been sent to him. He was a friend of the naturalist John Templeton of Cranmore, Belfast, who supplied him with most of the records from northern Ireland and to whom he inscribed one of the 350 printed copies: 'John Templeton Esq with Mr. D. Turner's best respects and thanks for his assistance.' This particular copy also has marginal notes by Templeton and an extra colour drawing, by Templeton, of *Dicranum tamarindifolium*, with the note 'from Dr. Stokes specimen'. The sixteen hand-coloured plates, containing 235 drawings by Sir William Hooker, mark the first extensive use of coloured plates in an Irish natural history book.

Under the aegis of the Dublin Society, botanists were encouraged to contribute to the improvement of agriculture in Ireland, and this led John White, one of the gardeners to the Dublin Society, to publish *An Essay on the Indigenous Grasses of Ireland* in 1808. The book contains a description of native Gramineae, with Irish names for each species, and where they can be found. There are two hand-coloured plates, engraved by Maguire, with a key to each of the twenty-seven different parts of a grass. In his introduction, White announces that he will publish, at a future time, an account of trees, shrubs, and herbaceous plants which are indigenous to Ireland, with their medicinal uses. This never appeared.

Also in 1808 was published Wade's *Sketch of Lectures on Meadow and Pasture Grasses, Delivered in the Dublin Society's Botanical Gardens, Glasnevin.* There may have been some friction between White and Wade concerning their two publications (Nelson, 1981). Wade is not listed by White as a subscriber, yet John Underwood, head gardener at Glasnevin, is. In a privately held copy of Wade's *Sketch of Lectures*, a printed slip bound in before the preface reads: 'Mr. John White, one of the gardeners at the Botanical Garden, must be considered as responsible, in a great measure, for the Irish names in this "Sketch".' Rev. Dr William Richardson's 'Memoir on Fiorin

Grass' was published in 1808 in the form of Select Papers of The Belfast Literary Society. Richardson pursued a vigorous and eccentric campaign to promote this type of grass as excellent 'for cattle grazing on it whether fattening or milch'. He claims that 'our harshest bottoms, and even our healthy mountains could be easily changed into valuable pastures and meadow, by the aid of this Grass' (Nelson, 1991).

In 1811 Walter Wade's most substantial book was published by the Dublin Society. Entitled *Salices or an Essay towards a General History of Sallows, Willows & Osiers, their Uses, and Best Methods of Propagating and Cultivating Them*, the book has 493 pages and contains descriptions of the *Salix* species and a list of those growing in the Botanic Garden. The coloured frontispiece of *Salix acutifolia*, or Caspian osier, was drawn by Richardson and engraved by Ford.

Nineteenth-Century Floras

The scientific study of botany in Ireland was firmly established by the second decade of the nineteenth century. Belfastman John Templeton 'advanced the cause of Irish botany more than any other', according to Praeger (1949). His manuscript 'Catalogue of Native Plants of Ireland' (now in the Royal Irish Academy, Dublin), with records to the end of 1801, supplied important information to many other botanists. He planned an elaborate 'Flora Hibernica' which remained in skeletal form only with notes and fine watercolour drawings; this material resides in the Ulster Museum, Belfast.

James Mackay, an industrious and talented Scot, was appointed Curator of the Trinity College Botanic Garden at Ballsbridge in 1806. He began that year to publish papers on the flora of Ireland that were to lay the foundations for his book *Flora Hibernica*, published in 1836. But he was beaten to laying claim for the first national flora by a small volume, *The Irish Flora Comprising the Phaenogamous Plants and Ferns*, published anonymously in 1833. Praeger (1949) described it as 'a modest and accurate book' while Moore and More (1866) said 'it is a portable book, containing short and clear descriptions of all the Irish plants then known, and deserves notice as the first Flora of Ireland'. John White of the National Botanic Garden is acknowledged in the preface as having supplied all the information on localities and habitats of the species. The author seems to have been Katherine Baily, later Lady Kane (wife of Sir Robert Kane), who crafted this inaugural book at the tender age of twenty-two (Praeger, 1949). There was a second printing of the book in 1846 with a new title-page. This edition is varyingly made up; some copies have no preface and some have an additional title-page with a hand-coloured engraving of the heath *Dabeocia*.

Mackay's *Flora Hibernica* was published in 1836. A handsome volume of some six hundred pages, it was the first comprehensive publication about the Irish flora, and its scope has not been equalled because no subsequent author has attempted to include the phanerograms and cryptograms of the entire island in one work (Nelson and Parnell, 1992). Although Mackay was named on the title page as sole author, Dr Thomas Taylor was responsible for the second part of the book, concerning mosses, liverworts and lichens, while Dr William Harvey wrote the third part, on algae. A total of 750 copies were printed, but though it was well received by the botanical community only 300 were sold within nine months (Nelson and Parnell, 1992). Despite exhortations by Taylor to Mackay, a second edition never materialized. The other available national flora, *The Irish Flora*, at six shillings, was a successful competitor – it went through a second issue in 1845 – to the sixteen-shilling *Flora Hibernica*.

In 1843 the British Association held its meeting in Cork, and for the occasion the Cuvierian Society of Cork brought together and published a small volume of 'communications' that had been made to the Society from time to time. The title was *Contributions Towards a Fauna and Flora of the County of Cork*. Dr Thomas Power was responsible for the section 'The Botanist's Guide for The County of Cork', which is a systematic catalogue of native plants together with 'their stations' arranged according to 'the natural system of botany'. While apparently an accurate recorder himself, Dr Power was too inclined to accept records from insufficiently qualified observers (Allin, 1883).

Ralph Tate published his *Flora Belfastiensis* in 1863, distinguished as the first published local flora in Ireland. It is a small book listing the flowering plants and ferns found within a radius of fifteen miles of Belfast, with notes on their habitats and distributions – and containing some incorrect nomenclature. In his preface, Tate says he hopes the book will be of assistance to the botanical members of the Belfast Naturalists' Field Club. The club, established by Tate in 1863, was a direct outcome of the interest and excitement aroused by his lectures on geology, zoology and botany at the Belfast School of Science, under the Committee of Lectures, Dublin Castle.

A year later, Dr George Dickie published *A Flora of Ulster*, another small, slim volume, which he 'offered as "Collectanea" towards a more complete Flora of the North of Ireland'. It was considered as a good flora but lacking attention to the critical species, and as a result some errors had crept in. Dickie spent eleven years in Belfast as Professor of Natural History at Queen's College, returning to Aberdeen University in 1860. There he wrote up his botanical notes on flora collected while in Belfast. Dickie's definition of Ulster was the area lying north of 54° N which included the northern portions of Leitrim, Sligo and Mayo belonging to Connacht and excluded the most southern portions of Monaghan and Cavan. He was one of the first to appreciate the importance of the distribution of plants. In his introduction he states: 'A mere list of species cannot afford any definite information respecting the peculiar features of the Flora.' He devotes some space to an analysis of the altitudinal range of species in Ulster, and comments on the flora of offshore islands.

The next major publication on Irish botany was *Contributions towards a Cybele Hibernica* (1866) by David Moore and Alexander More. Moore had been a pupil of Mackay's and was responsible for the botanical section of the remarkable and adventurous, but short-lived, scheme to include natural history as part of the work of the Ordnance Survey in Ireland. The fruits of the initial work were published in 1837 as *Memoir of the City and North Western Liberties of Londonderry: Parish of Templemore*, by Colonel Colby. After the project was wound up, Moore was appointed Curator of the Botanic Garden at Glasnevin in 1838 and remained so until he died in 1879. Alexander More was an exceptional all-round naturalist with prodigious energy for investigation, classification, and cataloguing flora and fauna. *The Life and Letters of Alexander Goodman More* edited by C.B. Moffat (1898) is ample testimony to this man. He was appointed to an Assistantship at the Natural History Museum, Dublin, and elevated to Keeper in 1881.

Cybele Hibernica broke new ground, putting emphasis on plant distribution rather than presenting the traditional species list. While living in England, Alexander More had collaborated with H.C. Watson in the preparation of *Cybele Britannica; or, British Plants and their Geographic Distribution* (1847-59). When he moved to Ireland, More launched himself into a companion volume for Ireland, which he divided into twelve botanical sectors. Plant distribution was analysed using this framework. In 1872 there was a forty-page supplement by More, bound at the end of the volume, entitled 'Recent Additions to the Flora of Ireland'. A second edition of *Cybele Hibernica* was published in 1898, edited by More's friends Nathaniel Colgan and Reginald Scully, who were to produce their own county floras a few years later, on Dublin and Kerry respectively.

The rarest and least known of all Irish county floras was published in 1883. It was *The Flowering Plants and Ferns of the County Cork* by Rev. Thomas Allin. Allin was born in Midleton, Co. Cork, educated at Trinity College, Dublin, and held curacies in counties Galway, Carlow and Cork. An active and and accurate observer (Praeger, 1949), he later moved to Somerset, where his book was printed and sold by J. Marche, Printer & Bookseller, Weston-super-Mare. He divided Cork into two districts, shown on a coloured map frontispiece, which did not coincide with the divisions in *Cybele Hibernica*. The systematic list, with distribution details of seven hundred flowering plants and ferns, covers 101 pages. James Britten, reviewing the book in the *Journal of Botany* (1884), wrote: 'We think many English botanists will share the regret which we feel on learning that the number of copies for sale – for which application should be made to the publisher – is very limited.' It is estimated that there are fewer than fifty existing copies today. The book is absent from many important libraries, including the British Museum and Trinity College, Dublin.

By now the county flora was well established, strongly influenced by the Watsonian approach to plant distribution featured in *Cybele Hibernica*. A regional flora destined for a long life was the *Flora of the North-east of Ireland* by Samuel A. Stewart and Thomas Corry, published in 1888. It has been the standard text for the region ever since, having been updated, revised, groomed and improved by different hands on six separate occasions, a record for an Irish flora. Its aim was to 'give a full and reliable account of the native vegetation of the Counties Down, Antrim and Derry'. Stewart, born in Philadelphia, returned with his father to Belfast, where he started work as an errand-boy at eleven, and was later a trunk maker. His interest in natural history, determination and hard work established him as a leading authority on botany, zoology and geology. He was Curator of the Museum of the Belfast Natural History and Philosophical Society from 1891 to 1907. His colleague Thomas Corry was a brilliant and diligent botanist, tragically drowned in 1883, aged twenty-four, when plant-hunting in Lough Gill, Co. Sligo. Corry was also a poet. A year before his death he published privately a collection of poems, *A Wreath of Wind-Flowers*.

The first edition of the *Flora of the North-east of Ireland* was updated by *A Supplement to the Flora of the North-east of Ireland* by Stewart and Robert Lloyd Praeger, published by the Belfast Naturalists' Field Club in 1895. *A Second Supplement to, and Summary of Stewart and Corry's Flora of the North-east of Ireland*, compiled by Sylvanus Wear with an introduction by Praeger, was published in 1923. The second edition of the *Flora*, prepared by Praeger and William Megaw, was brought out in 1938. This was followed by a *Supplement to the Vascular Section of the Second Edition*, compiled by Mary Kertland with Doreen Lambert (1972). The third and very handsome edition of the *Flora*, completely rewritten, compiled and edited by Paul Hackney with the assistance of Stan Beesley, John Harron and Doreen Lambert, was published in 1992 – bringing to a close, for the moment, the fruits of over a hundred years' intensive botanical study of the north-east of Ireland. The endurance and survival of this flora into the 1990s says something about the continuity and persistence of botanists in this region.

Having cut his teeth on a more modest volume, *Flora of Howth* (1887), Henry Chichester Hart published his *Flora of the County Donegal* in 1898. In the introduction, he salutes *Cybele Hibernica* (1866) as providing a great impetus to the study of field botany in Ireland. Most of the records in the

Flora of Donegal – twice as many as in *Cybele Hibernica* – are Hart's own, gathered from his explorations in his home county. The Donegal *Flora* is rare, as the bulk of the stock, according to Praeger (1949), was destroyed by fire during the uprising of 1916.

Robert Lloyd Praeger's own magnum opus, 'Irish Topographical Botany' was published in 1901 as Volume VII of the *Proceedings of the Royal Irish Academy*. It is remarkable that any person, single-handed, should have produced a national flora of such high quality. In many respects it represents a peak in Irish botanical research. It was the result of five years of intensive field-work throughout Ireland and the collation of thousands of records from the literature and individual botanists. Praeger considered that twelve geographic districts, adopted in *Cybele Hibernica*, were too large and unwieldy, so he divided the whole island up into forty botanical divisions, effectively creating forty county floras in his book. The book that followed, *A Tourist's Flora of the West of Ireland* (1909), is an excellent, well illustrated and practical guide. It is still used today by many botanists and visitors, as is *The Botanist in Ireland* (1934). Praeger was not only an outstanding investigative botanist but was also interested in spreading the word and wrote three educational books. The first was *Open-Air Studies in Botany: Sketches of British Wild-Flowers in Their Homes* (1897) – an enlightening textbook drawn from Praeger's field experience in Ireland. He followed with *Weeds: Simple Lessons for Children* (1913). Praeger's third textbook was *Aspects of Plant Life with Special Reference to the British Flora* (1921). The essays in the book have a strong emphasis on ecology and personal observation.

Unfortunately, Praeger's *The Natural History of Ireland* (1950), which had the potential of being an exciting book, turned out to be a great disappointment because the task was too great for the author, who was then quite old. However, his earlier *The Way That I Went* (1937) is the best book for the general reader on the natural history and topography of Ireland. *Floreat Hibernia* (1985) by Timothy Collins is a detailed and valuable biography of this great naturalist with a listing of his extensive publications.

The Modern Zoological Literature

From the early days of the writing of Irish natural history, botany received most attention, for a number of reasons. Herbs had a long tradition of being useful for medicinal purposes; plants do not walk, run or jump and could be easily captured and studied; flowers are beautiful; botany was a gentle art, pursued by people of learning and refinement. The study of animals is quite different. Although constituting fewer species for study, a mere fraction of the number of plants, they are extraordinarily difficult to observe because of their mobility and their shyness of man.

Some of the earliest and most original zoological investigations in Ireland were carried out by John V. Thompson, born in Berwick-on-Tweed in 1779 and posted to Cork in 1816 as Surgeon to the Forces and later Deputy Inspector-General of Hospitals. Fascinated by luminous creatures in the sea, he trawled a muslin hoop behind a boat, thereby accidentally discovering the hidden world of plankton in 1816, five years before Charles Darwin used a similar net. Thompson, working in relative isolation from zoological institutions, proved that the edible crab hatches from a larval form, a zoea, which had earlier been classified as a species unrelated to the crab. Also, until Thompson's work it had been thought that the fundamental difference between insects and Crustacea (crabs, lobsters, etc.) was that the latter did not pass though metamorphosis in their development. Thompson discovered the intermediate Crustacean forms in his plankton studies, and created a zoological revolution. He was also responsible for the re-classification of acorn barnacles from Mollusca to Crustacea, contrary to the accepted Cuvierian system of the time. Thompson published most of his work in *Zoological Researches, and Illustrations; or, Natural History of Nondescript or Imperfectly Known Animals*, a privately printed series of six memoirs which appeared between 1828 and 1834. Published in Cork, they are extremely rare as few copies were printed. A facsimile of the memoirs was published in 1968 by the Society for the Bibliography of Natural History.

The Industrial Revolution had the effect of throwing some people back into the arms of nature – not the mill workers but their masters, who congregated in nautral-history societies and spent days in the countryside looking for rare species. Those Victorian societies, with their paraphernalia of impossible attires, picnics and banquets, provided a social forum for new discoveries and scientific discussions. Within them debates on evolution were organized; 'cabinets of curiosities' were set up to display the collections ('to know and to have' was the motto of the age); libraries were established; and learned transactions could be published. *The Natural History Review* (1854-9) was a quarterly journal containing the transactions of the Cork Cuvierian Society, the Belfast Natural History Society, the Dublin Natural History Society, the Dublin University Zoological Association and the Literary and Scientific Institution of Kilkenny. It was an essential reference text and survived through seven volumes before its demise. The two indispensable works of this century for Irish natural history bibliophiles are: 'Periodical Publications of Science in Ireland' by Kirkpatrick (1921) and *Some Irish Naturalists* by Praeger (1949).

Ten years after the foundation of the Belfast Natural History and Philosophical Society in 1821, The British Association for the Advancement of Science was formed in Britain. Their annual meetings provided a forum for scientists to exchange information. For each meeting, a publication was produced on the natural history of the area in which the meeting took place. These writings are important sources of zoological and other natural history information. *Contributions to the Fauna and Flora of the County of Cork* was prepared for the 1843 meeting (Harvey *et al.*, 1843); *Guide to Belfast and the Adjacent Counties* for the 1874 meeting (BNFC, 1874); *Guide to the County of Dublin* for the 1878 meeting (MacAlister and M'Nab, 1978); *Belfast and Adjacent Counties* for the 1902 meeting (Bigger, 1902); *Handbook to the City of Dublin and the Surrounding District* for the 1908 meeting (Cole and Praeger, 1908). The tradition was continued this century with *Belfast in its Regional setting: A Scientific Study* for the 1952 meeting (Evans, 1952); *A View of Ireland* for the 1957 Dublin meeting (Meenan and Webb, 1957); and *Province, City & People* for the 1987 Belfast meeting (Buchanan and Walker, 1987).

William Thompson's *The Natural History of Ireland* was a zoological landmark. Thompson was born into a Belfast linen family but decided to pursue natural history rather than the loom. Together with John Templeton he was the most outstanding naturalist produced by Belfast. His first three volumes on birds (1849–51) appeared before he died in 1852, aged forty-seven. Containing an astonishing amount of detailed and original information, this large opus was based on his own original observations and information from an extensive network of correspondents. It is still used today as a source of reliable information. As directed by his will, his notes on the remaining vertebrates and all invertebrates were edited by James Garrett and Robert Patterson, to make up the fourth volume (1856). Patterson himself was also an outstanding naturalist and published *The Natural History of the Insects Mentioned in Shakespeare's Plays* (1841) as well as several textbooks, including *Introduction to Zoology* (1845) and *First Steps in Zoology* (1848).

William Thompson had wanted an inexpensive work on the birds of Ireland. His friend John Watters obliged with a small, popular book for the general reader: *The Natural History of the Birds of Ireland* (1853). The book concentrates on descriptions of bird habitats, migrations and occurrences of the 261 species listed but adds very little new knowledge. Watters also laced his text with the occasional romantic poem.

Following in the tradition of the Belfast merchant naturalists, Robert Lloyd Patterson, son of the Robert Patterson above, published *The Birds, Fishes and Cetacea of Belfast Lough* (1880). Derived mainly from a series of papers read to the Belfast Natural History and Philosophical Society, it is a detailed and accurate account of the natural history of the lough.

The Fowler in Ireland (1882) by Ralph Payne-Gallwey is a lively, authoritative book on wildfowl and seafowl in Ireland and on how to shoot and capture them. An essential reference text, it is enlivened by engravings by Charles Whymper (*see p. 533*). Four years later *Our Irish Song Birds*

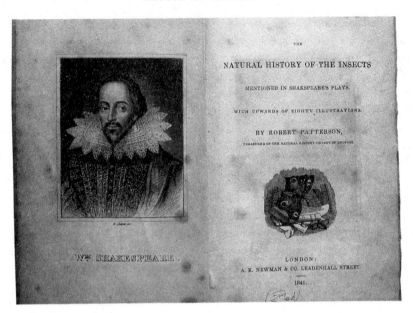

(1886) by the Rev. Charles Benson was published, a charming volume with an evangelical flavour, written for those with a general interest in natural history. Benson was a schoolmaster and clergyman. *Song Birds* was the first Irish book to have coloured plates of birds. There is a series of interesting and curious appendices, such as 'Odds and ends of bird life for my youthful readers'.

The systematic study of bird migration was never attempted in Ireland until 1881. Under the guidance of the British Association, special recording forms were sent to all lighthouse keepers in Britain and Ireland. Richard M. Barrington and Alexander Goodman More, of *Cybele Hibernica* fame, were the Irish members on the BA Committee. In 1884, to guard against misidentification, More suggested that the lighthouse keepers cut off a wing and leg from each bird that had died striking the light at night. The recording scheme was stopped in 1887 as the BA felt they had enough data. Barrington, realizing the importance of a long-term survey and annoyed that such a valuable exercise had been terminated, continued the scheme in Ireland until 1897 at his own expense. In 1900 he published *The Migration of Birds as Observed at Irish Lighthouses and Lightships*, most of it in the form of raw data. Only 350 copies were printed. The book is an invaluable source of information on bird migration, quarried many times by later Irish ornithologists.

The Birds of Ireland (1900) by R.J. Ussher and Robert Warren is a masterly text, full of original and accurate observations and drawing upon an extensive network of correspondents. The quality of information on the status and distribution of birds, including much material from Barrington's work, has ensured the book's value throughout the century. It was intended that Barrington and More would be joint authors but Barrington's commitment to his migration studies and More's ill health precluded this. Most of the work was done by Ussher, a fearless fieldworker, who climbed the most dangerous cliffs, swam out to islands, and relentlessly pursued the peregrine falcon. Warren was strategically placed near Killala Bay and Bartragh Island to contribute valuable observations on waders and wildfowl in northern Connaught to the survey. Fifty copies of *The Birds of Ireland* were printed on large paper, royal octavo, but these are seldom encountered. Ussher and Warren's masterpiece is a fitting title, and its year of publication a fitting year, with which to bring to a close this annotated bibliography of essential texts in Irish natural history.

References

Allin, T. 1883. *The Flowering Plants and Ferns of the County Cork.* Weston-super-Mare: J. Marche.

Anon. [Katherine Sophia Baily]. 1833. *The Irish Flora Comprising the Phaenogamous Plants and Ferns.* Dublin: Hodges and Smith.

Barrington, R. 1900. *The Migration of Birds as Observed at Irish Lighthouses and Lightships.* London: Porter.

Belfast Naturalists' Field Club. 1874. *Guide to Belfast and Adjacent Counties.* Prepared for the 1874 Meeting of the British Association. Belfast: Marcus Ward.

Benson, C. 1886. *Our Irish Song Birds.* Dublin: Hodges, Figgis.

Bigger, F.J. (ed.). 1902. *A Guide to Belfast and the Counties of Down & Antrim.* Prepared for the Meeting of the British Association by the Belfast Naturalists' Field Club. Belfast: McCaw, Stevenson & Orr.

Boate, G. 1652. *Irelands Naturall History.* London: Hartlib.

Bottigheimer, K.S. 1971. *English Money and Irish Land: The 'Adventurers' in the Cromwellian Settlement of Ireland.* Oxford: Clarendon Press.

Browne, P. 1774. 'A Catalogue of the Birds of Ireland, Whether Natives, Casual Visitors, or Birds of Passage, Taken from Observation; Classed and Disposed According to Linnaeus.' *The Gentleman's and London Magazine: or, Monthly Chronologer.* Dublin: Exshaw, 385-7.

Browne, P. 1774a. 'A Catalogue of Fishes Observed on our Coasts, and in our Lakes and Rivers, Classed and Disposed According to Linnaeus.' *The Gentleman's and London Magazine: or, Monthly Chronologer.* Dublin: Exshaw, 515-16.

Buchanan, R.H. and B.M. Walker (eds). 1987. *Province, City & People: Belfast and its Region.* Prepared for the Meeting of the British Association. Antrim: Greystone Books.

Cole, A.J. and R.L. Praeger (eds). 1908. *Handbook to the City of Dublin, Its Geology, Industries, Flora, and Fauna.* Prepared for the Meeting of the British Association, 1908. Dublin: British Association.

Colgan, N. 1904. *Flora of the County Dublin.* Dublin: Hodges, Figgis.

Collins, T. 1985. *Floreat Hibernia: A Bio-Bibliography of Robert Lloyd Praeger 1865-1953.* Dublin: Royal Dublin Society.

Dickie, G. 1864. *A Flora of Ulster and Botanist's Guide to the North of Ireland.* Belfast: Aitcheson.

Doogue, D. and J. Parnell. 1992. 'Fragments of an Eighteenth-Century Herbarium, Possibly that of Caleb Threlkeld in Trinity College, Dublin (TCD).' *Glasra* 1: 99-109.

Evans, E.E. (ed.). 1952. *Belfast in its Regional Setting: A Scientific Survey.* Prepared for the Meeting of the British Association by the local Executive Committee. Belfast: Nicholson & Bass.

Fairley, J. 1972. *Irish Wild Mammals: A Guide to the Literature*. Galway: author.

Fairley, J. 1975. *An Irish Beast Book: A Natural History of Ireland's Furred Wildlife*. Belfast: Blackstaff Press.

Harris, W. 1744. *The Ancient and Present State of the County of Down*. Dublin: A. Reilly for E. Exshaw.

Hart, H.C. 1887. *Flora of Howth*. Dublin: Hodges, Figgis.

Hart, H.C. 1898. *Flora of the County Donegal*. Dublin: Sealy, Bryers & Walker.

Harvey, J.R. et al. 1845. *Contributions Towards a Fauna and Flora of the County of Cork Read at the Meeting of the British Association Held at Cork in the Year 1843*. London: John van Voorst for the Cuvierian Society of Cork.

Hoppen, K.T. 1964. 'The Dublin Philosophical Society and the New Learning in Ireland.' *Irish Historical Studies 14*: 99-118.

How, W. 1650. *Phytologia Britannica*. London.

K'Eogh, J. 1735. *Botanalogia Universalis Hibernica, Or, A General Irish Herbal*. Cork: George Harrison. 2nd ed. 1986. Dublin: Anna Livia Press.

K'Eogh, J. 1739. *Zoologia Medicinalis Hibernica*. Dublin: S. Powell.

Kertland, M. 1972. *Supplement to the Vascular Section of the Second Edition of A Flora of the North-east of Ireland* (S.A. Stewart and T.H. Corry). Belfast: for the Belfast Naturalists' Field Club.

Kirkpatrick, T.P.C. 1921. 'The Periodical Publications of Science in Ireland.' *Bibliographical Society of Ireland 2*: 33-58.

Krutch, J.W. 1976. *Herbal*. Oxford: Phaidon Press.

Lhwyd, E. 1712. 'Some Farther Observations Relating to the Antiquities and Natural History of Ireland.' *Philosophical Transactions 22*: 524-6.

MacAlister, A. and W.R. M'Nab (eds). 1878. *Guide to the County of Dublin*. Prepared for the Meeting of the British Association. Dublin: Hodges, Foster and Figgis.

McCarthy, M. and C. Sherwood-Smith. 1992. *The Enchanted Herbs*. Dublin: Marsh's Library.

Mackay, J. 1836. *Flora Hibernica ... Arranged According to the Natural System with a Synopsis of the Genera According to the Linnaean System*. Dublin: William Curry Jun.

Meenan, J. and D.A. Webb (eds). 1957. *View of Ireland*. Prepared for the Meeting of the British Association. Dublin: Hely's Ltd, East Wall.

Mendyk, S. 1985. 'Gerard Boate and Irelands Naturall History.' *Journal of the Royal Society of Antiquities of Ireland 115*: 5-12.

Meyer, K. (trans., ed.). 1903. *Our Old-Irish Songs of Summer and Winter*. London: Nutt.

Mitchell, M.E. 1974. 'The Sources of Threlkeld's Synopsis Stirpium Hibernicarum.' *Proceedings of the Royal Irish Academy 74B*: 1-6.

Mitchell, M.E. 1975. 'Irish Botany in the Seventeenth Century.' *Proceedings of the Royal Irish Academy 75B*: 275-84.

Moffat, C.B. 1898. *The Life and Letters of Alexander Goodman More*. Dublin: Hodges, Figgis.

Moore, D. and A.G. More. 1866. *Contributions towards a Cybele Hibernica*. Second 'issue' 1872 with Supplement, 'Recent Additions to the Flora of Ireland' by A.G. More; Dublin: Hodges, Smith. Second ed. 1898, Nathaniel Colgan and Reginald Scully (eds); Dublin: Ponsonby.

Nelson, E.C. 1978. 'The Publication Date of the First Irish Flora. Caleb Threlkeld's *Synopsis Stirpium Hibernicarum*, 1726.' *Glasra 2*: 37-42.

Nelson, E.C. 1979. '"In the Contemplation of Vegetables" – Caleb Threlkeld (1676-1728), his Life, Background and Contribution to Irish Botany.' *Journal of the Society for the Bibliography of Natural History 9*: 257-73.

Nelson, E.C. 1981. 'A Select, Annotated Bibliography of the National Botanic Gardens, Glasnevin, Dublin.' *Glasra 5*: 1-20.

Nelson, E.C. 1991. 'David Moore's Fasciculi of Grasses to 1843, 1856.' *Long Room 36*: 21-36.

Nelson, E.C. and J. Parnell. 1992. '*Flora Hibernica* (1836): Its Publication, and Aftermath as Viewed by Dr. Thomas Taylor.' *Taxon 41*: 35-42.

Nicholson, H. 1712. *Methodus Plantarum in Horto Medico*. Dublin: A. Rhames.

O'Flaherty, R. [1684] 1846. *Chorographical Description of the Territory of West or H-Iar Connaught.* Dublin: Irish Archaeological Society.

O'Meara, J. (trans.). 1951. *The First Version of the Topography of Ireland by Giraldus Cambrensis.* Dundalk: Dundalgan Press.

Patterson, R. 1841. *The Natural History of the Insects Mentioned in Shakespeare's Plays.* London: A.K. Newman.

Patterson, R. 1845. *Introduction to Zoology for the Use of Schools.* London: Simms & McIntyre.

Patterson, R. 1848. *First Steps in Zoology.* 2nd ed. Belfast: Mullan.

Patterson, R.L. 1880. *The Birds, Fishes and Cetacea of Belfast Lough.* London: David Bogue.

Payne-Gallwey, R. 1882. *The Fowler in Ireland.* London: John van Voorst. Rpt. 1985. Southhampton: Ashford Press.

Praeger, R.L. 1897. *Open-Air Studies in Botany: Sketches of British Wild-Flowers in Their Homes.* London: Charles Griffin.

Praeger, R.L. 1901. 'Irish Topographical Botany.' *Proceedings of the Royal Irish Academy 7.* 3rd series. 7: i-clxxxviii, 1-410.

Praeger, R.L. 1909. *A Tourist's Flora of the West of Ireland.* Dublin: Hodges, Figgis.

Praeger, R.L. 1913. *Weeds: Simple Lessons for Children.* Cambridge: Cambridge University Press.

Praeger, R.L. 1921. *Aspects of Plant Life with Special Reference to the British Flora.* London: SPCK.

Praeger, R.L. 1934. *The Botanist in Ireland.* Dublin: Hodges, Figgis.

Praeger, R.L. 1937. *The Way That I Went.* Dublin: Hodges, Figgis.

Praeger, R.L. 1949. *Some Irish Naturalists.* Dundalk: Dundalgan Press.

Praeger, R.L. 1950. *The Natural History of Ireland.* London: Collins.

Praeger, R.L. and S.A. Stewart. 1895. *A Supplement to the Flora of the North-east of Ireland.* Belfast: Belfast Naturalists' Field Club.

Richardson, W. 1808. 'Memoir on Fiorin Grass.' Select Papers of the Belfast Literary Society. Belfast: Smyth and Lyons.

Rutty, J. 1772. *An Essay Towards a Natural History of the County Dublin.* Dublin: Author.

Scully, R. 1916. *The Flora of Kerry.* Dublin: Hodges, Figgis.

Smith, C. 1746. *The Ancient and Present State of the County and City of Waterford.* Dublin: Author.

Smith, C. 1750. *The Ancient and Present State of the County and City of Cork.* Dublin: Exshaw.

Smith, C. 1756. *The Ancient and Present State of the County of Kerry.* Dublin: Author.

Stephens, W. 1727. *Botanical Elements.* Published for the Use of the Botany School in the University of Dublin. Dublin: Risk.

Stewart, S.A. and T.H. Corry. 1888. *A Flora of the North-east of Ireland.* Cambridge: Macmillan and Bowes. 2nd ed. 1938, R.L. Praeger and W. Megaw (eds). Belfast: Quota Press. Third ed. 1992, P. Hackney (ed.). Belfast: Institute of Irish Studies, Queen's University.

Stringer, A. 1714. *The Experienced Huntsman.* Belfast: James Blow. 2nd ed. 1977, J. Fairley (ed.). Belfast: Blackstaff Press.

Tate, R. 1863. *Flora Belfastiensis.* Belfast: G. Phillips.

Templeton, J. 1801. *MS Catalogue of Native Plants of Ireland.* Royal Irish Academy, Dublin.

Thompson, J.V. 1828-34. *Zoological Researches, and Illustrations; or, Natural History of Nondescript or Imperfectly Known Animals in a Series of Memoirs.* Cork: King and Ridings. Facs. rpt. as *Zoological Researches and Illustrations 1828-1834.* 1968. London: Society for the Bibliography of Natural History.

Thompson, W. 1849-56. *The Natural History of Ireland.* London: Reeve, Benham and Reeve (vol. 4: Henry G. Bohn).

Threlkeld, C. 1726. *Synopsis Stirpium Hibernicarum.* Dublin: Davys, Norris and Worrall.

Turner, D. 1804. *Muscologiae Hibernicae Spicilegium.* Yarmouth: J. Black.

Ussher, R.J. and R. Warren. 1900. *The Birds of Ireland.* London: Gurney and Jackson.

Wade, W. 1794. *Catalogus Systematicus Plantarum Indigenarum in Comitatu Dublinensi Inventarum. Pars Prima.* Dublin: Dublin Society.

Wade, W. 1802. 'Catalogus Plantarum Rariorum in Comitatu Gallovidiae.' *Transactions of the Dublin Society 2*: 105-27.

Wade, W. 1804. *Plantae Rariores in Hibernia Inventae; or Habitats of Some of the Plants, Rather Scarce and Valuable, Found in Ireland; with Concise Remarks on the Properties and Uses of Many of Them.* Dublin: Graisberry and Campbell.

Wade, W. 1808. *Sketch of Lectures on Meadow and Pasture Grasses, Delivered in the Dublin Society's Botanical Gardens, Glasnevin.* Dublin: Graisberry and Campbell.

Wade, W. 1811. *Salices or an Essay towards a General History of Sallows, Willows & Osiers, their Uses, and Best Methods of Propagating and Cultivating Them.* Dublin: Dublin Society.

Wear, S. 1923. *A Second Supplement to, and Summary of Stewart and Corry's Flora of the North-east of Ireland.* Belfast: Belfast Naturalists' Field Club.

Watters, J. 1853. *The Natural History of the Birds of Ireland.* Dublin: McGlashan.

Webster, C. 1974. 'New Light on the Invisible College: the Social Revelations of English Science in the Mid Seventeenth Century.' *Transactions of the Royal Historical Society.* Fifth Series. 24: 19-42.

White, J. 1808. *An Essay on the Indigenous Grasses of Ireland.* Dublin: Graisberry and Campbell.

The Art of Nature Illustration

MARTYN ANGLESEA

The boundary between 'fine art' and 'illustration' has always been a vexed question. This strange but fascinating no-man's land, particularly in the area of natural-history illustration, has been explored from various angles by several recent writers (Dance, 1978; Pointon, 1979; Mengel, 1982; Potts, 1990). At some time during the late seventeenth century, and in that most theoretically minded country, France, academic thinking about the visual arts became crystallized into a 'hierarchy of genres'. Thus 'history painting' was reckoned superior to 'portrait painting' or 'landscape painting', and both of these were considered to be a cut above 'still-life painting', and certainly well above 'low-life painting'. 'Illustration', whether literary or scientific, would have been regarded as a lowly mechanical craft. Such a situation persists to this day. Yet there are instances, such as the drawings of Leonardo da Vinci, or the anatomical engravings of George Stubbs, where even the most hermetic aesthetes would have to concede a high artistic status. Such incidental aesthetic qualities may also be found in Irish examples of scientific illustration, as I hope to demonstrate.

One of the earliest Irish drawings of modern times – dating from somewhere between 1588 and 1597 – depicts the skull and antlers of a Giant Irish deer (*Megaceros giganteus*). It is an outline pen drawing purporting to be nothing more than a straightforward, almost diagrammatic, full-face image of a spectacular, newly discovered natural curiosity (*plate 18*). The drawing would seem to have been commissioned by Adam Loftus, a Yorkshireman who became Archbishop of Armagh and Dublin, Queen Elizabeth's Lord Chancellor of Ireland, and, briefly in 1591, the first Provost of Trinity College, Dublin. The unknown draughtsman might have been an Irishman. Fortunately the drawing is quite well documented, both in inscriptions on the sheet itself and in a letter Loftus wrote to Sir Robert Cecil in 1597.*

---

* This drawing is now in the Natural History Division of the National Museum of

497

The sheet gives measurements, and an account of the finding of the object which reads:

About the year of our Lord God 1588 there was found by certain labourers (by the occasion of the making of a ditch about some new enclosure) near unto a great bog within the county of Meath in Ireland the head of a Deer of this form and quantity here described, blemished in diverse parts by the breaking off of sundry tines ... before it was conceived what the same might be, for the same was overgrown with the said bog – wherein it had lain beyond the memory of man: whereby and by reason of the hugeness thereof it could not be taken up whole. Nevertheless the broken parts being conjoined to the main and fastened thereto with plates of iron ... This head is to be seen in the house of the Right Hoble. Adam Loftus, Lo. Chancellor of Ireland, called Rathfarnham about four miles distant from the city of Dublin and is fastened to the screen of the hall there.

Loftus's letter to Sir Robert Cecil, dated Rathfarnham 27 September 1597, attempts to curry favour with his English magnate bosses by presenting the deer skull as a prestigious gift. Luckily, the skull has survived; reaching Cecil's country house in Hertfordshire, it was placed on display there. It has since migrated to the Provincial Museum of Alberta, Canada, where it is displayed.

Though probably born a Catholic, Adam Loftus saw his duty in Ireland as the implementation of the Reformation, and therefore he was regarded by the Irish Catholics as an enemy; he saw his close relatives killed by Catholics at his front door. Ireland's turbulent seventeenth century began with England's ruthless cleaning-up operations after suppressing the rebellion against Queen Elizabeth by Hugh O'Neill (Earl of Tyrone) and Red Hugh O'Donnell, and the consequent exile of Tyrone and Red Hugh's son Rory (Earl of Tyrconnell): the famous 'Flight of the Earls'. The few graphic depictions of Ireland during the first half of this century generally fall into the categories of cartography and military topography.

After the English Civil War and the regime of Cromwell – with all its sad repercussions for Ireland – Charles II's Restoration ushered in a period of comparative sanity, albeit enjoyed chiefly by those fortunate enough to be on the winning side. It was at this time that the Royal Society was founded in London, laying the foundations of empirical science. And it was in this climate that English or Anglo-Irish investigators such as Sir William Petty and Thomas Molyneux, both of whom had studied medicine at the liberal

Ireland, Dublin. Loftus's letter to Robert Cecil is in a *Calendar of State Papers Relating to Ireland, 1596-7*, in the London Public Record Office, PRO 1893, 406. I am grateful to Professor Anne Crookshank of Trinity College, Dublin, for telling me about this drawing, and to Nigel Monaghan of the Geological Section of the National Museum for providing more information.

Dutch university of Leyden, communicated their Irish findings to the Royal Society. Early illustrated communications to the Royal Society concerned that extraordinary geological feature, the Giant's Causeway in Co. Antrim.

Early Geological Illustrations of the Giant's Causeway

Topographical draughtsmanship of the seventeenth and eighteenth centuries impinges upon natural history through interest in the infant science of geology. This new interest stemmed in particular from the discovery of the Giant's Causeway (Rudwick, 1976; Stafford, 1977; Pointon, 1979). The Causeway was not marked on any printed map of Ireland before 1714, when it appeared on Herman Moll's map. It is marked on Senex, Maxwell and Price's map of the same year, and on Senex's map of 1720.

The Causeway enters scientific literature only in the 1690s, in the years of comparative peace immediately following the Williamite wars. The first published description of it is a letter written by Sir Richard Bulkeley, a Fellow of Trinity College, Dublin, published in 1693. A long geological dispute, the Neptunist-Vulcanist controversy, was sparked off in 1694 by the publication of the earliest graphic depiction of the Giant's Causeway in *Philosophical Transactions*. The original drawing is lost; what we have is an engraving done second-hand, probably in London, by someone totally unfamiliar with the site. Bishop Samuel Foley of Down and Connor commissioned this drawing by one Christopher Cole of Coleraine, whom he describes as 'Collector in those parts' – the Crown's local agent for the collection of taxes and customs duties. Foley's paper of 1694 is in fact a rejoinder to Bulkeley's notice, using an anonymous engraving after Cole as an illustration. Foley writes of Cole:

He tells me he has not drawn the Causway as a Prospect, nor as a Survey or Platform, which he thought would not answer his Design, and that he has no other name for it but a Draught, which he took after this sort: he supposed the Hills and Causway &c., epitomised to the same height and bigness the draught shews them, and this he fancied the most Intelligible way to express it.

The Thomas Molyneux papers in Trinity College Library include a letter written by Cole to the Dublin Society, which concludes: 'The discripcon of the Cawsie dos not Please me Ile Draw it better by next Post & send it up with some thing Els that I design for the Society.'

Thomas Molyneux (1661-1733) soon realized that Cole's 'Draught' was inadequate as an illustration of a geological curiosity:

Perceiving then I could not so well rely on the Draught of the Giant's Causeway that was first taken ... as, being done by the Hand of one who was no extraordinary Artist, tho' the best that could then be had; I proposed the last summer to some

Philosophical Gentlemen here in Dublin, that we should imploy, at the common charge, one Mr Sandys, a good Master in Designing and Drawing of Prospects, to go into the North of Ireland, and upon the Place take the genuine and accurate Figure of the whole Rock, with the natural Posture of the Hills and Country about it for some distance. Accordingly we sent him away with such instructions as I drew up for him, and he returned soon after with a fair and beautiful Draught very expressive of each Particular we desired; an exact Copy of which my Brother lately sent over to the Royal Society.

The original drawing by this Edwin Sandys was for a long time lost. The image was known only in the form of an engraving which would have been done in London, far from the actual subject. Thus it was natural to blame its strange inaccuracies on the London engraver rather than on Sandys himself. However, the original drawing in pen and watercolour surfaced in a book sale at Sotheby's in London in December 1994. Though the British Library would have liked it, they graciously withdrew from the bidding to enable the Ulster Museum to buy it. It is a large, impressive sheet, drawn in a cartographic style, and exceptionally well preserved (*plate 4*). Nevertheless, it proves Sandys's responsibility for the houses and trees on the cliffs, ridiculed by later geologists, despite Molyneux's enthusiasm. Perhaps it is best to quote the eloquent contempt for it expressed by the Rev. William Hamilton, writing in 1786 in his *Letters Concerning the Northern Coast of the County of Antrim*:

Neither the talents nor the fidelity of the artist seem to have been at all suited to the purpose of a philosophical landscape .... In this true prospect, the painter has very much indulged his own imagination at the expense of his employers, insomuch that several tall pillars, in the steep banks of this fanciful scene, appear loaded with luxuriant branches, skirting the wild and rocky bay of Port Noffer with the gay exhibition of stately forest trees. In the background he discovered a parcel of rude and useless materials which his magic pencil soon transformed into comfortable dwelling-houses; and for chimneys he has happily introduced some detached pillars of basaltes, which, from their peculiar situation, and the name given to them by the peasants of the country, naturally excited the attention of this extraordinary artist. And thus were concluded the labours of the last century concerning this curious work of nature. (Hamilton, 1822)

Hamilton was a very able geologist; a spot on the cliffs near the Giant's Causeway, where he liked to sit in philosophic contemplation of nature's wonders, is still known as 'Hamilton's Seat'. Hamilton was murdered in Donegal in 1797 'by an armed banditti'. The 1822 Belfast edition of his *Letters* is illustrated by an obscure but underrated landscape artist named Donald Stewart.

It was not until 1740 that a trustworthy image of the Giant's Causeway was produced, and that by a Dublin artist, Susanna Drury, of whom we know little. The diarist and draughtswoman Mrs Delany tells us she 'lived three months near the place, and went almost every day'. In the words of the igneous petrologist John Preston, formerly Reader in Geology at the Queen's University of Belfast, Susanna Drury had 'a real eye for basalt' (Anglesea and Preston, 1980). Two pairs of beautifully finished gouache paintings on vellum by her are now known, one pair belonging to the Knight of Glin in County Limerick, the other to the Ulster Museum. In 1742/3 two fine line-engravings were executed after Drury's paintings by the distinguished London-based French Huguenot engraver François Vivarès. Though they take some minor liberties with the surrounding topography, mainly for compositional effect, the importance of these prints for the development of igneous petrology cannot be overestimated. In their circulation throughout Europe, they provoked new interest and discussion of the site among geologists. Most importantly, they led the French savant Nicolas Desmarest to the 'Vulcanist' conclusion that the Causeway was comparable to the volcanic basalt cones of the Auvergne, and was consequently of volcanic rather than aqueous origin (Anglesea and Preston, 1980; Anglesea, 1991). Susanna Drury's brother, Franklin Drury, a Dublin miniature painter (of whose work, unfortunately, nothing is at present identified), visited the Causeway in 1753 at the behest of Dr Richard Pococke, then Archdeacon of Dublin, later Bishop of Ossory. Pococke, a geologist of the 'Neptunist' camp, had already visited the place twice, making careful observations. Franklin Drury made two maps of the Causeway, one by pacing at sea level, the other by viewing the site from the cliff-top. He also made cork models of some of the Causeway stones, which Pococke presented to the Royal Society.*

Early Botanical Illustration

Mrs Delany (Mary Granville) was one of the most informative diarists of the eighteenth century. Born in England, she spent happy years in Ireland, at Delville and Downpatrick, married to Dr Patrick Delany, Dean of Down, from 1743 until his death in 1768 (Llanover, 1861-2). She was a prolific amateur draughtswoman as well as a diarist, and is rightly celebrated for a series of nearly a thousand botanical pictures in ten volumes now in the British Museum, made in cut paper or 'paper mosaick', as she called it. Mrs Delany frequented the Physick Garden at Chelsea and was personally acquainted with the botanist Daniel Charles Solander and the German

---

* Drury's maps illustrate a letter from Richard Pococke in the *Philosophical Transactions of the Royal Society 48* (1753): 238.

flower-painter Georg Dionysius Ehret, who worked at Kew. She was familiar with Linnaeus's new classifications. Unfortunately, Mrs Delany's flower pictures have only a tenuous connection with Ireland. After her husband's death, Mrs Delany returned to high society in her native England. She did not take up her flower collages until 1772, when she was seventy-three, but she worked at them until she was eighty-two (Hayden, 1980).

At least in modern times, botanical illustration has always had a practical justification. Plants were used in herbal medicine, and it was vital that they be identified and classified. It was also necessary to know which were poisonous. Therefore plants needed to be meticulously studied and described. Such was the purpose of the great Renaissance herbals like John Gerard's *The Herbal or Generall Historie of Plantes* (1597). As travels and explorations increased, new plants were discovered, brought home for cultivation, drawn and described. The Linnaean Society in London has a collection of botanical and zoological notes and drawings by a naturalist believed to be Irish-born, John Ellis (c. 1705-76), whom Linnaeus himself described as 'the main support of natural history in England'. Ellis's entry in the *Dictionary of National Biography* states that his Irish birth was 'admitted' by Sir J.E. Smith in *Linnaean Correspondence 1*. A merchant by trade, Ellis succeeded in gaining an importing agency for West Florida in 1764, and for Dominica in 1770, thus enabling him to import a quantity of hitherto unknown American seeds. Ellis published *An Essay towards a Natural History of the Corallines* in 1754, which earned him the Copley Medal in 1768, and Linnaeus thought so highly of him as to name a group of borage-related plants *Ellisia*. Ellis's work on zoophytes was completed and published by his friend Daniel Charles Solander of the British Museum.

William Kilburn (b. Dublin 1745, d. Wallington, Surrey, 1818) must be cited as one of the earliest Irish-born botanical illustrators. Having received his initial apprenticeship as a woodblock printer on linen in Dublin and at Lucan, Co. Kildare, Kilburn left Ireland for London following his father's death about 1766, never to return. He was obliged now to support his mother and sister. He must have had some formal training in drawing, perhaps at the Royal Dublin Society Schools, as his draughtsmanship is sophisticated. In London, Kilburn sold his designs to calico printers as well as, significantly, drawing and engraving flowers from nature for sale in print shops. He came to the attention of his neighbour, the botanist William Curtis, who employed him to illustrate his three-volume work *Flora Londinensis*, of which twenty-five of the plates bear Kilburn's signature as draughtsman and engraver. The first volume was published in 1777, the other two at the end of the 1790s. The volume of *Kilburn's Designs* in the Victoria and Albert Museum contains thirty working designs for floral textile patterns dated between 1787 and 1792 (Longfield, 1981; Butler, 1990).

Although Ellen Hutchins (b. Ballylickey, Co. Cork 1785; d. Ardna-gashel House, Bantry Bay 1815) only lived to be thirty, she along with the Fitton sisters was a pioneer among Irish women artists in the illustration of scientific books. Encouraged by her physician, Dr Whitley Stokes, to take up botany, she became a specialist in the cryptogams, that is, mosses, liverworts, lichens and seaweeds, of the Bantry Bay area. *Hutchinsia alpina*, an Alpine cress, and *Jungermannia hutchinsiae*, a liverwort, are among the many species that European naturalists named in her honour. Hutchins was particularly remarkable for her drawings of the unglamorous unflowering plants, like seaweeds, which are easily perishable and require an accurate scientific drawing to be made as soon as possible after collection. Some of these were used as illustrations to *Historia Fuci*, by the English botanist (and prolific draughtsman) Dawson Turner (1775-1858), with whom Ellen Hutchins corresponded. Her drawings are in the collections at Kew and at Sheffield City Museum (Nelson, 1987).

Early Depictions of Animals and Birds

If the plant painters found their practical justification in the use of herbs as medicines and poisons, what then was the reason for describing, painting or drawing animals or birds? On the one hand, there was hunting and sport, and many of the early zoologists were keen sportsmen who needed to be able to identify the correct birds to shoot. Travel and the discovery of new species was also an important stimulus, but there always seems to be a more pedestrian approach with the ornithological painters. Quite early on, there appeared the convention of drawing a bird (from a stuffed specimen more often than from life) in rigid profile, for this showed the characteristics of each species more clearly, to the satisfaction of a taxonomic master – that is, a natural philosopher who specialized in the naming and description of species.

The bird painter Charles Collins (c. 1680-1744) gets his entry in Strickland's *Dictionary of Irish Artists* (1913) on the strength of a sale notice in the *Dublin Evening Post* of May 1786, advertising the sale of the collection of Sir Gustavus Hume, which included 'two pictures most admirably executed, one of live fowl, the other of a dead hare, etc., by an Irish master, Collins'. A signed oil painting by Collins, a still life of *Dead Game*, is in the National Gallery of Ireland. It is likely, however, that much of his obscure career was spent in London, as an obituary notice describes him as 'bird-painter to the Royal Society'. Despite the impressive quality of his work, Collins was served badly by the early compilers of art reference books. Horace Walpole's *Anecdotes of Painting in England* (1765-71) and Samuel Redgrave's *Dictionary of Artists of the English School* (1878) are very dismissive.

His work did not receive acclaim until a quantity of it appeared in London in the sale of the collection of Taylor White FSA at Sotheby's on 16 June 1926. The Victoria and Albert Museum acquired four of his large water-colours: *Curlew Sandpiper*, signed and dated January 1789; *A Rook*, signed and dated 'Cha. Collins Fect. April 10 1740'; *Great Crested Grebe*, dated December 1740; and *White-headed Sea Eagle*, dated July 1742. Other examples are in the British Museum and at Leeds City Art Gallery, which has the largest single group of Collins's work.

Five signed albums and one small sketchbook by the Dublin artist Mary Battersby are known. One album is in the Ulster Museum; the rest are in the National Library of Ireland, having been given to the Royal Dublin Society by the artist in 1820 and 1836.* Battersby's bird paintings, thoroughly eighteenth-century in style, appear to have been done mostly from stuffed specimens. The give-away sign in many of them is the droop of the tail, resulting from storage in cramped cupboards. Some were painted from 'a collection of stuffed birds in the Dublin Museum', others, dated 1810, were from birds shot in Meath, and yet others were taken from birds shot in Pennsylvania by Dr Robert Battersby, presumably the artist's nephew. The Ulster Museum's volume contains many exotics, such as birds of paradise, parakeets and hummingbirds. Two of the drawings are stated to be from pets – an African whidah (weaverbird) and, surprisingly, a collared dove, dated 1807. Before its mass colonization of western Europe, as late as the 1950s the collared dove would have been considered a rare Asiatic species. This volume also includes an American robin, dated 1809 and marked 'migratory thrush' (its scientific name is *Turdus migratorius*), some woodpeckers (not found in Ireland), and a 'butcher bird', or great grey shrike. There is also a smew, dated 1814, noted as 'shot on the Dublin coast'.

A considerable figure as a naturalist and illustrator was John Templeton of Belfast (1766-1825), wholesale merchant by trade and father of the much-travelled Dr Robert Templeton. He lived at Orange Grove, later named Cranmore, off the Malone Road, the oldest house in Belfast, now ruined. Principally a botanist, Templeton corresponded with Sir Joseph Banks, Sir William Hooker, William Turner, and the botanical illustrator James Sowerby. He was a friend also of Dr Walter Wade (1760-1825), from 1795 first curator of the Royal Botanic Gardens at Glasnevin; having visited Kew, Templeton as early as 1809 advocated the creation of a Botanic Garden in Belfast. He worked for years writing and illustrating a *Flora Hibernica*, which was never finished.

The Ulster Museum has a large collection of watercolours and drawings of mammals, plants, fish, sea-urchins, starfish, mollusca and crustaceans, and

---

* Anne Crookshank generously provided me with extra information on Battersby. See A. Crookshank and the Knight of Glin, 1994.

128 drawings of birds, all of which seem certain to be by John Templeton. Purely taxonomic illustrations, they are for the most part lifeless, though some of them have a certain charm. On the other hand, Templeton's pencilled notes on his drawings are of great scientific significance. It is clear that not all of them were painted from dead specimens. A pair of 'mumruffins' (long-tailed tits) were 'taken through a spy-glass'. A little grebe is inscribed 'caught before 1798 in the spring and after taking its picture let go in the Lagan'. His drawing of a brambling is inscribed:

One caught at Strandmills [Stranmillis, a suburb of Belfast] during a deep snow and hard frost Feb. 3 1799. Became in a short time familiar with a cage, went out and in. It often quarrelled with a chaffinch, principally about a piece of loaf bread, cracking its bill, but in strength and courage the chaffinch seemed its equal. When the spring came I set both at liberty. In the Autumn of 1801 I saw a bird of this kind in the Avenue probably this bird.

There is also a drawing of a hobby, which deserves comparison with Richard Parker's painting and report (noted presently). Templeton's specimen was found 'building at Ballynascreen Mountains ... July 10 1802'. He puzzlingly states Ballynascreen to be in County Wicklow, whereas it is actually in County Derry. Many of the dead birds were found by Templeton in the Belfast markets, including teal, shoveller, redshank and turnstone.

John Templeton's son Robert (1802-92), who graduated in medicine at Edinburgh in 1831, obtained a commission as Assistant Surgeon in the Royal Artillery in 1833, and soon after was posted to Mauritius. There he continued to pursue his early interest in insects and spiders. He was back in London in 1835, but soon set out again for Rio and then for Colombo for a short visit. In 1839 he returned to Ceylon for a twelve-year period. As one of the remarkable Belfast fraternity present in colonial Ceylon (along with Emerson Tennent, Andrew Nicholl and others), Robert Templeton made his incomparable coloured drawings of Ceylonese lepidoptera, which are now in the Ulster Museum (Nash and Ross, 1980.) Only the dorsal side of the body and right wing of each specimen is drawn, a labour-saving device with objects that are bilaterally symmetrical. The drawings are enclosed within a neatly-ruled pencil rectangle, outside which is a wide margin for scribbling scientific notes. There is no attempt to illustrate the food-plant or the immature forms of the insects, though in some cases the ventral surfaces of the wings are drawn. These are entomologists' working drawings *par excellence*, their artistic quality being only incidental. But this does not negate their undeniable intrinsic beauty. Robert Templeton was certainly involved with John Blackwell's lavishly illustrated *History of the Spiders of Great Britain and Ireland*, published by the Ray Society in 1861, and probably drew some of the illustrations, though it is impossible to tell which ones.

Andrew Nicholl

Mention of the Irish presence in Ceylon necessarily invokes the name of the self-taught Belfast painter Andrew Nicholl (1804-86). Precocious in drawing as a youth, he early came to the attention of local *cognoscenti* such as Dr James Macdonnell, an enlightened surgeon who was one of the founders of the Linen Hall Library, and Dr James Lawson Drummond, surgeon, anatomist and amateur botanist, who invited the young Nicholl to stay in his house and help illustrate his books. Apprenticed originally as a compositor with the *Northern Whig* newspaper, Nicholl was discovered about 1830 by the Belfast MP James Emerson (later Sir James Emerson Tennent), who took him to London and became his main patron. Early in the 1830s, Nicholl travelled as draughtsman with an expedition to the Isle of Staffa. This resulted in some sketches of basalt rock formations (*Clam Shell Cave* and *Fingal's Cave*) which complement Nicholl's many studies of the north Antrim coast and the Giant's Causeway.

In July 1845 Emerson Tennent was appointed Colonial Secretary for Ceylon. Nicholl followed him there the next year to take up a position as 'teacher of landscape painting, scientific drawing and design' at the Colombo Academy, an institution modelled on the English public school. He remained there until 1849. It would seem likely that Tennent's real purpose in bringing Nicholl to Ceylon was to illustrate his own book *Ceylon*, a comprehensive, scholarly and well-written account of the geography, history and natural history of the island. The revised fifth edition of 1860 contains thirty-one engravings after Nicholl (Tennent, 1860.) This book is still regarded with high esteem by Sri Lankans (though this opinion does not extend to Tennent's administration, which is seen by the natives as a disastrous period of insensitivity). Tennent's verandah tax and dog tax did not endear him to the local population, and it is possible that he was instrumental in causing the rebellion of 1848 in the central province of Kandy. Tennent and Nicholl were on an exploratory expedition to Kandy when this rebellion broke out, and had to flee for their lives, an episode Nicholl described in a long article in the *Dublin University Magazine* in 1852.

A lot of Nicholl's drawings remain in the National Museum in Colombo. It was in Ceylon that Nicholl produced a set of botanical water-colours of native plants, which resurfaced on the London market in 1981 (Spink, 1981). It is not usual to think of Nicholl as a botanical painter, but these are straightforward taxonomic drawings, quite different from the sort of flower watercolour perfected by Nicholl in his Dublin period during the late 1830s, which are picturesque rather than scientific. Attractive examples showing a bank of poppies and daisies in the foreground, with a recognizable

Irish landscape in the background, still turn up in the salerooms, and are greedily sought after by collectors.

The Ulster Museum's files contain an interesting letter from Tennent to Nicholl, dated 17 March 1859, requesting help with an illustration of *Noosing Wild Elephants*, to be used as the frontispiece to *Ceylon*. The elephants were drawn from life in the Regent's Park Zoo by one of the greatest of nineteenth-century animal and bird artists, Joseph Wolf (1820-99), who provided four illustrations. Tennent writes to Nicholl:

A scientific draughtsman, Woolf *[sic]* is employed by Longman's to make 3 drawings of the attitudes of the elephants during their struggles in the Kraal. The animals, he will do well, as he makes studies from the living elephants in the Zoological Gardens, but he is at a loss for foliage. He has no sketches of Ceylon trees, and especially of creepers and climbing plants, and straggling roots above ground. Now it occurs to me, that you may have some rough sketches of these that would enable Woolf to make the foregrounds in character with Ceylon vegetation. And if you would lend them to me, for that purpose, you see what an advantage it would be to me. If you can oblige me in this matter, please would you put the sketches in a packet and send it by Post – addressed to me, Board of Trade, Whitehall, London – marking it in the corner *Private* ... I will be responsible for the safe return of the sketches to you.

Evidently, Nicholl was able to comply with this request, as the engraved illustration contains a luxuriant array of trees and creepers (Anglesea, 1981a).

Richard Dunscombe Parker

One of the pleasantest experiences of my curatorial career thus far was the finding of the 'Illustrations of the Irish Birds' by the amateur painter Richard Dunscombe Parker (1805-81). This remarkable ornithological painter, who has no entry in Strickland's *Dictionary*, was a gentleman-farmer, sportsman and naturalist, who lived a bachelor life with his brothers at Landscape House, Sunday's Well, on the western outskirts of Cork city. He had been completely forgotten until the rediscovery of his 170 large watercolour bird paintings in the Ulster Museum in 1976. They had been bequeathed to the Museum by Parker's niece in 1932, and had lain neglected, but safe, in a store. Consequently their condition for the most part was as fresh as when they were painted (*see plate 18*).* The Ulster Museum put on a large exhibition of all 170 of Parker's watercolours in 1980, with a catalogue compiled

---

* I was grateful to Mr C.J.F. McCarthy, a Cork local historian, who did much valuable research on the Parker family in the Cork Record Office, and generously placed his findings at my disposal.

by the present author (Anglesea, 1980). Four years later, a hand-bound limited edition was published, reproducing in colour forty of Parker's paintings (Anglesea, 1984). This selection was subsequently exhibited at the Crawford Municipal Art Gallery, Cork, in 1986.

Parker must be considered as the only Irish rival to John James Audubon (1785-1851). It is possible that he knew the American bird-painter's work; his younger brother, Dr Noble Dunscombe Parker, was a medical graduate of Glasgow University, one of the four British universities (Oxford, Cambridge, Glasgow and Edinburgh) that subscribed, along with many private individuals and societies, to the printing costs of Audubon's 'Double Elephant Folio', i.e. *The Birds of America*, the largest and most famous bird book ever printed (four volumes, each volume standing four feet high, containing over four hundred hand-coloured aquatint etchings).

When some of Parker's bird paintings were shown in 1843 to the Natural History Section of the British Association for the Advancement of Science, then holding its meeting in Cork, the reaction was enthusiastic. 'Mr Strickland' – i.e. H.G. Strickland FGS, an eminent English authority on the birds of Madagascar; he must not be confused with W.G. Strickland, author of the *Dictionary of Irish Artists* – 'expressed his gratification at Mr Parker's paintings; in fact, they were only second to Mr Gould's, of London, and fully equal to Audubon's. He pointed out particulars in which they far excelled the continental drawings, especially in familiarity with the living habits of the birds and of their plumage. Mr Thompson [i.e. William Thompson, the Belfast naturalist] would go even further than Mr Strickland. In lifelike appearance they excelled even Mr Gould's, beautiful as the latter were.'* Appropriately, the forty paintings reproduced in the 1984 Blackstaff limited edition were shown again to the British Association when it held its meeting in Belfast in 1987.

Parker always made a real attempt to show the habitat of each bird. When the whole series of 170 paintings was put on display, it was realized that Parker was also an excellent botanical painter. The plants and flowers he includes as environmental details are always appropriate; they may be seen at their best in his pictures of the moorhen, water-rail and corncrake. As with most bird painters, Parker is not successful with all the species. His small passerines lack the conviction of his vigorously drawn ducks, gulls and birds of prey. Also, when he attempts to show flying birds as background detail, he sometimes fails, as they tend to be ill-observed and badly articulated.

---

* A cut-out notice from a Cork newspaper of 1843, quoted in the printed advertisement to Parker's *Illustrations of the Irish Birds*.

The two perennial difficulties besetting an ornithological painter are identified by a witty American writer (Mengel, 1982) as the 'taxonomic problem' and the 'faunistic problem'. The taxonomic problem arises from the expectation of naturalists that each bird illustration should be fully descriptive of the species, that every point of recognition should be shown. This accounts for the convention of drawing the bird in rigid profile, allowing the maximum number of field-markings to be included. Taken to its logical extreme, the ideal would be more like a diagram or a map than a picture, the analogy being, for instance, an engineer's drawings of a car. One is reminded of the 'bird-maps' of the twentieth-century ornithological painter Charles Tunnicliffe. On the other hand, the faunistic problem stems from another expectation, which is hardly ever fulfilled: that the artist should be master of every species in a geographical area. A single artist can never have the time to study in detail not only the external form and markings, but the stance, movement and habits of every species. It is evident that, like Parker, most bird artists have their strengths and weaknesses. In contrast to Parker, the English bird illustrator P.D. Selby (1788-1867) is more comfortable with the small sparrow-like birds than with eagles. Some of the greatest ornithological painters actually specialized in certain groups or families, such as Edward Lear's parrots or Joseph Wolf's raptors. Mengel names one ornithological painter who, he claims, fulfils both ideals of taxonomic exactitude and faunistic comprehensiveness: the American Louis Agassiz Fuertes (1874-1927).

Richard Parker and his brothers are mentioned many times throughout the three *Birds* volumes of William Thompson's unfinished masterpiece *The Natural History of Ireland* (1849-51). The great Irish naturalist was also very interested in art. In 1843 he was President of the Belfast Society for the Promotion of the Fine Arts, a body that organized some quite ambitious exhibitions and pressed the government to set up of a School of Design in the city. On the committee of this society, he would have fraternized with Francis McCracken, the Belfast cotton-mill manager who was later to become one of the earliest patrons of the English Pre-Raphaelite painters. McCracken was friendly with the Dublin painter and antiquary George Petrie, who was Librarian of the Royal Hibernian Academy. In the section of *The Natural History of Ireland* dealing with the heron, Thompson describes in some detail a large 'gallery watercolour' called *The Home of the Heron*, which Petrie exhibited at the RHA in 1846. It was painted at Lough Athry, near Clifden in Connemara. Thompson writes: 'It may be observed that Petrie's style approximates to that of Copley Fielding more than to any other; both artists being remarkable for a depth of fine poetic feeling in their treatment of landscape.' This watercolour is now in the National Gallery of Ireland. Strickland, by the way, considered Petrie's watercolours overpraised in his lifetime.

Nineteenth-Century Scientific Illustrators

The pioneering English geologists William Conybeare, later Dean of Westminster, and William Buckland, first Professor of Geology at Oxford, undertook a detailed study of the north coast of Ireland which was published in 1816. By this time, Werner's 'Neptunist' theory of the aqueous origin of all rocks, including basalt, had lost ground in Europe. The study, entitled *Descriptive Notes Referring to the Outline of Sections Presented by a Part of the Coasts of Antrim and Derry*, is illustrated by outline sections, coloured by hand. Diagrammatic though they are, they occupy an important place in any account of scientific draughtsmanship in Ireland. These drawings may have been made by Conybeare and Buckland themselves. This was not an unusual practice. Drawing at this time was a social accomplishment, like speaking French or playing the piano. It was also taught in military academies for use in the field. We have already seen the quality of the entomological drawings of Robert Templeton; Major-General Joseph Ellison Portlock (1794-1864), the geologist, and William Henry Harvey (1811-66), the botanist, also made their own drawings.

Other very able amateur scientific draughtsmen and draughtswomen are too numerous to examine in detail (such as the Fitton sisters, Mary Ward, Robert, Anne and Mary Ball, the Plunkett sisters and Lady Cuffe). The example of Alexander Henry Haliday (b. Holywood, Co. Down 1806, d. Italy 1870), one of the greatest of nineteenth-century entomologists, may stand as typical of the exemplary collaboration among that class of dedicated people. Haliday met the famous entomologist John Curtis of Norwich, fifteen years his senior, in 1827 (Nash, 1983). As the son of an engraver, Curtis was able to draw and engrave his own plates. In 1835 Curtis made an entomological tour of Ireland, accompanied by Haliday. Curtis's *British Entomology*, a monumental work that appeared in sections between 1823 and 1840, has as plate 596 the wasp *Stenocera walkeri*, dated by Curtis 'May 1 1836'. Each of these finely engraved plates is embellished with an illustration, hand-coloured and varnished, of a plant on which the particular insect might be found. In this case the plant is *Rosa hibernica* (the Belfast Rose), for the 'beautiful drawing' of which Curtis acknowledges his debt to 'Miss Haliday', who was Haliday's sister.

In other instances professional artists were employed. The topographical department of the Ordnance Survey consisted entirely of civilians, with the artist George Petrie as superintendent. During its brief existence, from 1833 to 1842, the department, as J.H. Andrews (1975) tells us, operated from Petrie's house in Great Charles Street, Dublin, so as to be close to the libraries for research into placenames. Petrie had as his assistant one of his many pupils, George Victor Du Noyer. Petrie and Du Noyer's studies of topography and antiquities do not concern us, but after the topographical department was closed down, Portlock found Du Noyer employment for the rest of his life in the Geological Survey (Coffey, 1993, 1993a). Du Noyer also produced extremely accurate ornithological and botanical drawings and watercolours, many of which are at Glasnevin (Scannell and Houston, 1980). According to Du Noyer's obituary notice, 'his watercolour drawings of objects of natural history, Irish roses, grains, birds, &c., possess a charming truthfulness; but it is as a geological landscape painter that his productions show so much of poetry and truth – his brilliant colour brightening, and giving, so to speak, life to his pictures' (Gages, 1869).

An example of a highly skilled specialist scientific illustrator from abroad working in Ireland is Joseph Dinkel, a Munich art student employed by the great Swiss naturalist Louis Agassiz. The task of classifying the fossil fish of the world brought Agassiz in contact with the owners of the two best collections of fossil fish in the British Isles, Sir Philip Egerton at Oulton Park, Cheshire, and William Willoughby Cole, 3rd Earl of Enniskillen, at Florence Court, Co. Fermanagh. These two obsessive collectors had become friends at Oxford in the 1820s, where they had attended Buckland's lectures on geology and gone on his field excursions to quarries. They met Agassiz in Munich in 1830, and Agassiz visited them in the summer of 1834. The coloured drawings on which Dinkel laboured for months, in London, at Oulton Park, and at Florence Court, are almost photographic in their accuracy. Some of them were used as illustrations to Agassiz's major work *Recherches sur les Poissons Fossiles*, published in five volumes between 1833 and 1844. Lord Enniskillen adapted one of the flanking pavilions at Florence Court (now a National Trust property) as a private museum for his collection, top-lit by a skylight, and insulated from the kitchen below by metal sheets. One of its many distinguished visitors, Reverend W.S. Symonds from Worcestershire, described it:

The museum is an octagon room lighted from the roof, and contains with the exception perhaps of Sir P. Egerton's, the finest private collection of fossil-fishes in Great Britain. On a platform in the centre there towers the perfect skeleton of the gigantic elk, Megaceros Hibernicus, and the walls are surrounded by glass-cases filled with the choicest fossils.*

Dinkel returned later to paint fossils in the collections of Egerton and Lord Enniskillen. Many of his original drawings were presented to the Geological Society of London in Burlington House. Towards the end of his

---

* James, 1986, 14-15. The title 'Damned Nonsense!' reflects the 3rd Earl's father's opinion of his son's collecting.

life, having gone blind, Lord Enniskillen sold his collection of fossil fish to the British Museum (Natural History), where they are kept adjacent to Egerton's collection (James, 1986). From the cultural point of view, it should be noted that the third Earl of Enniskillen was one of Ireland's leading unionists, and the first Imperial Grand Master of the Orange Order.

An odd nineteenth-century parallel to Susanna Drury in tantalizing obscurity is found in the case of Philip Brannon (Rowan, 1980). It is not known when or where this artist was born, but he may have lived for a time in Belfast, as his earliest known work is a small watercolour, 'The Commercial Buildings, Belfast', dated 1841, now in the Local History Department of the Ulster Museum. The following year he produced a drawing of Devonport Town Hall, and seems to have spent his working life in the south of England. He wrote and illustrated a number of guidebooks, such as *Southampton and Netley Abbey* in 1850, and *Poole and Bournemouth* in 1856. By 1875 the latter volume had gone through eighteen editions. Brannon evidently had a scientific bent as well as financial means, as in 1875 he published at his own expense an illustrated account of his invention of a 'gas-less air-boat': 'making aero-navigation rapid, safe and certain'. Whether this contraption ever flew is not recorded.

In 1880, when he must have been in his sixties, Brannon lent twenty of his paintings of Irish views to an Irish exhibition in London (Stewart, 1990). He was then living at Walton-in-the-Naze in Essex. Though it is by no means certain that these paintings were executed that year or even a short time before, the titles indicate that Brannon had travelled in counties Dublin, Wicklow, Mayo, Donegal, Tyrone, Down and Louth. One of them, *Black Sod Point, Co. Mayo*, a large watercolour, was acquired in 1980 by Professor Alistair Rowan for the collection of University College Dublin. This Victorian 'gallery watercolour', intended to be displayed in a heavy gilt frame, shows Brannon's intensive and accurate observation of the fractured, jointed granite shelf, which takes up most of the composition. Part of the Termon granite, an intrusion of about four million years ago, later revealed by erosion, this rock was known to nineteenth-century geologists as 'Black Sod Granite'.

Brannon took more than a passing interest in geology; his publications include *The Geologic Scenery of Purbeck* (1858), an illustrated guide to the coastal rock features of Dorset. The full title of the Mayo view is *Black Sod Point, with Saddle and Achill Head to the Left, Black Rock and Other Islands in the Distance, with the Hill and Tower of Glask and Falmore Village to the Right*. Like Susanna Drury at the Giant's Causeway over a century before, Brannon has taken some topographical liberties to bring some of the distant features into the picture, but has nevertheless succeeded in making geological sense of the foreground granite mass. Despite perspectival infelicities in linking the foreground to the middle distance, and a weakness in drawing the tiny figures of children playing on the rocks, Brannon's scientific landscape deserves greater recognition than it has received.

The horse-painter Michael Angelo Hayes (b. Waterford 1820; d. Dublin 1877) lectured to the Royal Dublin Society in November 1876 on the subject of the conventions of drawing horses galloping. The conclusions expressed in Hayes' paper anticipate the photographs of animals in rapid motion made by the Anglo-American Eadweard Muybridge (1830-1904), and the later invention of cinematography. Muybridge started photographing moving horses in the 1870s, and published his book *The Attitudes of Animals in Motion* in 1881. Hayes had to rely on his own careful observation of horses, either in military reviews in the Phoenix Park or at race meetings. Using his own drawings as illustrations, Hayes demonstrated that the Greeks had correctly observed the position of the legs of a galloping horse in the Parthenon frieze. The seventeenth-century convention of planting both hind hooves of a horse on the ground, with the forefeet high in the air, was shown to be untrue, and so was the convention, introduced by Henry Alken in the early nineteenth century, of showing the forelegs stretched out fully in front, and the hind-legs stretched out behind, with the body of the horse reduced in height. While Alken's convention gave a convincing illusion of speed, it was misleading. Hayes observed that there was no difference between the height of a standing horse and that of a galloping horse. This was made obvious, he saw, when a body of cavalry was executing a wheel; the riders on the inside walked their horses, those in the middle trotted, and those on the outside galloped, but the three ranks of horses remained equal in height. Hayes's drawings correctly analyzed the rapid movements of a horse's legs in galloping and walking. At the end of his lecture, Hayes demonstrated a set of drawings he had prepared for the phenakistiscope or zoetrope, a revolving French toy which was a hand-made precursor of the cinema. Hayes reported that 'the revolving phenakistiscope was looked at and examined by most of those present, and was generally pronounced to be a faithful and accurate representation of the action of a living animal in full gallop' (Hayes, 1878).*

Some remarkable early photographers worked in Ireland; of these, the Belfast photographer Robert John Welch (1859-1936) should be singled out. Welch was accustomed to travelling throughout Ireland from an early age with his father, a professional photographer. His father's death in 1875 left Welch as the family breadwinner, so he had to give up his intention of entering Queen's College and taking a degree. The collection of glass negatives he built up as a professional should be regarded as one of the national treasures

---

* I am grateful to Helena Chesney for drawing my attention to this.

of Ireland. Welch bequeathed them to the Belfast Naturalists' Field Club, which in turn passed them to the Ulster Museum. They depict antiquities, folk-life, buildings, industry, botany and geology, testifying to Welch's wide-ranging interests. Particularly outstanding are his geological photographs, taken mainly during the 1880s and 1890s with a cumbersome full-plate camera. His clear, sharp images of the Giant's Causeway and Fair Head have never been bettered, and are still used as illustrations in geological textbooks. One beautiful close-up study shows the tessellated pavement of the Causeway, with sea-water lying in the depressions. Another photograph shows the cliffs of Port Noffer with the red lateritic inter-basaltic bed picked out in red ink. But the most memorable image is of Welch himself, in his stockinged feet, seated precariously on the collapsed basalt column that spans the Grey Man's Path above Fair Head. This was taken about 1892, Welch having bribed a local boy to remove the lens-cap (Evans and Turner, 1977; James, 1985).*

During the second half of the nineteenth century there appeared a new class of illustrators, female and professional, as distinct from the older but still well-established class of amateurs who were fortunate enough to have the economic independence to pursue their scientific interests. An early example of this new phenomenon is Lydia Shackleton (b. Ballitore, Co. Kildare 1828; d. 1914), who was possibly the foremost Irish botanical painter of the nineteenth century. The bulk of her work, about fifteen hundred drawings, remains at Glasnevin (Morley, 1979), where she was employed for twenty-three years by the Keeper of the Royal Botanic Gardens, Sir Frederick Moore, starting at the age of fifty-six. One of the groups of plants she was employed to paint, in 1885, was the carnivorous pitcher-plants, native to North America, of which the first artificial hybrids were bred at Glasnevin. As early as the 1880s, Shackleton travelled extensively in the United States on two occasions, collecting and recording plants.

She was succeeded by Alice Jacob (b. Dublin 1862; d. Dublin 1921), one of the first women to teach in the Schools of Design in Dublin and Cork. While she won herself considerable fame as a designer of lace, textiles and ceramic decoration (for the Beleek Pottery in Co. Fermanagh), she merits inclusion here because of the series of more than fifteen hundred water-colour studies of orchids, commissioned from her by Moore at Glasnevin, between 1894 and 1920. Moore built up the largest orchid collection in the world at Glasnevin. Some of Alice Jacob's drawings are executed in gouache

---

* Reproduced on the cover of Evans and Turner, 1977. The *Irish Naturalists' Journal* 6 (6) (1936) contains obituaries and reminiscences of Welch written by Robert Lloyd Praeger, A.W. Stelfox, A.R. Hogg (photographer) and J. Wilfred Jackson of the Manchester Museum.

on tinted paper, a technique that gave the artist the middle tones ready-made, and enabled her to build up the highlights with white paint. Charles Nelson, author of 'Orchid Paintings at Glasnevin' (1981), has written brief biographies of Lydia Shackleton and Ellen Hutchins, and, with Nicola Gordon Bowe, a brief biography of Alice Jacob, all in *Irish Women Artists* (Ryan-Smolin et al., 1987).

Nelson also provides a biography of Edith Osborne (b. Clonmel, 1845; d. 1926), a belated example of the industrious amateur draughtswoman, who from the time her husband, Henry Arthur Blake, was knighted in 1888, was known as Lady Blake. Blake was a British colonial diplomat, serving successively as Governor of the Bahamas, Newfoundland, Jamaica, Hong Kong and Ceylon. Between 1888 and 1907 Lady Blake accompanied her husband to all these places, where she collected, drew, and painted plants and especially insects. The Natural History Museum in London has a series of 195 paintings by her of Jamaican Lepidoptera, which include, as well as the adult insect, the caterpillar, chrysalis and food-plant. The bulk of her botanical watercolours made in Jamaica and Hong Kong are in private collections.

Though in no sense a scientific illustrator, Mildred Anne Butler (1858-1941) of Thomastown, Co. Kilkenny, took nature as a theme for much of her work. Her father, Captain Henry Butler, widely travelled in South Africa and South America, was yet another of those assiduous amateur draughtsmen of botany and zoology. He wrote and illustrated with lithographs *South African Sketches, Illustrative of the Wild Life of a Hunter on the Frontier of the Cape Colony*, published by Ackermann of London in 1840. Some of his watercolours and lithographs were placed at the end of the sale of *Watercolours by Mildred Anne Butler* at Christie's in London on 13 October 1981. In contrast, Mildred Butler's artistic training and attitude were definitely those of 'gallery art'. She worked with Norman Garstin (an Irish-born painter) as part of the artistic colony at Newlyn in Cornwall in 1894 and 1895, where she absorbed the Newlyn School's habit of painting out-of-doors. She exhibited regularly in London with the Royal Academy and the Royal Society of Painters in Water-Colours.

Although she travelled on the Continent a great deal, Mildred Butler had a particular affection for her own home, Kilmurry, where she spent all her life recording the gardens, the cattle and the birds. Her reputation was established in 1896, when her large watercolour *The Morning Bath*, featuring the white fantail pigeons at Kilmurry, was picked out from the Royal Academy Summer Exhibition for purchase by the Tate Gallery through the Chantrey Bequest. The Ulster Museum has another large watercolour, *A Sunshine Holiday*, dated 1897, which again shows fantail pigeons bathing in a water-trough in the yard at Kilmurry. Her diploma piece, presented on election to the Ulster Academy of Arts about 1931, is *The Dust Bath*, one of her many studies of the Kilmurry peacocks (reproduced in Anglesea, 1981). In her bird paintings Mildred Butler shows particular sensitivity to the crow family, warming to the challenge of rendering the glossy sheens of their feathers. These pictures tend to have whimsical, anthropomorphic titles; perhaps the most spectacular of them is a study of rooks, a large watercolour dated 1893 and entitled '*And straight against that great array/Went forth the valiant three*' (Macaulay, *Lays of Ancient Rome*), which was bought in 1981 by the National Gallery of Ireland. Despite their whimsicality, these bird pictures of Mildred Butler attain what Richard Dunscombe Parker never quite achieved – a sense of life (Crookshank and Glin, 1981; Pyle *et al.*, 1987).

Several technical manuals on scientific drawing and painting have been produced in Ireland. One of the earliest of these must be *The Art of Botanical Drawing*, published in 1873 by Frederick William Burbage (b. Leicestershire 1847; d. Dublin 1905), who came to Ireland in 1879 to take up the post of Curator of Trinity College Botanic Gardens. Even earlier, Mary Ward (d. 1869) of Castle Ward, Co. Down, a cousin of the astronomer Earl of Rosse, identified Halley's Comet at the age of eight, and, through the use of her cousin's telescope at Birr, published *Telescope Teachings* in 1859. Many of her watercolours remain at Castle Ward. Perhaps her most influential book, *Microscope Teachings*, resulted from her early acquisition of what may have been the best microscope in Ireland, which also may be seen at Castle Ward. She took a particular interest in insects.

One of the poet William Butler Yeats's sisters, Elizabeth Corbet Yeats (1868-1940), wrote two instruction books, including *Brushwork Studies of Flowers, Fruit and Animals*, published in 1896. It is interesting to recall that W.B. Yeats himself, besides being a trained and accomplished draughtsman, had been a keen entomologist as a schoolboy. He was known as an 'insect-collector' who carried cardboard boxes 'filled with his victims', and, unlike his fellow-pupils, was familiar with the ideas of Darwin (Murphy, 1978). Yeats was later to turn his back on empirical science in favour of magic and the occult.

Rosamond Praeger (b. Holywood, Co. Down 1867; d. 1954), though principally a sculptor of somewhat sentimental subjects, was forced through economic necessity to work as an illustrator, and wrote and illustrated more than fifteen delightful picture books for children. In 1913 she drew the line illustrations for a book by her naturalist brother, Robert Lloyd Praeger, entitled *Weeds, Simple Lessons for Children*, of which some of the original drawings are at Glasnevin.

Sculpture, Taxidermy and Wood-engraving

Sculpture is not a medium normally associated with wildlife. In nineteenth-century France there developed a tradition of animal sculptors, *les animaliers*, of whom the most famous was Antoine-Louis Barye (1796-1875). This tradition is recalled by the work of the London-trained sculptor Morris Harding (b. Stevenage, Hertfordshire 1874; d. Holywood, Co. Down 1964).* Harding was brought to Belfast in 1925 by the architect Sir Charles Nicholson to execute the decorative sculpture for St Anne's Cathedral, which was then under construction. He worked for twelve years on the nave capitals and corbels, and liked Ulster so much that he settled for the rest of his life in Holywood. There he had a studio in the same building as Rosamond Praeger, who worked alongside him at St Anne's. Harding was a prolific sketcher of zoo animals in movement, usually in the rapid medium of coloured chalks on tinted dark blue paper. The forty-seven animal drawings by him in the Ulster Museum all predate his coming to Belfast, and were apparently done in the London Zoo around 1919-24. But some of the twelve sculptures of leopards and polar bears in plaster, stone and alabaster carry the dates of 1936 and 1940, by which time Harding had been elected a Member of the Royal Hibernian Academy and President of the Ulster Academy of Arts. Harding's daughter, Miss Rita Morris-Harding, gave her father's animal sculptures and drawings to the Ulster Museum in 1966.

The question arises whether taxidermists should be regarded as sculptors, and I believe that the best of them should be so regarded. Certainly all the taxidermists I have known have possessed artistic temperaments. Displays of stuffed birds and animals, usually shot on the estate, formed an important feature of the Victorian country house in both Britain and Ireland. Sometimes even the glass cases were made an architectural feature, as at Crom Castle, Co. Fermanagh, for which the Earl of Erne in the 1840s commissioned Gothic-revival bird-cases from Arthur Jones, a Dublin furniture-maker (Knox, 1993). During the nineteenth century James Sheals of Belfast ran an important business in taxidermy, carried on and expanded by his sons Alfred and Thomas to the point of world fame. The Sheals brothers produced dramatically posed and vividly lifelike tableaux that merit consideration as a three-dimensional equivalent to the bird paintings of Richard Dunscombe Parker (McKee, 1983).

Wood-engraving has a long and distinguished history as a means of portraying nature. The pioneer of the modern (white-line) method of

---

* There is a biography of Morris Harding by Theo Snoddy in Hewitt, 1977. Harding's activities with the Royal Ulster Academy are chronicled by Anglesea, 1981.

engraving with the burin on the end-grain of hard boxwood, Thomas Bewick of Newcastle-upon-Tyne, left as his masterpieces *The General History of Quadrupeds* (1790) and *The History of British Birds* (1797 and 1804). After Bewick's time, the tradition of wood engraving in England lost its white-line purity and degenerated into a mechanical means of reproducing pen-drawings; the caricatures in the Victorian issues of *Punch* magazine are familiar examples. The engravers who carved such blocks constituted the true proletariat of nineteenth-century art. Early in the twentieth century, however, a small reformist movement brought about a revival of the craft of wood engraving in England, resulting in the foundation of the Society of Wood-Engravers in 1920. A significant number of the artists involved were Irish, including Robert Gibbings from Cork and E.M. O'Rorke Dickey from Belfast. Their beautiful productions were based on private presses and small editions.

The Ulster Museum owes its rich collection of modern wood engravings to Lady Mabel Annesley (1881-1959), of Castlewellan, Co. Down, who herself was trained as a wood engraver by Noel Rooke at the Central School of Arts and Crafts in London. Annesley knew all of the major figures in the movement, including Gibbings, Eric Gill, John Farleigh, Gertrude Hermes and Blair Hughes-Stanton, and generously gave her distinguished collection of their works to the museum in 1932 and 1939. Robert Gibbings (b. Cork 1889, d. London 1958) followed the Bewick tradition by writing and illustrating many works of which nature is the main subject. The son of the Church of Ireland Rector of Carrigrohane (coincidentally the place where Richard Dunscombe Parker spent his boyhood), Robert Gibbings first studied at University College Cork. In 1912 he went to the Slade School of Art in London, and joined Noel Rooke's classes in wood engraving at the Central School. After receiving a serious neck wound while serving with the Royal Munster Fusiliers at Gallipoli, Gibbings was invalided out of the army, and in 1920 founded the Society of Wood-Engravers. Between 1924 and 1933 he ran the private Golden Cockerel Press, based at Waltham St Lawrence, Berkshire. He visited Tahiti in 1929 and the West Indies in 1932. From 1936 to 1940 be lectured in book production at Reading University under Professor Allen Seaby, who himself produced some beautiful images of birds and fish using the Japanese medium of colour woodcut. (Allen Seaby's son, Wilfred Arthur Seaby, was Director of the Ulster Museum from 1953 to 1971.) In 1937 Gibbings visited Bermuda, and in 1938 went to the Red Sea to draw underwater.

Gibbings's output was phenomenal. He illustrated sixty-one books, fourteen of which he also wrote. During the 1930s he took up sculpture. 'I was always a close-to-nature man,' Gibbings writes in his published recollections, edited by Patience Empson (1959). When he illustrated Lord

Grey's *Fallodon Papers* for Constable (1926), and the same writer's *The Charm of Birds* for Hodder and Stoughton (1927), he 'began to see not only the decorative quality of birds but the suitability of wood engraving for their clearly defined textures'. But by the time Gibbings produced the engravings of fish for his own book *Iorana* (1932), inspired by his visit to Tahiti, his technique had gained an unprecedented subtlety while remaining true to the quality of the woodblock. Llewelyn Powys's *The Glory of Life* (1934) has large and impressive animal, bird and insect engravings by Gibbings. Also in 1934 Gibbings illustrated the Belfast-born Helen Waddell's translations from medieval bestiaries, *Beasts and Saints*. This was followed by *A Bird Diary* and *The Insect Man* in 1936, *A Book of Uncommon Prayer* in 1937, and *The Microbe Man*, *Blue Angels and Whales*, and *Marvels of the Insect World* in 1938. Gibbings's style finally attained a mature simplicity in the illustrations to the eight 'river' books that he wrote himself from his own explorations in a boat, beginning with *Sweet Thames Run Softly* (1940), and including his tributes to his homeland, *Lovely is the Lee* (1945) and *Sweet Cork of Thee* (1951).

Contemporaries

At the moment, Ireland is the working-place of two of the most distinguished botanical artists alive: Wendy Walsh, who lives near Dublin, and Raymond Piper, who lives in Belfast. Both are of English origin, but have strongly identified with Ireland. Walsh is something of a cosmopolitan, having been born in Westmorland, England, and having received instructions from a Japanese painter while living in Japan. She has designed postage stamps for the Gilbert Islands and for the Republic of Ireland. Since about 1970 she has been specializing in botanical painting, working largely at the National Botanic Gardens at Glasnevin. She was awarded the Gold Medal of the Royal Horticultural Society in 1981. I have heard her say she enjoys painting white flowers, which is a matter of technical mystery to those untrained as painters. Walsh has illustrated a number of books, including *The Native Dogs of Ireland* (Irish Kennel Club, 1984), *An Irish Flower Garden* (1984), the two handsome volumes of *An Irish Florilegium: Wild and Garden Plants of Ireland* (Walsh, 1983, 1987), and *Trees of Ireland* (Nelson and Walsh, 1993).

Piper, born in 1923 in London, was brought to Belfast by his father at the age of six. He is a man of many parts, having combined a career as an academic portrait painter and a topographical draughtsman with an obsessive interest in Irish orchids, which earned him election as a Fellow of the Linnaean Society. He has painted every Irish species of orchid (*plate 20*). In 1974 he was awarded the John Lindley Medal of the Royal Horticultural

Society for his watercolours of Irish orchids, which until then were not widely known outside Northern Ireland. Piper exhibits regularly with the Royal Ulster Academy, of which he is an Academician. A tribute to Raymond Piper was made in 1991 by Rowel Friers, draughtsman and cartoonist, in a large pencil drawing called *The Botany Lesson* (now owned by the Ulster Museum), which is loosely based on Rembrandt's *Anatomy Lesson* of Dr Tulp. Piper is shown, scalpel in hand, explaining the intricacies of an orchid to a rapt audience of five Royal Ulster Academicians. The Ulster Museum's Department of Botany and Zoology has eight of Raymond Piper's botanical watercolours, as well as a pencil portrait by him of Norman Carrothers (1970).

Over the years, several Irish painters who are normally regarded as 'gallery artists' rather than scientific draughtsmen have tried their hand on occasion at treating wildlife subjects. Here may be mentioned Edward Murphy (c. 1796-1841), a Dublin painter who committed suicide and who is known today by only one picture, a creditable oil painting of *Parroquets* in the National Gallery of Ireland. He is recorded as exhibiting pictures of animals, flowers and still life in both Dublin and London, so the remainder of his work must be mistakenly attributed to other painters (Crookshank and Glin, 1978). The tradition in which Murphy worked has persisted into the present century, sometimes in the form of still life painting of dead game. Sir William Orpen (1878-1931), born and brought up in Ireland, who succeeded Sargent as Britain's richest dandified society portrait-painter, painted one of his numerous self-portraits holding up a dead ptarmigan (Dublin, National Gallery of Ireland). More recently, the Dublin painter Edward McGuire (1932-86), a reclusive figure with an obsessive fascination with painting technique, painted detailed studies of birds, mostly dead or stuffed. McGuire devised an appliance for controlling the mixing of paint using scales of fourteen tones. Working very slowly, producing only about four pictures a year, he became celebrated in Ireland as a portrait-painter, mainly of literary figures and academics (Fallon, 1991). Stuffed birds appear in the background of McGuire's oft-reproduced portrait of Seamus Heaney (1974, Ulster Museum).

One last contemporary artist who does not belong to the illustrative or taxonomic tradition, but who is definitely a 'fine' or 'gallery' artist, is Barrie Cooke (b. 1931). He is a transplant, born in Cheshire, brought up in the West Indies and educated at Harvard. There he initially studied biology, Chinese poetry and art history, but eventually chose art history after finding that he 'didn't have a scientific mentality' (quoted by Dunne, 1992). He re-crossed the Atlantic in the 1950s, intending to settle in London, but, finding the austere atmosphere of his native England restricting, he took a ferry to Dublin, where he immediately felt much more relaxed, and he has lived in Ireland ever since. He first went to Co. Clare, then worked in Co. Kilkenny for many years, and has now moved to Sligo.

Much of Cooke's painting is, at first sight, abstract. Its subject-matter, however, is nature itself, portrayed instinctively and immediately. Cooke has been an expert angler since childhood, and in his youth seriously considered studying fish management at Cornell University. His paintings of fish can be as objective as the *Portrait of the Lough Derg Pike, Life Size, with Relics*, in the Crawford Art Gallery, Cork. Many of his paintings are about the movement, flow and depth of water. In fact, he has inscribed on the wall of his studio, in the original Greek, Heraclitus's dictum 'everything flows' (Heaney, 1983). In the 1970s he added a sculptural dimension by constructing perspex boxes containing fired-clay objects that represent bones. Cooke's work conveys an almost tactile sense of nature (whether inspired by the rivers and lakes of the Irish midland plain, the bog-bodies of Denmark, or the tropical rain-forests of Borneo), through saturated colour and the brushing and dripping of paint. In this sense, he appears to have much in common with poets such as Ted Hughes and Seamus Heaney, who express themselves in tactile language. With Heaney he shares a fascination with bogs – their vegetative, preservative qualities, and the treasures they conceal.

This brings us again, full circle, to the 'Irish Elk', or giant Irish deer, which Cooke has used in paintings like *Megaceros Hibernicus* (1983, Gordon Lambert Collection, Irish Museum of Modern Art, Dublin), and *Elk Meets Sweeney* (1985, Kerlin Gallery) as a symbol of the potent, primeval life-force of pre-Christian Ireland. Cooke's more recent work, after a series of idyllic, optimistic paintings inspired by a visit to New Zealand, strikes a darker note by reference to the threat of nuclear contamination. *Death of a Lake* (1989, private collection, California) is a visual commentary, or elegy, on the destruction of the aquatic environment of Irish rivers by the dumping of industrial waste. In our own troubled times, concern for nature, even in art, is literally a matter of life or death.

References

Andrews, J.H. 1975. *A Paper Landscape: the Ordnance Survey in Nineteenth Century Ireland*. Oxford: Oxford University Press.

Anglesea, M. 1980. *Richard Dunscombe Parker's Irish Birds*. Belfast: Ulster Museum.

Anglesea, M. 1981. *The Royal Ulster Academy of Arts: a Centennial History*. Belfast: Royal Ulster Academy.

Anglesea, M. 1981a. 'Andrew Nicholl and his Patrons in Ireland and Ceylon.' *Studies 71*: 130-51.

Anglesea, M. (ed.). 1984. *Birds of Ireland by Richard Dunscombe Parker*. (250 hand-bound copies.) Belfast: Blackstaff Press.

Anglesea, M. 1991. 'The Iconography of the Antrim Coast,' in G. Dawe and J.W. Foster (eds), *The Poet's Place: Essays in Honour of John Hewitt*. Belfast: Institute of Irish Studies.

Anglesea, M. and J. Preston. 1980. 'A Philosophical Landscape: Susanna Drury and the Giant's Causeway.' *Art History 3*: 252-73.

Butler, P. 1990. 'Designers of Distinction: William Kilburn and Samuel Dixon.' *GPA Irish Arts Review Yearbook*: 176-89.

Coakley, D. 1992. 'Anatomy and Art: Irish Dimensions,' in *The Anatomy Lesson: Art and Medicine* [exhibition catalogue]. Dublin: National Gallery of Ireland.

Coffey, P. 1993. 'George Victor Du Noyer 1817-1869: Artist, Geologist and Antiquary.' *Journal of the Royal Society of Antiquaries of Ireland 123*: 102-19.

Coffey, P. 1993a. 'George Victor Du Noyer 1817-1869.' *Sheetlines* (Journal of the Charles Close Society) *35*: 14-26.

Conybeare, W. and W. Buckland. 1816. 'Descriptive Notes referring to the Outline of Sections presented by a Part of the Coasts of Antrim and Derry.' *Transactions of the Geological Society*, 1st series, *3*: 196-216.

Crookshank, A. and the Knight of Glin. 1978. *The Painters of Ireland c.1660-1920*. London: Barrie and Jenkins.

Crookshank, A. and the Knight of Glin. 1981. *Mildred Anne Butler*. Dublin: Bank of Ireland.

Crookshank, A. and the Knight of Glin. 1994. *The Watercolours of Ireland*. London: Barrie & Jenkins.

Curtis, J. 1823-40. *British Entomology, Being the Illustrations and Descriptions of the Genera of Insects Found in Great Britain and Ireland: Containing Coloured Figures from Nature of the Most Rare and Beautiful Species and in Many Instances of the Plants on which they are Found*. London: author.

Dance, S.P. 1978. *The Art of Natural History*. London: Cameron Books.

Dunne, A. 1992. 'Barrie Cooke, Change and Decay,' in *Barrie Cooke* [exhibition catalogue]. The Hague: Gemeentemuseum.

Empson, P. (ed.). 1959. *The Wood Engravings of Robert Gibbings, with some Recollections by the Artist*. Introduction by Thomas Balston. London: Dent & Sons.

Evans, E.E. and B.S. Turner. 1977. *Ireland's Eye: the Photographs of Robert John Welch*. Belfast: Blackstaff Press.

Fallon, B. 1991. *Edward McGuire*. Dublin: Irish Academic Press.

Gages, M. 1869. 'Biographical Notice of the late George V. Du Noyer, M.R.I.A., read January 11, 1869.' *Proceedings of the Royal Irish Academy*.

Hamilton, W. 1822. *Letters Concerning the North Coast of the County of Antrim ... with the Natural History of the Basaltes*. Belfast: Simms and McIntyre.

Hayden, R. 1980. *Mrs Delany: Her Life and Her Flowers*. London: Colonnade Books.

Hayes, M.A. 1878. 'On the Pictorial Delineation of Animals in Rapid Motion, with Illustrations.' (Read Monday evening, 20 November 1876.) *Royal Dublin Society Journal 7*: 73.

Heaney, S. 1983. 'Barrie Cooke,' in *Six Artists from Ireland* [exhibition catalogue]. Dublin: Department of Foreign Affairs.

Hewitt, J. 1977. *Art in Ulster I*. Belfast: Blackstaff Press.

James, K.W. 1985. 'A Hungry Lens.' *Belfast Review 10*: 18.

James, K.W. 1986. *'Damned Nonsense!'* – the Geological Career of the Third Earl of Enniskillen. Belfast: Ulster Museum.

Knox, T. 1993. 'Flights of Fancy.' *Country Life*, 10 June 1993: 120.

Llanover, Lady (ed.). 1861-2. *Autobiography and Correspondence of Mary Granville, Mrs Delany*. 6 vols. London: Richard Bentley.

Longfield, A.K. [Mrs H.G. Leask]. 1981. 'William Kilburn (1745-1818) and his Book of Designs.' *Irish Georgian Society 24*: 1.

McKee, M. 1983. *James Sheals, Naturalist and Taxidermist: the Story of Victorian and Edwardian Taxidermy*. Ulster Museum Publication no. 253. Belfast: Ulster Museum.

Mengel, R.M. 1982. 'Beauty and the Beast: Natural History and Art,' in *The Living Bird*. Ithaca: Cornell University Press.

Mitchell, G.F. and H.M. Parkes. 1949. 'The Giant Deer in Ireland.' *Proceedings of the Royal Irish Academy 52B*: 291-394 [pl. 17].

Morley, B. 1979. 'Lydia Shackleton's paintings in the National Botanic Gardens, Glasnevin.' *Glasra*

2: 25-6.

Murphy, W.M. 1978. *Prodigal Father: the Life of John Butler Yeats*. Ithaca and London: Cornell University Press.

Nash, R. 1983. 'A Brief Summary of the Development of Entomology in Ireland during the Years 1790-1870.' *Irish Naturalists' Journal 21(4)*: 48.

Nash, R. and H.C.G. Ross. 1980. *Dr. Robert Templeton, Naturalist and Artist*. Ulster Museum Publication no. 234. Belfast: Ulster Museum.

Nelson, E.C. 1981. 'Orchid paintings at Glasnevin.' *Orchid Review 89*: 373-7.

Nelson, E.C. 1987. 'Irish Women Artists as Natural History Illustrators,' in Wanda Ryan-Smolin, Elizabeth Mayes and Jenni Rogers (eds), *Irish Women Artists*. Dublin: National Gallery of Ireland.

Nelson, E.C., and W. Walsh. 1993. *Trees of Ireland: Native and Naturalized*. Dublin: The Lilliput Press.

Nicholl, A. 1852. 'A Sketching Tour of Five Weeks in the Forests of Ceylon. Its Ruined Temples, Colossal Statues, Tanks, Dagobahs, etc.' *Dublin University Magazine 40*: part 1, 527, part 2, 691.

Piggott, S. 1976. *Ruins in a Landscape*. Edinburgh: Edinburgh University Press [p. 11, fig. 2].

Pointon, M. 1979. 'Geology and Landscape Painting in Nineteenth-Century England.' *British Society for the History of Science: monograph 1*: 84-108.

Potts, A. 1990. 'Natural Order and the Call of the Wild: the Politics of Animal Picturing.' *Oxford Art Journal 13.1*: 12-33.

Pyle, H., A. O'Connor and O. Walsh. 1987. *Mildred Anne Butler (1858-1941)*. Cork: Crawford Municipal Art Gallery.

Rowan, A. 1980. 'Philip Brannon Watercolour.' (With a Geological Note by Dr Seamus Kennan.) *UCD News*, March 1980: 12.

Ryan-Smolin, W., E. Mayes and J. Rogers (eds). 1987. *Irish Women Artists*. Dublin: National Gallery of Ireland.

Rudwick, M.J.S. 1976. 'The Emergence of a Visual Language for Geological Science 1760-1840.' *History of Science 14*: 149-95.

Scannell, M. and C. Houston. 1980. 'George V. Du Noyer (1817-1869): a Catalogue of Plant Paintings at the National Botanic Gardens, Glasnevin, with Aspects of his Scientific Life.' *Royal Dublin Society Journal of Life Sciences 2(1)*: 1-13.

Spink & Son (dealers). 1981. *Andrew Nicholl and the Plants of Ceylon* [sale catalogue]. London, 4-28 August.

Stafford, B.M. 1977. 'Towards Romantic Landscape Perception: Illustrated Travels and the Rise of "Singularity" as an Aesthetic Category.' *Art Quarterly*: 89-124.

Stewart, A.M. 1990. *Irish Art Loan Exhibitions 1765-1927*. Dublin: Manton Publishing.

Strickland, W.G. 1913. *A Dictionary of Irish Artists*. 2 vols. Dublin and London: Maunsel & Co. Repr. with an Introduction by Theo Snoddy, 1968. Shannon: Irish Universities Press.

Tennent, J.E. 1860. *Ceylon: an Account of the Island, Physical, Historical and Topographical, with Notices of its Natural History, Antiquities and Productions*. 2 vols. London: Longmans.

Thompson, W. 1849-56. *The Natural History of Ireland*. 4 vols. London: Longmans.

Walsh, W. 1983, 1987. *An Irish Florilegium*. (With Introduction by R.I. Ross and Notes by C. Nelson.) 2 vols. London: Thames and Hudson.

Wild Sports and Stone Guns

MICHAEL VINEY

The Nobility of the Hunt

In the drawing-room of some Irish Big House there may exist (but probably does not, so much of this sort of history having gone up in flames) a painting of the Curragh of Kildare, circa, say, 1690. It is a panoramic picture with a big, windy sky, and its painter has echoed the white puffs of cloud in flocks of sheep which graze among the heather. There is a great sense of openness and atmospheric distance.

The picture has to be big to accommodate all that is happening in it. In the foreground, prominent in a mounted group of gentlemen and ladies, the Lord Lieutenant of Ireland gazes raptly skywards, following the mounting flight of a falcon after larks. In the distance beyond his raised hand three horsemen are engaged in what is quite clearly a race, cheered on by knots of friends. And far off, in a frieze of even smaller figures, another mounted group are urging their horses after a pack of hounds, the fox a mere dab of russet in the heather.

All these things did, indeed, go on concurrently at the Curragh at that time, if perhaps at a greater separation across the plain. It was 'a place naturally adapted to pleasure', and even at seventeen miles' ride from Dublin it attracted 'all the nobility and gentry of the Kingdom that either pretend to love, or delight in, hawking or hunting or racing' (MacLysaght, 1950). As painting or snapshot, our imaginary scene makes some topical points. At the end of the seventeenth century, hawking was well on its way out as a top people's recreation, superseded by shooting and, latterly, by fox-hunting with special breeds of hounds. But the scene has other resonances. The very openness of the Curragh, without hint of fence or forest, suggests the physical landscape that shaped so much of Ireland's field sport. And the lordly dash of the mounted gentlemen, with their mingling of military uniforms, suggests its social landscape. In Ireland, as in England, such recreation was not for the poor: a statute of Richard II was headed unequivocally, 'None Shall Hunt But They Which Have A Sufficient Living'. But in Ireland, by 1698, not only did one need property worth £1000, or commensurate income, to be qualified to kill a hare or pheasant, but 'no Papist ... shall be employed as fowler for any Protestant, or under colour or pretence thereof shall have, keep, carry or use any such gun' (Levinge, 1860). Thus, for long periods, a good part of Irish field sport was the preserve of an uneasy colonial elite.

For the native Irish, hunting, fishing and – a little – shooting were always more urgently connected with getting enough to eat. In the early Ireland of fern and wildwood and Gaelic poets,

> They'd gnaw the haunch of a stag
> Hard and hungry and houndlike;
> They'd not leave a jot or a joint
> That they would not mince.

But that taut, explicit poetry was also marked by a striking love of nature ('I hear the stag's belling/ Over the valley's steepness/ No music on earth/ Can move me like its sweetness'), and a similar sensibility ran through early Irish hagiology, in which saints had pet deer to attend them – 'Two stags, obeying the sound of the bell of St Fintan, came and carried his satchel ...' (Wilde, 1860). The honour and respect that pagan hunters accorded their animal prey, and that made the Deer God so important in Celtic mythology, was thus absorbed into early Christianity. A close look at the carvings of Clonmacnois, or high crosses like that at Kells, for example, finds deer being hunted by men with spears and dogs (Henry, 1963).

The Pursuit of Animals

The introduction of deer parks from medieval England by the Normans, and the importation of fallow deer 'to stock the King's park of Glencry' (Glencree, Co. Wicklow, south of Dublin) in 1244, began a parallel world of hunting as private property. In the wildwood to the west, and the bogs, moors and mountains beyond, a scattered population of red deer continued to be harried much as they had been by Eochy the Huntsman, the pagan king. Others were collected into deer parks like that of the O'Flahertys at Glinglass in County Galway, visited by John Dunton at the end of the seventeenth century. He was awed at the sight of 'some hundreds of stately red deer' on the hillsides, and describes a hunt with his host: 'Eighteen long greyhounds and above thirty footemen made up the company ... O'flaghertie gave the word and immediately the company with the doggs surrounded a large thicket, whilst he and I with two hunting poles enter'd it to rouze the game' (Lewis, 1975; MacLysaght, 1950).

More than a hundred deer parks are listed among the townlands of Ireland and others survive as smaller pieces of the map. They occur in at least twenty-nine of the counties, their high walls and deep ditches now often subsumed into farmland (Gibbons, 1991). Many of the Anglo-Norman lords maintained their own hunting forests, and some of these matured into outstanding landscapes. In 1296, for example, Eustace le Poer of Curraghmore, Co. Waterford, was given twelve fallow deer from the Royal Park at Glencree. By the time Arthur Young visited Curraghmore, in the 1770s, the deer park was 'truly a forest one, without any other boundary in view than what the stems of trees offer from mere extent, retiring one behind another until they ... form a distant wall of wood' (Young, 1780).

Dublin's Phoenix Park was the largest and most famous single deer park, of more than two thousand acres, but some rural estates may have contrived to combine even larger areas. Arthur Stringer, in his remarkable manual, *The Experienced Huntsman* (1714), wrote of Lord Conway's parks beside Lough Neagh as containing 'three thousand acres of land, with a thousand brace of red and fallow deer therein ... I killed 54 brace of [fallow] bucks, and four brace of [red deer] stags in a season'. He was not greatly impressed by hunting buck in a park: 'it is what every pretender can perform if he has staunch hounds'. Among landowners, it nonetheless remained the most popular way of hunting deer. Around 1750, around the foot of the Galtee Mountains in Co. Limerick, some twenty packs of buck hounds were to be found, each for a separate deer park (Wyndham-Quin, 1919).

Even by Stringer's time, enough fallow deer had escaped the parks, or had been liberated by the peasantry, to become a second wild species in many parts of the island. 'In the late war of 1688', he wrote, 'most of the parks in Ireland were broke and the deer beat out into the country, so that after the peace there was hardly any place, either mountain or lowland, that had not plenty of fallow deer.' He described the bucks lying up by day in the coppices and brambles of the 'fairy forts' left uncultivated in the middle of cornfields, and coming out to feed at night. By the 1880s escaped fallows were still roaming unchecked. 'In Counties Galway and Clare, and across the Shannon, every large cover holds its two or more. In the spring they descend at night from the woods and uplands, and make sad havoc in the gardens of the peasantry' (Payne-Gallwey, 1882).

The native red deer, meanwhile, harassed by hunting and deforestation, had been in steady and final retreat to the wilder reaches of the mountains. O'Flaherty, in his descriptive inventory of West Connaught in 1684, recorded the frequent hunting of 'fat deere' in the Joyce Country hills. But in Ireland generally, as Sir Thomas Molyneux noted by 1715, the deer 'is much more rare with us ... than it has been formerly, even in the memory of man. And though I take it to be a creature naturally more peculiar to this country than to England, yet, unless there be some care to preserve it, I believe, in the process of time, this kind may be lost like [the giant red deer]' (Wilde, 1860). A century later, in his hunting saga *Wild Sports of the West* (1832), William Maxwell found the deer 'diminished sadly' in the hills of west Mayo and seldom seen in numbers beyond 'a few bracc'. Hc blamcd thc pcasantry, armed with guns they had managed to keep from the French landing at Killala in 1798. But as his chronicle proceeds, news that 'three outlying deer are at this minute in a neighbouring glen' brings an immediate expedition with three guns and a dozen beaters.

The 'long greyhounds' John Dunton saw bringing deer to bay in County Galway of the 1690s were synonymous, for him, with 'wolfe doggs'; both were the very large, fast, coursing hound, hunting by sight (or 'gaze'), which seems to have evolved uniquely in Ireland and which made gifts for early Romans, the Great Mogul and Cardinal Richelieu. For centuries they had been among the island's exports to the Continent: there were Celtic hounds in the cargo of the boat that took St Columba from Ireland to France (Apsley, 1936).

'The long, shaggy-haired great-boned greyhounds', as a soldier in the Irish campaigns noted, 'are held most proper for vermin or wild beasts – the wolf, fox and such like.' Yet they became cherished companions for many of the gentry and travelled with them abroad – a custom checked by an order of 1652, lest the hunting of the wolf should suffer. Although deforestation had greatly reduced its refuges, the wolf had gained from the disorder of the Cromwellian wars, so that by the middle of the seventeenth century it was seen right up to the outskirts of Dublin (MacLysaght, 1950). In more settled periods, hunting the wolf had been a fashionable sport, but now there were more organized and single-minded campaigns. In 1653 a Captain Piers obtained a lease of forfeited lands in Meath in return for hunting wolves three times a month. Elsewhere, common huntsmen were appointed and bounties were paid for heads. What finally drove the wolf to its last mountain retreats was, however, none of this, but the destruction of the wildwood. By 1750 Lord Chesterfield could write: 'I have been trying these two years to get some of those large dogs of Ireland; but the breed has grown extremely rare there by the extinction of their enemies, the wolves.'

In the hunts retailed in the heroic poems of Fionn in the first millennium AD, there were two kinds of dog: the *cu*, which was swift, and the *gadhar* which was 'sweet-voiced' and probably a kind of beagle. The introduction of deer parks, and the need to flush the fallow deer from cover, favoured the development of packs of hounds that hunted by scent and could be followed through dense woods by their cry. In 1525 Piers, eighth Earl of Ormond, kept '24 personnes with 60 grehowndes and howndes for Dere hunting, another nombre of men and doggse for to hunt the Hare and a thirde number to hunt the Martyn'. The scenting packs tended, as C.A. Lewis (1975) believes, to be 'large, heavy, loud-voiced, like bloodhounds'. By the 1700s, as fox-hunting became the prevailing passion of the gentry, huntsmen began to seek smaller and more active hounds and the first Belvoir bred foxhounds were imported from Britain.

Under the statute of Richard II, no layman or peasant could be so bold as to keep sporting dogs of any sort, and the Game Law of 1662 prohibited the keeping of setters by persons of less substance than £100 a year. Hounds or even spaniels could not legally be kept by the ordinary small farmer or cottier. Richard's concern was that 'divers artificers, labourers and servants, and grooms, keep greyhounds and other dogs, and on the holydays, when good Christian people be at church, hearing divine service, they go hunting in parks, warrens and connigries of lords and others, to the very great destruction of the same ...'. (Levinge, 1860).

Mere laws did little, of course, to check poaching in either country, and many of the most assiduous poachers of the newly planted Ireland were the soldiers of Charles II's army. 'There is scarcely a partridge left in these parts,' complained the manager of the new Phoenix Park. 'Trammels are carried out every night under red coats.' In the 1690s the penal laws reduced still further the amount of land retained by native owners, so the 'mere Irish' had even less cause to cease netting or snaring on estates leased to alien soldiers, farmers and adventurers (MacLysaght, 1950).

Looking over the old game laws, the modern reader is struck by the priority accorded to the hare. In most lists, only the deer precedes it; in a statute on the burning of mountain, it comes ahead of grouse. 'No one to trace any hares or other game whatsoever in the snow', and no one without £40 a year to shoot hares, partridge, pheasant, grouse or quail. Even in the mid-1800s, a legal commentator was citing 'hare-holes dug in the beaten track of hares across the bogs' as a typical aggravation of poaching by the lower classes (Levinge, 1860).

Arthur Stringer considered that, 'Although there be a great heroic gallantry in the chace of the stag, buck and fox ... I think there is a mellow sweetness and kind friendly chearfulness peculiar to the chace of an hare that nothing can equal ....' In *The Experienced Huntsman*, the first treatise on hunting in Ireland and the first serious work on the wild mammals of these islands, his observations on the biology and behaviour of the hare are, as James Fairley observes in his introduction to the 1977 edition, 'in stark contrast to the absurd credulity regarding animals which prevailed at the time'.

Here and there in Stringer's essays can be glimpsed the profound changes in Ireland's wild landscape brought about by deforestation. He describes 'boggy fenny grounds full of high banks of earth ... the woods being all cut away' where 'the [pine] marterns do still remain and and are to be found there at any time of day as you would unkennel a fox, and, for want of trees to lie in all day, will lie in an old blackbird's nest or throstle's nest in a holly or briar bush within two foot of the ground ...'.

Stringer's empathy with animals was born of a lifetime's close observation and he felt bound to defend the otter, for example, against charges of lamb-killing: 'I have in my time killed near one hundred brace of otters and never could find any thing in their belly but fish.' He had no sentiment about how a hunt should end: 'When an otter is killed, you cannot be too kind to your hounds in clapping and encouraging them, and let them bite him as long as they please. Then hold him up on a pole, quarter-staff, otter-spear or pitch-fork, and let them bay him.'

Wildfowling

The Conway estate for which Stringer worked exemplified a way of life in which hunting was part of a massive provision of food for household, servants and guests: a self-contained and largely self-sufficient world within the boundary walls. Among the innovations at Portmore was one of the first duck decoys in Ireland. These were traps of a most ingenious kind, constructed on secluded ponds to which ducks could be attracted to feed. At the edge of the pond, long channels or 'pipes' curved away under tunnels of netting. Wild duck were enticed to swim along the channels, sometimes by following tame duck used to being fed but also by the antics of the 'piper', a dog trained to show himself at gaps between screens, skipping about but never barking, until the duck were far enough up the pipe for the decoyman to cut off their retreat. More than twenty estates had duck decoys during the eighteenth and nineteenth centuries, some of them highly successful as commercial operations. One at Kellyville, near Athy in County Kildare, caught almost 26,000 duck in twenty-four seasons from 1880 to 1904 (Fox, 1986). But another, at Mountainstown near Navan in County Meath, which in its time caught 'immense quantities' of teal, ceased to be worked much earlier, its owner remarking in 1845 that 'the country has been so drained and improved, that all kinds of wildfowl are now very scarce, and a decoy is among the things we read of, rather than see' (Thompson, 1851).

At the other end of the scale from decoys were the pitfall traps by which the Irish peasantry captured wintering geese. Sir Ralph Payne-Gallwey, in *The Fowler in Ireland* (1882), spoke of these traps as 'in constant use by the peasantry in parts of Ireland, though only Bean Geese [actually Greenland white-fronted geese] were caught in them'. Cut in meadows where the geese were used to grazing, the holes were shaped 'somewhat like a flower-pot' and were just deep enough for the goose to touch the bait, overbalancing and wedging itself tight. 'A man in County Monaghan ... has been known to capture a dozen in a day.'

Netting of plovers, liming of larks, digging of pits for deer – there were many ways of trapping wildlife for food that did not involve the gun and that continued long after its general introduction. But the gun did put an end, almost entirely, to a sport that had obsessed the nobility. Ireland's falcons were prized by kings: Roderick of Connacht sent peregrines to Henry II, and Henry IV put a heavy export duty on any not intended for his choice (Watters, 1853). 'A gift of hawks could sometimes smooth the way to a grant of land in Ireland' (Ussher, 1900).

Hawking is mentioned frequently in the Irish State Papers of the early seventeenth century – combat with herons was especially popular – but the development of the light flintlock gun rewarded hunting with greater pleasures at the table. Charles II was very fond of hawking, but the 'perching' of pheasants by stalking them and shooting them where they sat was a growing recreation for gentlemen, and it was already not unusual to 'shoot flying'. This was regarded as a difficult art, the more so as it was sometimes practised from horseback (Trevelyan, 1944).

The early guns were clumsy and often erratic in performance. As late as the 1830s William Maxwell was pitying the obstinacy of 'antique gunners' who still preferred the flint-spark to the copper percussion cap. 'The misery entailed upon the man who in rain and storm attempts to load and discharge a flint gun may be reckoned among the worst in the human catalogue; and if he who has suffered repeated disappointments of eternal misses and dilatory explosions, from a thick flint and a damp pan, tried the simple and elegant improvement now in general use, he would abandon the stone gun forever.'

For the wildfowler of the marshes and estuaries, the temperamental mechanism of the early guns was often accompanied by great physical discomfort, especially for the men who now made this shooting their winter livelihood. On Belfast Lough they squeezed themselves into barrels sunk in the mud banks and spent long night hours waiting for the feeding wigeon to come within range of their muskets (Patterson, 1881). In Wexford Harbour the shooters lay in scrapes dug in the sand to ambush the brent geese by night with the 'long Shelmalier', aiming at the farthest bird so that the dropping shot might wing the nearest risers (Watters, 1853). Even with the advent of the double-barrelled shotgun, the poorer coastal fowlers often faced an endurance test of the kind described by Sir Ralph Payne-Gallwey in the 1880s: 'These men, chiefly for profit, and from the Irish love of sport, go out night after night on the flats in the severest weather, and, with a small shovel they carry with them, throw up a shelter of mud. They then lie prostrate for hours, waiting for the fowl to feed up in shot with the flowing tide.

Thus do these mudsquatters remain in slime and ooze.'

The commercial rewards of wildfowling were vastly multiplied by the advent of the heavy artillery of shooting, the swivel-gun (or stanchion-gun) and the punt-gun, in the early 1800s. The mounted swivel-gun, with a barrel up to eight feet long and a bore of, perhaps, one and a half inches, fired up to one pound of large shot at a usual distance of about one hundred yards. Payne-Gallwey used it to shoot at grey-lag geese on the Shannon marshes 'and have even known fowlers to kill, in this fashion, forty to fifty at one discharge'.

On Belfast Lough the swivel-gun put an end to the more primitive shooting from barrels. In a winter of hard frost, which brought great flocks to the lough, a fowler with the first of the new guns killed 336 birds in one week – brent geese, teal, wigeon and mallard. A fowler on Larne Lough told Thompson of killing over ninety wigeon with one discharge of his swivel gun. There were more great kills of wigeon at Clontarf, in Dublin Bay, where 'after the report of the swivel the flocks become so wild that for that day all further approach would be impossible' (Patterson, 1881; Watters, 1853).

Such heavy casualties, and the disturbance of daytime shooting made possible by the greater range of the swivel-guns, were bound to have an impact. 'The wigeon is so much persecuted in Belfast Bay', wrote Thompson, 'that before the dawn of morning multitudinous numbers rise from the banks on which they have been feeding all night and betake themselves to Strangford Lough, as a place of comparative security ....' Teal, too, were 'very much diminished' in the Lough by 1850. But Thompson, as an ornithologist, was also careful to consider the changes in the Lough's environment: enclosure of feeding grounds for the railway, reclamation of the slobs, disturbance of the wigeon by the gas-lights of the town, and by the increase in shipping – 'the steam vessels with their black smoke particularly alarming them' (Thompson, 1851).

Engine of destruction as the swivel-gun may have been, the punt-gun was even bigger and more mobile. In his evocative memoir *The Wildfowler* (1982) Roger Moran described the gun he used to fire on the Shannon in the 1930s, tugging a string in the bottom of the punt when cued by a kick from his father. The gun was double-barrelled, nine feet long and weighed sixteen stone. It was loaded with slow-burning, coarse black powder and the recoil drove the punt back several feet. One and a half pounds of snipe shot would mow through a flock of golden plover 'like a scythe through corn ... [Once] we picked up ninety-six golden plover, three curlew and four redshank'.

The Morans were cottiers, shooting for the market and their own pot (lapwing boiled with turnips). A century earlier, their counterparts at Wexford were firing rather smaller guns ignited by flint and mounted on cockle-shell punts. 'Dark or light nights, out they all go', wrote Payne-Gallwey. 'If they cannot actually see the birds, they fire to the sound of their guzzling, so well do they know the creeks and where to find their game.' And just as the Morans despised the 'poppers' shooting from the shore, the punt-gunners of Wexford Harbour were so banded together that 'any stranger, to obtain sport, would have to empty his bag for their benefit'.

Sir Ralph Payne-Gallwey, a wealthy English baronet, is one of the most intriguing figures in the history of Irish field sports – and, indeed, of the island's ornithology. His book *The Fowler in Ireland* is an industrious blend of natural history and sporting instruction, and his personal observation of 'wildfowl and seafowl' extends to the habits of gannets, kittiwakes or herons as readily as those of quarry species. He had the naturalist's instinct for experiment ('I have placed live trout in a very shallow glass dish, with just sufficient water for them to swim in. The Heron, though now and then darting his bill like lightning to obtain the food, never strikes the bottom of the vessel, though but two inches depth of water be in it') and his instruction ranges from the secrets of plover netting ('an art little understood, save by the few who make a living by it') to the specifications of the ideal double handed fowling-punt.

Although he writes as one of a confraternity of gentleman fowlers, there cannot have been many prepared to spend whole winters dodging from estuary to estuary in a fowling-cutter and braving fierce weather in return for occasional calm mornings with the punt-gun. 'A wildfowl shooter's existence is often tinged with melancholy,' he writes, while riding out an easterly gale, 'by reason of the broad expanse of waste and shipless water whereupon his favourite sport is pursued' – but then, enthusiastically, 'What a scene is this compared to the never-varying turnip-field, the leafless, dripping wood!'

In the remoter western bays that he frequented, from Kerry to Donegal, he needed to maintain good relations with the scores of professional shore-shooters. 'To keep these men in pleasant temper, and prevent their spoiling sport by firing up the fowl, they must be liberally dealt with in the way of a good share from the bag.' But the shoremen had his sympathy: 'These poor shooters trudge to the nearest town of a Saturday to sell what birds they may happen to have killed during the week. A stranger visiting their estuary with his fowling-punt is looked upon, more or less, as a thief come to rob them of their living; especially when they see him with great, and to them unappreciated, skill go forth and obtain in a few hours more than they can kill in a week.' He felt, too, that the new Wildfowl Preservation Act (1880), with a close season from 1 March to 1 August, bore harshly on the coastal fowlers: 'On the 15th April, 1881, I saw upwards of two thousand Brent geese in a bay off the Kerry coast; their presence, by Act of Parliament, being of no service to the local fowlers. These poor men,

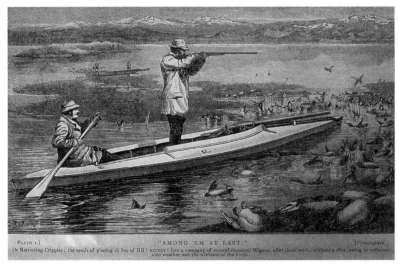

Engraving by Charles Whymper from Payne-Gallwey's The Fowler in Ireland *(1882)*

though at times starving for want of a shilling, view a source of profit, the gift of Providence, before their eyes from day to day. There can be no object in protecting Brent Geese, for they never nest in the British Islands.'

Wounded, then tamed, geese were sometimes pegged down as decoys on the last mud-bank to be covered by the tide, but Payne-Gallwey's punt-gunning was never so unsporting. His own favourite cannon had an oval bore, to send the shot in a lateral swathe ('for general work, twenty ounces is a handy charge'). And since he was prepared to follow the birds several miles out to sea off the larger rivers, a large, safe punt for two men was indispensable. 'One of the best day's shooting I ever had was far from shore in a calm like glass: the Wigeon when fired at pitched again at no great distance, and sat so thick on the water that until they were within shot one bird could not be distinguished from another; but merely living black islands of from three to five thousand fowl each.' On one occasion of this sort, accompanied by a Captain Gould, RE., the day yielded 139 mallard and wigeon – 'the heaviest shot stopped sixty birds, and four shots were fired'. In the winter before he wrote his book, living on a fishing-smack and 'running at times great risks', he killed fifteen hundred duck on the estuaries (and, one must presume, sold most of them to defray his expenses).

He lists comparable triumphs by his peers: Captain Kinsey Dover, with single-handed punt and small swivel-gun killing 671 duck in Mulroy and Sheephaven Bays in 1860/61; Mr Vincent and his man 'Sambo' killing 106 teal with a single punt-gun shot on a southern estuary. The figures amaze, but eventually grow tedious. More enduring are the images of the winter duck flocks off the Irish coast, so immense 'that though the wind be from you to them, I have heard the roar of sound transmitted a full mile and more as they rose or pitched'.

Like most educated fowlers of his time, Payne-Gallwey was always on the watch for unusual species: 'Let the fowler or shore-shooter never miss the chance of securing a rarity. If a rich man, the pleasure afforded when presenting his capture to a collecting friend, or to some public museum, will amply repay his trouble; if a poor man, directors of museums and naturalists will often pay as much, and more, for a rara avis as a good day's sport would have put in his pocket.'

After Game and Other Birds

Payne-Gallwey tells of shooting three hooded mergansers, rare vagrants from America; these were the only nineteenth-century records of this species in Ireland. Shooting and preserving were the standard means of obtaining specimens, and the naturalists of the time were also, very often, enthusiastic fowlers. William Thompson of Belfast was often out night-shooting on the marshes and 'felt a kind of wild joy in hearing the ringing of the pinions through the air. From the sound of the wings alone the mallard, wigeon, teal, pochard &c, could be distinguished ...'. Robert Warren, in Richard Ussher's *Birds of Ireland* of 1900, tells of shooting 'the sixth specimen of the Surf-Scoter captured in Ireland', near Killala on the north Mayo coast. It escaped the blast from his big punt-gun and several shots from his 'cripple stopper' and was finally ambushed by a friend 'with a charge of No. 6 shot from his 4-bore'.

Many of the rarities shot during this period passed through the skilful hands of the Sheals family in Belfast, whose taxidermy particularly enriched the collections of the Ulster Museum. Among them were the last white-tailed eagle to be obtained in Ulster, shot at Mountstewart in 1891 (McKee, 1986; Ussher, 1900).

In Payne-Gallwey's winters of roaming the west, white-tailed and golden eagles were already growing scarce. 'Mr Evatt states that before the days of strychnine he has seen from five to six Sea Eagles at one time, hovering over the island of Inishbofin, off the Galway coast. Mr Sheridan of Achill also blames this deadly poison ... [A gamekeeper told him] that one year he poisoned eleven Eagles on the island.' Payne-Gallwey quotes, with evident approval, the protection of eagles on Colonel Cooper's estate at Collooney, Co. Sligo.

William Maxwell, visiting Achill fifty years earlier, did not hesitate to shoot 'a beautiful specimen of the sea-hawk' (probably an osprey) which he intended to preserve with salt, pepper and alum. A white-tailed eagle would have been equally acceptable; '[it] is extremely destructive to fish, and particularly so to salmon'. Maxwell had been teased into undertaking his sporting expedition among the 'primitive people' of west Mayo by a letter from an Irish kinsman: 'You talk of exercise: pshaw, what is it? ... You shoot a score of rascally pigeons within the enclosures of Battersea, or make a grand excursion to slaughter pheasants in a preserve; last and proudest feat comes the battue, when, with noble and honourable confederates, you exterminate a multitude of semi-civilized fowls, manfully overcoming the fatigue of traversing an ornamented park and crossing a few acres of turnips ....' In west Mayo, Maxwell spent many days tramping over bog and tumbled rock in pursuit of grouse ('not being exterminators, we ceased shooting at three o'clock, and returned to our cabin with two-and-twenty brace of birds') and memorable nights in the company of poteen-makers and other colourful natives. All this was a strange and zestful interlude in Maxwell's life, and provided, in *Wild Sports of the West* (1832), a classic record of the rougher kind of rough-shooting.

It seems likely that Irish red grouse were never as plentiful as the birds of the Scottish bogs and moors, but Giraldus Cambrensis noted, at the end of the twelfth century, 'immense flights of snipes, both the larger species of the woods [woodcock] and the smaller of the marshes' and also an abundance of capercaillie in the woods. This turkey-sized bird seems to have survived in Ireland until the eighteenth century, when a combination of hunting and the devastation of the woodlands finally rendered it extinct. Capercaillie may well have been the 'turkeys' listed among game conserved at Portmore in the late 1700s, and the Conways were also among the first landowners in Ireland to plant a glen specially for woodcock (Stringer, 1714).

Pheasants were introduced in the late 1500s, initially from the Caucasus; the Chinese pheasant predominated from the late 1700s onwards. By 1900, as Ussher noted, there were very few 'old, brown pheasants' uncrossed with Chinese ring-necked birds. The pheasants introduced to the wild have occasionally survived for long periods; indeed, the great majority of cock birds shot today are wild. Substantial releases of hand-reared pheasants continue among the local gun clubs, but less than ten per cent of these survive to be shot (Robertson, 1987).

The pheasant shoots at the big houses in Ireland followed the social pattern developing in England, where game books (in which were entered each day's shooting party and each day's bag) seem to have appeared towards the end of the 1700s, and the 'grand battue' of driven pheasants, of the sort for which Maxwell was teased, reached its zenith about 1820. Payne-Gallwey, who might have been expected to despise driven shoots, actually defended them strongly: 'Pheasants flushed before dogs are the very easiest of marks as they flap up ... [but] stand in a narrow ride with dark-foliaged firs, like a wall, on either side of you, a small lane of sky overhead corresponding in width to the space below; a high and perhaps favourable breeze, and some distance to gain speed; then, as the pheasants (those much-despised fowl) pass skimming above with extended and almost motionless wings, bring them down if you can! "Rocketers", "collar-bone crackers" and driven birds are what we seek for nowadays when pheasant-shooting ...' (Payne-Gallwey, 1882).

In the early 1800s the English pattern of farming, with increasing acreages of root crops and more intensive growing of cereals, favoured pheasant and partridge, and buoyant landed incomes paid for elaborate hatcheries and gamekeeping (Thompson, 1963). In Ireland around the same time, it was largely the peasants who benefited from game birds attracted to the weedy stubbles and potato-gardens of a closely tilled and densely populated countryside. Quail were netted on a large scale, along with partridge, and the decline of both species followed hard upon the Famine and the reversion of tilled land to pasture (Ussher, 1900; Butler, 1985; Hutchinson, 1989).

The pride of Irish 'big house' shooting continued to be the challenge of rough shooting for the abundant snipe and woodcock. Watters, in 1853, noted that 'in the county of Cork fifty brace [of snipe] have been shot with a single gun, in one day, an occurrence which no preserve of equal extent in England or Scotland could produce'. A Limerick shooter, cited by Payne-Gallwey, shot a thousand snipe in a thousand hours within ten miles of the city.

Rough shooting for woodcock had a challenge and excitement of the sort captured by Somerville and Ross in their barely fictional *Experiences of an Irish R.M.* (1899): 'The Aussolas woods were full of birds that day. Birds bursting out of holly bushes like corks out of soda-water bottles, skimming low under the branches of fir-trees, bolting across rides at a thousand miles an hour, swinging away through prohibitive tree tops .... Hit or miss, a good day with the cock comes very near a good day with the hounds.'

But Ireland has also had its own 'grand battue' for woodcock and the only driven shoot for these birds of any significance in Europe. At Lord Ardilaun's estate at Ashford, near Cong in County Galway, woodcock were already so numerous in the 1870s that five guns bagged 106 in a day. By the turn of the century, the tree plantings by Ardilaun were attracting such an influx of the birds that the first driven shoot was organized in 1905 with the Prince of Wales as one of the guns. With some interruptions, the shoots have continued annually under successive owners and lessees, but the British and Irish record for one day's shooting for seven guns (236 birds on 10 January 1910) seems never to have been surpassed (Campbell, 1984).

The game books of Lord Sligo's estates at Westport, County Mayo, convey the intensity of 'big house' shooting in the Edwardian years. Between 1900 and 1914 the bags totalled 13,184 birds, including 2267 grouse, 1964 woodcock, 7037 snipe and 589 pheasants. In the same county, in the 1930s, a mere four days' shooting on Lord Oranmore's land at Castle MacGarrett yielded 518 pheasants and 147 woodcock. But the years between had been enormously eventful for the control of land and the conservation of game birds. Thousands of acres of demesne land had been acquired by the Land Commission and broken up into small farms, often with the destruction of woodland, fresh drainage and an end to heather management. World War I and Ireland's own upheavals for independence produced a period of almost a decade in which keepering and game-rearing went by the board. Woodcock found new haunts and spread themselves more widely; grouse and pheasant were freely poached; predators forgot they were 'vermin' and took up old relations with their prey. 'When shoots of 10,000 acres are advertised to let at £30 the season', wrote the Shooting Editor of *Country Life*, 'the price is the measure of the game they harbour' (Drought, 1940).

Fox-hunting

Not only the ownership of land, but the way it was used and laid out have influenced Irish field sport. In the colonization of the island, almost the whole country was divided into large and compact estates, but until the late 1700s great stretches of farmed land were open or 'champain' landscape, on which farmers made temporary fences with bushes in summer. In Kildare, in 1758, ditches and hedgerows were still rare and large areas lay in grassy fields of more than a hundred acres. When John Power began a pack of fox-hounds in Kilkenny in 1797 he 'found the country so much unenclosed that he declared that he was often able to ride from the "Welsh" mountains [around Mount Leinster] to Waterford Bridge without having to jump a single fence' (Aalen, 1970; Lewis, 1975).

When the enclosure movement arrived from England, in the late 1700s and early 1800s, it took most rapid effect in the more autocratic and 'scientifically' minded farm estates of Leinster. One after another, as Arthur Young (1780) saw in the 1770s, estates were 'throwing down and levelling old banks, making new ditches, double ones six feet wide and five deep, with a large bank between for planting [of hawthorn quicks]'.

Thus fox-hunting, as a general obsession of the Irish gentry, took on very different styles from one region to another. The country's first successful subscription pack, the County Galway Foxhounds, began hunting in 1839 over an area almost forty miles square and later, as 'The Galway Blazers', roamed out across a welcoming landscape laced with 'single' limestone walls, easily displaced and rebuilt. In east Mayo, too, William Maxwell enjoyed his freedom to gallop for miles – but 'when one does meet fences they are generally raspers ...'. The ploughed land of Leinster, on the other hand, demanded stout, strong horses and the ability, when leaping the new double ditches, to alight, momentarily, on the bank between. In west Cork, walls of sharp slate were a deterrent (even Edith Somerville's West Carbery Hunt found them 'horrid'), while in Monaghan, the fields were so small that the fox was left to the linen weavers, hunting on foot, with 'dwarf fox-hounds' (Wakefield, 1812).

Although the fox seems to have been hunted in Ireland since at least 1200, its role as the quarry of gentlemen arrived only in the late 1600s. By the time Arthur Stringer was writing, in 1714, the hunting season was fixed (from Michaelmas Day, September 29th, to Lady-day, March 25th) and the sport 'very well known to be a general advantage to the inhabitants of that part of the country where it is used'. As time went by, however, the low-land hunting areas repeatedly ran short of foxes. In 1861 seventy-six brace of Kerry foxes were released in County Limerick. A decade later, the Galway Blazers' country was becoming denuded of foxes through the wide-spread use of gin-traps to catch rabbits. In the early 1900s, foxes were imported from Wales for hunts in Cork. A further rearrangement of nature, widely adopted, was to create new coverts, some with artificial earths, at convenient galloping intervals and to stock them with foxes as one stocked other kinds of wildlife. Thus, vixens with cubs – or cubs alone – found themselves displaced into horseshoe-shaped earths under newly planted gorse (Lewis, 1975; Mahony, 1979). Spinneys and thickets planted as fox cover have survived to enrich the country's vegetation; so, alas, has the inva-sive shrub *Rhododendron ponticum*, planted for pheasant-cover, as well as for ornament, on many estates in the south and west.

The early private packs of kennelled hounds, followed on horseback, were divided in their quarry between deer and fox. By 1750 they had been formed in a dozen counties and were then augmented or succeeded by sub-scription packs, in which the members guarantee the Master a set sum, while he keeps the hounds and foots the rest of the bill. The hunts sustained the social life of families who otherwise would have lived in considerable isola-tion, and bonded a whole Ascendancy caste. 'Any man who is utterly uncon-cerned with the fox,' said Lord Dunsany, 'lives a little apart from the rest of us' (Lewis, 1975).

While mounted fox-hunting, with stag-hunting, remained an upper-class or at least 'county' occupation, the hunting of the hare attracted both landowners and army officers, hunting on horseback, and very many ordi-nary people following packs of harriers on foot. Individual countrymen kept their own hounds for coursing hares. On 12 March 1831 Humphrey O'Sullivan, a Kilkenny hedge-school teacher, 'spent the day hunting hares with two hounds, one white and the other spotted. We raised eight hares, although we killed only two' (De Bhaldraithe, 1979). Such dogs became the basis of the dozens of 'trencher-fed' footpacks which still assemble on

Sundays and Holy Days, especially in counties Cork, Kerry and Clare and the border drumlin counties. Some hunt the fox, others the hare, while still others set their foxhounds, beagles, harriers or basset hounds on the scent of an aniseed 'drag'.

It becomes obvious in any review of the plain Irishman's field sports that the hound, of whatever breed or permutation, has been the prime focus of pleasure and pride, and that the quarry species has been almost incidental. Lewis, in his *Hunting in Ireland*, thinks it likely that footpacks have existed in Kerry and Cork since pre-Elizabethan days, if not since before the Normans, and that the mounted packs of harriers, so noteworthy in County Cork, also follow a tradition that predates fox-hunting (but they now, very often, hunt foxes rather than hares). He finds the extraordinary dominance of County Cork and west Waterford in hunting difficult to explain: 'Perhaps it was due to the absence of any one dominant landlord family and the consequent rise of a squire class which, in fertile agricultural surroundings, became sufficiently wealthy to support the sport.' Whatever the cause, County Cork now supports more than seventy packs of hounds – foxhounds, harriers and beagles, both kennelled and trencher-fed (looked after at home). At least six of the packs operate out of Cork city itself, and 'together with coursing and bowling, hunting is the principal Sunday afternoon activity throughout the county' (Twomey, 1985).

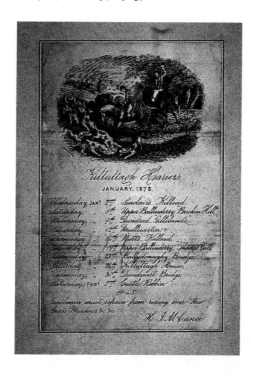

Coursing

Although the word 'coursing' was originally synonymous with hunting in relation to the hare, it took on extra connotations of testing dog performance when greyhounds were used in the chase. The organized release of greyhounds after hares was launched with formal rules in England in 1776 and the first record in Ireland is of a meeting of the Loughrea Coursing Club in County Galway in 1820. An outstanding Irish greyhound, Master McGrath, won the Waterloo Cup in England on three occasions, beginning in 1868, and the first enclosed meeting in Ireland took place at the new racecourse at Tralee in 1893. Enclosed meetings, controlled by the Irish Coursing Club, still command much rural support, especially in Munster. They have been strongly disapproved of, however, by a large majority of people polled in opinion surveys. A widespread objection to the apparently frequent killing of hares resulted, in the early 1990s, in the introduction of muzzles for the dogs. Greyhound owners who wish to race their dogs at tracks are bound by the industry's regulations to register as members of a coursing club.

The vigorous hunting traditions of Cork show up again in the recent history of otter hunting, since the last otters legally pursued in Ireland were tracked by hounds along rivers in that county as late as 1989. The otter is certainly among the most ancient of the island's quarry, hunted originally for its fur. Old Antony the otter-killer, with his terriers, gin-traps and fishspear, is one of the vivid portraits in Maxwell's *Wild Sports of the West*, and Payne-Gallwey speaks of knowing Irish otter-hunters 'who have spent their lives trapping these animals'. Until the otter was protected in the Republic by the Wildlife Act of 1976, advertisements for otter skins appeared frequently in local newspapers, and Fairley, in *An Irish Beast Book*, says that gin-traps were used, illegally, to take otters in Galway 'at least up to 1975'.

Like many other predators whose true diet was unknown or misunderstood, the otter was widely persecuted for bounty payments – especially, in more modern times, by fishing interests. This policy was abandoned when otters came under the protection of the Act, but, as with stags and hares, the protection was provisional. Otters could still be hunted, with packs of hounds, under licence – a concession to a sporting tradition surviving at that time only among a few packs in west Limerick and County Cork. Stringer's references to otter hunting in Antrim in 1714 are to a well-established gentlemanly pursuit in which 'a water spaniel is very requisite and useful' as an adjunct to the otter hounds themselves. In the 1800s the Irish rivers were also hunted by English otter packs, whose activities were reported in periodicals such as *Land and Water*. In this century, hunting under licence by the four Munster clubs finally ceased in 1989, partly in response to public feeling against the harassment of a species increasingly rare in Europe if not in Ireland. The number of kills had, in fact, been small – nine otters between the four packs in 1987 (Boazman, 1988).

Some wildlife scientists actually regretted the end of licensed hunting because, as monitored by local Wildlife Rangers, it provided regular and valuable information on the otter population. Other naturalists objected to the hunts because they disturbed the nests of water-birds along the river banks. Following the English example, the Munster packs have continued in existence for 'mink hunting', following the same hounds along the same rivers on Sundays and Wednesdays. Feral mink are not a protected species and the clubs make no return of kills.

Stag-hunting with hounds is another exception licensed by the Republic's Wildlife Act, and it survives both north and south of the border. The County Down hunt, with a deer park outside Hillsborough, was founded in 1881. Its members ride after stags which have had their antlers removed and they hunt each stag, on average, twice a season. The Ward Union hunt, based at Ashbourne, Co Meath, dates from 1854 and similarly seeks to capture its quarry to run again another day. For almost a century the hunt had the freedom of farmland north-west of Dublin and it fielded, at times, well over a hundred riders. In the early 1900s, Eric Craigie recalls in his *Irish Sporting Sketches* (1984), a special train from Kingsbridge each Wednesday took city riders and their horses to the meet where the deer was released. Most of Meath was then under grass: 'Here we had a country which was given to stag hunting.' But from the 1940s onwards, the advance of tillage and barbed wire, stud farms and commuter housing has steadily circumscribed the running of the deer.

Craigie relates that, in the early part of the Second World War, many English and Irish army officers came to Ireland on leave to hunt with Ward Union. They leaped so recklessly at Meath's high, double-ditched fences that many horses were killed and the livery stables refused to hire out more. The episode is a reminder of the presence of army officers in certain branches of hunting over long periods, a reflection partly of the numerous British garrisons in Irish towns, partly of the career traditions of so many gentry families.

An intriguing example of military enthusiasm was the role of British officers in the revival of falconry in nineteenth-century Ireland. In the 1850s, when the regiment of Captain Francis Salvin was posted here, he and his professional falconer, John Barr, perfected the art of magpie hawking with peregrines in the country around Cahir Barracks. They advertised their meets in the local papers 'to encourage a field, so necessary as an aid in magpie hawking' and took 184 magpies in about four months. The Old Hawking Club, founded in Britain in 1864, launched 'many campaigns ... against the cunning magpies of Kildare and Fermoy'. A Colonel Brooksbank recorded that the meets at Fermoy 'were large, and graced by a good sprinkling of ladies who ... crossed the country on foot in a marvellous manner'. A hawking lodge in Ireland was among the attractions of The Falconry Club, a rival group launched in England by a Captain Dugmore in 1877. In the following summer 'there was a great scrabble for eyas peregrines in Ireland, Captain Dugmore having taken all the young hawks in 1877, to the exclusion of the Irish falconers'; among those seized was 'a nest of three from Horn Head in County Donegal' (Upton, 1987). Irish peregrine eyasses are still taken (under licence, and with a Wildlife Ranger in attendance) by members of the Irish Hawking Club. The highlight of their hunting year is to fly a falcon at grouse in September, using radio telemetry to locate the kill (Morris, 1984).

Angling

The stationing of British troops in Ireland was highly significant for the development of another field sport: coarse fishing. All of Ireland's major coarse fish species – pike, perch, tench, carp, bream and rudd – were introduced in the sixteenth and seventeenth centuries (roach and dace came much later and accidentally). Of these, only pike and perch seem to have figured to any extent in the diet of the native Irish. Young notes in the 1770s that perch 'appeared in the Shannon for the first time about ten years ago, in such plenty that the poor lived on them'. Maxwell, sixty years later, describes angling for pike and perch as 'usually an amusement of the peasantry' but makes it plain that fishing for pike was also a serious occupation: 'By meshnets, immense numbers of pike are annually taken.' On Mask and Corrib, 'It is no unusual event for pikes of thirty pounds weight to be sent to their landlords by the tenants; and fish of even fifty pounds have not unfrequently been caught with nets and night-lines.' Pike, undoubtedly, continued to be fished for food, but the abundance of native trout and salmon, caught legally and by poachers, together with a general improvement in diet, diminished the status of coarse fish, even among the rural poor.

Thus, when the Second World War stationed new regiments of British troops in Northern Ireland, they 'found that the lakes and rivers of the Erne catchment contained stocks of coarse fish beyond their wildest dreams. Many of these anglers were accustomed to catching gudgeon, small roach and bleak in murky, polluted canals and waterways. In contrast, the Erne provided hundreds of thousands of unfished acres of pure water containing coarse fish of (as it must have seemed to them) gargantuan proportions ...'. In their excitement lay the foundation of the present coarse fishing tourist industry, both in Fermanagh and on lakes and rivers south of the border (Whelan, 1989).

The enthusiasm of pike anglers has produced an unlooked-for ecological impact in the extraordinary spread of roach. Although its accidental introduction dates to 1889 (on the Munster Blackwater), it was the widespread use of roach as live bait for pike in the 1960s that produced an extraordinary spread of the species. It is now established in many large catchments, including those of the Shannon, Erne and Corrib, and its abundance in lakes such as Lough Derravaragh has been known to strain the capacity of freshwater trawls.

Not only coarse fishing but Irish sea angling also, says Whelan, 'was really a British invention', being pioneered early this century by members of the British Sea Anglers' Society, later known as the Dreadnoughts. Fishing out of Ballycotton, Co. Cork, in particular, they discovered the great size and quantity of species such as skate and halibut. During the 1930s resident Irish anglers (Lord Sligo among them) devised new adventures by battling with porbeagle sharks from small open boats around Achill, but the attractions of Clew Bay and other western sea angling centres remained to be discovered until well after the Second World War.

Whatever of coarse or sea fish, the native Irish have not lacked appreciation of trout and salmon. From the twelfth century the Cistercian abbey of Mellifont had three fishing weirs on the Boyne, where the salmon were thought to be 'always fat and never out of season' (Went, 1953). Discussion of the decline of salmon in the rivers goes back to at least the early 1700s, when the Archbishop of Dublin concerned himself, most knowledgeably, with overfishing. The 'severe and strict' fishing, he said, was not letting enough salmon up to spawn, and 'the fishings are commonly farmed, and the farmers are for their present gain'. Further, 'the brooks and rivulets ... since the country has been thoroughly planted, are generally stopped up with mills and weir-dams'. When people could get salmon for sixpence each 'they endeavoured to preserve them, but since the revolution they either can't have them at all, or at what they count an excessive rate ... [so] they are eager to destroy them'. Finally, he noted that 'after the long intermission of fishing by the war in 1641, salmons have been taken in brooks, some six foot long ...' (in Boate et al., 1726).

At the time Arthur Young was touring Ireland, the commercial salmon fisheries at the river mouths were flourishing: at Coleraine, the catch in 1776 was the best ever – 1452 salmon at one haul of a net; at Ballina, they were salting seventy or eighty tons a year 'besides the fresh'. But over the next century, with the spread of stake-nets and other 'engines', it became necessary to set up boards of conservators and to licence all methods of capture, including rod and line.

In the history of angling for salmon and trout, the inventive imitation of the salmonids' natural food goes back a long way: in his *An Angler's*

Entomology (1952), J.R. Harris shows artificial flies tied in the 1780s and 1790s for use in particular months on lakes in Galway and Clare. In her novel *The Absentee* (1812), Maria Edgeworth depicts military enthusiasm for flies:

The count produced from an Indian cabinet, which he had opened for the lady's inspection, a little basket containing a variety of artificial flies, of curious construction, which, as he spread them on the table, made [Captain] Williamson and [Major] Benson's eyes almost sparkle with delight. There was the dun-fly, for the month of March, and the stone-fly, much in vogue for April ... 'And the green-fly and the moorish-fly!' cried Benson, snatching them up with transport ... 'Capital flies! capital, faith!' cried Williamson. 'Treasures, faith! Real treasures, by G__!' cried Benson.

The well-to-do Englishmen fishing western rivers in the nineteenth and early twentieth centuries contributed many books to the hundred or more dealing wholly or partly with angling in Ireland. Indigenous anglers came late to such writing (Went, 1953), but Niall Fallon, in his anthology of 1991, asserts that 'the solid heart of our angling literature is indisputably Irish – O'Gorman, Kingsmill Moore, Dick Harris, Luce, Gwynn, Greendrake [W. Coad], Gaffey'.

The books record enchanted landscapes and unforgettable seasons: in five weeks on the Erne in 1883, Mr E.P. Bates took 114 salmon weighing 1100 lb.; Kingsmill Moore, fishing the Connemara lakes in September, caught 245 white trout in fifteen days. They also enshrine the Irish ghillie in a fond fiction of devoted goodwill. 'Now look on this picture of rags, hearty interest, indefatigable zeal, and active good humour, all for two shillings a day ...'; 'Hour after hour over those broken, treacherous rocks, gun and game-bag weighing him down, he would go on and on until his companion, bathed in perspiration, was forced to beg for a rest ....' The ghillie was part 'good fairy in homespun' (though sometimes, on an empty stomach, a drunken one) and part faithful spaniel who, 'attached to a reasonably-minded master will serve him with unflagging fidelity' (Fallon, 1991). To which might be added Payne-Gallwey's encomium to the 'active, willing peasant ... who, should your tobacco be carelessly left behind, perhaps high up the mountain-side, whence you toiled for a well-won view, will step up for it after the day's fatigue with the nimbleness of a stag'.

How such relationships were seen from the other side it is not even possible to guess, but against the stereotype of the ghillie's tireless benevolence may be set Maxwell's glimpse of night poaching of salmon and sea trout with gaff and flaming torch: 'Hundreds of breeding fish are annually thus destroyed and although the greater fisheries may be tolerably protected, it is impossible to secure the mountain streams from depredation.' As Edward Fahy comments in his study of the sea trout, *Child of the Tides* (1985): 'In addition to the disorder following the 1798 rebellion and the agitation accompanying the Land War in the later years of the next century, the very real need for food in the later Famine years must have imposed a considerable stress on spawning and easily accessible salmonids.'

The Luxury of the Hunt

The reality of poverty, social oppression and exploitation keeps asserting itself as a shadow behind the bright, rich colours of the sporting art. Seán Lysaght (1991) alludes to it in a poem on the fate of the golden eagle:

> The ledges are cold,
> the eyries drenched
> in the great desert of Erris
> where the last ones
> flew into extinction a lifetime ago
> above ghillies and starvelings.

The extent to which the Irish countryside was the playground of a wealthy colonial class and a bored military garrison makes its own comment on cultural conclusions such as this, from G.M. Trevelyan's *Social History of England*:

There was no luxury about the field sports of those days. Hard exercise and spartan habits were the condition of all pursuit of game. This devotion took the leaders of the English world out of doors and helped to inspire the class that then set the mode in everything from poetry to pugilism, with an intimate love and knowledge of woodland, hedgerow and moor, and a strong preference for country over town life which is so seldom found in the leaders of fashion in any age or land. Indirectly, therefore, the passion for shooting game did much for what was best in our civilization.

What was 'luxurious' about the first four hundred years of field sports in Ireland was the privilege of hunting for recreation, however spartan its chosen mode. The same could be said about England for much of that time, since the weight of law protecting upper-crust privilege was, if anything, more rigorously enforced in the home country than the colony. But a self conscious 'intimate love' of nature and a preference for country living found a wider acceptance in the culture of English society, where it was filtered through a substantial rural middle class. In Ireland there were few social channels by which the values of the Ascendancy were likely to serve as models or bring about popular change, and when the really significant things were happening in English attitudes to nature, the Irish were otherwise and less happily engaged (Viney, 1986). In particular, the plain Irish did not experience the nineteenth-century English vogue for nature study, or the sentiment about animal welfare that was stimulated by living in cities.

Thus, the modern sensibilities of Irish field sports have been rooted more straightforwardly in a utilitarian view of nature. Occasionally, they have also taken on political overtones. The extent of private, and often for-eign, ownership of salmon fishing became a focus of agitation in the late 1960s, when 'colonels and captains and knights-in-arms' were still plentiful among Ireland's riparian owners. A National Waters Restoration League was formed, and in a pamphlet, *Stolen Waters* (1969), the Republican movement urged nationalization of the lakes and rivers and an interim support for poaching. In the 1980s came a much more widespread and successful pop-ular resistance to the government's attempt to licence trout anglers. The move was seen as a challenge to an immemorial 'right' to fish for nothing that even the Big House had never sought to curb, and it aroused an impres-sive display of hunter-gatherer solidarity.

Among the country's shooters, partially organized into about eight hun-dred local gun clubs, there was vigorous resistance in the 1970s to the with-drawal of the Greenland white-fronted goose (along with brent and barna-cle geese) from the list of quarry species. But there is general assent, at the same time, to the principles of conservation. Indeed, in objecting to promo-tion of winter shooting as a tourist attraction (in which snipe and woodcock are the prime quarries), the gun clubs have made much of the 'differing tra-ditions' of shooting in Ireland and on the Continent.

The ultimate English distaste for killing songbirds did, after all, rub off on Irish culture, and recent memoirs such as Eric Craigie's *Irish Sporting Sketches* (1984), Edmund Mahony's *Falcons and Foxhounds* (1984) and Jim Reynolds's *A Life By the Boyne* (1989), while vigorous and idiosyncratic, are almost indistinguishable in sensibility and literary texture from their coun-terparts in British sporting reminiscence. As with their colleagues in Britain, some Irish field-sports organizations are driven to alarm and even paranoia by the newer philosophical forces at work in British and European animal-welfare movements. In the activism of the 'antis' they see a progressive threat to all traditional activities in hunting, shooting and even angling.

In Ireland, the chief target of the well-supported Irish Council Against Blood Sports has been enclosed hare coursing, to which many traditional sportsmen also object. The pastime of badger-baiting with dogs, while still organized from time to time within a rural sub-culture, is illegal, clandes-tine and nowhere defended, but many killings of badgers (as carriers) have been encouraged by the State's campaign to eradicate tuberculosis in cattle. As articulated by Seamus Heaney (1966) in 'The Early Purges':

> 'Prevention of cruelty' talk cuts ice in town
> Where they consider death unnatural,
> But on well-run farms pests have to be kept down.

The direct impact of field sports on Ireland's quarry populations and their ecosystems has been generally benign, in order that sportsmen may have something to hunt, shoot or fish another day. Conservation of a wide range of habitats – woodland, scrub, peatland, marsh, river bank – gained from the sporting priorities of the landed gentry and afterwards from the interest of local hunters and fishermen. This has benefited many other species incidentally. Easy targets among the bigger birds of prey were harried into extinction, although farmers' and estate managers' strychnine certainly killed more sea eagles and buzzards than ever were shot. Some less considered birds on the 'vermin' hit-list were also greatly reduced at the height of the gamekeepers' activities in the 1800s. By the end of that century, ravens' nests had been eradicated from large areas of the lowlands and the bird was generally rarer than even the peregrine or chough (Ussher, 1900). Here again, the interests and prejudices of shooting and farming coincided, a factor that still costs buzzards their lives at the edge of their expanding range in northern Irish counties.

A wider impact of field sports is on attitudes: awareness of nature, ecological concern, ethical consideration of animal welfare and of human relations with other species. In many respects, hunting, shooting and fishing have proved an enriching cultural force in Ireland, promoting, as elsewhere, the scientific advance of natural history and an informed sensitivity to the countryside. On the other hand, in the way land was managed for more than two centuries, and in social organization, they expressed the colonial Ascendancy as sharply as anything else. Occasionally in those years, in the excitement of the hunt, or celebration of a profitable day on the lake, they must also have improved the island's stock of good feeling: a not inconsiderable cultural contribution.

References

Aalen, FH.A. 1970. 'The Origin of Enclosures in Eastern Ireland,' in N. Stephens and R.E. Glasscock (eds), *Irish Geographical Studies*. Belfast: Queen's University.

Anon. 1969. *Stolen Waters: The Case for Public Ownership of Ireland's Rivers and Lakes*. Dublin: Republican Publications.

Apsley, Lady. 1936. *Bridleways through History*. London: Hutchinson.

Boate, G. et al. 1726. *A Natural History of Ireland in Three Parts*. Dublin: Grierson.

Boazman, G. 1988. 'Otter Hunting: A Traditional Field Sport Under Threat.' *Irish Hunting, Shooting and Fishing* Sept-Oct: 24-5.

Butler, D. 1985. 'Quail.' *Field & Countryside* Dec.-Jan.: 345.

Campbell, P. 1984. 'Driven Woodcock Shoots at Cong.' *Irish Forestry* 41: 30-5.

Craigie, E. 1984. *Irish Sporting Sketches*. Mullingar: Lilliput Press.

De Bhaldraithe, T. (trans.). 1973. *The Diary of Humphrey O'Sullivan*. Dublin: Mercier.

Drought, Capt. J.B. 1940. *A Sportsman Looks at Eire*. London: Hutchinson.

Edgeworth, M. [1812] 1915. *The Absentee*, in *Selections from Her Works*, ed. Sir M. Cotter Seton. Dublin: Phoenix.

Fahy, E. 1985. *Child of the Tides: A Sea Trout Handbook*. Dublin: Glendale.

Fallon, N. 1991. *The Irish Game Angler's Anthology*. Dublin: Country House.

Fox, J. 1986. 'Kellyville Decoy and its Catches.' *Irish Birds 3*: 245-54.

Gibbons, M. and T. Clarke. 1991. 'Deerparks.' *Carloviana: Journal of the Old Carlow Society* (1990-1): 4-5.

Giraldus Cambrensis [c.1188]. *Giraldus Cambrensis in Topographiaa Hibernie*. Trans. J.J. O'Meara. *Proc. Roy. Irish Acad. 52 C*: 113-78.

Harris, J.R. 1952. *An Angler's Entomology*. London: Collins.

Heaney, Ss. 1966. *Death of a Naturalist*. London: Faber.

Henry, F. 1963. *Early Christian Irish Art*. Dublin: Three Candles.

Hutchinson, C. 1989. *Birds in Ireland*. Calton: Poyser.

Levinge, E. 1860. *Game Laws of Ireland*. Dublin: Hodges.

Lewis, C.A. 1975. *Hunting in Ireland: An Historical and Geographical Analysis*. London: Allen.

Lysaght, S. 1991. *The Clare Island Survey*. Oldcastle: Gallery Press.

McKee, M. 1986. *James Sheals, Naturalist and Taxidermist*. Belfast: Ulster Museum.

MacLysaght, E. 1950. *Irish Life in the Seventeenth Century*. Cork: Cork University Press.

Mahony, E. 1979. *Memoirs of the Galway Blazers: A Galway Sportsman's Notebook*. Galway: Kenny.

Mahony, E. 1984. *Falcons and Foxhounds*. Galway: Kenny.

Maxwell, W. 1832. *Wild Sports of the West*. London: Richard Bentley.

Moran, R. 1982. *The Wildfowler*. Belfast: Blackstaff.

Morris, J. 1984. 'Grouse Hawking.' *Field & Countryside*, Oct: 489.

O'Flaherty, R. (1684) 1846. *Chorographical Description of the Territory of West or H-Iar Connaught*. Dublin: Irish Archaeological Society.

Payne-Gallwey, R. 1882. *The Fowler in Ireland*. London: Van Voorst. Repr. 1985. Southampton: Ashford Press.

Patterson, R.L. 1881. *The Birds, Fishes and Cetacea of Belfast Lough*. London: Bogue.

Reynolds, J. 1989. *A Life By the Boyne*. Scariff Bridge: Zircon.

Robertson, P. and J. Whelan. 1987. 'The Ecology and Management of Wild and Hand-reared Pheasants in Ireland.' *Irish Birds 3*: 427-40.

Somerville, E., and M. Ross. 1899. *Some Experiences of an Irish R.M.* London: Longman.

Stringer, A. 1714. *The Experienced Huntsman*. Belfast: Blow. Repr. 1977, ed. James Fairley. Belfast: Blackstaff.

Thompson, F.M.L. 1963. *English Landed Society in the Nineteenth Century*. London: Routledge.

Thompson, W. 1849-56. *The Natural History of Ireland*. Vol. 3 (1851): Birds. London: Reeve and Bentham.

Trevelyan, G. 1944. *English Social History*. London: Longman.

Twomey, G. 1985. 'Keeping to the Trencher System.' *Field & Countryside*, March: 42-3.

Upton, R. 1987. *O, For a Falconer's Voice*. Marlborough: Crowood.

Ussher, R. and R. Warren. 1900. *The Birds of Ireland*. London: Gurney and Jackson.

Viney, M. 1986. 'Woodcock for a Farthing: the Irish Experience of Nature.' *The Irish Review 1*: 58-64.

Wakefield, E. 1812. *An Account of Ireland, Statistical and Political*. London.

Watters, J. 1853. *The Natural History of the Birds of Ireland*. Dublin: McGlashan.

Went, A. 1953. 'Material for a History of the Fisheries of the River Boyne.' *Journal of the County Louth Archaeological Society 13*.

Whelan, K. 1989. *The Angler In Ireland*. Dublin: Country House.

Wilde, W.R. 1860. 'An Essay on the Unmanufactured Animal Remains in the Royal Irish Academy.' Dublin: Gill.

Wyndham-Quinn, W.H. 1919. *The Foxhound in County Limerick*. Quoted in Lewis, 1975.

Young, A. 1780. *A Tour in Ireland 1776-1779*. London: Cadell.

The Natural History of Demesnes

TERENCE REEVES-SMYTH

Demesnes have been a dominant feature of the Irish landscape since medieval times and once occupied over 5 per cent of the country. Although dependent upon their surrounding tenanted estates, demesnes – the manor lands farmed directly by the lord – have evolved as separate social and economic areas with distinctive planned and managed layouts incorporating woodland, farmland, gardens and ornamental grounds, as well as a range of building types. Considering their central role in the development of Irish agriculture, horticulture, sylviculture and field sport, it is perhaps not surprising that demesnes have made a distinct contribution to the natural history of Ireland. Indeed, they continue to do so, for despite widespread devastation over the past eighty years, the demesne remains a significant component of the Irish landscape, offering suitable habitats to a wide range of flora and fauna.

Demesne Development

The term 'demesne' or 'demaine' is Norman French in origin and denotes that portion of the manorial estate not leased out to tenants but retained by the lord for his own use and occupation. Although long obsolescent in England, both the term and concept of demesne survived in Ireland until the early twentieth century when the estate system was finally dismantled. The term is still used today, although it is often wrongly understood to be synonymous with landscape parks around country houses. In fact, these parks, which were developed from the middle of the eighteenth century onwards, only covered parts of demesnes, and were invariably the culmination of successive landscape changes over many centuries. Indeed, the continuity of demesnes – many with origins going back half a millennium or more – is a striking characteristic of their development and contributes enormously to their rich variety of archaeological, architectural and botanical features.

Although demesnes were widespread in medieval Ireland, particularly in the eastern part of the country, our knowledge of their composition at that time remains surprisingly limited, partly because of a paucity of documentary material and partly because medieval archaeological research has been so concentrated upon military and ecclesiastical aspects of the period. However, it is evident that both the manorial and ecclesiastical demesnes in medieval Ireland were broadly compatible with their English equivalents, with fields for crops and livestock, an enclosed garden, an orchard and possibly a fish pond, a rabbit warren and deer park.* From an early period these demesnes would have constituted a distinct component of the landscape, their neat fields presenting quite a contrast to the surrounding unenclosed countryside.

During the post-medieval era, demesnes continued to function as manorial home farms, but their size and layouts were increasingly dominated by ornamental rather than economic considerations. After the Restoration of 1660, in particular, there was an increased desire to provide suitably impressive settings for the great mansions being built in Ireland (Loeber, 1973). Formal features, arranged axially upon the house on broad, controlled vistas, began to affect much of the demesne area. Tree-lined avenues, which sometimes marched out from the house for great distances, were a dominant feature of these layouts, serving as symbols of the authority and rank of the owners and emphasizing the importance of the mansion in the landscape. Demesne fields were laid out in a regular, often grid-like manner, together with small blocks of tree plantations. Other standard features included circular pools and canals, many of which served as fish ponds as well as being ornamental. Closer to the house there were formal garden areas, terraces, bowling greens and *bosquets* (ornamental groves pierced by walks), often wedged between a kitchen garden, orchard, haggard and outbuildings.

By the middle of the eighteenth century a new conception of man's place in nature began to transform Ireland's demesnes. The old formal geometric layouts, which sought to prove that man could subdue nature, now made way for 'naturalized' parklands, the planting and layout of which reflected a new appreciation that 'natural' features, such as woods, streams and hills, were beautiful in themselves and indeed good for the soul. It now pleased the optimistic spirit of the age to create Arcadian parkscapes of 'untouched' nature, secluded from the outside world by encircling walls and belts of trees that enclosed the mansion at their heart. The ideal now was smooth, open meadows dotted with clumps of oak or beech, sweeping lakes in which the house and park were flatteringly mirrored, and tree-lined glades with animals grazing peacefully in the shadow of romantic ruins, temples and pavilions.

---

* Most historical research has been focused upon specific manors, but a useful general account can be found in Down (1987).

Although the new landscape style emanated from England, it was ideally suited to the rolling Irish countryside. Nevertheless, parkland creation in Ireland was invariably a costly operation and involved considerable engineering skills, not least in selecting and accentuating the best existing landscape features – moving soil and rock, felling and planting trees, diverting rivers into the park, constructing dams to create lakes, building ha-has and other contrivances. Sometimes even villages were relocated and roads re-routed in the emparkment process. In sharp contrast to the old formal layouts, horticulture was now largely confined to walled gardens, sometimes at some distance from the house, while the home farm was invariably relocated on to newly acquired demesne lands lying beyond the parkland perimeter and out of sight of the house.

The 'natural style' landscape parks were so enthusiastically adopted by Irish landowners that by the close of the eighteenth century only a handful of the old formal layouts survived. By the middle of the nineteenth century, parkland occupied around 800,000 acres, or 4 per cent of Ireland, with over 7000 houses featuring associated ornamental or pleasure landscapes of ten acres or more.* Their popularity can be attributed to a variety of factors, not least their suitability to the Irish countryside, the comparatively low cost of their maintenance and the potential of parkland for allowing landowners to distance themselves physically from the economic realities that sustained them, whilst helping to convey the comforting notion that the contemporary social order was somehow natural, unchanging and inevitable. The process of park-making was also greatly aided by the availability of cheap labour and by the need to provide local employment for the poor in times of hardship. Once established, the new demesne parklands proved to be ideal for game shooting and were well adapted to accommodate the specialized plant collections, notably the newly introduced exotic trees and shrubs, that became such a feature of the Victorian era.

In the years following the Great Famine (1845-9), when money and labour were no longer so abundant, there was a sharp decline in the number of parklands being created in Ireland. Indeed, after 1849 hundreds of demesnes changed hands in the Encumbered Estates Courts; many were subsequently reduced in size and in some cases disappeared. The decline of the demesne's traditional social and economic role was greatly accelerated after 1885 with the Ashbourne Act and later with the Wyndham Act of 1903. These acts allowed agricultural tenants to buy out their farms using funds provided by the Treasury; by 1914 three-quarters of the country's former tenants had bought their holdings. The sale of estate lands meant that most demesnes could no longer continue to rely on rental income for their

---

* Figures based on the author's unpublished research.

maintenance and now had to survive as self-supporting units. Inevitably, a large number of demesnes and their mansions had to be sold as their owners could no longer afford to maintain them. Many were converted into hospitals, government research centres, schools or convents, but the majority had their lands subdivided among local farmers, their park and woodland trees uprooted and their buildings demolished or allowed to fall into ruin. The sad process reached its climax in the 1950s and continues to this day, though the pressures on demesne parklands now come mainly from housing and leisure developments, notably golf courses and their ancillary buildings. Yet despite the devastation wrought on demesnes over the past century (*plate 17*), they still remain the dominant man-made feature of the post-medieval landscape in Ireland.

Demesnes and Arboriculture

A visitor to Ireland in 1837 remarked: 'In Britain, it is frequently very difficult, when one cannot see the wall or fence, to discriminate between what is, and what is not, park. But in Ireland this is a matter about which there can be no mistake. They differ as widely as light and darkness.' This sharp contrast between demesnes and the immediately contiguous parts of their estates, noted so frequently by travellers in the eighteenth and nineteenth centuries, owed much to the cultivation of trees. As Wakefield (1812) observed, 'A traveller in Ireland finds timber as he does shrubs and exotic plants, merely as appendages to a gentleman's place of residence and after leaving a favoured spot of this kind, he at once loses sight of green foliage, so agreeable to the eye, and enters dreary wastes, where there is scarcely a twig sufficient to form a resting place to the birds fatigued with their flight.'

The scarcity of timber outside the demesne walls was due principally to the ruthless exploitation of Ireland's surviving woodlands during the sixteenth and early seventeenth centuries (Hore, 1858; McCracken, 1971; Hall, 1992). Despite the passage of seventeen Acts in the Irish Parliament between 1698 and 1791 to encourage planting and prevent illegal felling, most estate lands outside the demesne boundaries remained treeless 'dreary wastes', as the tenants were unable to establish adequate rights over the ownership of their plantations (Anderson, 1943; McCracken, 1971).

Until the mid eighteenth century the principal wooded areas in most demesnes lay in the deer parks, where remnants of ancient woodland often survived (Forbes, 1933). Irish landowners were generally slow to appreciate the value of trees and most early planting consisted of orchards, hedgerows, avenues and ornamental areas around the house rather than full-scale plantations. One Irish landowner, Sir John Percival, who was perhaps typical, imported in December 1683 one hundred limes, two hundred Dutch elms and a variety of fruit trees for his demesne at Ballymacow (Egmont) in Co. Cork. In April 1684 he obtained 'an ounce of Scotch fir seed, which cost 5 shillings' and the following year was sent 'a parcel of young elms, I think about 70 or 71, nor have I forgot my Lady's pippens' (Nelson, 1990). Less typical of the time was Lord Granard's demesne at Castle Forbes, Co. Longford, where a visitor in 1682 found 'growing there in great order large groves of Fir of all sorts with Pines, Juniper, Cedar, Lime trees, Beech, Elm, Oak, Ash, Asp [aspen] and the famous Platanous tree ...'. (Sherrard and Fitzpatrick, 1945).

Trees were, of course, an essential component of the formal layouts that dominated demesnes from the 1660s until the 1740s. Common limes were the most favoured choice for avenues because of their regularity of shape and because when planted close together their branches interweave without becoming stunted. Good lime avenues still exist at Huntington in Co. Carlow, Kilruddery in Co. Wicklow and Castletown in Co. Kildare. Lime was also frequently used to flank canals, as at Gaulstown (Malins and Glin, 1976) and Castle Ward (McErlean and Reeves-Smyth, 1990); at Antrim the limes along the canal were clipped into tall hedges (Jupp, 1993).

Another popular tree of the period was the Dutch elm, and until recent decades there was a fine avenue of these trees at Old Rossenarra in Co. Kilkenny planted in 1690 (Forbes, 1933). Dutch elms were planted along the walks at Castlemartyr, Co. Cork, in the 1720s,* while at Breckdenstone, Co. Dublin, Lord Molesworth was planting elms in 1720 about his great circular basin '30 or 40 foot asunder in double rows by which means all the fine prospects will appear under their branches and between the intervals of trees till they grow exceedingly old' (Malins and Glin, 1976). A mixture of 'fir and elm' was being planted along the grand avenues at Florence Court, Co. Fermanagh, between 1716 and 1719, while its demesne lands had been 'divided into large square parks, all planted with ash and elm' (Reeves-Smyth, 1990). Other trees used for avenues at this time included sycamore, walnut, Spanish chestnut and sometimes oak; the still impressive grand oak avenue at Castle Coole, Co. Fermanagh, was recently dated by dendrochronology to 1725 (McErlean, 1984). Beech was occasionally planted along avenues, though like hornbeam it was more commonly used for *bosquets* and arcades, as at Kilmore, Co. Cavan**. Beech in particular was favoured for hedging as it kept its leaf late into the winter and thus helped preserve the garden structure through the seasons; until recent years the gardens at Howth boasted magnificent beech hedges, planted in 1738 and claimed to be the tallest in these islands.

---

* Shannon Papers D2707 (Public Records Office, Northern Ireland).
** Henry Mss, pp. 111-12 (Public Records Office, Dublin).

Block planting in the formal demesne layouts of the 1660-1740 period was very limited, though most demesnes had at least one small plantation of a single species. At Eyre Court, Co. Galway, for example, there was a grove of beech present in 1697 (Boate, 1755, appendix) and at Belan, Co. Kildare, there were blocks of elm, oak and Scots pine amidst an elaborate layout incorporating canals and avenues (McCracken, 1971). Sometimes such woods were traversed by straight alleys and walks to form a 'wilderness'; one such still existing at Antrim comprised 'very tall and tapering elms, intersected with a few other trees and shrubs'.*

Some late seventeenth-century landowners were enthusiastic planters of pines and conifers, notably Lord Massareene, who had his 'greatest entertainment' planting different kinds at Antrim (MacLysaght, 1979). Many demesnes of the period consequently boasted a 'fir grove', usually a reference to Scots pine. At Burton, Co. Cork, one such 'Firr Grove' was laid out in March 1686,** and at Thomastown, Co. Tipperary, there were several 'large plantations of fir' (Loveday, 1790), while farther to the south at Coolnamuck Court, Co. Waterford, Pococke on his 1752 tour of Ireland noted that there were '20,000 firris which thrive much' along the banks of the Suir (Pococke, 1891). In 1723 at Castle Ward, Co. Down, a 'fir tree park' was planted in linear belts, giving the illusion of more extensive tree cover than in fact existed, and typically for the period it was confined to sloping land of little agricultural value (McErlean and Reeves-Smyth, 1990).

More extensive demesne planting in Ireland followed the introduction of 'natural style' landscape parks in the 1740s. Professional 'landscape gardeners' were widely employed to design the new parks; James Sutherland was the most celebrated (Bowe, 1977, 1980), while others included Peter Shanley and Thomas Leggett (Desmond, 1994). Great numbers of trees were now required, not for regularly shaped woods or avenues, but to frame views and make shadows in the belts and clumps of the new parks. While many magnificent avenues were felled in the creation of these new landscapes, it should be noted that many trees from the old formal layouts were often retained. At Carton, avenue trees were kept as isolated specimens in the new park; at Florence Court old woodland blocks were ingeniously incorporated into the new 'Brownian' park; and at Castle Coole, substantial portions of the old Queen Anne layout, including the oak avenue, were left largely untouched in the new 'naturalized' layout of the 1780s (Horner, 1975; Garner and Webb, 1977; Reeves-Smyth, 1990; McErlean, 1984). The practice of moving mature trees also helped give the new naturalized parks an aged

---

* James Boyle in the Ordnance Survey Memoirs for Antrim Parish (1835); see Jupp (1993) for full text.
** Egmont Papers 3: 739-47, 371, Historical Manuscript Commission Report.

appearance (Forbes, 1933); diagrams of transplanting machines were published in Hayes's *Practical Treatice on Planting* (1794), the first and perhaps only really important book available on Irish arboriculture in the eighteenth and nineteenth centuries.

The trees in demand for the new parks were predominantly oak, beech, chestnut, elm, lime and sycamore with a mixture of silver fir, pine and spruce. Popular nurse trees included Scots pine, birch, hazel and ash, while plenty of holly was often planted on the woodland fringes. Wide shelter screens on the western and south-western perimeters were a standard feature of the new parks. In the 1760s at Bellevue in Co. Galway, the owner selected 'hardy trees for the west side of his plantations; they are very much beech, hornbeam and sycamore'. Other trees he planted, notably larch, Scots pine and sweet chestnut, were 'bent by westerly winds', though his oak, spruce, silver fir and Weymouth pine were apparently unaffected (Dutton, 1824). Elsewhere in Ireland the trees most used for parkland shelter belts were sycamore, beech, silver fir, spruce and maritime pine.

Fences were normally used to protect the trees from livestock, though these were not always successfully maintained, and Irish demesne records are peppered with references to cattle breaking into the plantations. The young parkland plantations must have looked rather stiff behind their wooden fencing. In order to improve their appearance a variety of shrubs were often added to the underplanting to provide interest. At Downhill, Co. Derry, the Earl-Bishop's architect, Michael Shanahan, informed his patron in July 1778 that he had tried to procure for his plantations 'an ample store of tamarisk, laburnums, myrtles, roses of every kind, sweet briar etc etc, as your Lordship order'd ... the walks round the demesne being planted with shrubs of this kind will look very delightful' (Reeves-Smyth, 1991). At Gracefield Lodge, Co. Leix, in 1817, a profusion of hyacinths, primroses and violets were planted beneath the trees (Brewer, 1826).

Although the Dublin Society offered yearly premiums for tree planting and the stocking of nurseries from 1740 until 1807, landowners were slow to establish large-scale plantations. The absence of local nurseries certainly curtailed planting in many areas as transporting seedlings was expensive, but by the late eighteenth century many large demesnes were raising most of their own seedlings (McCracken, 1979). At Baronscourt, Co. Tyrone, for example, the Marquis of Abercorn had established by the 1790s a series of thriving nurseries for his demesne plantations (Gebbie, 1972), as had Lord Mountjoy nearby at Rash, outside Omagh. When planting first commenced at Rash large quantities of seedlings were imported from Scotland, but this ceased once those raised on the demesne's nurseries proved more satisfactory. More than 600,000 trees were planted at Rash between 1791 and 1800, while a further 300,000 plants were given to other gentlemen in the district

(Camblin, 1967). Such large numbers of trees were still quite unusual at the time, though after the Napoleonic wars demesne-planting operations increasingly started to assume a more economic aspect. By this time, however, most of Ireland's demesne parklands had already been created.

The Victorian era was marked by the introduction of numerous new exotic species from abroad – so many, indeed, that rare specimens were increasingly cultivated for their own sake rather than as part of the overall parkland scheme. Arboreta and pineta became a standard feature of demesnes – usually informal areas, arranged botanically or at random, traversed by paths, rides and vistas (Malins and Bowe, 1980). New tree varieties were occasionally displayed on avenues, such as the splendid monkey-puzzle avenues at Woodstock and Powerscourt or the mile-long avenue of Wellingtonias at Emo, Co. Leix (Fitzpatrick, 1933). After 1840 the block planting of conifers also became fashionable and they increasingly played an important role in commercial forestry.

Sadly, Irish demesne woodlands went into serious decline following the Land Acts of 1881 and 1885 (Forbes, 1933; Durant, 1979). Irish landowners were forced to fell their tree stocks prior to the sale of estate lands, while tenant purchasers were rarely interested in retaining 'even as few as one tree' (Edwards, 1908). By the 1920s Ireland's woodland had shrunk from 340,000 acres in 1880 to about 130,000 acres. Although by this time the State had started to become involved in forestry (Fitzpatrick, 1966), little was done to prevent the inexorable decline of demesne hardwood plantations, which have continued to diminish to the present day.

Demesnes and Garden Horticulture

The cultivation of vegetables, fruit and flowers was inevitably an important feature of demesne life from medieval times. The manor house always needed to be supplied with garden produce for culinary and medicinal purposes, while cut flowers were widely in demand from an early date to sweeten interiors. Ornamental plants played an increasingly important role as gardens were developed for pleasure purposes, and as they evolved, these gardens reflected their own generation's attitude to nature.

The documentary evidence for gardening activity in Ireland before the seventeenth century remains rather sparse (Nelson, 1990). It seems likely that Tudor and pre-Tudor manorial Irish gardens were broadly similar to those in England. They would have had formal grass or gravel paths, turf seats, raised flower and vegetable beds, and possibly trellised arbours or clipped knot hedging, all enclosed behind a sloping bank, surmounted by a wall, fence or hedge (Harvey, 1981). Garden areas were small; even the large Irish monastic gardens covered barely an acre when the inquisitions were taken in the mid sixteenth century, and much of this was generally orchard (Pim, 1979). Orchards were a standard feature of medieval and post-medieval Irish gardens (Lamb, 1951). In the seventeenth century the practice of cultivating named varieties of fruit trees was well established and there are many references to their importation from Holland (MacLysaght, 1979; Nelson, 1990). The trees were generally staggered in a quincunx pattern to allow maximum light and air to reach the fruit.

The choice of plants available was largely restricted to varieties of European origin, though Jon Gardener's late fourteenth-century work on gardening, the first of its kind in the English language, lists a substantial number of plants, most of which were probably available in Ireland, for both surviving manuscripts have Irish connections (Zettersten, 1967). More than a hundred herbs and vegetables are mentioned: colewort, parsley, onion, saffron, sweet-smelling herbs such as rosemary, lavender, chamomile, and flowers such as gladwin, red and white roses, hollyhock, peony, violet, daffodil and primrose (Harvey, 1985). While the emphasis was primarily on 'useful' plants, the best gardens must have made a splendid display, especially in the medieval monasteries where there existed a flourishing exchange network of seeds and cuttings throughout Europe (Hobhouse, 1992).

The development of gardening greatly accelerated in the late sixteenth century when exotic plants began arriving back in large quantities from newly discovered areas of the world. The damask rose came from Persia, marigolds from Mexico and potatoes from South America, the latter introduced, as tradition says, by Sir Walter Raleigh, who is also credited with the introduction to Ireland of edible cherries and a sweet-smelling wallflower from the Azores (Walker, 1799; Pim, 1979). The new plants were written up in publications such as Gerard's *Herball* (1597) and Parkinson's *Sole Paradisus Terrestris* (1629), the latter being among the first books to treat herbal plants separately from those used for 'ornament and pleasure'.

Plant collecting and an increased interest in the natural world led to a more scientific approach to botany and horticulture, as expressed in an attempt to create a physic garden in Dublin in 1654 and in the successful establishment of a botanical garden in Trinity College, Dublin, in 1687 (Nelson, 1990; Wyse Jackson, 1987; Nelson 1982). A few years later Sir Arthur Rawdon erected a 'large stove' (glasshouse) on his demesne at Moira, Co. Down, to shelter an astonishing collection of over a thousand tropical plants that he had imported from Jamaica (Nelson, 1983). This collection had been gathered by James Harlow, a gardener in Rawdon's commission, and transported to Ireland in a ship 'almost laden with cases of trees, and herbs, planted and growing in earth', a remarkable achievement that remained unmatched until the mid nineteenth century (Nelson, 1983a).

It is worth noting that Rawdon managed to pursue his gardening activities even though a war raged in Ireland at the time. The unsettled political situation during the seventeenth century meant that most substantial Irish manorial gardens were protected within fortified enclosures, often with impressive walls, turrets and terracing as at Lismore, Co. Waterford, and Burton House, Co. Cork. Sometimes they covered large areas: at Lemaneagh Castle, Co. Clare, over ten acres were enclosed (Westropp, 1900). Normally these gardens were designed in rectangles or squares with axially planned gravel paths, bordered with boxhedges or close walks of ashes (Loeber, 1973). Aside from fruit and vegetables, their walls often sheltered a wide range of trees and flowers, as Dowdall discovered when he visited Castle Forbes in 1682 to find 'lovely gardens of pleasure enclosed by high stone walls against which plenty of fruit of all sorts grow and in the said garden are all kinds of flowers and flower trees that grow in the kingdom as the Lelaps, Liburnum and many more, with Philarea hedges, Lawrel &c, and the Tubirosa beareth here which is not to be raised but with ye assistance of glasses' (Sherrard and Fitzpatrick, 1945). Plenty of flowerpots, no doubt, featured in this garden, probably of Irish manufacture (Loeber, 1973), while the term 'glasses' apparently denotes bell glasses, much used from 1650 onwards for rearing and forcing delicate plants.

The arrangement of Irish gardens started changing towards the end of the seventeenth century, especially following the Williamite wars, when the French use of long perspectives inspired the planting of rows of trees along radiating avenues and vistas. Pleasure grounds around the house, with axially planned geometric layouts, replaced the old fortified garden enclosures, and typically incorporated bowling greens, parterres, *bosquets*, flower yards, orchards and melon grounds, as at Castle Coole, Co. Fermanagh (McErlean, 1984). Features of such gardens may have included trees in vases, statues and topiary, the latter often framing parterres and grass *plats*. Normally the parterre 'possessed' the ground immediately below the main reception rooms and in some cases may have comprised intricate schemes of dwarf scrollwork set in coloured gravels, though most parterres probably contained flowers and box hedges, as at Thomastown, Co. Tipperary (Campbell, 1778), and Powerscourt, Co. Wicklow.

Popular flowers of the time, some of which were grown in parterres, included improved Dutch strains of tulips, pinks, carnations, ranunculus, hyacinths, auriculas and polyantha. At Kilruddery, Co. Wicklow, there are payments for seeds by the sixth earl of Meath in 1731 for thirty-one species of carnation from a Mr Bacon and seventeen from a Mr Chamney, while other lists of carnations include twenty kinds in one, nearly seventy in another and forty-two in a third. In 1731 there are lists of forty-two auriculas and another list in 1736 mentions seventy-four Irish and sixty-nine

English varieties. The lists also include ranunculas and tulips from Holland in 1739 and tulips from Lille and Brussels in 1739 (Knight of Glin and Cornforth, 1977).

This intimate relationship between garden and house, so striking a feature of the late seventeenth and early eighteenth centuries, disappeared with the advent of the landscape park, whose lawns now swept up to the windows of the mansion. The growing of flowers, fruits and vegetables now had to be confined to enclosures, usually walled, located out of sight of the house. Sometimes the distance between these enclosures and the mansion was considerable, though most owners preferred to keep them as conveniently close as the new parkland aesthetics would permit – usually on the edge of the pleasure grounds and often adjacent to the stable yard where a ready supply of manure was at hand. They ranged from about half an acre to several acres in extent and usually had perimeter and cross paths, a pond, glasshouses and potting sheds. Rectangular plans were standard in the nineteenth century, but during the previous century walled gardens tended to the more experimental and usually adopted irregular plans in attempts to provide as much sheltered and south-facing walling as possible. Their bounding walls, generally between ten and thirteen feet high, were principally intended to support fruit trees and were often lined with brick to absorb and retain the warmth of the sun. Shelter belts outside the walls provided essential protection against the winds; normally conifers were planted to give protection throughout the year, usually being mixed with hardwoods to blend into the parkland (Davies, 1987).

The walled gardens in some of the great demesnes were subdivided into separate areas for fruit, vegetables and flowers, as at Castle Coole, Co. Fermanagh, where early records of the garden from 1778 to 1795 mention the presence of two graperies, two peacheries, a melon house, a cherry house, an orangery, a greenhouse and list a wide range of vegetables and herbs (McErlean, 1984). Most Irish walled gardens of the late eighteenth and nineteenth centuries lacked any rigid subdivision and were characterized by a mixture of flowers, fruit and vegetables in a *potager* layout, in which rows of vegetables were discreetly hidden from view behind long flower or shrub borders. The popularity of this practical way of combining pleasure and utility may have owed much to the frequent employment of head gardeners from Scotland, where such layouts had a long tradition. One such garden still existed at Florence Court, Co. Fermanagh, until the 1930s; here the gravel paths were flanked by long beds of roses with dwarf box edgings, long iris and herbaceous borders and magnificent beds of begonias and large flowering gladioli, all backed by lines of espalier fruit trees, fuchsia or laurel hedges, screening the currant bushes and vegetables behind (Reeves-Smyth, 1990). The Florence Court layout also incorporated a herb garden, a long pergola, large shrub borders, extensive lawns surrounding beds of dahlias, two ponds and a rose garden – the last a frequent feature of late-Victorian Irish walled gardens. Also to be found were an apple store, a mushroom house, and heated greenhouses adroitly placed at the ends of paths in focal points, containing vines, peaches, apricots, nectarines, melons, tomatoes, chrysanthemums and a fernery.

Heated greenhouses were a standard feature of nineteenth-century walled gardens and played an enormously important role in the development of garden horticulture. With the introduction of hot-water heating systems, cast-iron skylights and curved metal glazing bars by 1820, it was possible to grow a vast range of plants in controlled conditions under glass, while the invention of the sealed 'Wardian case' in 1830 enabled large numbers of very tender exotics to be obtained from abroad. Many of the newly imported ferns, orchids and other tropical plants were housed in conservatories, which by the 1840s were being built all over Ireland, often attached to country houses where they served as ornamental or recreational rooms (Diestelkamp, 1981). A wide range of fruit could now be easily grown: vines, peaches, figs, lemons and pineapples among others, while the new hothouses also allowed head gardeners to rear vast numbers of new annuals as seedlings and cuttings, a process that was boosted enormously by the repeal of the glass tax in 1845, when glasshouses proliferated and became even larger in size.

The remarkable influx of new plants in the nineteenth century, both through introductions from abroad and through the work of plant breeders, created enormous pressures to find appropriate display areas outside the walled gardens to accommodate them. Imaginative ideas were forthcoming from the explosion of garden literature during the early nineteenth century, most notably from the books, encyclopaedias and magazines produced by the Scottish author John Claudius Loudon. In *An Encyclopaedia of Gardening*, first published in 1822, he wrote that the 'hand of man should be visible in gardens laid out in the natural style as in the most formal geometric styles, because both are equally intended to show that they are works of art, and to display the taste and wealth of the owner'. This philosophy encouraged the creation of the formal and architectural display gardens – so much a feature of the mid nineteenth century – located in areas close to the home, for Loudon believed that gardens should be seen as a natural, verdant extension of the house and not confined to some distant walled area.

Although Loudon's writings were aimed principally at the rising middle classes in England, he was widely followed in Ireland, notably by James Fraser and Alexander McLeish. It was mainly through his influence that floral parterres started making a reappearance on terraces around Irish country houses during the 1820s, notable early examples being at Merville, Co. Dublin (1824), and Caledon, Co. Tyrone (1827). At this time separate flower gardens were created within the extended pleasure grounds. Rose gardens were early favourites, as were 'American Gardens', made by preparing the ground for acid-loving plants such as heathers, rhododendrons and azaleas, usually set amidst mown lawns and a network of meandering paths; a good example survives at Florence Court (Reeves-Smyth, 1990). Further 'compartmentalization' followed during the early Victorian period with the creation of separate gardens devoted to different geographic or historical styles: Italian gardens, Dutch gardens, a whole range of eclectic 'revival' gardens as well as areas devoted to particular plant themes, such as evergreens or aquatic plants (Elliott, 1986). Some houses had a whole series of these compartmented gardens *en suite*, as for example at Knockdrin Castle, Co. Westmeath (Malins and Bowe, 1980).

Perhaps the most striking feature of mid-Victorian country-house gardens were the brightly coloured and often gaudy 'bedding out' schemes of annuals and tender plants, reared in their thousands from seeds or cuttings in the new glasshouses (Carter, 1984). The introduction of *Verbena venose* and other 'perfectly dazzling' plants from South and Central America in the 1830s triggered the style, followed by the hybridization of lobelias, verbenas, petunias, calceolarias and pelargoniuns. Lavish displays of massed annuals filled flower beds of every conceivable shape and form and normally were changed three times a year, in spring, summer and autumn, in some places more often. The number of flowers and succulents involved could be enormous; at St Helen's, Co. Dublin, the parterre required 72,000 plants a year (Malins and Bowe, 1980).

The inevitable reaction against high-Victorian formalism in gardening came during the 1870s. It was spearheaded by William Robinson, an Irishman who left for England in 1861, having worked as head gardener at Ballykilcavan, Co. Leix. Fed up with the 'dark ages of flower gardening', he launched a new philosophy of plant cultivation in his classic book *The Wild Garden* in 1870, advocating 'the placing of perfectly hardy exotic plants under conditions where they will thrive without further care'. His ideas found a large audience through his weekly journal, *The Garden*, established in 1871, and many of his themes were widely adopted in the demesnes of Ireland from the 1880s onwards with the creation of bog gardens, lakeside gardens, rhododendron and other forms of woodland gardens, mixed borders, grass paths and the massing of naturalized bulbs in grass, particularly daffodils. Natural rock gardens also became popular, while Robinson's admiration of the cottage garden in his book *The English Flower Garden*, first published in 1883, encouraged the creation of herbaceous borders, a feature later developed by Gertrude Jekyll.

While Robinson was advocating the re-creation of nature in gardening, various forms of formal gardens continued to be made during the late-

Victorian and Edwardian era, though not in any large number. At Killarney House, Co. Kerry, John D. Sedding laid out extensive gardens in the early Renaissance style (Malins and Bowe, 1980); Edwin Lutyens created a handful of gardens, notably at Heywood, Co. Leix (Nelson, 1985); and a number of Japanese gardens were also made, as at Tully, Co. Kildare. However, the desire to create or indeed maintain formal gardens declined in Ireland after the effects of the Land Acts began to be felt in the 1880s and especially after the post-1903 period. The comparatively less labour-intensive 'wild' Robinsonian themes were often preferred, not least because the temperate Irish climate is so suited to this form of gardening. After the Second World War, when virtually all the remaining walled kitchen gardens and formal display gardens disappeared from Ireland's demesnes, the Robinsonian legacy remained, as at Annes Grove, Co. Cork, Mount Usher, Co. Wicklow, and other places. Perhaps the most famous of these gardens was created by Sir John Ross of Bladensburg at Rostrevor, Co. Down, but it no longer exists. Some notable examples that survive include Rowallane, Co. Down; Altamont, Co. Carlow; Fernhill, Co. Dublin; and Derreen, Co. Kerry. Invariably, they were the creations of the owners themselves – often fine plantsmen – rather than garden designers or head gardeners, and although few in number, they still bear witness to the continuing role of demesnes in Ireland's horticultural development.

Demesnes and Fauna

The keeping of animals has always played an important role in the development of demesnes. Aside from cattle, sheep, pigs and horses, a variety of other animals were bred to ensure diversity in the demesne's economic resources. Deer, rabbits and pigeons were kept mainly to provide fresh winter meat, though such food also assumed a high status value, as did freshwater pond fish. A supply of wild birds came from decoys; some birds, such as pheasants, were bred for sport as well as food, while other fowl were retained for ornamental purposes only.

A dominant feature of the demesne landscape from an early period has been the deer park. Typically, a deer park consisted of an area of open country enclosed (in medieval times) by fences or banks or (from the seventeenth century) by walls. More than a hundred deer parks are listed as townlands, while there are records relating to more than three hundred across the country. The earliest were established in the early thirteenth century by the Normans, who were partial to venison and introduced the fallow deer, a gregarious breed native to southern Europe that needs little attention, breeds readily, fattens up well on indifferent land and produces excellent venison (Bond, 1993). Some medieval parks must have been quite large, for many also held red deer for hunting, an extremely popular activity that was normally conducted on horseback with helpers and packs of hounds (Prendergast, 1852). The Royal Park at Glencree, Co. Wicklow, had large stocks of red deer imported from Chester in 1246 (Le Fanu, 1893), while other parks no doubt had stocks of native red deer, a breed so noted for their large size that Giraldus Cambrensis, in his *Topographia Hiberniae* (1183-5), spoke of the stags as being too fat to run fast.

It is apparent from the scattered documentary records available that medieval manors had their own deer parks; indeed, the fashion seems to have been copied by native Gaelic lords beyond the Pale (Weir, 1986). The importance of these parks to their owners is underlined by the considerable expense, skill and care needed in their maintenance. Restocking had to take place regularly, and the deer often had to be fed in winter to avoid starvation, while park boundaries had to be constantly repaired (Birrell, 1992). Deer were frequently also poached; for example in 1305 Richard de Burgo, owner of a deer park at Ballydonegan in Co. Carlow, brought a case against one William Waspayl, accusing him of poaching deer with greyhounds and spears, breaking down some of the park's perimeter paling, stealing timber, digging a pit inside the park, threatening the parker and stealing a spear from the parker's son*.

There was a decline in the number of deer parks in Ireland after the mid fourteenth century, but during the seventeenth and early eighteenth centuries they became very popular again; indeed, by 1740, virtually every large house had its own walled deer park, usually located on the demesne's perimeter or as a detached unit half a mile or more distant. Some of these parks had medieval origins, for example, that at Ballydonegan mentioned above, lying on the fringe of the demesne at Oak Park, Co. Carlow. Like their medieval predecessors, these parks were stocked with fallow deer, some red deer and occasionally also swine cattle: at Portmore, Co. Antrim, Highland swine were imported for the deer park in 1680 (Loeber, 1973). Most deer parks ranged in size from fifty to two hundred acres and usually included areas of tree cover, access to water and a lot of grazing land, for deer are voracious feeders all year round (Whitehead, 1950).

The importance of deer parks declined in the late eighteenth century, with the advent of the turnip and other root vegetables for winter feeding. Many were absorbed into the new landscape parks, as at Tullymore, Co. Down, while others were contracted in size, as at Florence Court, where the old portion is typically labelled 'The Old Deer Park' (Reeves-Smyth, 1990). Feral deer that had escaped from the parks also suffered a decline during

---

* Gibbons (1989) from the Calendar of Justiciary Rolls, Ireland, 1295-1314 (Dublin: HMSO, 1904-5).

this period due to the invention of the breech-loading shotgun, the lack of tree cover and the very high human population levels (Delap, 1936).

During the Victorian era there was a determined attempt by landowners to reintroduce deer into Ireland; these were obtained for the purpose from many forests and parks in Britain, as well as native stocks in Kerry. Small enclosures with wire fencing were often created close to the house, so that the fallow deer could be admired from the windows, as at Crom, Co. Fermanagh, and Ballyfin, Co. Leix. Larger enclosures were created for red deer, as at Caledon, Co. Tyrone, where the herd was later crossed with a wapiti cow from Canada. The park at Colebrooke, Co. Fermanagh, contained both red and fallow deer and a variety of exotic species, notably sambur and sika deer, the latter having been imported from Powerscourt in 1870, where sika were first introduced from Japan in 1860. Sika deer were distributed widely over Ireland and still survive in large numbers, notably at Muckross, where they live alongside the native red deer. Attempts to introduce the roe deer, which has never been native to Ireland, were less successful, though a herd established in the 1870s at Lissadell, Co. Sligo, survived for about thirty years (Whitehead, 1964).

Most Irish deer parks were abandoned in the decade following the outbreak of war in 1914. During the war and especially during the Troubles of 1919-23, park walls were often breached, or as at Charleville, Co. Offaly, the park gates were opened deliberately to prevent the deer from being slaughtered by Republicans (Whitehead, 1964). As a result deer escaped to form the nuclei of small feral herds all over the country.

Deer parks invariably played host to other animals on the demesne, notably rabbits, which were bred in warrens to provide another source of fresh meat in winter. Like the deer, rabbits were introduced from southern Europe by the Normans, who regarded their meat as a great delicacy and considered their fur a valuable commodity (Bettey, 1993). They were kept in large enclosures, fenced to keep out predators, and their former presence on or near demesnes is often indicated by such placenames as 'coneyburrow', 'coneygar', 'coneybank', or occasionally simply 'the warren'. On the basis of comparative English evidence, it can be assumed that most of these warrens contained a group of long, straight or slightly curved banks known as pillow mounds thrown up between parallel ditches, to provide loose soil for the rabbits to dig into. The animals were usually caught in long nets, placed parallel to the bank after they had gone out to feed and intercepting them as they returned to their burrows when chased by dogs (Tebbutt, 1968). Seventeenth-century maps and documents contain many references to warrens, but it is unlikely that they supplied the manor with meat after the mid eighteenth century. Many coastal warrens, however, continued to produce large numbers of rabbits until the early nineteenth century for the fur market. Hares were also kept for food and sport until this period and lived entirely above ground within enclosures, the former presence of which is indicated by such placenames as 'hare warren' or 'hare park'.

Dovecotes or pigeon houses survive on numerous demesnes across Ireland, and their former presence is also frequently attested to by field names and documentary evidence. Aside from eggs and guano, these structures provided yet another supply of fresh meat during the winter months. The birds featured regularly in the menu of the great house from medieval times, and there were numerous recipes available for the cook. Most dishes used the young flightless birds, the squabs or squeakers, which were considered especially delectable (Buxbaum, 1987). The squabs were culled at about four weeks when the flesh was still tender, juicy and fat, without any trace of the toughness brought about by flying (Hansell, 1988 and 1988). The fact that pigeons are highly prolific, producing two chicks about nine or ten times a year, meant that there was a constant supply of food, especially from the seventeenth- and early eighteenth-century dovecotes, which generally had between three hundred and six hundred nesting pairs. By the late eighteenth century the keeping of pigeons for food had declined, but they continued to be kept, particularly for ornament, throughout the nineteenth century. Doves remained a decorative feature of Irish parks and gardens into the present century and were often depicted in contemporary garden paintings, for example, those of Mildred Anne Butler (1858-1941) of Kilmurry, Co. Kilkenny.

Freshwater fish were another important ready supply of food for the manorial table and remained a high-status food until the eighteenth century. In the medieval period there were fisheries all over Ireland, many in the control of monasteries, but most of these were for salmon and eels and only a small number supplied trout and possibly coarse fish (Went, 1955). For the most part, freshwater fish, mainly carp, pike and tench, appear to have been supplied by fish-ponds. These are often mentioned in medieval documents and were common during the seventeenth and eighteenth centuries. At Lismore during the 1630s, for example, there were no fewer than ten ponds in the deer park; these often suffered from flooding and had to be frequently repaired and restocked with tench and carp, some of the latter on one occasion being imported from the Netherlands (Grosart, 1886). Most of the many hundreds of ornamental canals that decorated the formal demesnes of the early eighteenth century served as fish-ponds and are usually labelled as such on maps.

A fish-pond normally comprised a vivarium or breeding pond and a *servatorium* or holding pond. The former was a large dammed area where the fish were allowed to grow fat on the underwater feeding available, while the latter contained the fish ready for eating (Currie, 1990). The fish were caught for the holding pond either by nets or by draining the *vivarium*; the latter method was a large operation, but had to be undertaken regularly to clean the pond. At Castle Ward the large canal known as the Temple Water had a problem with eels, as Michael Ward told his son in a letter dated October 1757: 'Vexed at ye tench being so destroyed but knew before ye eels destroyed ye spawn, if possible more ye pike, I thought I had destroyed all ye eels but find it impossible without draining ye pond every 5 or 7 years, which indeed ought to be done and which ye could now after preserving as many tench as ye can' (McErlean and Reeves-Smyth, 1990).

Fish were also stocked in the artificial lakes that graced many hundreds of landscape parks in the eighteenth and nineteenth centuries. Indeed, one of these lakes – at Montalto in Co. Down – was shaped in the outline of a fish. To improve the ornamental appearance of these lakes, a variety of fowl could be introduced. The mute swan, for example, was desired for its graceful beauty. As early as the 1820s a correspondent to the *Gardener's Magazine* noted the presence of the Australian black swan on the lake at Castle Martyr, near Youghal, together with a variety of what were called 'American geese'. The pinkfooted, Egyptian and Canada geese all arrived in Ireland as ornamental lake introductions.

An important source of food and profit for many demesnes were decoy ponds, devices that originated in Holland in the sixteenth century for catching migratory wildfowl, principally mallard, teal and wigeon (Tarrant, 1990). Evidence from maps, documentary records and aerial photography has to date revealed more than seventy decoy ponds in Ireland, mostly in the east and north of the country. They were located in remote areas, invariably in the deer park or outside the demesne boundary, and comprised a shallow pool, not more than two acres in extent, surrounded by woodland – normally a dense growth of hazel, willow and evergreens – so the wild ducks would not be disturbed by the sights and sounds of the surrounding countryside. A flock of semi-resident mallard ducks were often kept to encourage the wildfowl to use the pond as a daytime refuge; the mallards were usually white in colour so they could be distinguished from those to be slaughtered. Once resident, the birds were enticed into one of the curved channels or pipes that radiated from the pond; each of these had a covering of netting over circular hoops and were lined on one side with high overlapping hurdles to hide the decoyman from view. Bait was sometimes used, but usually the ducks followed or 'mobbed' a specially trained dog as it walked briskly in and out of the hurdles along the steep banks of the pipe, until most of the birds were drawn into the pipe's narrow end and caught (Payne-Gallwey, 1882).

The earliest decoys were built in Ireland during the 1660s (Loeber, 1973), but most belong to the period from 1680 to 1780, after which time there was a dramatic decline in their usage. A number continued operating into the nineteenth century; one at Kilcooley, Co. Tipperary, was discontinued in 1860 and another at Longueville, Co. Cork, survived until the 1920s, the last Irish example to remain in use. There were four pipes in the decoy at Longueville, but after 1865 it was reduced to two and by the 1920s only had one; a typical annual catch in the post-1870 period seems to have been two hundred to four hundred birds per annum (Fox, 1982). Four pipes was the norm for nearly all Irish decoys, the only real exceptions being two elaborate nineteenth-century examples – at Caledon, Co. Tyrone, and Kellyville, Co. Kildare, both built in the mid-1840s. The Caledon decoy had eight pipes and during the thirty years of its use netted 2000 to 3000 ducks a season. The Kellyville decoy had an annual catch of about 1400 ducks from 1872 to 1880, but after the number of pipes was increased from four to six, the wildfowl catch rose to 2500 per season. Most of these were teal and mallard, with no wigeon and only the occasional pintail and shoveller (Payne-Gallwey, 1887).

It may be no coincidence that the decline of the decoy in Ireland was paralleled in the late eighteenth century by the increased popularity of shooting, which was brought about by the introduction of the breech-loading shotgun with which game could be shot in flight. The rise of shooting saw pheasant hatcheries being established on numerous Irish demesnes during the early nineteenth century to meet the increasing demand for larger 'bags'. As the sport became organized, game books were kept and the expenditure on game preservation rose rapidly (Thompson, 1963). Winter feed had to be provided and a staff of gamekeepers employed to rear the birds and protect them from 'vermin', a term that covered foxes, badgers, pine martens, cats and even otters, all of which were ruthlessly trapped or shot. Gun dogs were kept and trained – mostly pointers and retrievers – usually in kennels close to the keeper's house, while the woods, which were planted with laurel and rhododendron to provide cover for the game, had to be intensively managed. Woodland strips were often specially planted for driven shoots and a number of new landscape parks were laid out with shooting rather than picturesque ideals in mind, for example Lisnavagh, Co. Carlow, and Shaen, Co. Leix.

Pheasants dominated the driven game shoots during the nineteenth century, while partridges never figured so prominently as in Great Britain. Some red grouse were shot on the uplands and bogs, but ptarmigan and black grouse seem to have been completely absent. The snipe population never fully recovered from the severe winter of 1854-5 (Payne-Gallwey, 1882), but Ireland had large wintering populations of woodcock and many demesnes maintained shoots specially for them, particularly in the mild western counties of Sligo, Mayo and Galway (McKelvie, 1984).

While gamekeepers waged war with the fox, landowners encouraged them to live and breed outside the demesne walls by creating coverts, usually small areas of trees and undergrowth, which provided shelter, seclusion and ready access by hounds. The fox replaced the stag as the fashionable object of pursuit around the mid eighteenth century, though it was not until the nineteenth century that fox-hunting was systematically organized and the countryside quartered out among regular hunts (Lewis, 1975). The sport absorbed much of the time of the Irish landed classes during the winter months and served as an enormously important social bond among its members during the eighteenth and nineteenth centuries. Many demesnes had their own kennels for hounds, usually located at some distance from the house, while considerable sums were directed towards breeding high-class hunters and bloodstock (Lewis, 1979).

The passion for hunting led to the emergence in eighteenth-century Ireland of 'steeple-chasing', where hunt members would race each other across country. By the early nineteenth century quite a few demesnes had developed their own racecourses. It should not be forgotten that steeple-chasing, like hunting, was a sport 'for the benefit of the participants rather than the spectators. The riders counted first, then the horses, while the onlookers, often literally, also ran' (Watson, 1969). This outlook reflected the wide social divisions between the gentry in their well-kept demesnes and the peasants outside the gates.

Conclusion

In Ireland, demesnes were not just delightful scenery around country houses; for many centuries they dominated developments in the Irish landscape. Their social and economic role has now gone, following the collapse of the estate system early this century, but despite the wholesale destruction that has so often followed their subdivision and sale over the past century, they remain the most significant man-made feature of the landscape.

The surviving residual features of the demesne's former arboricultural, horticultural and agricultural activities contribute to their high scientific and conservation value in the modern landscape. Their mature broad-leaved woodlands, wood pastures, parklands and lakes support rich communities of fauna and flora that are rarely found elsewhere in Ireland. This is perhaps best demonstrated by the detailed biological surveys carried out by the National Trust of its Northern Ireland properties, most notably that of the 1500-acre demesne of Crom, Co. Fermanagh. This survey revealed the presence of 146 lichen species in the demesne woods and parkland; eighteen species of bryophytes; nearly four hundred plant species, including many rare grasses and wild flowers; thirty-five species of *Diptera syrphidae* (hoverflies);

eight species of *Hymenoptera;* sixty-six species of *Lepidoptera* (butterflies and moths); seventeen species of *Micro-lepidoptera;* eleven species of *Odonata* (dragons and damselflies); nineteen species of *Hemiptera-heteroptera;* a variety of mammals and amphibians; and ninety-one species of birds, including wild-fowl, breeding waders and woodland birds (Whatmough and Nelson, 1989).

Had Crom demesne been sold to the Forest Service as originally envisaged in the late 1940s, this great wealth of wildlife would have completely vanished under a monoculture of spruce (Reeves-Smyth, 1989). Although not every demesne boasted such diverse wildlife habitats, it is perhaps sobering to contemplate how much the Irish landscape has lost with the devastation of over 400,000 acres of parkland during the present century. Sadly, the process still continues, for demesnes are seen as attractive locations for such environmentally sterile developments as golf courses and housing estates. Even Carton, Co. Kildare – historically the most important demesne park in Ireland – has recently been granted planning permission for hundreds of houses, two major golf courses and a hotel, while other important but lesser demesnes, such as Rockingham, Co. Roscommon, and Powerscourt, Co. Wicklow, have received permission for similar complexes. Such developments will continue into the foreseeable future, unless there is a greater awareness of the demesne's historical, archaeological and biological importance in the Irish landscape.

References

Anderson, M.L. 1943. 'Items of Forestry Interest from the Statutes Prior to 1800 AD.' *Irish Forestry* 1: 6-26.

Bettey, J.H. 1993. *Estates and the English Countryside.* Landscape Series. London: Batsford.

Birrell, J. 1992. 'Deer and Deer Farming in Medieval England.' *Agricultural History Review* 40: 112-26.

Boate, G., T. Molyneaux, et al. [1726] 1755. *A Natural History of Ireland in Three Parts.* Dublin: Ewing.

Bond, J. 1993. 'The Management of Medieval Deer Parks in England.' *Historic Garden* 6: 27-9.

Bowe, P. 1977. 'Mr Sutherland's Elegant Taste.' *Country Life* 162 (4176): 118-19.

Bowe, P. 1980. 'Some Irish Landscape Gardeners,' in G. Jackson-Stops (ed.), *National Trust Studies.* London: Sotheby Parke Bernet Publications.

Brewer, J.N. 1826. *The Beauties of Ireland: Being Original Delineations, Topographical, Historical and Biographical, of each County,* vol. II (2 vols). London: Sherwood, Gilbert and Piper.

Buxbaum, T. 1987. *Scottish Doocots.* Aylesbury: Shire Publications.

Camblin, G. [1951] 1967. *The Town in Ulster.* Belfast: W.M. Mullan.

Campbell, T (Rev.). [1777] 1778. *A Philosophical Survey of the South of Ireland in a Series of Letters to John Watkinson, M.D.* Dublin: W. Whitestone.

Carter, T. 1984. *The Victorian Garden.* London: Bracken Books.

Currie, C.K. 1990. 'Fishponds as garden features c.1550-1750.' *Garden History* 18: 22-46.

Davies, J. 1987. *The Victorian Kitchen Garden.* London: BBC Books.

Delap, P. 1936. 'Deer in Wicklow.' *The Irish Naturalists' Journal* 6: 828.

Desmond, R. 1994. *Dictionary of British and Irish Botanists and Horticulturalists.* Rev. ed. London: The Natural History Museum.

Diestelkamp, E.J. 1981. 'Richard Turner (c.1798-1881) and his Glasshouses.' *Glasra 5*: 51-3.

Down, K. 1987. 'Colonial Society and Economy in the High Middle Ages,' in A. Cosgrove (ed.), *Medieval Ireland II*. Oxford: Clarendon Press.

Durand, J.F. 1979. 'The History of Forestry in Ireland,' in E.C. Nelson and A. Brady (eds), *Irish Gardening and Horticulture*. Dublin: Royal Horticultural Society of Ireland.

Dutton, H. 1824. *A Statistical and Agricultural Survey of the County of Galway, with Observations on the Means of Improvement*. Dublin: University Press.

Edwards, T.S. 1908. *Irish Forestry Report*. London: Departmental Committee on Irish Forestry: 4857-4961.

Elliott, B. 1986. *Victorian Gardens*. London: Batsford.

Fitzpatrick, H.M. 1933. 'The Trees of Ireland: Native and Introduced.' *Scientific Proceedings of the Royal Dublin Society 20*: 597-656.

Fitzpatrick, H.M. (ed.). 1966. *The Forests of Ireland: An Account of the Forests of Ireland from Early Times Until the Present Day*. Bray: Society of Irish Foresters.

Forbes, A.C. 1933. 'Tree Planting in Ireland During Four Centuries.' *Proceedings of the Royal Irish Academy 41C* (6): 168-199.

Fox, J.B. 1982. 'Duck Decoys in Ireland.' *Irish Wildbird Conservancy News*, July 6.

Garner, W., and R. Webb. 1977. 'Survey of Carton.' *A Report for Kildare County Council*. Dublin: An Foras Forbartha.

Gebbie, J.H. 1972. *An Introduction to the Abercorn Letters As Relating to Ireland, 1736-1816*. Omagh: Strule Press.

Gibbons, M. 1989. 'Deers and Bunnies.' *Bulletin of the Irish Association of Professional Archaeologists 10*:14-16.

Glin, Knight of and J. Cornforth. 1977. 'Killruddery, Co. Wicklow I.' *Country Life 162* (4176): 78-81.

Grosart, Rev. A.B. (ed.). 1886-8. *The Lismore Papers*. 10 vols. London: Author.

Hall, V.A. 1992. 'The Woodlands of the Lower Bann Valley in the Seventeenth Century: The Documentary Evidence.' *Ulster Folklife 38*: 111.

Hansell, P. and J. 1988. *Dovecotes*. Aylesbury: Shire Publications.

Hansell, P. and J. 1988. *Doves and Dovecotes*. Bath: Millstream Books.

Harvey, J.H. 1981. *Medieval Gardens*. London: Batsford Ltd. Rev. ed. 1990.

Harvey, J.H. 1985. 'The First English Garden Book: Mayster Jon Gardener's Treatice and its Background.' *Garden History 13*: 83-101.

Hayes, S.H. 1794. *A Practical Treatice on Planting and the Management of Woods and Coppices*. Dublin: William Sleator. 3rd ed., 1822. Dublin: Samuel Jones.

Hobhouse, P. 1992. *Plants in Garden History*. London: Pavilion.

Hore, H.F. 1858. 'Woods and Fastnesses in Ancient Ireland.' *Ulster Journal of Archaeology 6*: 145-61.

Horner, A. 1975. Carton, Co. Kildare. 'A Case Study in the Making of an Irish Demesne.' *Bulletin of the Irish Georgian Society 19*: 1-45.

Jupp, B. 1993. 'Antrim Castle Gardens.' *Moorea 10*: 28-34.

Lamb, J.G.D. 1951. 'The Apple in Ireland; its History and Varieties'. *The Economic Proceedings of the Royal Dublin Society 4*(1): 1-61.

Le Fanu, T.P. 1893. 'The Royal Forest of Glencree.' *Journal of the Royal Society of Antiquaries of Ireland 23*: 268-80.

Lewis, C.A. 1975. *Hunting in Ireland*. London: J.A. Allen.

Lewis, C.A. 1979. *Horses, Hounds and Hunting Horses*. London: J.A. Allen.

Loeber, R. 1973. 'Irish Country Houses and Castles of the Late Caroline Period: An Unremembered Past Recaptured.' *Bulletin of the Irish Georgian Society 16*: 1-70.

Loudon, J.C. [1822] 1859. *An Encyclopaedia of Gardening*. Ed. Mrs [Jane] Loudon. London: Longman, Brown, Green and Longman.

Loveday, J. 1790. *Diary of a Tour Through Ireland*. London.

McCracken, E. 1971. *The Irish Woods Since Tudor Times: Distribution and Exploitation*. Newton Abbot: David and Charles.

McCracken, E. 1979. 'Nurseries and Seedshops in Ireland,' in E.C. Nelson and A. Brady (eds), *Irish Gardening and Horticulture*. Dublin: Royal Horticultural Society of Ireland.

McErlean, T. 1984. *The Historical Development of the Park at Castle Coole*. Unpublished: National Trust.

McErlean, T. and T.J. Reeves-Smyth. 1990. *Castle Ward Demesne*. 2 vols. Unpublished: National Trust.

McKelvie, C. 1984. 'Woodcock,' in Albert Titterington (ed.), *Irish Fieldsports and Angling Handbook*. Belfast: Appletree Press.

MacLysaght, E. [1950] 1979. *Irish Life in the Seventeenth Century*. Cork: Cork University Press.

Malins, E. and Knight of Glin. 1976. *Lost Demesnes: Irish Landscape Gardening 1660-1845*. London: Barrie and Jenkins.

Malins, E. and P. Bowe. 1980. *Irish Gardens and Demesnes from 1830*. London: Barrie and Jenkins.

Nelson, E.C. 1982. 'The Influence of Leiden on Botany in Eighteenth-Century Dublin.' *Huntia 4*: 133-45.

Nelson, E.C. 1983. 'Some Records (c.1690-1830) of Greenhouses in Irish Gardens.' *Moorea 2*: 2-28.

Nelson, E.C. 1983a. 'Sir Arthur Rawdon (1662-1695) of Moira: His Life and Letters, Family and Friends, and his Jamaican Plants.' *Proceedings of the Belfast Natural History and Philosophical Society 10* (Series 2): 30-52.

Nelson, E.C. 1985. 'Three Centuries of Gardening at Heywood, Ballinakill, Country Laois.' *Moorea 4*: 45-52.

Nelson, E.C. 1990. '"This garden to adorn with all varietie": The Garden Plants of Ireland in the Centuries Before 1700.' *Moorea 9*: 37-54.

Payne-Gallwey, Sir R. [1882] 1985. *The Fowler in Ireland*. Reprinted for the Field Library. Southampton: Ashford Press.

Payne-Gallwey, Sir R. 1887. *The Book of Duck Decoys. Their Construction, Management and History*. London: John Van Voorst.

Pim, S. 1979. 'The History of Gardening in Ireland,' in E.C. Nelson and A. Brady (eds), *Irish Gardening and Horticulture*. Dublin: Royal Horticultural Society of Ireland.

Pococke, R. 1891. *Pococke's Tour in Ireland in 1752*. Edited G.T. Stokes. Dublin: Hodges and Figgis.

Prendergast, J.P. 1852. 'Of Hawks and Hounds in Ireland.' *Transactions of the Kilkenny Archaeological Society 2*: 144-54.

Reeves-Smyth, T.J. 1989. *Crom Castle Demesne*. 2 vols. Unpublished: National Trust.

Reeves-Smyth, T.J. 1990. *Florence Court Demesne*. 3 vols. Unpublished: National Trust.

Reeves-Smyth, T.J. 1991. *Downhill Demesne*. 2 vols. Unpublished: National Trust.

Robinson, W. [1870] 1881. *The Wild Garden, Or, Our Groves and Gardens Made Beautiful by the Naturalisation of Hardy Exotic Plants*. London: The Garden Office.

Robinson, W. [1883] 1906. *The English Flower Garden and Home Grounds*. London: J. Murray.

Sherrard, G.O. and H.M. Fitzpatrick. 1945. 'Early tree planting in Ireland.' *Bulletin of the Royal Horticultural and Arboricultural Society of Ireland 1* (22): 346-58.

Tarrant, A. 1990. 'The Duck Decoy.' *Wildlife and Wetlands Trust 102*: 20-5.

Tebbutt, C.F. 1968. 'Rabbit warrens on Ashdown Forest.' *Sussex Notes and Queries 17*: 52-4.

Thompson, F.M.L. 1963. *English Landed Society in the Nineteenth Century*. London: Routledge & Kegan Paul.

Wakefield, E. 1812. *An Account of Ireland Statistical and Political*. 2 vols. London: Longman.

Walker, J.C. 1799. 'Essay on the Rise and Progress of Gardening in Ireland.' *Transactions of the Royal Irish Academy 4* (Antiquities): 3-19.

Watson, S.J. 1969. *Between the Flags: A History of Irish Steeplechasing*. Dublin: Allen Figgis.

Weir, W.L. 1986. 'Deerparks of Clare.' *The Other Clare 10*: 54-5.

Went, A.E.J. 1955. 'Irish Monastic Fisheries.' *Journal of the Cork Historical and Archaeological Society 60* (191): 47-56.

Westropp, T.J. 1900. 'Excursions of the Royal Society of Antiquaries of Ireland, Summer Meeting, 1900, Third Excursion.' *Journal of the Royal Society of Antiquaries of Ireland 30*: 392-445.

Whatmough, J.A. and B. Nelson. 1989. *Biological Survey for Crom Estate, Co. Fermanagh.* Unpublished: National Trust.

Whitehead, G.K. 1950. *Deer and their Management in the Deer Parks of Great Britain and Ireland.* London: Country Life.

Whitehead, G.K. 1964. *The Deer of Great Britain and Ireland: An Account of their History, Status and Distribution.* London: Routledge and Kegan Paul.

Wyse Jackson, P.S. 1987. 'The Botanic Garden of Trinity College, Dublin 1687 to 1987.' *Botanical Journal of the Linnean Society 10*: 3052.

Zettersten, A. 1967. 'The Virtues of Herbs in the Loscombe manuscript.' *Acta Universitatis Lundensis:* Sectio 1, 5.

Threat and Conservation:
Attitudes to Nature in Ireland

JOHN FEEHAN

Early Views of Nature in Ireland

This green island off Europe's north-west corner is the continent's farthest outpost. New and more efficient ways of exploiting the land, which originated in the European heartland, took longer to reach Ireland, and by the same token tended to survive here longer. For the first four thousand years of its human history, Ireland was inhabited by peoples who lived by hunting and fishing, and by gathering the plants of the wild. We know very little about these earliest inhabitants of Ireland because for them home was not centred on the fixed abode of the farming family, which must fix its place to the annual rhythms of crop and flock. Their impact on the evolving wildwood was little greater than that of the wild animals with which they shared this aboriginal world, and which we can scarcely even imagine today, because that world has disappeared.

The few woods that remain to us are not primeval woods. They merely hint at the wild complexity of the lost forests, but they are the last places that can awaken the sense of wonder that was the birthright of humankind for most of its history, and their conservation today is all the more critical on that account. The early inhabitants' relationship with nature did not centre on the idea of ownership of land necessary to those who farm, but on the sense of being part of nature. And because everything necessary for human life came directly from the natural world, it was understood with an intimacy that was gradually lost as people learned how to grow and rear food in the fields won from the wilderness.

The dominant theme in Irish history from that time on was the retreat of the wild. Fields were won at the expense of the wilderness, even if in the beginning they still retained much of the diversity of wild nature. The creation of this new landscape opened up new opportunities for plants and animals for which the wildwood provided few habitats. In response to the

573

spread of farming, birds like the swallow, the skylark and the corncrake multiplied, adapting their ways to barn and byre. Cowslips and primroses and waxcaps flourished, and at the edges of the fields, along the marches where farmland met the wildwood, hawthorn responded to the light with new riot of blossom at the entry of each summer, establishing a special place in rural lore that is reflected in the special role of the May tree in the custom and practice of Bealtaine (Wilde, 1852).

We know little about how the early farming communities of the Neolithic and Bronze Ages down to 600 BC, and the Celtic Iron Age which followed, valued or appreciated the natural world, beyond hints in the stone monuments and other surviving artefacts of how their world of husbandry revolved around the seasons. Belief and practice were fashioned to keep track of the sun and moon in the heavens, and to ensure their benign influence on the productivity of the earth. But productivity, since the beginnings of agriculture, was conceived in terms of the bounty of the fields won at the cost of such toil from nature: the flow of milk in summer and the golden harvest of autumn. The rest of the natural world was noticed only when it impinged in some way on man's agricultural activities. Larger animals whose ways of life conflicted with those activities could not be allowed the space they needed to live and were forced to the fringes of the cultivated world, to the brink of extinction and finally beyond. The wolf – which occupied a special place in the literature of the early Irish saints (Plummer, 1910) – survived at the edge of the human world until late in the eighteenth century, and only those mammals small or wily enough to adapt their ways survived.

The Celtic View of Nature

Celtic society was a rural society without cities or towns, and the religion of the Celts – and indeed of the peoples who were here before them – was essentially a nature religion, in which sacred places in the wilderness, usually associated with forests or water, took the place of temples. Large numbers of precious and valued objects were deposited in springs and lakes during the Bronze Age. The vast hoard of objects found at Dowris in the nineteenth century were cast into a lake which stood on the edge of the fertile cultivated lands of the rolling moraine country of south Offaly, beyond which lay the uncharted and treacherous wasteland of growing bog (Rosse, 1983-4). It seems likely that the hoard represents an accumulation of votive offerings, cast into the water during the eighth century BC in an annual ceremony connected in some forgotten way with the mystery and awe of the natural world that still framed the cultural life of the Celts and those who came before them. The veneration of wells and springs, water springing crystal-clear out of the earth, survived the conversion of the country to

Christianity to become the holy wells of later centuries, veneration for which has continued into our own time.

The lore of trees was highly developed and practical, because of their central role in the self-sufficient economy, but there was also a more personal and spiritual element in the Celtic attitude to trees. A good example of the two elements is given in the recitation of the Fire Servant in the tale of the Death of Fergus. Here is a version of this recitation in O'Grady's *Silva Gadelica* (1892):

Fer dédh or 'man of smoke' the fire-servant, as in Iubhdan's presence he kindled a fire, threw upon it a woodbine that twined round a tree, together with somewhat of all other kinds of timber, and this led Iubhdan to say: 'Burn not the king of trees, for he ought not to be burnt; and wouldst thou, Ferdedh, but act by my counsel, then neither by sea nor by land shouldst thou ever be in danger.' Here he sang a lay:

'O man that for Fergus of the feasts dost kindle fire, whether afloat or ashore never burn the king of the woods. Monarch of Innisfail's forests the woodbine is, whom none may hold captive; no feeble sovereign's effort is it to hug all tough trees in his embrace. The pliant woodbine if thou burn, wailings for misfortune will abound; drie extremity at weapons' points or drowning in great waves will come after. Burn not the precious apple-tree of spreading and low-sweeping bough: tree decked in bloom of white, against whose fair head all men put forth the hand. The surly blackthorn is a wanderer, and a wood that the artificer burns not; throughout his body, though it be scanty, birds in their flocks warble. The noble willow burn not, a tree sacred to poems; within his bloom bees are a-sucking, all love the little cage. The graceful tree with the berries, the wizards' tree, the rowan, burn; but spare the limber tree: burn not the slender hazel. Dark is the colour of the ash: timber that makes the wheels to go; rods he furnishes for horsemen's hands, and his form turns battle into flight. Tenterhook among woods the spiteful briar is, by all means burn him that is so keen and green; he cuts, he flays the foot, and him that would advance he forcibly drags backward. Fiercest heat-giver of all timber is green oak, from him none may escape unhurt: by partiality for him the head is set aching and by his acrid embers the eye is made sore. Alder, very battle-witch of all woods, tree that is hottest in the fight – undoubtingly burn at thy discretion both the alder and the whitethorn. Holly, burn it green; holly, burn it dry: of all trees whatsoever the critically best is holly. Elder that hath tough bark, tree that in truth hurts sore: him that furnishes horses to the armies from the *sídh* burn so that he be charred. The birch as well, if he be laid low, promises abiding fortune: burn up most sure – and certainly the stalks that beat the constant pods. Suffer, if it so please thee, the russet aspen to come headlong down: burn, be it late or early, the tree with the palsied branch. Patriarch of long-lasting woods is the yew, sacred to feasts as is well known: of him now build ye dark-red vats of goodly size. Ferdedh, thou faithful one, wouldst thou but do my behest: to thy soul as to thy body, O man, 'twould work advantage'.

Trees occupied a special importance in this Celtic experience of the world; they were the dominant voice in the living language of landscape. A reflection of this is seen in the way in which, at the time writing was introduced to Irish, at first as ogham and then through the Latin alphabet, the letters were imagined as trees – as though to reflect the idea that trees are the alphabet of landscape as letters are the alphabet of literature (Kelly, 1976, 1988; Meroney, 1949).

The aspects of nature that were most appreciated were those which cater to human needs, so that among invertebrates only bees were valued, for their honey. The way in which, in Irish as in the etymologies of other European languages, whole groups of creatures are represented by a single name – if at all – reflects the way in which human need and want frame our perception of nature. The uses of plants were widely appreciated – as food and for cures, dyes and other practical things. And not only by the old and experienced in the community: children abroad in the fields knew that *carra mhilis* (*Lathyrus montanus*: heath pea) had knobby liquorice-flavoured tubers that were good to eat, whereas the related *carra mhilis dogs* (*Vicia cracca*: tufted vetch) did not (Colgan, 1911); that the runners of *blioscán* (*Potentilla anserina*: silverweed) could be roasted and eaten; and the deeply-buried tubers of pignut (*Conopodium majus*) were as good as hazelnuts to eat. Such knowledge has been all but lost among their computer-schooled descendants of today.

Nature, however, was not unambiguously benevolent, and appreciation of its beauty was tempered by fear of the unknown. There was much about the processes of nature that was mysterious and unpredictable, and imagination was ever ready to attribute what was not understood to a mythical dimension of the natural world. The real world, therefore, was peopled not merely with the unseen communities of the *sidhe* (the 'good people' or fairies) and other twilight creatures in human form, but with strange creatures that inhabited corners of nature that were beyond the reach of the eye. Deep lakes were inhabited by the *piast*, a monster reptile or hairy beast depending on the particular geographical variant, while the sea was inhabited by the *rosualt*, a monstrous creature that could destroy life on land, in the sea and in the air in a three-year cycle. In the first year it would bury its head in the depths and evacuate the contents of its stomach so as to kill all the fish in its part of the sea and wreck all boats on the surface; the following year it lifted its head above the water and belched out breath so poisonous that all the birds dropped dead; and in the third year it turned towards the land and vomited, causing a pestilential vapour to creep across the country, killing man and animal. Perhaps the *rosualt* had its origins in a desperate human need to account somehow for the pestilence that at times befell crop, herd and shoal, and that defied explanation in an age that had not yet penetrated that microscopic otherworld where disease has its origins (Joyce, 1903).

The darker, threatening side of nature often found embodiment in the imagination as creatures with reptilian form: a universal and oft-debated feature of the human imagination having its origins in who knows what archetypal memories, but more surprising perhaps in a country which has only a single species of reptile – the common lizard – and three amphibians, frog, newt and natterjack. It is a mistrust prevalent to our own day, and our handful of amphibians are not immune to it. In the vegetable kingdom this tradition is well illustrated by Irish mycophobia (fear of fungi), a particularly marked variant of something found everywhere in these islands; it is not that long since Irish mycophobia reached the extremity of people's refusing to eat even the common field mushroom. In the 1870s there was an astonishing abundance of mushrooms about Drogheda after flooding of the Boyne, but although quantities of them were picked and packed in hogsheads and shipped to English markets, the local people refused to eat them on the grounds that, as cows refused them, they could not be good for human beings (Ramsbottom, 1943).

But when people could afford to raise their eyes from the labour of the fields to the natural world at its fringes, which ramified into the man-made world of fieldbanks and walls, hedges, lanes and rivers, the beauty of the manifest natural world, and the mystery it embodied, were deeply felt. This appreciation finds expression through the pens of poets and others whose lives permitted the leisure and provided the training to write. For one brief golden period in Celtic times a new perception broke through, and significantly it developed among a privileged elite whose brief life was not so directly linked to the seasonal cycle of the fields, with its incessant anxiety and worry, and who could therefore afford to lift their eyes and turn their ears to sounds beyond the edges of the fields, listening to the blackbird, the rustle of the leaves, the babbling of brooks, and expressing their new appreciation with an extraordinary freshness of expression in Europe's earliest nature poetry.

Nature in Early Christian Ireland

The pagan adoration of nature in the Irish psyche was severely pruned with the advent of Christianity early in the fifth century AD, but not in a way that would prevent more vigorous new shoots of life and meaning from bursting forth when the time came, nourished by elements of both traditions. That time was between (roughly) AD 800 and 1000, among the Céli Dé, the hermits of Early Christian Ireland. This was around the period of the great Irish anchorite movement sparked off by the inspiration of Maelruain, founder and abbot of Tallaght, and Duiblitir, abbot of Finglas. These men withdrew from the companionship of their fellow men to live lives of undistracted piety and ascetic purity; they lived on a diet of water and wild plants – apples, nuts, nettles, sorrel, garlic, wood-sorrel, and 'the roots of every herb that they could find' (Plummer, 1922) – rediscovering something of the diversity of food plants that the wilderness could provide, and finding communion and a new brotherhood with the beasts of the field. They developed a deep love of the woodland retreats in which they found separation from the world of men. Living this life they discovered God in his creation, the first revelation of his nature, and in harmony with it came closest, perhaps, to the union with God they sought.

The extraordinary poetry they produced is infused with the beauty of observed nature: the voices of birds, wind and sea, rain and storm. The denudation of the landscape in winter, and the green luxuriance and bounty and colour of summer and autumn, are recurrent themes. Birdsong in particular was the voice of nature, and Irish nature poetry is full of passages not only highly lyrical, but fresh in the detail of observation, and vivid with the poets' ability to use words whose very sound mirrors reality. Much of this poetry may seem ponderous in literal translation to English, but in the original it scintillates with sympathy and love for the life of the wild. What characterizes this poetry is its interest in nature for its own sake rather than as the mirror of the poet's subjectivity. What distinguishes it from nature poetry of the classical period and almost all of the other nature poetry of the Middle Ages is its imaginative vitality. Nature features in classical literature, but only as the furniture on the stage of human life (Jackson, 1935). Theocritus listened to the birds and noted the pleasure their song brought the poet, but the hermits lived with the birds; the natural world pervaded their way of life; they absorbed the experience and meditated upon its implications; they developed – centuries before Francis of Assisi – a deep consciousness of the kinship of all life, and of the significance of the divine revelation experienced in nature. Perhaps this early poetry has its roots in attitudes to nature developed and nurtured within the druidic tradition to which nature was so central.

However, the deep sensitivity of the hermits is the appreciation of an elite, and it may be quite different from the outlook and values of ordinary people, who left no record of their values in writing. The gap between the elite and the wider community is perhaps not all that different today, and the consideration of this distance between the reflective few and the many who have less opportunity for reflection is critical. It is usually the latter who most *effectively* relate to the land, are most closely and directly in contact with nature – in the sense that they are the ones who actually bring about most of the change; it is not so easy for them to idealize the natural world, since they are daily confronted with the tribute exacted from nature to make human comfort possible.

With the advent of Roman Christianity, a different view of nature dominates. The new view is grounded in an interpretation of Genesis that sees man's role on earth as subduing and conquering the wilderness; paradise is conceived as the cultivated land of a Garden (Eden), and man's life on earth as a brief sojourn through a valley of tears which is merely preparation for an eternity of happiness in a future life, beyond death, which is not on this earth. There is nothing peculiarly Irish about this perspective on nature. It is the vision that dominates throughout Europe. There were few ripples in Ireland of the brief twelfth-century interlude of Francis of Assisi, who 'discerned perfectly the goodness of God not only in his own soul ... but in every creature' (Okey et al., 1938).

The Celtic nature tradition bursts into poetic flame anew in the *Fiannaíocht* literature of the thirteenth and fourteenth centuries. This body of stories deals with the deeds of the mythical warrior band of the Fianna, and it is filled with vivid imagery of the natural world which was the stage of their adventures. A key figure in it is Oisín, son of Fionn, who had spent three hundred years without ageing in Tír na nÓg, before returning to Ireland, where all his years have caught up with him. Nowhere is this appreciation expressed more movingly than in the 'Song of Oisín', which expresses the change the coming of Christianity brought about, in the language of a contrast between appreciation of the beauty of the natural world and the beauty of a world centred around the man-made things of monastery and church.

> *Sgolghaire luin Doire an Chairn,*
> * búithre an daimh ó Aill na gCaor,*
> *ceol le gcodladh Fionn go moch,*
> * lachain ó Loch na dTrí gCaol.*

> *Cearca fraoich um Chruachain Chuinn,*
> * feadghail dobhrín Druim Dhá Loch,*
> *gotha fiulair Ghlinn na bhFuath,*
> * longhaire cuach Chnuic na Scoth.*

> *An tráth do mhair Fionn 's na Ghiann,*
> * dob ansa leo sliabh ná cill;*
> *ba binn leo-san fuighle lon,*
> * gotha na gclog leo níor bhinn.*

> Throat-song of the blackbird of Doire an Chairn
>   and the stag's call from Aill na gCaor
> were Fionn's music, sleeping at morn,
>   and the ducks from Loch na dTrí gCaol.

> The grouse at Cruachan, seat of Conn,
>   otters whistling at Druim Dá Loch,
> eagle cry in Gleann na bhFuath,
>   cuckoo's murmur on Cnoc na Scoth.

When Fionn and the Fianna lived
  they loved the hills, not hermit-cells.
Blackbird speech is what they loved
  – not the sound, unlovely, of your bells.
(O'Tuama and Kinsella, 1981)

A gleam of the earlier tradition survives in later folk poetry – though here the birds hover on the fringes of a world at whose centre is the garden, into which they sometimes venture, passing finally as an even paler echo into the stylized references of folk music.

But whatever the relationship between the outlook of the hermits and the place of nature in the pre-Christian Irish mind, and whatever the relationship between the few who took themselves apart from the world and the many who were immersed in its day-to-day concerns, attitudes to nature in Ireland in the modern period are essentially dominated by that antagonism towards the earth which has characterized the Western Christian world for most of its history.

Attitudes to Nature in Early Modern Ireland

The landscape of Gaelic Ireland was a highly varied one. Although there was a considerable amount of permanent enclosure, much of the countryside was open land, to accommodate the large herds of cattle with which the Gaelic chieftains measured their wealth and status. This came to an end with the imposition of the new model of agriculture after the sixteenth century, which imposed personal tenure as the norm, and introduced systematic enclosure – though enclosure of the open cattle lands was a gradual process. Ireland did not have a poet to chronicle the passing of the Irish openfield, but the bards of the old school bemoaned 'the open fields crossed by girdles of twisting fences' and 'fairs held in the places of the chase' (McLysaght, 1939).

Considerable areas of woodland survived until the end of the Gaelic period, but in the centuries that followed war was waged against the last woods – because of the refuge they offered outlaws and rapparees, and for short-term economic gain in the form of fuel for the ironworks and other industrial enterprises of entrepreneurs such as Richard Boyle, Earl of Cork, and later as a means of providing Cromwellian grantees with ready cash (McLysaght, 1939; McCracken, 1971). As one poet of the period lamented:

> *Cad a dhéanfaimid feasta gan adhmad?*
> *Ta deireadh na gcoillte ar lár ...*
>
> *Ní chluinim fuaim lachan ná gé ann,*
> *ná fiolar ag éamh cois cuain,*

ná fiu na mbeacha chun saothair
thabharfadh mil agus céir don tslua.
Níl ceol binn milis na n-éan ann
le hamharc an lae a dhul uainn,
ná an chuaichín i mbarra na ngéag ann,
ós í chuirfeadh an saol chun suain ...

Now what will we do for timber,
with the last of the woods laid low? ...

Ducks' voices nor geese do I hear there,
nor the eagle's cry over the bay,
nor even the bees at their labour
bringing honey and wax to us all.
No birdsong there, sweet and delightful,
as we watch the sun go down,
nor cuckoo on top of the branches
settling the world to rest ...
                    (O'Tuama and Kinsella, 1981)

A distinction is sometimes drawn between the new Protestant view of nature – which began to crystallize out after the sixteenth century – and the traditional Catholic view. While it is possible to make too much of the distinction, the modernizing and improving attitude that characterized the reformed religions certainly informed the outlook of the new owners of the land of Ireland, and the biblical injunction to 'subdue the earth and conquer it' took on a new vitality that was to play a key role in the growth of modern science and in shaping contemporary western attitudes to nature. In modern guise it still surfaces in attempts to explain aspects of the difference in the appearance of the countryside on either side of the border.

By our modern standards the most beautiful part of Ireland is perhaps the Atlantic fringe, yet this was settled extensively in modern times only when there was nowhere else to go, by people forced off their farms on the more productive lands and exiled 'to hell or to Connaught', creating a cultural landscape wonderfully harmonious to the outside observer but heartbreakingly difficult to make a living from. Areas such as Connemara have a long history of settlement, but they do not have continuity of settlement. Like many other areas settled in the halcyon days of the postglacial climatic optimum between nine thousand and five thousand years ago, the Tipperary hills were abandoned with climatic deterioration; blanket bog crept up to the edges of the silent megaliths. As the population rose steeply through the eighteenth century and on into the nineteenth, Ireland became a treeless country in a way we could scarcely credit were it not for the numerous contemporary accounts.

By the time of the Famine there was a population of eight million people dependent for their survival on the resources of the immediate environment in which they lived. In the face of such pressure of population upon the land, nature stood little chance. There was no kind of social security; the vast majority of people depended on the support and sustenance they could draw from the particular corner of Ireland in which they lived. Upland heath and bog – and bare rock – were made productive at the cost of very high inputs of fertilizer and labour. Vast amounts of seaweed and sand were hauled from the shore and spread on the bare limestone to create from nothing the little fields of the Aran Islands. Even deep bog was reclaimed. John Gannon may have been an exceptional early-eighteenth-century peasant, but he was certainly not unique. Gannon took on the challenge of reclaiming red *Sphagnum* bog in County Kildare – the most difficult and unpromising kind – with what can only be described as ferocious enthusiasm. His method of preparation was enormously laborious: he dug out the limestone gravel he needed as manure from under seven or eight feet of bog. The result of his labour, besides 'large and numerous clamps of turf' was 'large plantations of fine corn, great gardens affording prolific crops of potatoes, and fine grass, all upon the same black bog, so lately under water'; he also had a garden of cabbage and a bed of garlic, which he shared with his poor neighbours. The Royal Dublin Society's referee, John Wynn Baker, recounted in 1733 how Gannon told him that if by some miracle money ever came his way he would buy a bog with it, 'for that he had rather occupy bog, than "the best land in the nation"' (Baker, 1733).

Under such population pressure, areas of high heritage value that could be dug to grow potatoes had little chance of being left as they were. Inspired by the stories of hidden treasure that are part of the folklore of every part of Ireland, people dug into megalithic tombs and other archaeological monuments. Even the wild integrity of the hidden underworld of caves was not immune. Stalactites that had taken millennia to form and adorned the most silent and undisturbed corner of nature for all those tens of centuries, were torn from their moorings by peasants who sold them for a few shillings to adorn the gardens of a dilettante gentry. Many of the enormous stalactites in the Old Cave at Mitchelstown were removed at the time of the Great Famine in 1847-8 by the starving peasants who sold them to neighbouring landowners (Hill et al., 1909). The activities of zealous gamekeepers in preserving woods, heaths and bogs for the birds and mammals that contributed to their Victorian masters' sport played no small part in the decline of harriers and other birds of prey. Irish ripples of the tide of the egg-collecting hobby, which was so popular and passionately pursued in Victorian England, undoubtedly also played a part.

This despoliation did not stop at the surface. It extended over the edges of the steepest and most inaccessible cliffs. At great risk to life and limb, for example, the cliffsmen of Aran quartered the cliffs for the eggs of nesting sea-birds (Robinson, 1986). In the Burren – perhaps the best example of the way natural richness and diversity have survived in Ireland in spite of, or indeed because of, human activities – the intrepid and entrepreneurial Patrick B. O'Kelly (1852-1937) scoured the land for rare and interesting plants, which he sold. O'Kelly certainly added a good deal to our knowledge of the Burren flora, and attained a certain immortality through having his name tagged to the botanical name of the characteristic Burren orchid *Dactylorhiza fuchsii f. okellyi*. O'Kelly offered for sale an extraordinary variety of wild plants; in one of his later catalogues (1934), big clumps of spring gentians ('no collection [being] complete without this gem of the first water') could be bought for six shillings a dozen, and three bee orchids for half a crown (Nelson and Walsh, 1991). But what is almost as extraordinary as his enterprise is the mildness of the rebuke that greeted his depredations – which reflects the general absence of a sense that there was any real need for conservation at this time. Only below low tide did nature survive in a relatively natural state; and on the banks of the raths where forgotten farmers toiled in the early centuries of the Celtic era, badgers and morels and goldilocks survived, protected by their otherworldly guardians.

The impact of nature poets and of the Romantic movement were minimal in Ireland – except within the walls of the demesnes. Indeed, this identification of an interest and concern for natural and cultural heritage with the leisured class has persisted down to the present. The growth of natural-history societies in Britain and north-west Europe, and the development of a more democratic awareness of the natural world, were not paralleled in Ireland, except in a very limited way through the Naturalists' Field Clubs in the cities. Floras were written for a few special areas by a small group of dedicated naturalists, but the flora of most of Ireland was virtually unknown in any detail until the pioneering work of Praeger.

The identification of nature conservation in the rural mind with a privileged elite ('West Britons and Castle Catholics'), which could afford to spend its abundant leisure time in the collecting and recording of wild plants and insects or in visiting and drawing old forts and castles, has its origins in this period. The identification has survived to our own time, and has been one of the most stubborn of all obstacles in the campaign to educate the community to an environmental consciousness. It still surfaces from time to time, especially when individuals or organizations outside of Ireland voice their opposition to some development in this country, and it is an echo from the past which is still from time to time skilfully exploited by protagonists of development projects who seek to mobilize the political power of the multitude behind them.

A Modern Case-study: Bogs

With the growth in population of the eighteenth century and the great scarcity of wood that resulted from such enormous land pressure, attention focused increasingly on the potential of the last wilderness, the seemingly endless expanses of bogland on the edges of the cultivated world (Feehan and O'Donovan, 1995). In an earlier time the bogs had been less of a wilderness; during the Bronze Age the still pools of the fens and growing bogs had attracted the annual tribute of the community, who deposited their treasured tools and weapons of bronze, and the drier margins of the raised bogs seem to have been exploited for spring grazing. For millennia trackways had been constructed to provide passage across the waste or to give access to precious deposits of bog iron. But in the late centuries BC the growth of the peat accelerated as the climate became even damper, and people had less to do with the bogs: attention only focused on the bogs again as the dearth of wood led increasingly to the need to use peat as fuel. The bogs had been exploited for fuel for centuries, but in the eighteenth century a more systematic attack began. The fringing fens which circled most of the raised bogs were reclaimed for agriculture and people began to nibble away the turf around the edges, a few metres a year. This cutaway fringe would come to constitute a wide aureole around many bogs as decades lengthened to centuries.

The mechanical exploitation of the bogs was regarded as a triumph of the newly independent Irish Free State (established in 1922), ranking alongside the taming of the Shannon and Liffey, a demonstration of how much more efficiently self-determination could develop the indigenous resources of the country.

But eventually it was the disappearance of the bogs that woke the perceptive few – individuals such as John Jackson, J.J. Moore, David Bellamy and Bill Watts, organizations such as the recently established An Taisce (the National Trust for the Republic) – to the realization that the last wilderness in Ireland was disappearing, a parallel in microcosm of the accelerating decline in diversity in the world as a whole. Other areas of natural interest that are suffering continuing reduction and degradation because of activities that can be seen as a response to the availability of European Union funding include the coastal sand formations of machair and dune, and blanket bogs, especially those of the west.

The practice of stocking mountain commonage with sheep instead of cattle is essentially a post-Famine phenomenon. In our own time, one of the most negative environmental consequences of membership of the European Community has been the destruction of blanket bog through overstocking with sheep. This has resulted from the payment of headage premiums on

ewes, which has led to a situation where the value of mountain land is estimated in terms of the number of sheep it can hold, without any regard for
the carrying capacity of the land. ('Hold' is a more appropriate term than
'carry', which has the implication that the land can support them.) It has
also led to increased division of mountain commonage, a trend currently
being fostered by an Irish Farmers' Association campaign, which could have
a dramatic negative impact on the natural quality of hundreds of thousands
of hectares of mountain land in landscape and ecological terms. There is also
a generally disregarded *social* impact, because it may be claimed that the payment of headage premiums encourages individual advancement at the
expense of the community, undermining the spirit of co-operation that is
essential to good commonage management.

In the more vulnerable areas the result has been devastation, in the
most literal sense, leading all too often to the appalling 'deserts of black
slime' of which Michael Viney and Frank Mitchell write with such despair
(Mitchell, 1993; Viney, 1994): 'greasy black tongues and terraces of naked
peat, sometimes (as in the Maam Valley) a whole hillside of degraded commonage oozing down to the road', extending farther and farther into the last
corners of mountain wilderness all down the west coast. The peat mud is
washed away by rain; when it dries the hard flakes and nuggets of baked
mud are blown away or carried to the nearest stream by surface runoff,
exposing more and more of the bare rock beneath. In spring and summer
the silt clogs the spawning beds of trout and salmon, and in winter it often
stains the ocean off the mouths of the rivers that carry it from the land.

Contemporary Concern for Nature

Public concern for what is happening to the natural world is essentially a
post-World War II phenomenon, the product of growing awareness of the
devastating pollution of soil, water and the atmosphere and the consequences
for human living, especially since the Industrial Revolution; of the appalling
reduction of biodiversity and natural habitat that has made our brief human
era the greatest and swiftest era for the extinction of life the earth has ever
known; of the consequences of the growing greenhouse effect and ozone
depletion.

In Ireland there was increasing concern during the 1960s that sites of
scientific, historical, archaeological, architectural and cultural importance
were being seriously destroyed or degraded through many kinds of development on the one hand, and through neglect and ignorance on the other.
The first important milestones in the development of a modern awareness
of the need for nature conservation in the Republic of Ireland were the publication of two reports for An Taisce; the first of these was prepared in 1958

by Micheál Ó Ruadháin, the other in 1963 by John Jackson and others (Finlay et al.).

Northern Ireland's nature conservation policy was largely shaped by those devised in Britain after World War II, and relies on the twin strategies of designation and statutory control on the one hand, and acquisition into public ownership on the other. However, as in Britain, voluntary bodies such as the National Trust (established in Northern Ireland as a semi-independent regional organization in 1936), the Royal Society for the Protection of Birds (1966) and the Ulster Trust for Nature Conservation (1978) have been more active in the actual acquisition of land for protection. Public concern about nature conservation was, however, considerably less than in Britain; since the pressure on land was so much less than in Britain, there appeared to be less cause for anxiety over the impact of development on natural areas. The political atmosphere among local administrations, which did not see land-use planning as a proper function of government, reinforced this apathy (Buchanan, 1982). However, the Unionist government was committed to moving in parallel with Britain, and although the publication of the important *Report on the Ulster Countryside* (1947) had little impact at the time, it provided much of the inspiration for the 1965 Amenity Lands Act, which drew up a coherent policy of landscape protection and nature conservation for Northern Ireland. The Act provided for the designation of National Parks and Areas of Outstanding Natural Beauty, for the acquisition of land as Amenity Parks, and for the establishment of a network of National Nature Reserves and Areas of Scientific Interest.

The influence of bodies like the National Trust and the Royal Society for the Protection of Birds, as well as the work of field clubs and extramural courses (particularly those organized by Estyn Evans), was much more important in the shaping of public opinion in Northern Ireland than were bodies in the Republic. In the Republic, An Taisce is still frequently identified in the rural mind with the privileged naturalists of an earlier generation.

A report published in 1969 by An Foras Forbartha (Protection of the National Heritage) led to the setting up of a National Heritage Inventory working party to co-ordinate the preparation of a report on Areas of Scientific Interest (ASIs). This led to the compilation of the first attempt at a systematic national inventory of areas of scientific interest in the Republic, published in 1981. This report identified 1059 ASIs covering a total of 231,500 hectares of land, which is roughly 3 per cent of the country (including tidal mudflats). In the years following 1969, reports on ASIs in each county were prepared by An Foras Forbartha for local authorities, and much of the information in these surveys was incorporated into County Development Plans. A national report on the status of peatlands (*Peatland Sites of Specific Interest in Ireland*) was prepared from the county surveys by

An Foras Forbartha in 1980 at the request of the Wildlife Advisory Council.

Continued surveying in the ensuing years saw the number of sites grow to nearly 2000, but many sites listed in the original report had deteriorated or been destroyed in the interim; the number now stands at around 1650. In addition to the ASIs there are some 1300 Protected Flora Sites, although these overlap considerably with the ASIs. There are also various other kinds of environmentally related designations (An Taisce, 1993), but only about a tenth of the total designated area enjoys strict protection as Nature Reserves or in national parks. A small number of designations (such as Ramsar Convention Sites for the protection of wetlands) apply to the entire island.

The national survey (An Foras Forbartha, 1981) was a milestone of the greatest importance in the identification of the Republic's natural heritage, but it had a number of weaknesses. Little attempt was made to further public awareness, appreciation or support, and owners of land were not informed if they had ASIs on their property. This meant that a landowner who began a land-use development in the legitimate expectation of grant aid might find the project was ineligible because of ASI status. This happened in 1989, when planning permission was refused for an airport on Roundstone Bog in County Galway because it was an ASI of international importance. The ensuing controversy resulted in a High Court decision (later upheld by the Supreme Court) that ASIs had no legal basis because the Wildlife Service had failed to inform landowners.

In 1992 the Wildlife Service, funded partly by the Office of Public Works and partly through the EC LIFE programme, initiated a comprehensive re-survey of the Areas of Scientific Interest, with the dual aim of checking and reviewing the status and boundaries of these areas prior to their re-designation as Natural Heritage Areas, and to establish an up-to-date computerized Sites Database. One of the results of the NHA Survey is likely to be that the number of sites will shrink to something like 1600 from nearly 2000 because of the destruction or amalgamation of sites.

The drawing of boundaries on maps and describing of the biota inside the reserves is the easy part. The more difficult challenge is to convince those who own these precious pockets of land – those surviving patches where some whisper of the richness of this island as it was before our arrival still remains – that their tenure is not absolute, that they are guardians of a heritage that belongs to the whole community.

The systematic and detailed mapping of the country by the Ordnance Survey in the nineteenth century froze the cultural landscape, and transferred responsibility for the naming of place and the setting of boundaries and meanings from the tradition and experience of the community to an arm of the central government. The delineation of Natural Heritage Areas may do something similar for the natural inheritance of the landscape, setting fixed boundaries on map and landscape that are designed to protect that heritage, but that at the same time may carry the implicit message that everything outside the boundaries is of lesser value. But there are many areas outside the refuges of the reserves that are of greater importance than many of those protected within these 'Pales' of the natural world, and in any case the diversity of the landscape is too complex and continuous for such a simple dichotomy of natural value to do it full justice.

The concept of Environmentally Sensitive Areas (ESAs) goes some way towards recognition of the natural and cultural heritage of the landscape as a whole, and imbues the heritage landscape with an economic dimension. It has the capacity to provide a *context* for the Natural Heritage Areas, through which the values that define the latter can filter into the landscape through the network of hedges and walls, the wilder corners of fields, the fringes of lowland bogs, and the wild high lands of hill and mountain.

This scheme was devised as part of the re-evaluation of the EC Common Agricultural Policy (CAP), brought about by over-production and growing awareness of the economic inadequacy of the policy and of the environmental consequences of the policy's implementation. In parallel with the reduction of support for production-orientated systems, a series of measures designed to protect the natural and cultural heritage of the farmed landscape were introduced.

The most important of these was the ESA scheme, under which payments were made to encourage farming practices that maintain or enhance natural diversity and the cultural character and detail of the landscape. The scheme was outlined in the revision of the Agricultural Structures Directives published in 1985; payments to seven areas designated in the United Kingdom commenced in 1987. A review of the first five years of the scheme in 1992 showed that it has operated with considerable benefit both to the participating farms in designated areas and to the natural environment. The scheme was effectively implemented in Northern Ireland, where the Mourne Mountains and Slieve Croob were the first areas to be designated; the number of designated areas has now grown to five, covering some 20 per cent of the agricultural land area of Northern Ireland (DANI, 1993).

The opportunity to designate ESAs in the Republic was not taken up until 1991, when a small part of Slieve Bloom in counties Laois and Offaly, and Slyne Head in Co. Galway, were designated as the country's first ESAs. However, the decision to designate Slieve Bloom – or rather, three of the District Electoral Divisions in the area – was taken on political grounds, with little regard for the ecological criteria that should have been the determining factor in designation. The take-up of the scheme was slow in the beginning, partly because of lack of information and partly because of the inadequacy of the subvention – a maximum premium of £50 per hectare up to an overall maximum of £1000 per farm. Although this is not negligible in the context of the very low incomes of many farm households in the area, it is far less than the payments made under the scheme in Great Britain and Northern Ireland.

CAP reform provides the opportunity to define, on a bioregional basis, a proper management policy for the conservation of the natural and cultural landscape. But it needs to be defined in detail, with imagination and with adequate resources, and it needs to be tailored to the problems and opportunities of each particular region. The new Rural Environment Protection Scheme (REPS), the details of which were announced by the Department of Agriculture at the end of January 1994, and which came into effect later that year, provides a new opportunity. The aims of the scheme are as follows: (1) the establishment of farming practices and controlled production methods that reflect the increasing public concern for conservation, for landscape protection, and for wider environmental problems; (2) the protection of wildlife habitats and of endangered species of plants and animals; (3) the production of quality food in an environmentally friendly way.

The scheme will cost £230 million over its first three years, 75 per cent of it funded by the EU. Under the terms of the scheme, farmers are paid £122 per hectare (£50 per acre) up to a maximum of forty hectares (one hundred acres) for implementing environmental management plans, which must be approved by Teagasc (the Irish government's agricultural advisory and research service) or other accredited agencies, on their farms. The management plans include measures for waste storage, controls on the application of fertilizers and lime and on overgrazing, and the retention of wetlands and such cultural features as stone walls and traditional buildings. The scheme includes a ban on such practices as stubble and straw burning, the use of cereal growth regulators, and the use of pesticides and fertilizer on field margins. An additional 20 per cent is paid in certain areas for avoiding the degradation of commonage, preserving areas of natural heritage or scientific interest, setting aside land for twenty years, granting public access, and providing leisure facilities on farmland, organic farming and the keeping of rare breeds. Some of these measures only apply in NHA and other designated areas. The package also includes a payment of £100 to each farmer completing a twenty-hour training programme in environmentally-sensitive farming with Teagasc or other approved training agencies.

The nature and emphasis of the different practices to be carried out vary from region to region: for example, in areas where the maintenance of ecological diversity depends in large measure on the continuation of traditional farm practices such as hay-making on the Shannon callows, these would be continued. Along with such conservation measures, the scheme provides an opportunity for ecological enhancement schemes such as broadleaved planting and the upgrading of surviving woods and scrub areas.

If properly applied, other aspects of the scheme will also have significant implications for nature conservation. The provisions that relate to extensification could reduce or solve the problem of overstocking by sheep in hill areas by providing a counter-incentive to the ewe premium. Decreased fertilizer use may be expected to reduce problems of eutrophication (the ecological effects of increased nutrient input), while lower stocking rates in general (if they come about) will reduce pressure on semi-natural ecotopes. But it needs to be emphasized that the new scheme stands little chance of real success unless it is underpinned not merely by a serious campaign to inform and educate farmers about aims and methods of the scheme, but by a wider educational campaign about the role and importance of the natural heritage for the whole community.

In 1988 the first of a series of Red Data Books embracing the whole island of Ireland was published. These books, which list threatened species in various groups, are intended to provide necessary background to enable Ireland to meet its obligations under the EU Birds and Habitats Directives. The first volume dealt with rare and threatened flowering plants (Curtis and McGough, 1988), and was followed in 1993 by a volume for vertebrates (Whilde, 1993). A series of Red Data books for Ireland and Britain are also being produced; the first of these appeared in 1992 (Stewart and Church, 1992).

Community Awareness

The conservation of the natural and cultural heritage of the landscape cannot be achieved solely through the designation and management of individual sites and monuments as isolated museums or reserves. There is also a need for conservation and management of the countryside matrix in which the sites are set. As Ratcliffe (1977) has argued, a constellation of protected sites 'by no means satisfies the total requirement' for nature conservation. 'There is a need to conserve the much greater part of the national capital of wildlife and habitat which lies outside this relatively small sample.' The diversity and richness of the environment as a whole must be maintained and promoted, however important the special protection of key sites may be. The designated areas account for only a tiny percentage of total land cover, and populations of many plants and animals are unlikely to be viable unless these areas are maintained within a supporting larger population.

Designated key areas of special natural interest are best protected within the awareness, pride and sense of care of the entire community whose special heritage they are. At present we cannot pretend that such awareness is widespread, and so it is necessary that these sites be protected by law against individual ignorance or selfishness. But it would be wrong to think that if we manage to protect these sites like oases in the middle of a productive desert we have protected our material natural heritage. The essential process of designating focal areas needs to be balanced and supported by an intensive and extensive campaign to create an awareness of the enormous importance of these areas, and a growth in recognition that they are an essential part of the *common wealth of the community*. We may seek for inspiration for this new attitude to nature in the lives of the early Irish saints discussed earlier, for it needs to be a moral imperative. But how it is to be done is a larger question.

In one shape or another, the criteria that provide the guidelines for the selection of areas to be designated for conservation because of their natural interest follow those set out by Ratcliffe, but it may be argued that these are inadequate in the Irish context. In a country where so little of wild nature remains, there is a need to maximize the opportunities for the regeneration of ecological diversity. Many of the areas currently listed as ASIs or NHAs have regenerated from a stage of impoverishment within historic times – eskers and most woodlands, for instance. If the perspective is extended to a few millennia, even the Burren must be regarded as a regenerated area. Inadequate consideration is given to the identification on the basis of ecological vitality of areas that have realistic possibilities of re-acquiring natural diversity. Cutover peatlands – hand-cut bogs – are profoundly important in this regard, but there are many other situations – for example, overgrazed machair and sand dunes, eroded blanket bog and heath. It should also be possible to encourage regeneration on some mineral soils, since over-production within the EU means that less land is now needed for food production.

The New Value of Nature

One of the most important developments of recent years has been the acquisition of a monetary value by areas of special natural heritage. Very often the reason such areas were able to retain their natural diversity in the first place was because they were too difficult – too rocky, too boggy – to be made productive, or because they were marginal areas where less intensive or mechanized methods of management were not applied. In the thinking of traditional agriculture, these areas were looked on as underdeveloped, with little potential to contribute to farming income. With the payment of the new subsidies to farmers to leave important natural areas alone, or to manage their land in ways conducive to the maintenance or enhancement of their natural interest, such areas take on a new economic dimension, contributing by virtue of their natural interest to rural income.

Two developments give a new monetary dimension to natural areas: the payment of subsidies to owners of ESAs and NHAs (and, under the new REPS, the semi-natural farmed landscape as a whole), and the acquisition by natural areas of new value as a resource in rural tourism. The establishment of the NHA network is particularly important in this regard, because the new REPS set up as part of the reform of the Common Agricultural Policy includes a provision for the payment of subsidies to farmers whose lands include an NHA. This provides for the first time an economic incentive of widespread application to habitat conservation. It carries with it, however, two dangers: that this may be taken as the *real value* of these places (whereas it is in fact merely a 'lowest common denominator' form of shadow pricing), or that areas valued in this way are the *only* natural areas that matter for nature conservation.

The expansion of rural tourism reflects the growing concern for environmental heritage, particularly in the European Union. New standards in education, coupled with the pace of modern urban life, give natural living and traditional landscapes a new attraction and meaning. The countryside has become a place increasingly valued as a world to which people can escape, a world that is imagined to enshrine a simple life rooted in tradition and the past, where values and dimensions lost to the city dweller can still be experienced. The entire rural landscape thus becomes a potential resource which may be developed for this new market, with important natural and cultural features as focal points. An indication of the growing importance of rural tourism in Europe is the fact that in the most important sector of activity within the EU's LEADER programme, tourism is the dominant activity in the business plans of 71 of the 217 LEADER areas; it features to some extent in the majority of others (Requena and Avilés, 1993).*

To a considerable extent, government 'investment' in nature conservation is made in the expectation of enhanced revenues from tourism. There is a real danger that the ready availability of funds for tourism will result in unsustainable, inappropriate exploitation of the natural resource through short-sighted self-interest. But the resources provided to communities through such programmes as LEADER are enormously significant because they enhance the prospect for the preservation of areas of natural and cultural value – because of the new economic dimension these areas acquire – while at the same time increasing awareness in the host community of the nature and significance of these features. The vision of the host community may thereby be enhanced by that of the visitor (Feehan, 1992).

---

* LEADER is the most important programme for the direct support of joint development initiatives devised and implemented by local communities in Objective I areas – those with a development lag – and Objective 5B areas: fragile rural areas, which include the whole of Ireland.

The New Greening of Ireland

We are at a crossroads, as we look to the future nature of Ireland across the threshold of the new millennium, at a time when the world's biodiversity is being ravaged. The attitudes of the past, essentially pragmatic and utilitarian, tinged by superstition, have come down to our own day. However, the growth of a new sense of value and meaning in nature comes from two directions. There is, first of all, the powerful influence of the 'New Thinking' on environment in the world in general and the developed world in particular, focused in a particularly powerful way in our own case through the legislative impact of EC membership. Membership of the EC (which Ireland joined in 1973) has not always had a positive environmental impact; indeed, in the early years of intensification and agricultural expansion, it was profoundly damaging to wild nature through grant support for developments that were economically of marginal value (which was the main reason most of them had not already been carried out). For example, without the support of the Western Package (special EU measures designed to promote rural development in the most disadvantaged parts of western Ireland), such environmentally destructive arterial drainage projects as those of the Boyne, Corrib, Mask and Robe could hardly have been implemented. The drainage of countless small wetlands and the afforestation of blanket bog were also funded under the Western Package. More generally, farm intensification in general was encouraged, resulting in the appalling water pollution of the 1980s.

The second new source of respect for nature in the Republic of Ireland has come from the Catholic Church. Here the new thinking has ultimately the same source as has the vernacular environmental perspective of the EU, and early echoes of it (in the case of the Catholic Church) can be found in the documentation of the Second Vatican Council. The New Theology claims a moral perspective for environmental awareness, grounding it in our responsibility to appreciate the natural world as God's first revelation, before all written scriptures, and to respect and preserve the goodness and integrity of God's earth, for which we are answerable.

A number of Irish theologians have played a role in shaping the new thinking on creation, and spreading the new 'gospel of Ecology'. Foremost among these is Sean McDonagh, who takes the new story of creation so eloquently articulated in the writings of the French Jesuit Teilhard de Chardin and the American monk Thomas Berry (Berry, 1988) and gives it an Irish perspective (McDonagh, 1986).

Some few, especially among the young, seek a deeper ethical ground in the inherent rights of nature through the Deep Ecology movement, which accords to wild creatures rights to the earth as fundamental as our own. Or they seek a deeper ground in the rediscovery of the Celtic view of nature, or at least in a modern re-interpretation of it. This minority is at its strongest within the walls of academe and in conservation groups that are concerned about the reduction of natural and cultural diversity in the modern Irish landscape. It is often, however, a concern that is focused through the lens of an individual's or a group's special chosen interest, in the way concern for salvation is quite differently focused through the different religions. But the hearts that must be won beat outside the ivory towers of academe.

As Aldo Leopold pointed out three decades ago, the conviction and concern of the thoughtful few do not constitute a land ethic: it must evolve within the community as a whole (Leopold, 1966). But slowly the sea change is occurring, facilitated by changes in educational programmes, extended through the possibilities of the 'New Media' (telecommunications, computerization, multimedia, etc.), and directed through the EC's environmental policy.

The voices of ecological prophets, the campaigns of dedicated activists, and developments in formal education and in the thinking of the churches, are important catalysts in the promotion of community concern for the natural environment and in fostering an Irish environmental ethic. Only through the schools can such an ethic be widely promoted, and here much remains to be done. But the most important developments in bringing about a change of attitude to nature in Ireland include increasing interest from the media, the growth of rural community empowerment, and the new economic dimension to natural heritage. One of the outstanding contemporary developments in Ireland is this growing understanding and appreciation of new environmental values within rural communities.

The greatest challenge of the new millennium will be to shape a new Irish environmental ethic. This may be grounded in the new world view of global and universal ecology and environmental responsibility, but it will for some look in a special way to the Irish past, drawing inspiration from the countless holy ones who lived in the dawn of Irish Christianity, like Ciarán of Saighir whose first disciple was brother boar, later to be joined by brothers fox, badger and deer, or the nameless author of the twelfth-century poem in *Buile Suibhne* who wrote with love of the bushes in his wood – 'hazel bush, little branchy one', 'bramble, little humped one' – knowing in his spirit, as we now know in a different way through the marvellous insight of our new science, that we are truly kin with the badger and boar, the bramble and oak, even of sister fire and brother rock, and, indeed, have too the very stars for kin.

References

Baker, J.W. 1733. *The Reclaiming and Cultivation of a Bog in Co. Kildare, by Wentworth Thewles Esq., Viewed and Examined in August Last, by the Desire of the Dublin Society and Now Reported in Pursuance Thereof.* Dublin: S. Powell.

Berry, T. 1988. *The Dream of the Earth.* San Francisco: Sierra Club Books.

Buchanan, R.H. 1982. 'Landscape: the Recreational Use of the Countryside,' in J.G. Cruickshank and D.B. Wilcock (eds), *Northern Ireland: Environment and Natural Resources.* Belfast: Queen's University and the New University of Ulster.

Buchanan, R.H. 1992. 'Issues in Tourism and Environment in Northern Ireland,' in J. Feehan (ed.), *Environment and Development in Ireland.* Dublin: Environmental Institute, University College Dublin.

Colgan, N. 1911. 'Gaelic Plant and Animal Names, and Associated Folk-Lore.' *Proc. R. Ir. Acad. 31:* 1-29.

Curtis, T.G.F. and H.N. McGough. 1988. *The Irish Red Data Book. I Vascular Plants.* Dublin: Stationery Office.

Department of Agriculture, Northern Ireland. 1993. *Environmentally Sensitive Areas: Explanatory Booklet and Guidelines for Farmers.* Belfast.

Feehan, J. (ed.). 1992. *Tourism on the Farm.* Dublin: UCD Environmental Institute.

Feehan, J. and G. O'Donovan. 1996. *The Bogs of Ireland: An Introduction to the Natural, Cultural and Industrial Heritage of Irish Peatlands.* Dublin: Environmental Institute, University College.

Finlay, W., J.S. Jackson, D.A. Webb and A.E.J. Went. 1963. *Preliminary Report from the Sub-committee on Nature Conservation.* Dublin: An Taisce.

An Foras Forbartha. 1969. *The Protection of the National Heritage.* Dublin.

An Foras Forbartha. 1980. *Peatland Sites of Scientific Interest in Ireland.* Dublin.

An Foras Forbartha. 1981. *National Heritage Inventory: Areas of Scientific Interest in Ireland.* Dublin.

Hill, C.A., H. Broderick and A. Rule. 1909. 'The Mitchelstown Caves, Co. Tipperary.' *Proc. R. Ir. Acad. 27B:* 235-68.

Jackson, K. 1935. *Studies in Early Celtic Nature Poetry.* Cambridge: Cambridge University Press.

Joyce, P.W. 1903. *A Social History of Ancient Ireland.* 2 vols. London: Longmans.

Kelly, F. 1976. 'The Old Irish Tree-List.' *Celtica 11:* 107-24.

Kelly, F. 1988. *A Guide to Early Irish Law.* Dublin: Institute for Advanced Studies.

Leopold, A. 1966. 'The Land Ethic,' in *A Sand County Almanac.* New York: Ballantine.

McCracken, E. 1971. *Irish Woods since Tudor Times.* Newton Abbot: David and Charles.

McDonagh, S. 1986. *To Care for the Earth: A Call to a New Theology.* London: Chapman.

McLysaght, E. 1939. *Irish Life in the Seventeenth Century: After Cromwell.* Dublin and Cork: The Talbot Press.

Meroney, H. 1949. 'Early Irish Letter-Names.' *Speculum 24:* 19-43.

Mitchell, F. 1993. 'Who is Going to Shout STOP?' *Living Heritage 10:* 3-4.

Nelson, E.C. and W.F. Walsh. 1991. *The Burren: A Companion to the Wildflowers of an Irish Limestone Wilderness.* Aberystwyth and Kilkenny: Boethius Press and The Conservancy of the Burren.

O'Grady, S.H. 1892. *Silva Gadelica: A Collection of Tales in Irish.* 2 vols. London and Edinburgh: Williams and Norgate.

Okey, T., E. Gurney Salter and R. Steele. 1938. *'The Little Flowers' and the Life of St Francis with the Mirror of Perfection.* London: Dent; New York: Dutton.

Ó Ruadháin, M. 1958. *Preliminary Survey of Areas and Objects of Natural Beauty or Interest.* Dublin: An Taisce.

Ó Tuama, S. and T. Kinsella. 1981. *An Duanaire 1600-1900: Poems of the Dispossessed.* Mountrath: Dolmen Press.

Plummer, C. 1910. *Vitae Sanctorum Hibernae.* Vol. I. Oxford: Clarendon Press.

Plummer, C. 1922. *Bethada Náem nÉrenn: Lives of Irish Saints.* 2 vols. Rpt. 1968. Oxford: Clarendon Press.

Ramsbottom, J. 1943. *Edible Fungi.* London: Penguin.

Ratcliffe, D.A. 1977. *A Nature Conservancy Review.* 2 vols. Cambridge: Cambridge University Press for the Nature Conservancy Council and the Natural Environment Research Council.

Report on the Ulster Countryside. 1947. Belfast: Amenity Committee of the Planning Advisory Board.

Requena, J.C. and P.R. Avilés. 1993. 'Tourism: an Opportunity for Disadvantaged Rural Areas?' *LEADER Magazine. 4*: 6-9.

Robinson, T. 1986. *Stones of Aran: Pilgrimage.* Dublin: Lilliput Press in association with Wolfhound Press.

Rosse, A. 1983-4. 'The Dowris Hoard.' *Éile 2*: 57-65.

Spellerberg, I.F. 1981. *Ecological Evaluation for Conservation. Institute of Biology Studies in Biology No. 133.* London: Edward Arnold.

Stewart, N.S. and J.M. Church. 1992. *Red Data Books of Britain and Ireland: Stoneworts.* Peterborough: Joint Nature Conservation Committee.

An Taisce. 1993. *Evaluation of Conservation Designations in Ireland.* Interim Unpublished Report. Dublin: National Heritage Council.

Usher, M.B. (ed.) 1986. *Wildlife Conservation Evaluation.* London and New York: Chapman and Hall.

Viney, M. 1994. 'When Land Turns to Slime.' *The Irish Times*, 15 January.

Whilde, A. 1993. *Threatened Mammals, Birds, Amphibians and Fish in Ireland. Irish Red Data Book 2: Vertebrates.* Belfast: HMSO.

Wilde, Sir W. 1852. *Irish Popular Superstitions.* Rpt. 1972. Dublin: Irish University Press.

Wildlife Service. 1989. *Index to Areas of Scientific Interest.* Unpublished. Dublin.

The Culture of Nature

JOHN WILSON FOSTER

Perceiving Nature

The idea has lately taken hold among cultural theorists that our systematic understanding of nature owes as much to culture as to science. For example, the cultural coding in what might appear to be the objectivity of map-making is being increasingly recognized. Maps are now understood plurally as communication systems, models of reality, geopolitical claims, and gauges of cultural perception. A history of the influence of map-making on the perception and cultural representation of Ireland remains to be written, though Andrews (1975 and in this volume) has furnished much of the foundational data for such a history. There are some general questions that could be posed. How do maps influence the way non-cartographers see the 'real' three-dimensional landscapes of Ireland? Conversely, how, and how far, do *cultural* perceptions of Ireland influence the reading of a map? How do cultural and political perceptions interrelate in map-reading? How does the map-maker represent the connections on Irish maps between topographical, historical and political boundaries and features, and how does the map-reader interpret them? Has the cartographic evidence of the intimacy between Ireland and Britain (on a map of the British Isles, the larger island can seem to embrace benignly or threateningly the smaller) influenced a political and social sense of the relationship between the two sets of inhabitants and the two polities? (Seamus Heaney has in his poem 'Act of Union' offered in extended allegory some implications of an anthropomorphic connection between the two islands on the map.)

We know the military and political importance of maps to the English colonists and administrators of the sixteenth and seventeenth centuries: what was the nature of their importance thereafter, and to whom? The makers of maps since early settlement days include ordnance surveyors, antiquarians, linguists, mining and military engineers, naturalists, rebels, compilers of atlases and tourist boards, and all have had their readers. The charting of Ireland composes a largely uninvestigated history of a paper island (i.e. of perception and representation), but one that has lived fitfully and vividly in the imagination. Such charting accelerated in the nineteenth century and has continued, newly impelled by the revolution in computer graphics.

There are other ways than mapping of perceiving and representing the landscape and its life-forms. In a valuable study, Gifford (1990) has speculated on the cultural importance of the nineteenth-century technology of visual perception of the natural world, which produced an epistemological paradigm shift that occurred in Ireland as well as England. The telescope and microscope were, of course, of considerable age, and the Claude glass and camera obscura were invented in the eighteenth century, but the following century saw an astonishing sequence of optical instruments or techniques that reproduced images of nature: the camera lucida (1807), the graphic telescope (1811), the kaleidoscope (1816), the diorama (1822), and the stereoscope (1838). The binocular telescope and the microscope were re-invented around the time the stereoscope was developed. Photography is a mid-nineteenth-century invention (Schaaf, 1992), and in 1895 the kinetoscope (1891) was combined with a seventeenth-century invention, the magic lantern, to produce the motion picture. All along, these inventions were 'training the eye to the mediating presence of the optical instrument' (Gifford, 1990), fulfilling Coleridge's belief that we half-create, half-perceive the world.

Such instruments have clearly played an important role in natural history, increasing the naturalist's capacity to see nature at a distance or in detailed close-up. So too has the technical ability to reproduce the resulting images. But images are not merely helpful for purposes of teaching and illustration; they set up expectations over time in the observer which are then imposed on nature as surely as the observer's emotional state to which Coleridge alluded.

Also important has been the creation of images directly from nature. Drawings and paintings made in the field for purposes of record and identification have the greatest immediacy and utility of all images, and they increased in urgency and importance in exploration and expeditions. For example, 'importation of foreign species to Europe was haphazard', writes Jackson (1994),

until the organisers of voyages of exploration and discovery followed the example set by Sir Joseph Banks on Captain Cook's circumnavigations in the 1770s. The consequences of sending trained artists, botanists and zoologists on voyages of discovery were profound. The roles of the draughtsmen on board ship were clearly defined. The professional artist painted landscapes, topographical artists drew the shoreline and recorded the territory. The naturalists drew the plants, animals, insects, amphibians and fishes ....

But all of this artistic activity could take place at home and did. For many decades, the sounds of nature have also been recorded and have been valuable for purposes of identifying species, studying variation in calls and songs, and monitoring behaviour.

The reproduction of visual images also quickened in force during the nineteenth century, through wood-engravings of paintings, lithography (1798), and chromolithography (1837). These methods of reproduction took their place in the tradition of book illustration, especially in the literature of natural history, that began as long ago as the fifteenth century. Bridson and White (1990) have provided us with an exhaustive bibliographic guide to plant, animal and anatomical illustration from the sixteenth century both in science and in art. Ford (1992) has given us a short but lavishly pictorial history of scientific illustration that shows how illustration is a limb of scientific study; but Stephen Jay Gould goes further when he claims that 'pictures are not incidental frills to a text; they are essences of our distinctive way of knowing' (in Eldredge, 1996).

Illustrations also straddle the boundary between science and art; they can represent both art in the service of natural history and nature in the service of art. This valuable ambiguity accounts for the symmetry of such representative titles as *The Art of Natural History* (Dance, 1990), *The Art of Botanical Illustration* (Blunt and Stearn, 1994) and *The Art of Bird Illustration* (Lambourne, 1990). Birds, like flowers, have been especially attractive to scientific illustrators and artists alike, and the surveys by Jackson (1975, 1985, 1994) and Pasquier and Farrand (1991) cover a broad historical canvas.

In human history, nature would have been illustrated (in cave paintings, petroglyphs, etc.) for the purpose of worship or of providing identification guides for hunters or recording their kills. Afterwards came the visual cultivation of nature in images for the purpose of aesthetic appreciation, of turning nature into art, and this both predated and survived alongside illustration for the purpose of scientific knowledge of plant and animal physiology, anatomy and topography. Landscape painting became its own venerable tradition, nature in this tradition being very much in the service of art. The topographical tradition in visual art typically depicts historical buildings – ruined or whole – for the antiquarian record, but the buildings often reside amidst a fully rendered landscape with the whole aspiring to artistic composition. And there is a multifarious tradition of wildlife art, in which the artist attempts a balance between plausibly objective reproduction and his own aesthetic vision of what he is reproducing. Flower paintings can incline towards the art-study or, as some of those by Lydia Shackleton (1828-1914) from Ballitore demonstrate, towards the botanical study (Crookshank and Glin, 1994), though with a beauty of execution over and above the beauty

599

of the plant subject. The floral still life is a form, however, that requires fidelity to the truth of nature. Another favourite subject for the still life has been the hunter's bag. Two notable Irish examples that come almost randomly to mind are 'The Dead Ptarmigan' by William Orpen (1870-1931) and 'Four Snipe' by Edward McGuire (1932-86).

Irish artists have of course been practitioners of the tradition of nature art in all of its various guises. Harbison et al. (1978) and Crookshank and Glin (1994) offer rich accounts of Irish landscape painters, topographical artists, wildlife painters, still-life students, and flower illustrators, and Anglesea in this volume has surveyed the Irish work that has inclined towards the illustrative rather than the autonomously imaginative. The genres represented in these surveys are not just ways of choosing and arranging subject-matter but also ways of seeing, ways of interpreting and re-presenting nature. So too within genre is style, and style is often suggested by fashion. Between the late 1730s and the 1750s, for instance, there was a taste for chinoiserie in Britain, and Samuel Dixon, the son of a Dublin hosier, catered for this taste. In a method he claimed was new, basso relievo (moulding the surface of a metal plate so that the bird and flower images stood out in relief), Dixon advertised sets of flower pictures and bird pictures (Jackson, 1994). The bird images were pirated, it is said, from George Edwards, the great British bird artist and ornithologist, and they lack scientific accuracy (Crookshank and Glin, 1994), but they are decorative with charming Chinese motifs.

I mention Dixon chiefly to indicate a more general inclination in the depiction of landscape and wildlife towards the decorative, a rather different inclination from both the illustrative (or functional) and the autonomously imaginative, though the three overlap. Audubon's depictions of American birds are at once illustrative contributions to early American ornithology and representations that transcend illustration into decorative posture and colour; but their stylistic recognizability as the unique work of a single artist also lifts them into the realm of the truly imaginative. The same is not quite true of the Cork bird painter Richard Dunscombe Parker (1805-81), who has been likened to Audubon (Crookshank and Glin; Anglesea in this volume) but who perhaps more closely resembles Audubon's predecessor in America, the English painter Mark Catesby; neither Catesby nor Parker seems to reinterpret nature for artistic reasons.

It has been a human temptation to see nature in certain of its manifestations as itself decorative, not just as the pleasing setting for human life (an idea as old as the Garden that Milton's Adam and Eve inhabit before the Fall) but also as an aesthetic surplus to human life. Colourful birds are put in decorative cages to emulate visual arrangements such as Dixon's panels just as such arrangements emulate nature. And of course parts of birds and other animals (plumes, bills, claws, pelts, tails) have been used as decoration for human implements and accessories and even the human body itself, as though nature's function is to ornament as well as sustain human life.

In any case, the full history of landscape and wildlife art, decoration, and illustration in Ireland remains to be attempted. Such a history should include photography, which like painting or drawing can function variously. Framed photographs of landscape and wildlife vie as decorative art with framed paintings, engravings, drawings, etc., while the utility of photography for immediate or archival purposes of illustration and identification is beyond dispute.* The *Report of the British Association for the Advancement of Science* for the year 1908, when the Association met in Dublin, includes 'Photographs of Geological Interest – Sixteenth Report of the Committee'. This committee was chaired by Professor Geikie, and the Ulster photographer and naturalist R.J. Welch was a member. The Association had acquired six hundred new photographs since 1904 (giving a grand total of 4817), twenty-four of which were of Irish geological features; most of the twenty-four, one assumes, were from the camera of Welch. The decorative and even imaginative quality of Welch's photographs (be they of geology, rural life, or the *Titanic*) is well known in Ireland, and we can very nearly speak of a Welchian vision of Irish nature and culture.

The artistic representation of nature is a portion of the larger cultural processing of nature. Indeed, some students of culture have investigated the political ideology that they claim informs the picturing of wildlife – see Christie (1990) and Potts (1990); comparable analyses of landscape depiction by art historians of a political bent are too numerous to mention. The cultural transformation of nature into art in the nineteenth century – culminating in the counter-nature aesthetics of Oscar Wilde and the *fin-de-siècle* 'Decadent' writers, whose interest in the visual arts was intense – has been investigated by Woodring (1989). An aesthetics of nature had already emerged, of course, in the eighteenth century (see 'Encountering Traditions' in this volume), so that what transpired in the succeeding century was not new in principle. In both centuries, aesthetics furthered scientific study of nature as often as it hindered or obviated it; how nature was seen could influence what was chosen in nature for investigation. In this fashion, the traffic between the science of nature and the aesthetics of nature has been two-way.

More than this: it has appeared to most of us on occasion that nature is capable of being artistic in its own right, without the intervention of

---

* Yet there has been a debate about the respective merits of photographs and paintings for bird identification purposes in field guides; it is generally accepted that paintings expressly executed for such guides, though composite or ideal profiles and therefore not realistic, have a superior utility for the bird-watcher in the field.

human artists. (Ironically, the interpretation of nature as an artist – but one who is sometimes off form and often inferior to human artists, capable, for example, of an inferior sunset – was a somewhat whimsical aspect of late nineteenth-century aestheticism.) The noted scientist Ernst Haeckel tried to demonstrate natural art in his 1904 illustrated celebration, *Art Forms in Nature*.

Optical instruments have enhanced our sense of nature's artistry. Satellite photographs of weather patterns or natural formations, photographs of micro-organisms through microscopes, enlarged photographic images of what is small and undetailed to the human eye (such as the anatomical particulars of insects) – these have produced an endless body of nature's work, disclosing unsuspected designs of striking beauty and surprising structural intricacy. Except to the focused eye of a Gerard Manley Hopkins, who traced designs in nature most of us do not have the concentration or refined perception to see, it is only the macro-formations of nature that suggest the artist's canvas: the texture of trees, the penmanship of winter hedges (to borrow from Heaney), the geometry of mountain skylines, the engravings of rivers through a landscape. We seem to require technical mediation to see artlike forms beyond these; nor can we be sure to what extent the aesthetic appreciation of these macro-formations is the result of generations of artistic representation through the lenses of which we unavoidably see nature.

An idea that flourished during the eighteenth and nineteenth centuries, that nature resembled the painter's canvas, lay behind the natural theologian's conviction that nature as we saw it entailed a divine Artist. The notion, therefore, that nature produces her artforms is nothing new; indeed, to contemplate certain enhanced or enlarged images of nature is sometimes to feel the stirrings – presumably ancient, if not primitive – of a spiritual response to them, the suspicion that there are more things in earth than have been hitherto dreamt of in our philosophy.

Science and Literature

Verbal description of nature – another form of reproduction and mediation – was developed intensely (and in a way different from Renaissance and neo-classical writing) during the same Romantic period that saw the acceleration in optical invention. Romantic language, however, did not reproduce nature in a putatively objective way but expressly mediated between nature and the seeing individual. The neo-classical language of the eighteenth century did this too, but Romantic language also mediated between nature and the *feeling* individual who became a largely new product of culture when the feelings were foregrounded and orchestrated. Romanticism fertilized the unique achievement of Gilbert White's *The Natural History and Antiquities of*

Selborne (1789) to produce the modern literature of natural history. Fowler (1895) wondered aloud about the copious 'literature of the fields' that sprang up after White, mentioning Howitt, Wood, Kingsley and Jefferies among the English. Hagberg (1952) sees the influence of Linnaeus everywhere in White, and makes the larger claim that 'English literature's general development is to a large extent dependent on the view of life and nature which the English natural historians have possessed'.

White's book was presented as a collection of letters, and the use of the letter became as important to the natural-history text as to the early novel. In Ireland, James L. Drummond published *Letters to a Young Naturalist* (1831), Robert Patterson *Letters on the Natural History of Insects Mentioned in Shakespeare's Plays* (1838), and Sir Ralph Payne-Gallwey *Letters to Young Shooters* (1895). (This last was highly popular: there were three series of letters and the first series saw six editions.) This makes the term 'belles-lettres' when applied to fine natural-history writing particularly apt. From John Tyndall through R.L. Praeger, E.A. Armstrong and John Stewart Collis to Michael Viney, Ireland has contributed to a noteworthy Anglo-American tradition of nature writing. For selections from this tradition, see Finch and Elder (1990) and Mabey (1995). But Irish nature writing has been sadly neglected, and there is none represented in the three volumes of *The Field Day Anthology of Irish Writing* (Deane, 1991).

Given the immense importance of literature in Irish culture, it might be well to pause at the influential image of nature in Irish literature other than nature writing. Because nearly everyone who lives in Ireland is within sight of landscape, and because the island is modestly sized, Irish literature in its totality has composed over the centuries a detailed relief map of the country. Just as few features of the landscape are without commemorative names and associations, so few regions and towns are without literary connections, making the literature a guide to rural Ireland of surprising colour and detail in the matter of topography and scenery (Cahill and Cahill, 1979; Foster, 1991). A detailed chart of the representation of nature in Irish literature would be an enormous project, and below I have indicated only the major coordinates of such a chart and, even at that, only since the late nineteenth century.

Nature writing as such has been slighted in Ireland for reasons that apply to the cultural neglect of the study of nature itself. Even in England, the literature of the fields, 'open-air' literature, was consigned to minority status in literature in the middle nineteenth century, and has suffered that status ever since. This is regrettable since nature writing can effect a reconciliation between science and literature.

The contest in Victorian times between science and literature was one between an advancing discipline growing in confidence and a defensive classicism claiming itself as the seat of genuine culture. 'Polite Literature', as Newman still termed it in the eighteen-fifties, meant a 'perusal of the poets, historians and philosophers of Greece and Rome' which would enrich the intellectual powers, whereas 'the study of the experimental sciences' had not been shown to do so. Experimental sciences he defined as those which 'investigate facts by methods of analysis or by ingenious expedients' (Newman, 1982). There was also a class dimension to the contest, for classicism was the educational philosophy of the upper classes, while science was often viewed as a parvenu, associated with meritocracy and individualism. As defenders of the cultural centrality of the classics, Newman and Matthew Arnold on this issue were uneasy allies. Their chief opponent was T.H. Huxley ably assisted by John Tyndall, son of a Carlow policeman. It has been said that 'if Huxley became the statesman of nineteenth-century science, Tyndall became its knight-errant' (Irvine, 1963).

As the century progressed, literature increasingly meant modern English literature, which was emerging as a serious university subject. This did not affect the basic issue. Arnold championed modern literature as well as classical literature against the emerging claims of science; in his essay 'Literature and Science' (1885), he answered the criticisms levelled at his position in Huxley's own essay 'Science and Culture' (1882). The gap between Arnold and Huxley succeeded this century to that between F.R. Leavis and C.P. Snow, and it was the scientist Snow who regretted the duality of culture (Snow, 1959; Leavis, 1962).

Similarly, it has largely been the Irish naturalists who have attempted to cross the Great Divide. Curiously, three notable Irish naturalists were also Shakespeareans: Robert Patterson (1802-72) wrote *Letters on the Natural History of Insects Mentioned in Shakespeare's Plays* (1838); Henry Chichester Hart (1847-1908, profiled in this volume), was an editor of the prestigious Arden series of Shakespeare editions; and Edward A. Armstrong (1900-78) was the author of *Shakespeare's Imagination* (1946), a serious contribution to Shakespeare studies that helped to pioneer the analysis of what became known as cluster imagery in literary texts. William Thompson (1805-52), one of Ireland's greatest all-round naturalists, was President of the Fine Arts Society in Belfast and patronized the poet Francis Davis, one of the nineteenth-century 'rhyming weavers'. J.J. Murphy, the Christian evolutionist, author of *Habit and Intelligence* (1869), *The Scientific Bases of Faith* (1873) and other works (see Livingstone in this volume), was President of Belfast's Literary Society and published *Sonnets and Other Poems* in 1890. Thomas Corry, drowned as a young man like a botanical Shelley, published with S.A. Stewart the still standard (if much revised) *Flora of the North-east of Ireland* (1888) and was the author of several volumes of poetry, *A Garland of Song* (1880), *A Wreath of Windflowers* (1882), and *Songs in the Sunlight* (1883).

This apparently healthy obliviousness to the Two Cultures would of course have had an element of dilettantism in it (versifying is not the making of poetry, and Corry's titles are the titles of the poetaster), and Belfast's Victorian interdisciplinary culture would have had its Dickensian Gradgrinds and Bounderbys. Nevertheless, the history of intellectual Belfast – kin to intellectual centres in Britain, especially those in the industrialized midlands and north of England and lowlands of Scotland, discussed by Allen (1976) – has been unfairly driven underground and should be brought to the surface. For researchers in Belfast, William Gray's *Science and Art in Belfast* (1904) is the essential starting-point.

The apparently necessary choice between science and literature as the touchstone of culture has remained in effect, certainly in the English-speaking countries: as two literary critics lament, 'Our culture and criticism tends to pair literature and science as opposites' (Christie and Shuttleworth, 1989). This includes Ireland, where the tendency of writing since Thomas Davis, James Clarence Mangan and Sir Samuel Ferguson (to choose the nineteenth-century trio whose tradition of Romantic literary nationalism the youthful Yeats famously said he was following) has been anti-scientific. Meanwhile, the amateur literary efforts of the naturalists I have mentioned have little bearing on Ireland's world-famous literary achievement.

The situation can be deceptive, admittedly. We associate Oscar Wilde with hostility to science: he was an aesthete who wittily bemoaned 'Nature's lack of design, her curious crudities, her extraordinary monotony, her absolutely unfinished condition' (Wilde, 1989). Aestheticism, it has been said, 'is predicated on a swerve from nature' (Paglia, 1991) and by nature we might mean variously human nature, the subject of the natural sciences, or the nature of things. In a letter to the *Pall Mall Gazette*, Wilde claimed to despise the etymology of scientific nomenclature, but he clearly knew what the plant in question looked like:

Sir, I am deeply distressed to hear that tuberose is so called from its being a 'lumpy flower'. It is not at all lumpy and, even if it were, no poet should be heartless enough to say so. Henceforth there really must be two derivations for every word, one for the poet and one for the scientist. And in the present case the poet will dwell on the tiny trumpets of ivory into which the white flower breaks, and leave to the man of science horrid allusions to its supposed lumpiness and indiscreet revelations of its private life below ground. On the roots of verbs, Philology may be allowed to speak, but on the roots of flowers she must keep silence. We cannot allow her to dig up Parnassus. (Wilde, 1962, 172-73)

This was humorous affectation. Hagberg (1952) brings to our attention a more sombre passage by Wilde on flowers, from the long letter he wrote from prison, *De Profundis*: 'Linnaeus fell on his knees and wept for joy when he saw for the first time the long heath of some English upland made yellow with the tawny aromatic blossoms of the common furze; and I know that for me, to whom flowers are part of desire, there are tears waiting in the petals of some rose.'

Wilde's remarks about the design deficiencies of nature derived not from art criticism but from the scientists he read diligently at Oxford, including Huxley, Tyndall, Herbert Spencer and William Kingdon Clifford (Smith and Helfand, 1989; Foster, 1993/4). Wilde took enormous pleasure in science and was an ardent Darwinian. In his youth he was a keen fowler and fisherman; he had scientific correspondents, and of course his father Sir William Wilde was a practising scientist (opthalmologist, antiquarian, naturalist) through whom his son would have absorbed the scientific element of Anglo-Irish culture (Wilson, 1946). Elsewhere I have tried to demonstrate the lingering influence on Wilde's work of his youthful enthusiasm for science, including evolutionary theory, which after his conversion to aestheticism translated itself but did not disappear (Foster, 1993/4).

W.B. Yeats too was a keen naturalist as a youth (especially enthusiastic about lepidoptera) and read Haeckel, Darwin, Tyndall and Huxley; he planned to write a book about the changes undergone by rock-pool creatures over the year, and recalled having chided a boyhood friend for having an insuffcently scientific dimension to his butterfly-collecting (Yeats, 1955). He might, it would have seemed, have gone on to emulate one of those nineteenth-century Protestant clergyman-naturalists, or even become a Robert Lloyd Praeger, that younger contemporary who became the island's leading naturalist of his day. But by the 1890s Yeats had repudiated the study of nature and discovered Celticism and the works of the mystics.

Yet it is possible, as in post-conversion Wilde, to see Yeats as having retained the methods of science, applying them to non-scientific, or even anti-scientific, subject-matter. For example, he classified Irish fairies and fairy tales in an almost Linnaean system, made claims for the 'scientific utility' of the study of fairy belief, and lectured to the Belfast Naturalists' Field Club in 1893 on the subject.*

Moreover, whereas we think of Yeats's interest in the occult writers (including Cornelius Agrippa) as being utterly incompatible with natural history, such an interest appears to have been compatible with Linnaeus's own scientific activity, if credence can be given to the recent claim that the great Swedish naturalist was (like Yeats) a delver into Rosicrucianism and possibly

---

* The talk was given on 21 November; for reports of the talk, see *Proceedings of the Belfast Naturalists' Field Club* (1893-94): 46-8; *Irish News and Belfast Morning News*, 22 November 1893.

a believer. In 1725 Linnaeus acquired for his personal library the collected works of Cornelius Agrippa. 'In his encyclopaedism, his interest in practical applications, his apparent interest in hermeticism and alchemy, then, Linnaeus comes near to the Rosicrucians of the 1600s...' (Cain, 1992). Drawing on Yates (1972), Cain reminds us that

> the original Rosicrucians in the early 1600s ... were intensely pious Protestants, acutely aware of the necessity for a reformation of religion, science and society, and expecting it to be fulfilled soon partly by their own efforts. They looked to a vast survey of Nature, and to the development of experimental and especially technological science, to produce such benefits for all men that Mankind would in large measure regain the dominion over Nature exerted by Adam before the Fall, and the insight into the operations of nature which he had possessed.'

Yeats's own mysticism culminated in *A Vision*, which is a Theory of Everything and its own kind of science, a detailed classification system, an inductive as well as historical ordering of the universe, the human psyche and human culture. This is worthy of comment because the mystical strand in the Irish Literary Revival steered by Yeats was hugely influential in twentieth-century Irish culture (Foster, 1987), and because it seems we may have overestimated the Enlightenment's break with what we would now regard as pseudo-sciences.

Still, the reformation that Yeats envisaged was decidedly anti-scientific and anti-technological, and it would be stretching things (though not beyond all reason) to see his Celticism as disguised Protestantism of an intensely pious kind. By 1897 Yeats in 'The Celtic Element in Literature' was welcoming a widespread reaction 'against the rationalism of the eighteenth century', mingled 'with a reaction against the materialism of the nineteenth century', which the new 'symbolical movement' in literature could spearhead (Yeats, 1968). In the developing symbolism of his own poetry, he famously claimed in 'Sailing to Byzantium' (1926) to turn his back on the natural world ('The salmon-falls, the mackerel-crowded seas .../Whatever is begotten, born, and dies') in favour of 'the artifice of eternity'. In 1921 he recalled his detestation of Huxley and Tyndall for depriving him of his childhood religion, and in 1934 he explicitly repudiated Darwin, nominally because of the latter's 'exaltation of accidental variations' which 'our instinct repudiates' (Yeats, 1976; 1968).

Yeats believed that Ireland provided the most fertile and hospitable ground available for the counter-Renaissance and counter-Enlightenment. Yeats's attitude to science remained influential in Ireland (it broadly accorded with the attitude of the Irish Catholic Church), and the Irish Literary Revival that he led re-energized the pre-scientific 'Irish tradition' in the twentieth century, especially in Catholic and nationalist Ireland.

Not just Wilde's dandyism and his ambiguously perceived nationality (and perhaps even his peculiar socialism), but also his interest in science, excluded him from the Irish Literary Revival. Another major Irish writer, George Bernard Shaw, was excluded from Yeats's movement for much the same reasons. In 1900 Yeats told Shaw in debate that Shaw belonged 'to a bygone generation – to the scientific epoch – and was now "reactionary"' (Yeats, 1954), and irked the playwright whose plays demonstrate a sympathetic knowledge of evolutionism (though a distaste for Darwin). Shaw's most relevant drama in this regard is *Back to Methuselah: A Metabiological Pentateuch* (1921), but in *John Bull's Other Island* (1904) there is a knowing reference to 'the late Professor Tyndall'.

It is worth registering, however, that the Romantic cultural nationalism of the Irish Revival rested on the scientific efforts of philologists and antiquarians. Some of the scholars in question straddled the Two Cultures. Of particular interest in this regard is George Sigerson (1836-1925), who grew up near Strabane, Co. Tyrone, and lived long enough to witness both the Famine and the birth of the Irish Free State (in which he became a senator). He was educated as a medical doctor and became a practising neurologist but also wrote poems and assembled collections of traditional Irish songs and verse, the most influential being *Bards of the Gael and Gall* published in 1897 during the Revival. Sigerson was appointed to the Chair of Zoology in Newman's Catholic University and still occupied it when the National University was established; James Joyce attended Sigerson's class as a student in the early 1900s (Lyons, 1979). It was presumably as a cultural nationalist of Romantic bent (and a believer, like many Revivalists, in Irish exceptionalism) that Sigerson found gratification in the idea that human evolution had not taken place in Ireland: 'And it may be a comfort in view of prevalent hypotheses', he wrote in the 1890s, 'that the stock of the Anthropoids never went through evolutions in this country. Whatever may have happened elsewhere, the beings who first leaped upon our shores must have been among the foremost in the developed attributes of manhood' (Duffy et al., 1894).

We find a rich Romantic depiction of Irish nature in writers of the Irish Revival, and I would pick out Padraic Colum, James Stephens and J.M. Synge as among the most gifted observers of landscape and wildlife. Such Romanticism gave way to the more knowledgeable naturalism of Liam O'Flaherty (1896-1984), who wrote extensively about animals and the rugged landscape of the western seaboard. Yet even O'Flaherty managed by his anthropomorphism and 'pathetic fallacy' (the attribution of human feelings to nature) to reinforce the Romanticism with which the non-scientific tend to perceive Irish nature to this day.*

---

* There have been Irish fiction writers since O'Flaherty who have demonstrated in their

The same paradox attended the poetry and prose of Patrick Kavanagh (1904-67). Kavanagh was a close observer of nature and a harsh painter of the begrudging landscape he had known intimately as a small farmer: 'O stony grey soil of Monaghan/The laugh from my love you thieved' ('Stony Grey Soil'). His long poem 'The Great Hunger' renovates and localizes the Famine and translates it into spiritual and sexual terms while faithfully, if resentfully, re-creating the country life of a husbandman and the 'sleety winds' and 'rushy beards', the snipe-forsaken and 'hungry hills' ('Shancoduff') that surrounded him in southern Ulster (Kavanagh, 1973; Foster, 1991a). But Kavanagh (thankfully) was also given at times to a poignant Wordsworthian lyricism – see, for example, his lovely and observant poem, 'Bluebells for Love' – and it is this by which he is chiefly and rightly remembered.

Kavanagh was an early and important influence on Seamus Heaney, and it is Heaney who has brought to fulfilment the Romantic Irish depiction of nature that is hostile to science, despite an evident knowledge of nature accumulated during a country boyhood. The titular poem of the poet's first book (1966), 'Death of a Naturalist', is a fanciful obituary of the boy Heaney who might have studied the countryside around him as a naturalist but who instead fled in fear from the dark underfoot powers of nature. The mature Heaney would revisit the fearful sites and probe them, but as a poet, not a naturalist. In a later volume (1979), Heaney imaginatively appropriated the naturalist's activity with the title *Field Work*. For Heaney, Irish nature is a mythic-aesthetic-female-nationalist complex. His engagement with this complex, examined at length elsewhere (Foster, 1995), has caused Heaney to dismiss Praeger's nature writing because it does not rest on a mythopoeic relationship to Irish nature. But Lysaght (1989 and in this volume) has staked a claim for the cultural and aesthetic significance of Praeger's kinship with nature, and this claim is the more convincing, coming as it does from the pen of a poet as well as historian of natural history. It is abundantly clear from a biography of Linnaeus, a figure associated with dry classification, that science can consort at times with poetry as well as with religion: Linnaeus had a strong poetic and even anthropomorphic bent and had (as was once said disapprovingly of Aristotle) 'an everlasting *magia naturalis* in his blood' (Hagberg, 1952).

---

work an intimacy with nature while going about their human and humane business. I would draw attention to the stories and novels of Benedict Kiely (b. 1919), an expansive painter of the Ulster landscape and its creatures, and a virtual laureate of rivers. The strenuous tales of Patrick Boyle (1905-82) include 'Meles Vulgaris', an unblinking story about a badger-baiting that uses the animal's Latin name as a punning comment on the behaviour of the men involved.

Michael Longley, a contemporary of Heaney's, is a very fine poet whose work, though it could be loosely described as Romantic, nevertheless displays in its knowledge of nature nothing but admiration for sensitive scientific observers of the land and its creatures and plants. *Gorse Fires* (1991) and *The Ghost Orchid* (1995) are full of delicate observation derived from both field and library. Other Irish poets have, like Longley, celebrated animals and been anthologized for doing so (Johnstone, 1984), but in their love of natural history (i.e., the discipline) Lysaght and Longley are not typical of Irish poets.

The Romantic landscapes of the Irish Revival were repudiated by James Joyce. The famous last paragraph of the last story ('The Dead') in Joyce's first book, *Dubliners* (1914), proved that Joyce could brilliantly depict the Irish landscape in Romantic style, but even this depiction is edged with irony. Meanwhile, Joyce's early persona, Stephen Dedalus (*A Portrait of the Artist as a Young Man*, 1916), is terrified of the countryside at night and his creator largely eschewed it in his fiction. Joyce's fictional method began as a form of naturalism but in its maturity became systematized out of recognition, in a way that is almost scientific. Joyce was a voracious reader and consulter of all kinds of books, including medical textbooks, and the maternity hospital episode of *Ulysses* (1922) recruits gynaecology for detailed allegorical service. But as a comparably self-conscious artist, Joyce rejected Darwinism as Wilde accepted it: in *A Portrait of the Artist*, Stephen contemplates and jettisons Darwin's theory of organic evolution as an explanation of aesthetic attraction. To this extent, Joyce exemplifies the late Victorian tension between scientific sense and literary sensibility.

In Joyce, nature is absorbed – to the point of invisibility – into cultural scheme in the manner of literary modernism, which tends to the urban and international. In the post-modern fiction of Samuel Beckett and Flann O'Brien, landscape returns, but in a deliberately unreal form. Beckett's countryside aspires to the unreal ambiguous nationality of both France and Ireland, more a dreamlike than an actual landscape. In *The Third Policeman* (completed 1940), O'Brien's landscape resembles stage properties and like Beckett's has an obscure nationality. Elsewhere, O'Brien was much given to parody of the Irish tradition, be it the modern Gaelic peasant autobiography or the venerable Gaelic saga. In *An Béal Bocht* (1941, trans. *The Poor Mouth*, 1973), he darkly duplicates the cruel landscape and hunted wildlife of Tomás Ó Crohan's celebrated Blasket Islands reminiscence, *An t-Oileánach* (1929, trans. *The Islandman*, 1934). Ó Crohan's view of nature as a hostile recalcitrance is an exalted realism that has more in common with the style of Daniel Defoe or Jonathan Swift than with that of Synge, who suffuses the harshness of the western islandscape with Romantic elegiac poetry (Foster, 1987).

O'Brien's most famous novel, *At Swim-Two-Birds* (1939), contains a multitude of parodies. Here is O'Brien's playful imitation of the nature catalogue of the ancient Cycle stories, in which Fionn Mac Cumhail intones his fellowship with the wild creatures in what we might call the pre-Famine, pre-scientific, anthropomorphic attitude to nature of the Irish tradition, filtered through O'Brien's post-Revivalism:

I am friend to the pilibeen, the red-necked chough, the parsnip land-rail, the pilibeen mona, the bottle-tailed tit, the common marsh-coot, the speckle-toed guillemot, the pilibeen sleibhe, the Mohar gannet, the peregrine plough-gull, the long-eared bush-owl, the Wicklow small-fowl, the bevil-beaked chough, the hooded tit, the pilibeen uisce, the common corby, the fish-tailed mud-piper, the cruiskeen lawn, the carrion sea-cock, the green-lidded parakeet, the brown bog-martin, the maritime wren, the dove-tailed wheatcrake, the beaded daw, the Galway hill-bantam and the pilibeen cathrach. A satisfying ululation is the contending of a river with the sea. Good to hear is the chirping of little red-breasted men in bare winter and distant hounds giving tongue in the secrecy of god. The lamenting of a wounded otter in a black hole, sweeter than harpstrings that.*

The increasing refraction of nature through the prism of literature is itself a reflection of the increasing human influence on the Earth and its inhabitants. The difficulty of distinguishing nature itself from the cultural meanings imposed upon it in Ireland is a theme of Brian Friel's celebrated play *Translations* (1981). The play is set in Donegal in 1833 and dramatizes the impact and implications of the early nineteenth-century Ordnance Survey as recounted by Andrews in *A Paper Landscape* (1975), a book on which Friel drew in writing his play. Friel re-creates the vestigial classical tradition in Ireland, the better to depict the Irish landscape as a recurrently translated text whose inhabitants have to be in a cultural sense multilingual (like the schoolmaster of the play) and multicultural. *Translations* advances the idea of cultural nationalism for post-colonial and post-modern Ireland.

The Language of Natural History

One of the urgent items on the early modern scientific agenda was the generation of an adequate and appropriate language by which to describe, identify, and classify nature. Science had to challenge and displace extant languages that tacitly purported to have already performed these tasks. For

---

* A glossary for this comic *reductio ad absurdum* may be useful. The pilibeen is the lapwing, the pilibeen sleibhe the mountain lapwing, the pilibeen uisce the water lapwing, the pilibeen cathrach the city lapwing, the pilibeen mona the bog lapwing. The little red-breasted men are robins. Cruiskeen lawn, meaning the little brimming jug, is the name O'Brien gave his brilliant and addictive *Irish Times* column (written under the name of Myles na gCopaleen): a soon to be public private joke, in other words (his column began the year *At Swim-Two-Birds* was published).

example, local plant names that Ray and Linnaeus wished to replace often derived from pre-Reformation Catholicism, incorporating the names of Christ, the Virgin Mary and other biblical figures (Hagberg, 1952). A study of the role of Protestant natural theologians-cum-scientists in the early project of a new systematic nomenclature might be useful. Of further interest might be a study of how long in Catholic Ireland such pre-Linnaean nomenclature survived; in scientific circles did Linnaean nomenclature and taxonomy gain firm purchase in England and Ireland simultaneously, or was there a time lag?

Secular and pre-Christian oral tradition also used language for nature that the new scientists had to ignore or challenge, especially in Ireland where folklore had strenuously persisted. Persistence is indeed one of the twin capacities and features of oral tradition, the other being variation. Local, regional and national variation is a characteristic of names for the parts of nature – for species and features of the landscape. For example, the English or Scottish terms 'copse', 'dingle', 'dell', 'coppice', 'down', 'fell', 'moor' and 'burn' are not common in Ireland, while 'whin' (furze or gorse), 'sheugh' (wet ditch), 'ditch' itself (as embankment), and 'moss' (bog) are uncommon in Britain.

When Irish names vary locally or regionally, they are dialectal and may or may not involve an Irish-language etymology. To some extent they reflect a local or regional perception of landscape and wildlife. There have been glossaries of dialect words for the parts of Irish nature. These have been contributions to, and products of, folklore studies, ethnographic studies, and linguistics (all immensely popular in Victorian times), but they have also been a minor branch of natural history. W.H. Patterson published *A Glossary of Words in Use in the Counties of Antrim and Down* in 1880, and many of his words were names of creatures. There is a strong Scottish strain in the dialect vocabulary of these north-eastern counties that remains to this day. In publishing over the years (1965-78) a list of local bird names in Ulster, John Braidwood had recourse to Patterson's glossary. Braidwood's 1965 glossary (part two) contains all the northern Irish items from Rev. Charles Swainson's *The Folk-Lore and Provincial Names of British Birds* (1885, 1886), and Swainson seems to have drawn on Thompson's *Natural History of Ireland* (1849-56) and Watters' *Natural History of the Birds of Ireland* (1853) for his Irish dialect names.

Folklore collection and study (including dialect word study) were aspiring to the status of science at a time when natural history was taking to the field in a similarly vigorous and scientific way through the agency of the naturalists' field clubs. Of course, folklorists were collecting and studying material that appeared to be the product of a mentality utterly opposed to that which had wrought the Scientific Revolution and the Enlightenment. Yet natural historians and folklorists were both in pursuit of standardized international classification of, respectively, nature and folklore, each of which was regarded as existing in constant variation and alteration. Antti Arne and Stith Thompson were in one sense the Ray and Linnaeus of folklore, with their type categories and type texts equivalent to the Linnaean species (and what after Linnaeus became known as type specimens); in another sense they were the Darwin and Wallace of folklore, recognizing the dynamic nature of variation. The recording of variation and the notion of existence as survival link folklore study, dialect study and naturalist fieldwork, and the heyday of all three was the three or four decades after Darwin's *Origin of Species* (1859).

However, the survival in Ireland of the Gaelic language, and its two revivals in the nineteenth century (in the 1830s and 1890s), represented a massive variation from what might otherwise appear to have been a regional Irish version of the British picture in the folklore and dialects of natural history. During and after the seventeenth century, when modern British science begins, the English language expanded its geographical and demographic spread as a result of exploration and colonization. In that century, vernacular English was officially blessed as the language of science in Britain, so long as it tried to remake itself according to a scientific severity and plainness, eschewing the oratory and 'fantastical terms' that Thomas Sprat in his *History of the Royal Society* (1667) – an early wedge between the Two Cultures – thought had been imported into the language by translators and religious sectarians (Collins, 1957; Horne, 1957). Sprat was a future Bishop of Rochester; this is an early instance of the Anglican input into modern English (and Anglo-Irish) science, and of hostility to the Dissenters, who did not come into their own in science until the nineteenth century and then (in north Britain and Ulster) in naturalist fieldwork rather than the hard or exact sciences.

Tymoczko (1990) has shown how Old and Middle Irish terms for black birds spill over modern scientific nomenclature. This implies a non-scientific, cultural perception of the natural world, a way of dividing and understanding nature that modern science cuts athwart. I leave others to question how far Modern Irish is a suitable medium for a scientific perception and description of the natural world, in light of the structure or principles of the language, of its cultural and historical practice, and of the centuries-old development of science in English in Britain and Ireland alike. How far is this a linguistic issue, and how far merely a cultural one?

There have, of course, been lists of Irish names for species, some of them arranged into scientific nomenclature: of plants and trees (Cameron, 1883, 1900; Hogan, 1900; Colgan, 1911/13); of mammals, birds, fish, insects, reptiles (Forbes, 1905; Colgan, 1911/13; Scharff, 1915, 1916); birds (Ussher and Warren, 1900; Mac Giollarnath, 1954; Nicolaisen, 1963). Many of the dates of these citations are revealing. Apart from its natural use in Irish-speaking areas of the island, Irish has tended to function in three cultural contexts.

One is nationalist or nativist enthusiasm. Just as the colonist will name an area or topographic feature (possibly without considering that he is indulging in re-naming), so the nationalist or nativist will often re-name the re-named, re-appropriating the name for the Irish tongue (symbolically for the Irish nation – the national topography – or native tradition). It is fitting that the nationalist or nativist should concern himself with nature, since one of the cognate derivations for the Latin *natura* is 'native'; it seems that *natura* originally signified *nativitas* or 'birth' (Weishepl, 1982). Between the 1880s and the creation of the Irish Free State, there was great interest in matters Celtic and Gaelic among cultural and political nationalists, and Irish nomenclature is a sign of those times.

The second context is Celtic scholarship, which was active but non-politically so during the same period: hence we have Gaidoz's 'Flora Celtica' (1886) and Forbes's *Gaelic Names of Beasts (Mammalia), Birds, Fishes, Insects, Reptiles, etc.* (1905). The third context is the practical desire of the Irish Free State (later Republic of Ireland) to maintain the Irish language as a distinguishing feature of the culture, thereby justifying political independence, and as part of the educational curriculum. In both regards, it is felt desirable for Irish names for nature to be available, though arranged by the Linnaean system; hence we have An Rionn Oideachais (Department of Education) in the Republic publishing a flora and fauna nomenclature in Irish for use in schools (Anon., 1978). Such a publication has as much relationship to the venerable English-language textbook tradition of natural history in Ireland as it has with cultural nationalism, and such a publication has also distanced itself from any possible reservations about modern science by Irish speakers.

Touring Nature

Among the visual perceptions and representations of nature discussed at the outset of this chapter, there is one specific kind that has had an enormous impact on our attitude to our natural environment. Photographs and film of the Earth from satellites and space stations have allowed us routinely to visualize the planet as a whole, and to see it suspended (as it were) vulnerably in space, as though it too were a fragile spaceship. Within a generation, nature has been radically transformed in our imagination. Heretofore nature was regarded as resilient, mysterious, formidable, indifferent or even hostile to humanity; this perception derived for Westerners chiefly from the Judeo-

Christian story, in which human dominion over nature was an original good and nature (after the Fall) threatening and imperfect. The state of nature could be seen as one of relentless competition, as Thomas Hobbes brutally saw it, and humanity was in competition with nature. Darwinism's agonistic interpretation of nature did not disturb this fundamental religious conception.

The virtue of human dominion over nature paradoxically became harder to maintain as nature seemed to offer less resistance to it. Nowadays, nature is increasingly seen as a friend or host (or for some a mother-goddess), not an enemy, and a friend whom in the past we have ill-treated (or a host to whom we have been destructively ungrateful). That McKibben (1990) can write of 'the end of nature' is indicative of a cultural (and to some extent ecological) reality as well as of a millennial anxiety. The remote has become the accessible, the untrodden the trodden, the wild the cultivated, the forested the cleared, the unknown the probed and monitored.

Indeed, we now seem to resemble the human beings of H.G. Wells's science-fiction novella, *The War of the Worlds* (1898), 'serene in the assurance of their empire over matter' (Wells, 1983). (Empire over matter is what Bacon envisaged when he ushered in the epoch of modern inductive science.) This new-found human amicability and custodial attitude towards the Earth could, of course, prove to rest on the illusion of the essential passivity of the Earth and proffer further proof of humankind's hubris. (This hubris is the theme of Wells's story.) The assumption of a fragile Earth whose fate is entirely in our hands could be easily undermined: a meteorite in collision with the Earth, cataclysmic earthquakes, widespread famine, critical global pollution, melting of the ice-caps or pandemics might drastically change the present attitude to the planet held by the enlightened.

Meanwhile, the mediated perception of nature has been accompanied by direct interference in nature. Since 1974, when Whittow referred to the survival of relatively unmolested landscapes in Ireland, the human impact on nature has intensified, as it has almost everywhere on the planet. The progress of civilization, with its incursions into neglected areas, has continued apace in Ireland – in the form of building, agriculture, road-making, removal of land for development from the agricultural zone – even if land-clearance and drainage have slowed down.* Modern accounts of the natural

---

* The claiming of acreage in itself is not always responsible for the negative human impact on animals; technological improvement in agriculture has apparently been sufficient to threaten the survival, for example, of the corncrake in Ireland. The desire to conserve individual species and species diversity has recently compelled a rethinking in agriculture. The corncrake and other birds have suffered through the intensive management of re-seeded grassland, and conservationists have called for a return to extensification: low-density grazing requiring less livestock or more land, for which farmers need financial compensation or inducement.

resources of the island date from Arthur Young's famous *A Tour in Ireland* (1780) through Robert Kane's celebrated handbook, *The Industrial Resources of Ireland* (1845) to Bishopp (1943), Wheeler (1945), Cranley (1976), Gillmor (1979), and others. And those resources were tallied the more vigorously, perhaps, in the Irish Free State, when a fragile independent economy permitted little ethical luxury in the matter. The danger has always been that utilization would become unconscionable exploitation of unrenewable natural resources.

But now to traditional industrial and commercial uses of nature have been added the demands of the expanding business of leisure. Habitats are being changed by the building of golf courses and marinas and disturbed by proliferating water sports. Tourist destinations are often leisure resorts set in natural surroundings. Although the word 'tourist' was coined as early as 1800, it is only recently that tourism has seriously joined industrial utilization to exert joint pressure on nature in Ireland. Indeed, tourism is itself an industry, the largest in the world due to increased widespread affluence and technical advances in transit, and one of the biggest in Ireland.

Tourism has been defined as 'the mass circulation of the middle classes around the globe' (Wilson, 1992). This mobile impingement of human groups on wild habitats has helped to endanger wildlife and its environment. At the same time, tourism has required nature to become a renewable resource. Some field sports, such as coarse fishing, have become economically beneficial Irish tourist attractions and therefore have spawned conservation efforts for their own continued existence.

Nature tourism and eco-tourism (controlled itineraries into protected or undisturbed areas) are not just utilizations of nature but means of justifying natural protection and conservation, if on no other grounds than economic self-protection and self-conservation. The history of conservation – at first an amateur and altruistic affair – overlaps England and Ireland, so that Evans (1992) is of relevance to Ireland; but see also O'Ruadháin (1956), Orme (1970) and Feehan (in this volume).

One traditional tourist attraction has also redefined itself in order to combine leisure with conservation. Zoological gardens (there are two major examples in Ireland, in Dublin and Belfast) got into their stride as exhibitions of imperial exotica for the enjoyment of the populace – displays of natural curiosities. Gradually zoos broadened their appeal while restructuring themselves from cages to larger enclosures that began to mimic the animals' natural habitat; many zoos now are in extent and philosophy somewhere between government reserves and Victorian cage-displays.

Begun by naturalists, zoos were appropriated by municipalities and even entrepreneurs (Blunt, 1976), and in turn frowned upon by the next generations of naturalists until the threat to individual species (and biodiversity generally) began to make itself felt. Now zoos are defended on grounds of their value for behavioural research, such as the recent study of tamarin monkeys at Belfast Zoological Gardens (see H.M. Buchanan-Smith in Rushton, 1996), but more importantly on grounds of their captive breeding programmes – once thought reprehensibly artificial – that enable endangered species to be bred and released into the wild to replenish their numbers. One observer has even insisted that 'we need to make the next millennium the age of the zoo' (Tudge, 1996). Indeed, Tudge describes a scenario for immediately future zoos that requires them to become substitutes for nature, with nature being accorded secondary importance pending the levelling off of human population. Whether this strategic promotion of culture over nature will prove to be temporary or permanent is something no one alive today will survive to find out.

As their enclosures get bigger, zoos and safari parks become exotic versions of the refuges for indigenous wildlife that have likewise become tourist destinations and leisure spots. Eco-tourism, interpretive and conservation centres (all to be found in Ireland) and wildlife parks, are often defended on the grounds that they bolster the local economy. But they are also justifiable on grounds of environmentalism, and in order to exist they cannot by definition be self-destructively exploitative. Nevertheless, there are those who prefer a policy towards the environment of benign neglect and oppose the 'soft' exploitation of a sensitive wildlife area – such as the Burren in Co. Clare (Ryan, 1994) – by those who would absorb it into the tourist itinerary.

There are also those who oppose interventionist conservation measures from the opposite direction, i.e. when those measures infringe upon livelihood or profit. Retroactive conservation, for example in the guise of re-introductions of species extinct in former habitats, can also provoke opposition, as when Scottish farmers oppose the setting free of Norwegian white-tailed sea-eagles, once native to Scottish coasts. Such programmes represent the imposition of human culture on nature but can be justified on grounds that human culture (in this case the desire in previous centuries to kill birds of prey, not just for economic reasons but for reasons of culturally inherited revulsion) caused the ecological deficit in the first place, and that these programmes are forms of reparation.

A more indirect way of maintaining a threatened nature is by redefining nature to include what would previously have been regarded as cultivation, for example coniferous plantations, many of which now occupy Irish wildlife sanctuaries. Indeed, if a recognition of the fragility of nature is one recent change in our relationship to the Earth, then another is the intensified acculturation of nature, the accelerated transfer of nature from the category of the 'raw' to the category of the 'cooked', to adapt Levi-Strauss (1969). The ecological inter-relations of a natural system have their cultural and economic equivalents, and the systems increasingly interpenetrate. A large and well conserved area (e.g. Strangford Lough in County Down) involves land zoning, building regulations, road transportation, tourist facilities, licensing of restricted recreational shooting, organized water sports, associated tourist attractions, advertising (brochures, signs, television 'infomercials'), administrative centres (and therefore employment), shared jurisdiction (e.g. of the National Trust and borough councils) and education (lectures, guided tours).

The Culture of Nature

Whereas nature has always in fact been part of culture, i.e. always been culturally perceived by human beings, it was in Western society perceived as being outside culture *in its essence*. Nowadays, however, nature is increasingly perceived as *essentially part of culture*. Each country now regards its wildest areas or animals as cultural or national 'treasure' to be managed as stately homes and grand gardens and famous birthplaces are managed. (When wildlife refuges and country parks seek funds from the private sector – which they occasionally do in Ireland in order to finance habitat improvement or the building of observation hides – their resemblance to formerly private, now public estates is closer.) Indeed, nature, like culture itself, is more and more being tacitly understood as *the representation of itself*, and 'itself' is often understood as *its former self*: the designated wildlife area can try to maintain the faunal and floral status quo in terms of biodiversity, population and distribution; certain species will be favoured as the main 'attractions' of the refuge and therefore their presence must be assured by whatever conservation measures are necessary.

The refuge can even devote part of itself to commemoration of its flora and fauna as if they were 'heritage', a past to be strictly conserved. The cultivated equivalent of this is the zoo or aquarium that specializes in native fauna, such as the large and popular aquarium in Portaferry, Co. Down, dedicated to Irish Sea fishes, molluscs and crustacea. Both refuge and aquarium in this regard move in the direction of a wildlife museum and become a portion of what began as the heritage movement and became the heritage industry (connected to the tourist and entertainment industries). Lowenthal (1997) has identified the factors involved in the making of this industry in the Western world, including our deepening sense of change (more worrisome as we see out or greet a millennium) and our countering wish to preserve and restore; our increased tendency to move away from our birthplace and our compensating need to cherish roots; our increased leisure and the easy availability of advanced transport to heritage sites; the decline of agricultural labour and an enlargement of the urban (often sentimental) perspective on nature. Heritage and conservation support each other and coalesce in An Taisce and the National Heritage Council in the Republic of Ireland, and in the National Trust, begun in 1894 in Britain and continuing to expand, in Northern Ireland as well as the rest of the United Kingdom.

Yet another factor, according to Lowenthal, is a decline in the Christian belief in a personal God, as a result of which we turn for ideas of our most authentic and meaningful selves to the cultural past. It may be possible to draw an analogy between this idea of the spiritual importance of culture and the idea of the spiritual importance of nature to our individual and collective humanity. In *Biophilia* (1984), the naturalist Edward O. Wilson defined his title concept as 'the innately emotional affiliation of human beings to other living organisms', and Wilson and others have recruited the idea in the service of conservation: conservation is good because it satisfies a deep need in us.* The validity of the biophilia hypothesis aside, it does seem that in the West at least, permanently or temporarily, the cathedral of nature rather than the cathedral of religion is now the site of our anxieties, the place where (to adapt the English poet Philip Larkin) our compulsions meet and robe themselves as destiny.

Heritage has involved the enlarged importance of historical spectacle, the entertainment guise of history. Museums, of course, were always occasions of visual display, places of spectacle. Most natural history museums up to thirty years or so ago were simple exhibitions of specimens in glass cases, with minimal attention paid to the specimens' appearance within the cases and with only the simplest of taxonomic relationships represented in the display. Of course, the real scientific value of the museum was, and is today, invisible to the public, in the undisplayed specimens or specimen parts available only to scientific workers. Still, this writer confesses to a nostalgic feeling for those over-stuffed Victorian period cases; the cultural origins of these were displays of imperial exotica and booty, but this writer learned from these cases much of what skill he has in the identification of a large number of indigenous bird species.

A couple of decades ago, natural history museums felt the competition from television, with its dynamic display of living animal images. As well, a certain unease about museums seemed to infect the public, comparable to that aroused by zoos: in the latter it arose from the notion of captive animals, in the former from the notion of taxidermy, in both from the doubt

---

* It has been pointed out by Mark Ridley, in a review of *The Biophilia Hypothesis* (1994), edited by Wilson and Stephen R. Kellert, that if human beings evolved 'with an exploitative, rather than a globally conservational, relationship with nature', the value of nature, as the biophiliacs posit it, would be 'a historical and culturally contingent invention' (*Times Literary Supplement,* 9 September 1994).

about the genuine scientific value in these places of spectacle*. Stuffed creatures, necessary staples in natural history museums, had unfortunate associations with household decorations in over-furnished Victorian drawing-rooms, not to speak of zealous trophy hunting in the Empire. These reservations ignored the role of taxidermy in nature study education and in zoological research, as well as the capacity of stuffed and mounted specimens to approach art in their verisimilitude and the artfulness of their pose (Ireland has in modern times produced taxidermists of great and artistic skill: the Williams family in Dublin and the brothers Sheals in Belfast).**

Museums have responded to public unease with a shift away from crude specimen display to dioramas, multi-media displays, and visitor participation. The chief justification is now explicit educational display from a primarily ecological viewpoint. In doing so, the museum both benefits from and advances the current absorption of nature into culture. The museum attempts to combine its educational mission with its entertainment mission (it is quick to exploit the public's fashionable interests, for example that in dinosaurs), thereby hoping to put behind it its imperial (not to say plunderous) Victorian heyday.

Zoos and museums require signs and labels, but in an age of infomercialism the urge to label and inscribe is increasing in our culture at large. Signage now proliferates in controlled natural areas and is a visual and verbal interference in the experience of nature: the semiotic mediation between

---

* Around the same time, spectacle in culture (with its associations of male voyeurism and dehumanizing objectification) came under hostile scrutiny from cultural theorists of an anti-bourgeois and feminist persuasion.

** Taxidermists' shops were at once systematic and serendipitous sites for the discovery of rare and unusual birds and mammals. They became less important towards the middle of the twentieth century when their numbers declined, and when the development of advanced cameras and binoculars decreased the value of dead specimens (which most accepted rarities were in the days when the shotgun was the chief field apparatus). In a series of articles for the Belfast newspaper *The Northern Whig* (late 1921, early 1922), Alfred Sheals published entries from his notes, furnishing details of specimens of rare species of birds brought to his shop by shooters and naturalists for preserving, including glossy ibis, green sandpiper, buff-breasted sandpiper, Wilson's petrel, eared grebe, Pallas's sandgrouse, ferruginous duck and black tern. Sheals's 'Nature and Antiquarian Notes' are useful also for reminding us that now-common species were unusual enough seventy-five years ago (at least in certain localities) to be worth recording by him, including fulmar and eider duck, while others have since shrunk their range alarmingly (for example, chough, a specimen of which was procured on Divis mountain beside Belfast). Some of Sheals's preserved specimens went to the Ulster (then Belfast Municipal) Museum, suggesting an interesting co-operation between museums and private-sector taxidermists.

nature and the observer grows more obtrusive and less innocuously facilitative. Wildlife refuges now require interpretive centres, which do educate the public about nature but also tell visitors what they are about to see, anticipating the experience itself and threatening to render it anticlimactic, disappointing (if the animals or plants on the explanatory displays do not materialize), or merely replicative. The experience of *discovery* threatens to be replaced by the lesser experience to be enjoyed at zoos, that of *confirmation*.

It is obvious that signage affects the way we perceive what is being signed. This is the more significant when we consider that traditionally nature was regarded as existing on the far side of our cultural borders. Of course, the general culture (especially tourism and public conservation) is doing what modern scientists have always done: classifying and labeling the parts of nature. This too seems to this weekend naturalist to have accelerated; the official vernacular names for bird species, for example, seem to be changing (often reverting to previous names) more rapidly than before, as professional international ornithologists meet to decide upon speciation and subspeciation and the appropriateness of the names. A faint presumption of ownership of nature on the part of professional naturalists can even suggest itself to the amateur. The registering of the new names in field guides can help to popularize the changes, but while they do so the guides gain commercially by inducing among amateur naturalists an anxious need to keep abreast of developments in nomenclature, which in turn helps the field-guide book industry since the latter needs to publish new lucrative editions.

Very often the nature reserves that the public can visit are also research areas where biologists trap, tag, count, ring, breed, cull and otherwise manage animals. Increasingly, nature is professionally supervised, literally 'looked over'. Nature is subjected to a vigilance comparable to the bureaucratic vigilance to which citizens can be subjected. Indeed, in a latter-day extension of Enlightenment liberalism, animals are treated as though they are citizens of a country and therefore have rights and needs that must be met. (At its most bathetic, such an attitude results in garden birds in winter being regarded as resembling human welfare recipients.)* However, these rights can by definition be removed if wildlife management deems this desirable in the light of an enhancement or conservation strategy. For example, wild species deemed pests can be actively discouraged and even 'culled' by

---

* A less 'socialist', more consumerist attitude can be found among the legion of 'twitchers' – fanatical listers of birds – who are uninterested in the welfare (or behaviour) of birds, especially common birds, but rather regard nature as a vast supermarket whose species are to be consumed (i.e. ticked off the Wetmore order of bird species, which in turn is regarded as a grocery list); in this 'bourgeois' view the rarest species are like exotic items in the supermarket's delicatessen.

wildlife managers. Eggs can be removed from birds' nests and eggs of a different species substituted, in order to move or shrink populations of species; this can be justified on grounds of conservation, though it is clear that on occasion an ecological situation is not being conserved, since the situation being 'rectified' has arisen naturally, without prior human intervention. At such times, management is really engineering.

Beyond the necessities of conservation, the physical space of the wildlife refuge (ignoring the wildlife programmes being conducted therein and the anticipatory displays in the interpretive centre) is often renovated for visitor convenience. Car parks, public conveniences and safety lighting have to be provided. Trees and plants are often labelled, feeding tables erected to attract as well as nourish birds or animals, nest-boxes put up, permanent hides erected (often named after a donor or naturalist) that are capacious enough to accommodate visiting parties as well as the solitary bird-watcher of yesteryear. Platforms are built to create viewpoints and bench-seats provided for lunch or viewing, in a latter-day version of the 'stations' established by demesne landscape gardeners for the contemplation of 'vistas' and 'prospects'. In place of the classical quotations demesne owners would sometimes display at the 'stations' to encourage contemplation and interpret allegorically the view, we now find information about the visible or invisible creatures or plants we are to see; if we are to contemplate, it is biodiversity and ecological interrelationship we are encouraged to contemplate. The refuge now aspires, it seems, to a democratic version of the elitist demesne, and it happens that many country parks in Ireland were in fact demesnes.

These 'improvements' suggest the entertainment value of the wildlife refuge and point it in the direction of an open zoological garden.* In North America there are annual festivals to signal large-scale migration, the laid-on

---

* A recent development in North America (and one that might well spread to Europe) has been the opening of wild bird stores, which combine the functions of the outdoors stores (selling elaborate field equipment for the economically significant pastime – one might almost say sport – of bird-watching) with garden stores. Wild bird shops sell food for wild birds, but also nestboxes, feeders, bird-tables and other contrivances for attracting birds to the garden. Unsurprisingly, these accessories grow ever more diverse and decorative, so that the garden is encouraged to resemble an aviary. Also, because the shops need to do business all year round, customers ('bird-lovers') must be encouraged to provide food for birds even in the summer, and the previous advice from ornithologists that we desist from feeding birds during the breeding season (when parent seed-eaters need to provide their nestlings with the protein from insects) has now been reversed for commercial purposes. The aim now is not only to attract and aid birds but to *maintain* a population of birds for as long as possible, for purposes of customer entertainment (and ultimately of vendor profit).

tourist equivalent of ancient Native American commemorations of the return of migratory food animals. (One of these in Ireland is being inaugurated beside Strangford Lough to celebrate the return in autumn of the pale-bellied brent goose.) Such events are part of the larger phenomenon of what we might call the 'festivalization' of culture.

The idea of wildlife management, even when determined by exclusive biological criteria and not by the criteria of economics and leisure, is strictly speaking a contradiction in terms since the definition of wildness is that which is outside or beyond control. Management retains a vestigial sense of benign 'supervision' or 'stewardship' but is giving way to the more interventionist sense of 'control', even the hegemonic sense of 'total control'. The danger is that management will become to wildlife what development is to contemporary human communities in the capitalist democracies, i.e. the commercially and economically driven appropriation of urban, suburban and, alas, agricultural zones with built-in leisure or 'festival' components for the sake of public relations.

There is no doubt that management is preferable to the extinguishing of species and the lessening of biodiversity, and the survival of a semblance of wildlife requires us to ignore the contradiction by a species of redefinition. Ironically, the acceptance of greater human control of nature has coincided with the emergence of benign attitudes towards it, some of them discussed in the Irish context by Feehan in this volume, including 'deep ecology', a branch of environmental ethics that confers value on the environment considered independently of its effects on its inhabitants (thereby differing from biophilia which for tactical reasons emphasizes the importance of the human inhabitants' viewpoint and the ultimate dependence of human happiness on nature). Deep ecology stands alongside biophilia and resource management (conversation and protection made into an applied science) as one of the three currently significant branches of conservationist ecology.

Interpretive and conservation centres often employ video monitors and visual displays which show images the visitor is otherwise unlikely to see (because of the rarity, furtiveness or seasonal absence of the species) as well as images the visitor will duplicate beyond the door in the protected area proper. The presentation of images of 'things you'd never see in a thousand walks in the wild' (Siebert, 1993), the 'traffic in images that are ordinarily invisible' (Wilson, 1992), is a feature of nature programming on television, which is hugely popular in Ireland as elsewhere. (Ireland has its own nature film-makers, including Michael Viney and David Cabot.) These involve the editing of nature to achieve a script, often a narrative. This manipulation by others of images that are not originally the viewer's doubles back, as Siebert suggests, to influence how we see nature later, 'in the wild', and it ironically gives mechanized life to Coleridge's observation which Siebert silently appropriates: 'Today, the natural world is for us a place of reticent and reticular wonders that command our coaxing, our active exposure and editing; a world made up of what we half create and what, even when we're there, we fully expect to see' (Siebert, 1993). But at least, according to Mills (1997), the editing of nature is performed according to a code of ethics: 'Wildlife film-makers ... seem to have developed a collegiate view, amounting to a code of conduct, that any scene can be staged provided it depicts a scientifically observable fact.' Yet Mills finds this small comfort, set against the sad reality that nature films can be 'period-piece fantasy' by which the truth of wild habitat shrinkage and human impingement on remaining habitats is disguised by framing. The dilemma as Mills sees it is that the myth of wild nature sustains the entertaining and educative wildlife film industry (and, we might add, keeps the idea of wilderness alive: thereby helping to satisfy the biophiliac need) but further endangers the wild by avoiding narratives and footage of its diminishment.

Nature films, says Siebert, 'appease our increasing impatience with nature's gradualness'. This is hardly surprising given the importance of television in our lives and the fact that television, as Postman (1985) has argued, is a species of knowledge, a way of perceiving that sets up rhythms of reception and expectation: the average camera shot on American television, for example, is three and a half seconds and the habitual viewer comes to anticipate the fresh angle and image and is subliminally frustrated when it does not come. (The recent fashion for time-lapse photography in television nature programmes may in part be an obedience to the viewers' televisual desires.) This epistemology, Postman has shown, has influenced our culture beyond television, including politics, education and sport (so that one cannot escape the effects of television by choosing not to watch it), and I would add, following Siebert, that our anticipatory experience of nature has likewise been influenced and shaped.

One wonders how far interpretive centres, conservation areas, wildlife parks and zoos are being prodded in the direction of entertainment (drama, narrative, whimsy, poster-art), 'programming' nature under the unwitting stimulus and tutelage of television nature programmes. Our culture may in fact be spiralling back towards Victorianism in this regard.*

---

* Recently, the favourite script of nature programmes has dramatized endangerment and ecological interaction, mirroring the concerns of our time. Before that, the script dramatized the Darwinian struggle for survival and reproduction. Even when they are not made by Disney (which corporation anthropomorphizes nature shamelessly), American nature films tend to be allegorical and still favour the older script, which covertly sees nature as justifying as 'natural' the cut-throat corporate and political systems of capitalist America, including its foreign policy.

In the most spacious context, it might be worth pondering not just the re-perception and implied re-definition of nature that the regulating, monitoring and celebrating of nature result in, but also the individual and collective psychological effect of this continuous human 'signing' of nature. How important to the Western sense of well-being are our ideas of the wildness, remoteness, 'freedom', 'neglectedness' and 'otherness' of nature? The answer involves in part the history of the perception of nature in particular cultures, such as Ireland's, but in *The Time Machine* (1895), Wells suspected that in the future 'things will move faster and faster towards the subjugation of Nature'. He imagined a remote time from which, looking back, his Time Traveller recognized that 'One triumph of a united humanity over Nature had followed another' and wondered about 'the patient readjustments by which the conquest of animated nature had been attained' (Wells, 1953). He famously believed that once Nature had been conquered and 'the whole earth had become a garden', fear and hardship would diminish in the human experience and the species would begin to decay in 'indolent serenity' and the garden become 'waste'.* Meanwhile, the process is already under way whereby nature, once vaguely thought to be 'infinite' (and eternal), is 'finitized'; we seem less to explore nature (by moving outwards from our domestic, urban, cultivated centre) than to study it by working inwards from the boundaries known or thought to be known.

As for wild creatures themselves, there will be adaptive responses to increased human presence: for example, the fox in Ireland, like the coyote in western North America, has latterly become a denizen of the very suburbs that have encroached upon its habitat. (As has, to take an avian example, the hooded crow, a wary country dweller in my boyhood.) Under a different human pressure, a relentless regime of monitoring, counting, tagging, artificial selection, culling, re-introduction, replenishing and genetic engineering, the species changes are harder to predict. We recall Goldsmith's belief, borrowed from Buffon, that domestication meant degradation of the

---

* Of course, Wells's Time Traveller discovers that fear has not vanished, since the human species has evolved into two, one species living underground except when preying on the 'Over-worlders'. Darwinian evolution might seem to have ensured that the struggle for survival has survived. But the decay is irreversible for those who live in what we normally regard as nature, i.e. the floral and faunal surface of the Earth, because the Over-worlders have lost the will and wherewithal to work the 'garden' that their ancestors made of the Earth. And since the subterranean humans have like the Over-worlders suffered what Wells elsewhere (Philmus and Hughes, 1975) called 'zoological retrogression' (1975), Darwinian evolution has reversed itself as Wells, taking his cue from T.H. Huxley, thought it eventually would.

Between now and Wells' remote future, it is likely that wars will survive our subjugations of nature and keep fear and hardship alive.

species, a belief that was absorbed into the cultural politics of Romanticism. But what is at stake for animals and humans in the management of nature is largely a matter of vague speculation.

Nature and Natural History Today

A challenge to our very idea of the natural has recently come from feminist theorists who argue that human gender is not biological but rather the social construction of sexual identities. Schiebinger (1994) has tried to demonstrate how male assumptions about gender influenced eighteenth-century taxonomy, especially in botany and primate studies (Linnaeus's system was, of course, radically sexual). Schiebinger's work succeeds the pioneering work of Keller (1985) and Harding and O'Barr (1987) on the role of gender and sex in the scientific study of nature; see also Shuttleworth (1990) and Kirkup and Keller (1992). The nature of scientific investigation has come for feminists to constitute what is known as 'the science question in feminism', the title of a book by Harding (1986), and the subject of a study by Tuana (1989) and of the first issue of *Women: A Cultural Review* (1990).

But the science question in feminism has also been posed because of the limited role historically played by women in scientific progress. There is no doubt that the exclusion of women from many early scientific societies was a custom that came to seem natural. The more learned societies in the United Kingdom excluded or ignored women up until the late nineteenth century because, Allen (1976) remarks, 'science was a man's business and the club a kind of intellectual stag-party where a male rattled his antlers'. When admitted, women were frequently patronized.

If it seemed natural to exclude women, it may have been in part because women were themselves associated by men with the natural, not with the intellectual or cultural, so that the scientific study of nature by women could seem like an exercise in gratuitousness. The Earth for a long time was thought to be female, specifically a mother (Mother Earth, Mother Nature), presumably because the phenomenon of fertility was held to define nature. The Earth itself could be seen as a womb; recently, the Gaia hypothesis has reaffirmed the femaleness of the Earth, the attribution of sex reinforced by the proliferation of space photographs of the globular planet with its subliminal suggestion of permanent pregnancy or lactation.

Whereas the traditional sexing of the Earth and of nature has been occasionally interpreted as an example of male sexism and patronage, it is not a conceptual practice to which every feminist takes exception. Indeed, it has been warmly embraced in some quarters and has helped some feminists to transfer blame for the destructive exploitation of nature from human beings in general to men in particular. A cognate notion is that there is a special relationship between feminism and environmentalism (Warren, 1996). And Lowenthal (1997) believes that for a number of reasons, including maternalism, women have been notably influential in the heritage movement.

Despite frequent discouragement, women in Ireland, England, North America and elsewhere have contributed to natural history; their contribution can be assessed in Kahle (1985), Ogilvie (1986), Abir-am and Outram (1989), Phillips (1990), Weisbard and Apple (1993) and Shteir (1996). Several of these studies outline the social context of women's scientific participation. For example, women scientists were until this century usually from the leisured classes. Shteir has studied at some length the attraction of women to botany in the eighteenth and nineteenth centuries (the story involved the education of young women as well as polite unease with aspects of nature and natural reproduction) and her studies are relevant to Ireland. I would add that the imitation of flowers and plants was a venerable component of what one anthropologist (Goody, 1993) has called 'the culture of flowers' and of home crafts practised by women, and in Ireland flowers were such common motifs in embroidery and lace-making that those who practised the craft were called 'flowerers' (Boyle, 1971).

It has been claimed that women faced less discrimination in Ireland than in England (Ross and Nash, 1986). The record of accomplishment is still modest, but there are notable achievers. The astronomer Agnes Mary Clerke (1842-1907) was a contributor to the ninth and eleventh *Britannica*s. Raised in Cork, she began to write a history of astronomy when she was fifteen. Her family moved to Dublin and wintered in Italy, where young Clerke used the Florence Public Library. She was a major contributor to the *Dictionary of National Biography*, wrote several books on astronomy, and was an honorary member of the Royal Astronomical Society (Thomas, 1992). But she also straddled the Two Cultures – publishing nearly fifty articles in the *Edinburgh Review* and writing *Familiar Studies in Homer* (1892) – and paid the price for it, having to refuse an invitation to go to Nova Zemblya to watch a solar eclipse because of her literary deadlines. She and her sister (another prolific contributor to the *Edinburgh Review*) were remembered in an appreciation by Margaret, Lady Huggins (c. 1849-1915). Huggins, an Irish astronomer specializing in spectroscopy and author of the *Atlas of Representative Stellar Spectra* (1899), was also something of a Renaissance woman. Ross (1982) has noted the Irish women naturalists of the nineteenth century but has also (1983) outlined the difficulties presented to the Irish historian of natural history who wishes to research the contribution of women.

If the Earth-mother is an example of anthropomorphism, so might be the cause of animal rights, rights which are held to parallel or even arise from human rights. Yet the animal rights movement often opposes itself to

the exploitative anthropomorphizing of animals. Like certain environmentalists, animal rights proponents base their views on ethics. Even natural events
(such as extinction, which occurs all the time in nature) are increasingly
regarded as ethical phenomena whatever the degree of human involvement;
indeed, the prevalence of natural ethics helps define our society and culture
today, and is a component of the cultural absorption of nature. Equally
defining are the high-profile politics of these two issues, environmental protection and animal rights.

The politics of environmentalism are well known (they emerged in the
whole-earth movement and counter-culture of the 1960s), with many political parties making conservation a plank in their platform. But the politics
of animal rights have a different and longer history, appearing in British parliamentary debate as early as 1800. The late eighteenth-century, early nineteenth-century concern with sentience, freedom and innocence in human
beings – concepts extendible to animals – was one cultural root of the animal rights cause, so it is not surprising that several literary figures were
prominent, two of whom were born in Ireland: Laurence Sterne (1713-68)
and Richard Brinsley Sheridan (1751-1816).

The Galway landlord and parliamentarian 'Humanity' Dick Martin
(1754-1834) – a cousin of the mineralogist Richard Kirwan – was very
prominent in the early movement against cruelty to animals. This compas-
sionate but combative figure was an active supporter of Catholic
Emancipation (as well as the Union) and a liberal reformer of criminal justice, but his campaign on behalf of animals has been his most enduring legacy, and his story is well told by Lynam (1989).

Martin roamed his estate (the largest property in fee simple in the
British Isles) watchful for animal abuse among his tenants, who treated animals with scant regard and sometimes brutality. An episode of cruelty to a
pet seal in Mayo (visited on the creature by its owner under the superstitious instruction of a 'wise woman' or medium) convinced Martin that the
purview of an animal-rights campaign extended far beyond his estate. He
joined forces with John Lawrence, author of *Philosophical and Practical
Treatise on Horses and the Moral Duties of Man towards the Brute Creation*
(1796). Lawrence based animals' rights on their possession of feelings and
intelligence, although he made a distinction that Martin accepted: between
wanton cruelty and hunting, the latter activity being viewed as honouring
'the scheme of universal providence', which permits man to kill animal
under certain circumstances. Behind the animal-rights campaign lay the old
issues of the relative status of human beings and animals in the scheme of
things, and the moral extent of human dominion over the animal kingdom.

Martin supported Lawrence's proposal for legislation, and the Society
for the Prevention of Cruelty to Animals (SPCA) was formed in 1824, after

the Ill-Treatment of Cattle Bill (a modest opening gambit), known as 'Martin's Act', successfully passed into British law. Martin actively if unsuccessfully campaigned against animal-baiting, cockfighting, vivisection and wanton cruelty to pets, work animals and wild animals. He was a tireless vigilante, scouring London for practitioners of animal abuse and, as a lawyer, bringing the culprits to book. The SPCA (later RSPCA) and its Irish branches can thus be traced to the efforts of, among others, a colourful Galwegian, the 'King of Connemara' as he was called.

Lawrence's *Treatise* was the ancestor of Peter Singer's *Animal Liberation* (1975), a book that brought animal rights to the fore in the Western world. The ensuing movement has been highly active and even extra-legal, and has chosen to rest its philosophy on secular and political grounds, rather than, as in Martin's day, moral and spiritual grounds.

Many branches of the study of the Earth and its creatures now depend upon technology that extends the capacity of human perception beyond the optical instruments with which this essay opened. This technology is usually transnational, and computers, for example, have made it possible for the same kind of research to be carried out in various countries and even by multinational groups of researchers. Irish micro-biologists are engaged in projects of international significance and their results are shared with co-workers abroad. Irish biologists who travel abroad nowadays are as likely to be attending an international conference as conducting exotic fieldwork. Micro- and molecular biology can work at levels above the local, regional or national, on a stratum of perception connecting all places and habitats on the Earth.

The most obvious extension of our ability to see and survey is aerial photography, now almost (but not quite) superseded by satellite photography. Imagery beamed from the American Landsat satellite helped geoscientists and surveyors from the Ordnance Surveys of Ireland and Northern Ireland to provide a common database of land cover, including farmland, forests, mountains and moorland. Details from the survey can be reproduced by computers in minutes for farmers and environmentalists; in six months the two Ordnance Survey agencies produced a road atlas of Ireland accurate to the last by-road.*

Computer technology does not simply reproduce images of nature but can engage in its own artificial version of natural reproduction. Artificial life

---

* International technology and the cross-border nature of habitats and animals have encouraged co-operation between natural scientists in both political parts of Ireland. As well as the joint projects of the Ordnance Survey agencies, a forestry plan was recently produced by the Royal Society for the Protection of Birds (UK) and the Irish Wildbird Conservancy (Republic of Ireland): *Ireland's Forested Future: A Plan for Forestry and the Environment* (1994).

('A-life') is, in the words of Rotman (1994), 'the newest wave of computer-driven science threatening to produce as deep an upheaval in biology as that effected by fractal geometry and chaos theory in the physical sciences'. It represents, too, another profound challenge to our notion of the natural. The computer's assemblages of pixels, bug-like, bird-like, or plant-like, undergo electronic versions of growth, procreation, death, birth and evolution. One scientist has tried to simulate natural selection by defining an artificial environment and releasing into it 'creatures' – pieces of code with built-in sources of mutation and built-in rewards for fitness – that evolve biological characteristics the scientist did not plan or predict. Scientists at the University of Toronto have generated 'virtual fish' on computer which began as aids to movie animators; now the fish 'remember' swimming technique, and the researchers hope to create 'an artificial ecology' in which predators constantly improve hunting strategies to deal with prey that evolves better ways of escaping. The scientists entertain the possibility that their fish will eventually imitate spawning and that traits 'would be passed on to future generations via an exchange of DNA-like software' (Strauss, 1994). In the meantime, these computer experiments are of interest to icthyologists.

At the very least, then, A-life may produce new understandings of natural mechanisms. However, according to Rotman (1994), some believe that A-Life de-natures life, liberating it from carbon-based and water-based forms 'to include all manner of manufactured organisms'. 'Could A-life creatures, chunks of code enjoying the benefits of electro-evolution, get so complex', he wonders, 'that consciousness might be one of their emergent properties?'

The possibility of a self-reproducing machine – an idea that stimulated students of A-life – is the possibility of technology as an end as well as a means. Some believe that there have been three blows to anthropocentrism: the discovery by Copernicus that the Earth is not the centre of the universe; the theory of Darwin that human beings evolved from lower life-forms; and the theory of Freud that human sexual instincts are not entirely controllable and that our mental processes have unconscious origins. To this, some say, we can now add a fourth blow: the 'discipline' of Artificial Intelligence. But whereas the first three blows promoted nature at the expense of human culture, the fourth blow would demote humankind in favour of a culturally produced mechanism.

'We are now on the threshold of erasing the boundary between human and machine' (Rabinbach, 1994), of having set in motion a mechanical 'second nature'. This would fulfil itself when simulations of nature evolve autonomous and unforeseen functions and characteristics; and this prospect has evoked the figure of Frankenstein. The prospect is as old as the conjunction of Darwinism and industrialization in the late nineteenth century. (Wells's Martians in *The War of the Worlds* have degenerated as organisms in all but their hypertrophied brains and manipulative limbs and have developed machines of such versatility that the boundary between machine and Martian has become blurred.) However, computers have stimulated the development of robotic machines to the extent that Mazlish (1994) contemplates the evolution of a new species that he calls 'homo-comboticus'. Whether this comes to pass is less important in the context of a volume such as *Nature in Ireland* than the changes even the very attempt will create in our attitude and relationship to nature, changes at present unforeseeable.

References

Abir-am, P.G. and D. Outram (eds). *Uneasy Careers and Intimate Lives: Women in Science 1789-1979*. New Brunswick: Rutgers University Press.

Allen, D.E. 1976. *The Naturalist in Britain: A Social History*. London: Allen Lane.

Andrews, J.H. 1975. *A Paper Landscape: The Ordnance Survey in Nineteenth Century Ireland*. Oxford: Oxford University Press.

Anon. 1975. 'Ireland's Natural Resources.' *Business and Finance 11*. Supplement.

Anon. 1978. *Ainmneach Plandai agus Ainmhithe/Flora and Fauna Nomenclature*. Baile Atha Cliath/Dublin: An Roinn Oideachais.

Anon. 1994. Review of L.S. Temkin, *Inequality* (1994). *Times Literary Supplement*, 24 June.

Armstrong, E.A. 1946. *Shakespeare's Imagination: A Study of the Psychology of Association and Inspiration*. London: Drummond.

Arnold, M. 1885. 'Literature and Science,' in *Discourses in America*. London: Macmillan.

Bishopp, D.W. 1943. *Natural Resources of Ireland*. Dublin: Royal Dublin Society.

Blunt, W. 1976. *The Ark in the Park: The Zoo in the Nineteenth Century*. London: Hamish Hamilton.

Blunt, W.S. and W.T. Stearn. [1950] 1994. *The Art of Botanical Illustration*. Woodbridge: Antique Collectors' Club.

Boyle, E. 1971. *The Irish Flowerers*. Cultra and Belfast: Ulster Folk Museum and Institute of Irish Studies, Queen's University.

Braidwood, J. 1965, 1966, 1971, 1978. 'Local Bird Names in Ulster.' *Ulster Folklife 11*: 98-135; 12: 104-7; 17: 81-4; 24: 83-7.

Bridson, G.D.R. and J.J. White. 1990. *Plant, Animal and Anatomical Illustration in Art and Science: A Bibliographical Guide from the Sixteenth Century to the Present Day*. Winchester: St Paul's Bibliographies.

Cahill, S. and T. Cahill. 1979. *A Literary Guide to Ireland*. New York: Charles Scribner's Sons.

Cain, A.J. 1992. 'Was Linnaeus a Rosicrucian?' *The Linnean 8*: 23-44.

Cameron, J. 1883. *The Gaelic Names of Plants (Scottish, Irish and Manx) Collected and Arranged in Scientific Order, with Notes on their Etymology, Uses, Plant Superstitions, etc*. London. Rev. ed 1900. Glasgow.

Christie, J. 1990. 'Ideology and Representation in Eighteenth-Century Natural History.' *Oxford Art Journal 13*: 3-10.

Christie, J. and S. Shuttleworth (eds). 1989. *Nature Transfigured: Science and Literature, 1700-1900*. Manchester: Manchester University Press.

Collins, A.S. 1957. 'Language 1660-1784,' in B. Ford (ed.), *The Pelican Guide to English Literature*. Harmondsworth: Penguin.

Colgan, N. 1911/1913. 'Gaelic Plant and Animal Names and Associated Folk-Lore.' *Proceedings of the Royal Irish Academy 31*: 1-17.

Corry, T.H. 1880. *A Garland of Song*. Belfast: Author.

Corry, T.H. 1882. *A Wreath of Wind-Flowers*. Belfast: Author.

Corry, T.H. 1883. *Songs in the Sunlight*. Belfast: Wm. Mullan.

Cranley, M.J. 1976. 'The Natural Resources of Ireland.' *Administration 24*: 50-75.

Crookshank, A. and Knight of Glin. 1994. *The Watercolours of Ireland: Works on Paper in Pencil, Pastel and Paint c. 1600-1914*. London: Barrie and Jenkins

Dance, S.P. [1978] 1990. *The Art of Natural History*. New York: Arch Cape Press.

Deane, S. (ed.). 1991. *The Field Day Anthology of Irish Writing*. 3 vols. Derry: Field Day Publications.

Duffy, C.G., G. Sigerson and D. Hyde. [1894] 1973. *The Revival of Irish Literature*. New York: Lemma.

Eldredge, N. and M. Alcosser. [1991] 1996. *Fossils: The Evolution and Extinction of Species*. Princeton: Princeton University Press.

Evans, D. 1992. *A History of Nature Conservation in Britain*. London: Routledge.

Finch, R. and J. Elder (eds). 1990. *The Norton Book of Nature Writing*. New York: Norton.

Forbes, A. 1905. *Gaelic Names of Beasts (Mammalia), Birds, Fishes, Insects, Reptiles, etc. Two Parts: Gaelic-English, English-Gaelic*. Edinburgh.

Ford, B.J. 1992. *Images of Science: A History of Scientific Illustration*. London: The British Library.

Foster, J.W. 1987. *Fictions of the Irish Literary Revival: A Changeling Art*. Syracuse: Syracuse University Press; Dublin: Gill and Macmillan.

Foster, J.W. 1991. 'The Geography of Irish Fiction,' in *Colonial Consequences: Essays in Irish Literature and Culture*. Dublin: Lilliput Press.

Foster, J.W. 1991a. 'The Poetry of Patrick Kavanagh,' in *Colonial Consequences: Essays in Irish Literature and Culture*. Dublin: Lilliput Press.

Foster, J.W. 1993/4. 'Against Nature? Science and Oscar Wilde.' *University of Toronto Quarterly 63*: 328-46.

Foster, J.W. 1995. *The Achievement of Seamus Heaney*. Dublin: Lilliput Press.

Fowler, W.W. 1895. *Summer Studies of Birds and Books*. London: Macmillan.

Friel, B. 1981. *Translations*. London: Faber and Faber.

Gaidoz, H. 1886. 'Flora Celtica.' *Revue Celtique 7*: 162-70.

Gifford, D. 1990. *The Farther Shore: A Natural History of Perception, 1798-1984*. New York: Atlantic Monthly Press.

Gillmor, D. (ed.). 1979. *Irish Resources and Land Use*. Dublin: Institute of Public Administration.

Goody, J. 1993. *The Culture of Flowers*. Cambridge: Cambridge University Press.

Gray, W. 1904. *Science and Art in Belfast*. Belfast: The Northern Whig.

Haeckel, E. [1904] 1974. *Art Forms in Nature*. New York: Dover.

Hagberg, K. 1952. *Carl Linnaeus*. London: Jonathan Cape.

Harding, S. 1986. *The Science Question in Feminism*. Ithaca: Cornell University Press.

Harding, S. and J.F. O'Barr (eds). 1987. *Sex and Scientific Inquiry*. Chicago: University of Chicago Press.

Heaney, S. 1966. *Death of a Naturalist*. London: Faber and Faber.

Heaney, S. 1979. *Field Work*. London: Faber and Faber.

Hogan, F.E., J. Hogan and T. MacErlean. [1883] 1900. *Luibhleabhran: Irish and Scottish Gaelic Names of Herbs, Plants, Trees, etc*. Rev. ed. Glasgow.

Horne, C.J. 1957. 'Literature and Science,' in B. Ford (ed.), *The Pelican Guide to English Literature*. Harmondsworth: Penguin.

Huxley, T.H. 1882. 'Science and Culture,' in *Science and Culture and Other Essays*. New York: Appleton & Co.

Irvine, W. 1963. *Apes, Angels, & Victorians: The Story of Darwin, Huxley, and Evolution*. New York: Time Inc.

Jackson, C.E. 1975. *Bird Illustrators: Some Artists in Early Lithography*. London: Witherby.

Jackson, C.E. 1985. *Bird Etchings: The Illustrators and Their Books, 1655-1855*. Ithaca: Cornell

University Press.

Jackson, C.E. 1994. *Bird Painting: The Eighteenth Century*. Woodbridge: Antique Collectors' Club.

Johnstone, R. (ed.). 1984. *All Shy Wildness: Anthology of Irish Animal Poetry*. Wolfeboro: Longwood.

Joyce, J. 1914. *Dubliners*. London: Grant Richards.

Joyce, J. 1916. *A Portrait of the Artist as a Young Man*. London: Egoist Press.

Joyce, J. 1922. *Ulysses*. Paris: Shakespeare & Co.

Kahle, J. B. (ed.). 1985. *Women in Science: A Report from the Field*. Philadelphia: The Falmer Press.

Kavanagh, P. 1973. *Collected Poems*. New York: Norton.

Kane, R. [1845] 1971. *The Industrial Resources of Ireland*. Shannon: Irish University Press.

Keller, E.F. 1985. *Reflections on Gender and Science*. New Haven: Yale University Press.

Kellert, S.R. and E.O. Wilson (eds). 1994. *The Biophilias Hypothesis*. Washington, D.C.: Island.

Kirkup, G. and L.S. Keller (eds). 1992. *Inventing Women: Science, Gender and Technology*. Oxford: Polity Press.

Lambourne, M. 1990. *The Art of Bird Illustration*. London: Collins.

Leavis, F.R. 1962. *Two Cultures? The Significance of C.P. Snow*. London: Chatto and Windus.

Levi-Strauss, C. 1969. *The Raw and the Cooked*. Trans. J. and D. Weightman. New York: Harper and Row.

Longley, M. 1991. *Gorse Fires*. London: Secker & Warburg.

Longley, M. 1995. *The Ghost Orchid*. London: Jonathan Cape.

Lowenthal, D. 1997. *The Heritage Crusade and the Spoils of History*. London: Viking.

Lynam, Shevawn. 1989. *Humanity Dick Martin, 'King of Connemara' 1754-1834*. Dublin: Lilliput.

Lyons, J.B. 1979. 'Sigerson, George,' in R. Hogan (ed.), *Dictionary of Irish Literature*. Westport, Ct.: Greenwood Press.

Lysaght, S. 1989. 'Heaney vs Praeger: Contrasting Natures.' *The Irish Review* No.7.

Mac Giollarnath, S. 1954. 'List of Irish Names of Birds,' in P.G. Kennedy, R.F. Ruttledge and C.F. Scroope, *The Birds of Ireland*. Edinburgh: Oliver and Boyd.

McKibben, W. 1990. *The End of Nature*. New York: Anchor Books.

Mabey, R. (ed.). 1995. *The Oxford Book of Nature Writing*. Oxford: Oxford University Press.

Mazlish, B. 1994. *The Fourth Continuity: The Co-evolution of Humans and Machines*. New Haven: Yale University Press.

Mills, S. 1997. 'Pocket Tigers: The Sad Unseen Reality behind the Wildlife Film.' *Times Literary Supplement*, 21 February.

Murphy, J.J. 1890. *Sonnets and Other Poems*. London: Kegan Paul.

Newman, J. (Cardinal). [1873] 1982. *The Idea of a University, Defined and Illustrated*. Notre Dame, Indiana: University of Notre Dame Press.

Nicolaisen, W.F.H. 1963. 'A Short Comparative List of Celtic Bird Names of the British Isles,' in D.A. Bannerman and G.E. Lodge, *The Birds of the British Isles*. 12: 405-23.

O'Brien, F. [B. O'Nolan]. [1939] 1967. *At Swim-Two-Birds*. Harmondsworth: Penguin.

O'Brien, F. [1940] 1968. *The Third Policeman*. London: MacGibbon and Kee.

O'Brien, F. [1941] 1973. *The Poor Mouth*. Trans. from *An Béal Bocht* by P.C. Power. London: Hart-Davis, MacGibbon.

Ó Crohan, T. [1934] 1974. *The Islandman*. Trans. R. Flower from 1929 Irish version. Oxford: Clarendon Press.

Ogilvie, Marilyn B. 1986. *Women in Science: Antiquity through the Nineteenth Century: A Biographical Dictionary with Annotated Bibliography*. Cambridge: MIT Press.

Orme, A.R. 1970. 'Conservation in Ireland.' *Geographical Viewpoint 2*: 105-16.

Ó Ruadhain, M. 1956. 'The Position of Nature Protection in Ireland in 1956.' *Irish Naturalists Journal 12*: 81-104.

Ousby, I. 1990. *The Englishman's England: Taste, Travel and the Rise of Tourism*. Cambridge: Cambridge University Press.

Paglia, C. 1991. *Sexual Personae: Art and Decadence from Nefertiti to Emily Dickinson*. New York: Vintage Books.

Pasquier, R.F. and J. Farrand. 1991. *Masterpieces of Bird Art: 700 Years of Ornithological Illustration.* London: Murray.

Patterson, R. 1838. *Letters on the Natural History of Insects Mentioned in Shakespeare's Plays With Incidental Notices of the Entomology of Ireland.* London: W.S. Orr and Co.

Patterson, W.H. 1880. *A Glossary of Words in Use in the Counties of Antrim and Down.* London: English Dialect Society.

Payne-Gallwey, Sir R. 1895 (4th ed.). *Letters to Young Shooters.* London: Longmans & Co.

Phillips, P. 1990. *The Scientific Lady: A Social History of Women's Scientific Interests 1520-1918.* London: Weidenfeld and Nicolson.

Philmus, R. and D.Y. Hughes (eds). 1975. *H.G. Wells: Early Writings in Science and Science Fiction.* Berkeley: University of California Press.

Postman, N. 1985. *Amusing Ourselves to Death: Public Discourse in the Age of Show Business.* New York: Viking.

Potts, A. 1990. 'Natural Order and the Call of the Wild: The Politics of Animal Picturing.' *Oxford Art Journal 13*: 12-33.

Rabinbach, A. 1994. 'Automata, Evolution and Us.' *Times Literary Supplement*, 13 May.

Ross, H.C.G. 1982. 'Irish Women Naturalists in the Nineteenth Century.' Unpublished lecture at Royal Irish Academy, Dublin.

Ross, H.C.G. 1983. 'Problems Researching Irish Women Naturalists.' Unpublished lecture to the Society for the History of Natural History, Belfast.

Ross, H.C.G. and Robert Nash. 1986. 'The Development of Natural History in Early Nineteenth Century Ireland,' in *From Linnaeus to Darwin: Commentaries on the History of Biology and Geology.* London: Society for the History of Natural History.

Rotman, B. 1994. Review of S. Levy, *Artificial Life: The Quest for a New Creation* (London: Jonathan Cape, 1992). *Times Literary Supplement*, 15 April.

Rushton, B.S. (ed.). 1996. *Abstracts of Papers and Posters and List of Contributors, Systematics and Biological Collections.* Belfast: Ulster Museum.

Ryan, S. 1994. 'The Battle of the Burren.' *The Sunday Times.* 2 January.

Schaaf, L.J. 1992. *Out of the Shadows: Herschel, Talbot, and the Invention of Photography.* New Haven: Yale University Press.

Scharff, R.F. 1915. 'On the Irish Names of Birds.' *Irish Naturalist 24*: 109-29.

Scharff, R.F. 1916. 'On the Irish Names of Invertebrate Animals.' *Irish Naturalist 25*: 140-52.

Schiebinger, L. 1994. *Nature's Body: Gender in the Making of Modern Science.* Boston: Beacon.

Shteir, A.B. 1996. *Cultivating Women, Cultivating Science: Flora's Daughters and Botany in England 1760-1860.* Baltimore: Johns Hopkins University.

Shuttleworth, S. (ed.). 1990. *Body/Politics: Women and the Discourses of Science.* New York: Routledge.

Siebert, C. 1993. 'The Artifice of the Natural.' *Harper's Magazine*, February.

Singer, P. [1975] 1990. *Animal Liberation.* Rev. ed. New York: Avon.

Smith, P.E. and M.S. Helfand. 1989. *Oscar Wilde's Oxford Notebooks: A Portrait of Mind in the Making.* New York: Oxford University Press.

Snow, C.P. (Sir Charles). 1959. *The Two Cultures and the Scientific Revolution.* Cambridge: Cambridge University Press.

Strauss, S. 1994. 'Artificial Life: Virtual Fish are the Catch of the Day.' *The Globe and Mail* (Toronto), 10 September.

Swainson, Rev. C. 1885. 'The Folk Lore and Provincial Names of British Birds.' *English Dialect Society 18*: 1-243. 1886. *The Folk Lore and Provincial Names of British Birds.* London: Folk Lore Society. Swainson has been updated by F. Greenoak. 1979. *All the Birds of the Air: The Names, Lore and Literature of British Birds.* London: André Deutsch.

Thomas, G. 1992. *A Position to Command Respect: Women and the Eleventh Britannica.* Metuchen, N.J.: Scarecrow Press.

Trapnell, D. 1991. *Nature in Art: A Celebration of 300 Years of Wildlife Painting.* London: David and Charles.

Tuana, N. (ed.). 1989. *Feminism and Science*. Bloomington: Indiana University Press.

Tudge, C. 1996. 'Captive Breeding is their Only Hope.' *The Times*, 29 July.

Tymoczko, M. 1990. 'The Semantic Fields of Early Irish Terms for Black Birds and their Implications for Species Taxonomy,' in A.T.E. Matonis and D.F. Melia (eds), *Celtic Language, Celtic Culture: A Festschrift for Eric P. Hamp*. Van Nuys, Ca.: Ford & Bailie.

Warren, K.J. (ed.). 1996. *Ecological Feminist Philosophies*. Bloomington: Indiana University Press

Weishepl, J.A. 1982. 'Aristotle's Concept of Nature: Avicenna and Aquinas,' in L.D. Roberts (ed.), *Approaches to Nature in the Middle Ages*. Binghamton, New York: Center for Medieval and Early Renaissance Studies, State University of New York.

Weisbard, P.H. and R.D. Apple. 1993. *The History of Women and Science, Health and Technology: A Bibliographic Guide to the Professions and Disciplines*. Madison: University of Wisconsin Women Studies.

Wells, H.G.1975. 'Zoological Retrogression,' in R. Philmus and D.Y. Hughes (eds), *H.G. Wells: Early Writings in Science and Science Fiction*. Berkeley: University of California Press.

Wells, H.G. [1895] 1953. *The Time Machine*. London: Pan.

Wells, H.G. [1898] 1983. *The War of the Worlds*. New York: Fawcett.

Wheeler, T.S. (ed.). *The Natural Resources of Ireland*. Dublin: Royal Dublin Society.

Whittow, J.B. 1974. *Geology and Scenery in Ireland*. Harmondsworth: Penguin.

Wilde, O. [1889] 1989. 'The Decay of Lying', in I. Murray (ed.), *The Writings of Oscar Wilde*. Oxford: Oxford University Press.

Wilde, O. 1962. *The Letters of Oscar Wilde*. Ed. R. Hart-Davis. New York: Harcourt, Brace.

Wilson, A. 1992. *The Culture of Nature: North American Landscape from Disney to the Exxon Valdez*. Cambridge, Ma.: Blackwell.

Wilson, E.O. 1984. *Biophilia*. Cambridge: Cambridge University Press.

Wilson, T.G. 1946. *Victorian Doctor; Being the Life of Sir William Wilde*. New York: L.B. Fischer.

Woodring, C. 1989. *Nature into Art: Cultural Transformations in Nineteenth-Century Britain*. Cambridge, Ma.: Harvard University Press.

Yates, F. 1972. *The Rosicrucian Enlightenment*. London: Routledge & Kegan Paul.

Yeats, W.B. 1954. *The Letters of W.B. Yeats*. Ed. A. Wade. London: R. Hart-Davis.

Yeats, W.B. 1955. *Autobiographies*. London: Macmillan.

Yeats, W.B. 1968. *Essays and Introductions*. New York: Collier.

Yeats, W.B. 1976. *W.B. Yeats: Selected Prose*. Ed. A. Norman Jeffares. London: Pan.

Young, A. 1892. *Tour in Ireland 1776-1779*. Ed. A.W. Hutton. 2 vols. London: Bell.

Notes on Contributors

JOHN H. ANDREWS graduated from the University of Cambridge and the University of London (PhD). From 1954 to 1990 he was Lecturer and later Associate Professor of Geography at Trinity College, Dublin. He is the author of *A Paper Landscape: The Ordnance Survey in Nineteenth-Century Ireland* (1975), *Plantation Acres: An Historical Study of the Irish Land Surveyor and his Maps* (1985), and *Shapes of Ireland: Maps and their Makers 1564-1839* (1997). He was secretary to the editorial board of the Royal Irish Academy's *Atlas of Ireland* (1979) and from 1981 to 1992 co-editor of the Academy's *Irish Historic Towns Atlas. Dublin City and County: From Prehistory to Present: Studies in Honour of J.H. Andrews* (1992) was edited by F.H.A. Aalen and Kevin Whelan.

MARTYN ANGLESEA was born in Wales and educated at the universities of Leeds and Edinburgh. In 1972 he joined the Ulster Museum (Northern Ireland) where he is now Keeper of Fine Art. From 1992 to 1995 he was Chair of the Irish Museums Association. He is the author of *Kenneth Shoesmith 1890-1939: Paintings and Graphics* (1977), *The Royal Ulster Academy of Arts: A Centennial History* (1981) and *Portraits and Prospects: British and Irish Drawings and Watercolours from the Ulster Museum, Belfast* (1989).

DAVID CABOT was born in Boston, Mass., and educated at Oxford, Trinity College, Dublin, and University College Galway. He has been a lecturer in Zoology (Galway), a BBC television and radio presenter, and for twenty years Head of Conservation and Amenity Research at the State Research Institute (Dublin). From 1990 to 1994 Dr Cabot was Special Advisor on Environmental Affairs in the Department of the Taoiseach, Dublin. In 1988 he formed Wildgoose Films; he has produced documentaries including *Valley of the Geese*, *Wild Islands*, and *The Irish Country House*. He is the author of *Collins Guide to Irish Birds* (1995) and *The Natural History of Ireland*, to be published by HarperCollins in 1998.

HELENA CHESNEY, originally from Doagh, Co. Antrim, is Keeper of Zoology at the Ulster Museum, Belfast, where as a malacologist she specializes in the study of bivalve molluscs. Her publications relate mainly to malacology and the history of Irish natural history. Gardening and wide-ranging interests in nature and the arts occupy much of her leisure time.

JOHN FEEHAN is a lecturer in the Department of Environmental Resource Management at University College Dublin. His main areas of interest include the maintenance of rural diversity, conservation biology, environmental education and landscape history. His most recent book is *The Bogs of Ireland* (1996), written with Grace O'Donovan. His earlier published work includes studies of the landscape of Slieve Bloom and County Laois as well as numerous papers and articles on aspects of environmental science and heritage. His television series *Exploring the Landscape* won a Jacobs Television Award in 1988.

PETER FOSS is the Director of the Irish Peatland Conservation Council, a position he has held since 1987. He is a graduate in Botany and Zoology from University College Dublin, where he also undertook doctoral research on Mediterranean heather in Ireland. He was involved in the national studies of peatlands in 1982 and 1986. He has written over thirty-five scientific papers. He is editor of *Irish Peatlands, the Critical Decade* and co-author of the *Irish Peatland Conservation Plan 2000*. He is the founder of IPCC's Save the Bogs Campaign, the longest-running conservation campaign in Ireland, and is active in the International Mire Conservation Group.

JOHN WILSON FOSTER was born in Belfast and educated at The Queen's University of Belfast and the University of Oregon (PhD). He is Professor of English at the University of British Columbia and is the author of *Forces and Themes in Ulster Fiction* (1974), *Fictions of the Irish Literary Revival* (1987), *Colonial Consequences: Essays in Irish Literature and Culture* (1991), *The Achievement of Seamus Heaney* (1995), and *The Titanic Complex* (1997).

MICHAEL GUIRY was born in Youghal, Co. Cork, and is a graduate of University College Cork and the University of London (PhD and DSc). He is Professor and Head of Department of Botany, University College Galway. He has been Visiting Research Fellow, University of Melbourne and James Professor in Pure and Applied Science, St Francis Xavier University, Nova Scotia. He is a member of the Royal Irish Academy and in 1996-97 was President of the International Phycological Society. *A Consensus and Bibliography of Irish Seaweeds* appeared in 1979, and in 1991 Dr Guiry co-authored *Seaweed Resources in Europe: Uses and Potential*. He has published more than 150 scientific papers on marine algae.

PAUL HACKNEY was born in Manchester but has lived in Northern Ireland since 1968. He is Keeper of Botany at the Ulster Museum and specializes in the floristics of vascular plants and bryophytes. He has an additional interest in the eighteenth- and nineteenth-century voyages of exploration.

IAIN HIGGINS was born in the Hebrides but grew up in Canada. Before switching to the humanities, he was a science student. His doctorate in English is from

Harvard University. He is the author of *Writing East: The 'Travels' of Sir John Mandeville* (1997) and a translator of contemporary Polish poetry. He is Assistant Professor at the University of British Columbia.

CLIVE HUTCHINSON was born in Cork and graduated in History and Political Science from Trinity College, Dublin. He then trained as an accountant and set up in practice in Cork in 1979. Meanwhile he wrote *The Birds of Dublin and Wicklow* (1975). He organized the Irish Wildbird Conservancy wetlands inquiry from 1971 to 1975 and published as a result *Ireland's Wetlands and their Birds* (1979). He began the journal *Irish Birds* and edited it for eight years. His textbook on the status of Irish birds, *Birds in Ireland*, appeared in 1989.

SHEILA LANDY graduated from Birmingham University in Russian Language and Literature. After gaining a diploma in Library and Information Studies, she was appointed Science Librarian at Queen's University of Belfast in 1991. She has organized a number of Science Library exhibitions on Irish scientists and engineers and contributed to *Some People and Places in Irish Science and Technology* (1985), ed. Charles Mollan et al.

DAVID LIVINGSTONE is Professor of Geography at The Queen's University of Belfast. He is the author of *Nathaniel Southgate Shaler and the Culture of American Science* (1987), *Darwin's Forgotten Defenders* (1987), *The Preadamite Theory* (1992) and *The Geographical Tradition* (1992). He is a Fellow of the British Academy.

SEÁN LYSAGHT was born in Cork and grew up in Limerick. He graduated in Anglo-Irish Literature from University College Dublin. After living in Switzerland and Germany, he returned to Ireland in 1990 to teach at St Patrick's College, Maynooth. He received his doctorate from St Patrick's College (NUI) for a critical biography of Robert Lloyd Praeger. He now lectures at the Regional Technical College – Castlebar Campus. He is best known as a poet, author of two collections, *Noah's Irish Ark* (1989) and *The Clare Island Survey* (1991).

MARY G. MCGEOWN graduated in Medicine from The Queen's University of Belfast in 1946. She spent eight years in research posts, graduating as MD in pathology and PhD in biochemistry, and later worked in the Department of Medicine at Queen's on the pathogenesis of kidney stones and on calcium metabolism. In 1959 she established a unit for the treatment of acute renal failure at the Belfast City Hospital, and later established units for the treatment of chronic kidney failure and for transplants. Professor McGeown was Chairman of the United Kingdom Transplant Service Management Committee from 1983 to 1990. In addition to over 250 articles and book chapters, she is author of *Clinical Management of Electrolyte Disorders* and edited *Clinical Management of Renal Transplantation*. She has received *Doctorates Honoris Causae* from the New University of Ulster and the Queen's University of Belfast. Her work was recognized in 1985 by the award of the CBE.

BRENDAN MCWILLIAMS joined the Irish Meteorological Service in 1964, and spent many years as an operational weather forecaster, including an extended period as an RTÉ weatherman. Since 1990 he has been Assistant Director of Met Éireann. He represents Ireland on the Council of EUMETSAT, the European Meteorological Satellite Organisation, and has been Chairman of the European Commission's COST Technical Committee on Meteorology. He writes a daily column, *Weather Eye*, on meteorological, astronomical and environmental matters, in *The Irish Times*.

CHRISTOPHER MORIARTY has been engaged in fishery research since 1958. His PhD was awarded for a thesis on the eels of Ireland, on which he is an international expert. His first book, *A Guide to Irish Birds*, was published in 1967, and his latest, *Exploring Dublin: Wildlife, Parks, Waterways*, in 1997. He is Chairman of the European Inland Fisheries Advisory Commission, Secretary of the National Committee for Biology (Ireland), a member of the National Committee for the History and Philosophy of Science (Ireland) and former Chairman of the Science Committee of the Royal Dublin Society. The Institute of Biology of Ireland and the Institute of Fisheries Management have both honoured him with their fellowships.

ROBERT NASH is Curator of Entomology at the Ulster Museum. He has studied Irish insects for a quarter century but is also interested in insects collected abroad by Irish entomologists in the nineteenth century. He is a Fellow of the Royal Entomological Society. One of the greatest of nineteenth-century entomologists, A.H. Haliday, is of especial interest to him.

EOIN NEESON's *A History of Irish Forestry* was published in 1991. That year he retired early from the Civil Service as Assistant Secretary and Director of Special Projects with the Department of Energy, having also served in that rank in other departments including the Department of Agriculture. He is a former head of Government Information Services. He is the author of fifteen books, including *The Civil War* and *The Life and Death of Michael Collins*. He is also a playwright. As a journalist he held senior positions with national papers and was editor of *The Kerryman* and *The Munster Tribune*.

CATHERINE O'CONNELL is the Head of Education with the Irish Peatland Conservation Council. She is a graduate in Botany and Zoology from University College Dublin, where she also undertook doctoral research on the palaeoecology of subfossil pine woodlands on Irish raised bogs. She was involved in the national surveys of peatlands from 1982 to 1984. A former teacher, she has pioneered the educational use of peatlands since 1985 through publication of resource materials and the provision of professional in-service training. She is the editor of the *IPCC Guide to Irish Peatlands*, the *Peatland Education Pack* and *Peatlands in the Primary School Curriculum*, and co-author of the *Irish Peatland Conservation Plan 2000*.

JAMES O'CONNOR was born in Dublin and was educated at University College Dublin. He is in charge of the Natural History Museum (Dublin) and the Natural History Division of the National Museum of Ireland. The Museum's entomologist, he curates a collection of a million specimens dating from 1792. He has written over

150 scientific papers on Irish and foreign insects and is joint author of *A Bibliography of Irish Entomology*. He has recorded many species new to Ireland and described several new to science. He is Editor of the *Bulletin of the Irish Biogeographical Society* and a Sectional Editor of *The Irish Naturalists' Journal*. A Fellow of the Royal Entomological Society, he is also a Life Member of the Freshwater Biological Association and the Royal Zoological Society of Ireland.

DORINDA OUTRAM teaches History at University College Cork. She was recently Landon Clay Visiting Associate Professor of the History of Science at Harvard University, and has also held a Visiting Chair at Griffith University, Queensland. In 1995-96 she was a guest scholar at the Max-Planck-Institute for the History of Science, Berlin. She has taught at universities in Britain and Canada. In 1989 she co-edited *Uneasy Careers and Intimate Lives: Women in Science 1789-1979*. She is the author of *The Body and the French Revolution* (1989) and *The Enlightenment* (1995).

TERENCE REEVES-SMYTH is an archaeologist and architectural historian employed by the Environment and Heritage service (DOE) in Northern Ireland. He has published books on architecture, gardens and archaeology.

PATRICK SLEEMAN holds a degree in Ecology from the University of Ulster and did his doctoral research at University College Cork on the Irish stoat. He has studied mammals in Ireland, Britain, Spain, France, New Zealand and Tanzania. He is currently studying the link between badgers and tuberculosis.

DONAL SYNNOTT studied botany at University College Dublin. Since 1963 he has worked as a herbarium botanist, first at the National Museum of Ireland and later at the National Botanic Gardens, Glasnevin, where he is Director. His research into the Irish flora focuses on the vascular plants and the bryophytes. His interests extend to plants in Irish archaeology, folklore and literature. He is co-author of *Catalogue Census of the Flora of Ireland* (1987).

MICHAEL VINEY lives in County Mayo. He has contributed a weekly column on nature and ecology to *The Irish Times* since 1977. He is a filmmaker and has directed several wildlife and landscape films for television. His book, *A Year's Turning*, was published in 1996.

PATRICK WYSE JACKSON is Curator of the Geological Museum, Trinity College, Dublin, where he carries out research on Carboniferous bryozoans, the use of building materials in Ireland and the history of geology in Ireland. He is a member of the International Commission on the History of Geology (INHIGEO) and past President of the Irish Geological Association and of the Dublin Naturalists' Field Club. His recent books include *The Building Stones of Ireland: A Walking Guide* (Dublin, 1993) and *In Marble Halls: Geology in Trinity College Dublin* (Dublin 1993).

Index
